Selected Papers of CHARLES H. BEST

The career of Charles H. Best needs no introduction to medical or lay readers. His great achievements are here signalized in a large and splendid volume which brings together over sixty of his important research papers in the fields of insulin, heparin, and choline. It is fitting that this volume should be produced at a time when the fortieth anniversary of the discovery of insulin is being celebrated. Dr. Best has on this occasion looked back over the record as given in these papers and provided informative and informal bridges between them which place them in historical perspective. All the references in the original papers have been reassembled in a master bibliography which is a new and full storehouse of references.

CHARLES HERBERT BEST (1899–1978), C.B.F., M.D., D.SC., LL.D., F.R.S., was Professor and Head of the Banting and Best Department of Medical Research and the Department of Physiology, University of Toronto, and was co-discoverer of insulin with F.G. Banting in 1921.

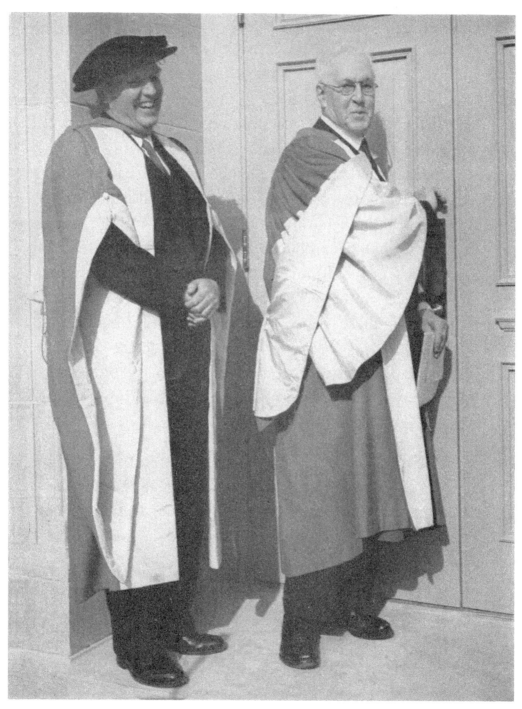

Professor C. H. Best and Sir Henry Dale at the opening of the Charles H. Best
Institute in 1953.

Selected Papers of
CHARLES H. BEST

C.B.E., M.A., M.D.(Tor.), D.Sc.(Lond.)

F.R.S.C., F.R.C.P.(C), F.R.C.P., F.R.S.

Head of the Department of Physiology

Director of the Banting and Best Department of

Medical Research, University of Toronto

University of Toronto Press

This book is dedicated to my wife

MARGARET MAHON BEST

who has helped me more than anyone, to all the fine colleagues whose names are mentioned in our joint papers, and to two of these in particular, Professor C. C. Lucas and Dr. Jessie H. Ridout, without whose efficient and unselfish contributions this volume could not have been prepared for publication

Publisher's Note

We are proud to have two special contributors to this volume, one from Great Britain and the other from the United States. Sir Henry Dale has graciously provided a Foreword and Dr. Elliott P. Joslin accepted with enthusiasm our invitation to write an Introduction.

SIR HENRY DALE, O.M., G.B.E., F.R.S., M.D., LL.D., D.SC., the first Director of the National Institute for Medical Research, London, Hampstead, 1928–1942, Secretary of the Royal Society 1925–1935 and President 1940–1945. He has been Director of Laboratories of the Royal Institution, and Chairman of the Wellcome Trust. He shared the Nobel Prize in Medicine and Physiology (1936) with Professor Otto Loewi for their work on acetylcholine as a chemical transmitter of nerve impulses. This and many other achievements have led to his universal recognition as one of the greatest physiologists and pharmacologists of this era.

ELLIOTT PROCTOR JOSLIN, M.D. (1869–1962) was the doyen of the diabetic specialists of the world. He undoubtedly had more experience with diabetic patients before and after insulin became available than any other physician had or ever can have. Dr. Joslin was the first Honorary President of the International Diabetes Federation, and of the American Diabetes Association.

Foreword

SIR HENRY H. DALE

I am glad to respond to the request from the University of Toronto Press, for a word of introduction from me to this collection of original scientific publications by Professor Charles Best. It will be seen that, for a large proportion of these, he has shared the responsibility of authorship with various colleagues and collaborators. Such collaboration has long been common, of course, in scientific researches, and more so, perhaps, in the general field of medicine than in those of the more fundamental disciplines. It must be clear, in any case, that the need for such teamwork has been growing, and will continue to do so, as more and more of the conceptions of biological, organic, and physical chemistry, using many of the new experimental resources and instruments which the electronic age is now making available, are pressed into the service of nearly all the aspects of medical research, in the laboratories now attached to the clinics, as well as in those of the pre-clinical departments.

Professor Best, however, had already given evidence of the gifts and qualities which would qualify him especially for such a sharing of activities, when he had his first experience of medical research more than forty years ago, even before he had graduated, and at a time when some of the cardinal discoveries in the medical sciences were still waiting to be made, and might even be accessible without any of the modern wealth of methods and instruments. It was under such conditions that the now historic partnership of Frederick Banting and Charles Best enabled them, with all the untarnished eagerness of their inexperience, to solve, in a few months of intense devotion to their common enterprise, a problem in physiology and practical medicine which had baffled more than one generation of practised investigators.

The whole story of this discovery of insulin, of the still heroic effort required for its first production under conditions of emergency and improvization, of its ultimate purification and world-wide application, of the elucidation of its mode of action, and even of its complex chemical structure —all this and much more, especially of the records of its success in giving new prospects of life and activity to millions, has recently been recorded in simple outline for the general reader, by a trio of Charles Best's friends, pupils and colleagues.[1]

There will be many others, however, who will welcome the opportunity which Professor Best has here given us, of direct access to those of the original documents to which he has been directly a contributor, concerned with the discovery of insulin and the subsequent forty years of investigation which have now been devoted to its properties and its significance. These constitute, of course, a large proportion of the publications in this field of research. Frederick Banting was early planning to extend his enterprise into other fields, and, as all the world knows, died on service in World War II. So that, of the original pioneers, Charles Best remained, to give a co-operative leadership in a large proportion of the subsequent researches on insulin. He has enriched the collection here made with the addition of his own detailed comments.

A large part of this collection is, naturally, thus concerned with his collaborative contribution to the development and expansion of knowledge concerning insulin, and its many-sided significance; and we may welcome his decision to add to this part of the collection an otherwise unpublished short essay, giving us an insight into his own present ideas on "The Future in the Field of Diabetes." It should particularly be observed, however, that, although the series dealing with insulin and diabetes extends to dates as recent as 1960, it by no means represents the whole of his interest, or of his important contributions to knowledge in the general field of experimental medicine. There were two short periods when I had the proud privilege of welcoming Charles Best in my own laboratory, and of joining him, with others, in research; and on the second of these occasions our work was concerned with histamine, on which he continued his investigations for a few years after he left us. During World War II, again, he and his colleagues were busy with researches on heparin, with results of which the importance has extended far beyond that of their contribution to immediate, wartime needs. Of much wider interest than either of these, however, are the impressive contributions which Professor Best and his co-workers have been making, as presented in some fifteen publications from 1932 onwards, and surveyed and discussed in his Croonian Lecture to the Royal Society of London in 1956, on the nutritional factors which promote the pathogenic deposition of fat in the cells of the liver, and the preventive, lipotropic action of lecithin, and of its simple component, choline. There will be many, again, to welcome the collection here of this important series, and to look for the possibility of its further extension.

[1]G. A. Wrenshall, G. Hetenyi, Jr., and W. R. Feasby, The Story of Insulin (London: The Bodley Head, 1962).

Altogether, apart from a scientific and closely personal friendship over now more than forty years, I am proud of the opportunity to greet this collection of Professor Best's scientific publications, rich already in historical significance, as well as in promise for years of continued activity, still happily in prospect for him.

July 1962

Preface

Several of my colleagues and representatives of the University of Toronto Press have urged me to reprint some of my papers and to make this collection somewhat more personal by including a series of notes introducing or commenting on the various articles.

In making a choice for such a volume, one must try to achieve a balance between what appeals particularly to the author and what will serve the probable interests of the readers. The number of papers that can be included is, of necessity, restricted. It has been difficult to decide what to leave out. The happy memories of hours spent with former associates in the laboratory, or in writing papers, often made the resulting publication appear more important to me than it may have seemed to others. Half-forgotten memories of successes, and disappointments too, crowded my mind during the re-reading of the early papers. Sometimes observations took on new significance in the light of more recent discoveries. The temptation to "correct" some paragraphs or conclusions has been resisted. The reprints show the state of knowledge at the time of publication. Obvious errors have been amended and some repetitious protocols of experiments have been eliminated. Certain figures that were in the original papers have had to be omitted. Some of the figures in the early papers have been left, for historical reasons, as they were drawn by Dr. Banting in spite of the inevitably limited legibility of certain features in the reproductions. A few have been redrawn (by C.C.L.). For the convenience of the reader the text figures here printed have been renumbered to progress consecutively through the book.

The journals in which these Papers originally appeared have been most kind in giving consent for this new appearance.

Affiliations of the authors of these Papers are with the Department of Physiology or the Banting and Best Department of Medical Research, University of Toronto, unless otherwise indicated.

I am grateful to Dr. Lucas and Dr. Ridout for taking the References as given in the original papers and collating them into a new Bibliography, printed at the end of the book. References in the text to items in this bibliography are indicated by numbers in square brackets.

I am very greatly indebted to Professor W. Stanley Hartroft and to Professor John Logothetopoulos for their expert help in making the coloured illustrations available.

Over the past forty years Mr. Eli Lilly of Indianapolis has gone even beyond the call of friendship in facilitating some of our scientific adventures, and, more recently, Mr. Donald Gilmore of Kalamazoo has generously helped us. A portion of the extra secretarial assistance necessary in the preparation of parts of this book has been provided by the Kalamazoo Civic Fund.

My warmest thanks are extended to the University of Toronto Press, particularly Mr. Marsh Jeanneret and Miss F. G. Halpenny, for their invaluable advice. I would also like to thank my secretary, Miss Linda Mahon, for the many hours outside the regular University day which she has spent in the preparation of manuscripts and reports on our scientific work.

C. H. B.

Contents

PART II: CHOLINE AND LIPOTROPIC PHENOMENA

PART III: OTHER PHYSIOLOGICAL STUDIES

PART IV: GENERAL PAPERS

PART V: EPILOGUE   699

Introduction

ELLIOTT P. JOSLIN

How pleased the friends of Professor Best will be to see this collection of his papers on insulin! Busy doctors will be thankful that here they can find a condensation of more than 70,000 articles on the same subject. Indeed how indebted will be the whole world, because, by his journeys to fifty lands, he has so publicized diabetes that most nations have become vitally concerned with its control. His later publications I shall label "Volume II," thereby protecting him from the dangers of retirement and a pension.

I suspect no one living can appreciate these articles as much as I because when I began practice in 1897 the life of a diabetic child was measured in days and adults with diabetes lived less than five years. One must lose a life really to feel what it is to save one. When I learned on August 7, 1922, that I was to receive insulin for Miss Mudge, whose weight had fallen from 157 to 72 pounds in five years, I stayed awake all night.

As far back as 1896 I had good reason to anticipate what the Best family stock, with its six generations, invigorated by a Canadian climate, could produce, because Charles Best's Aunt Anna, a nurse, and I, a house pupil, worked together in the wards of the Massachusetts General Hospital. She won the respect of all the house officers. I know what she did for his education. His feeling for her was confirmed when during an address in Philadelphia I saw he wore her watch. This trait of acknowledging help received from others has pervaded all of the papers he has written.

What an asset it was for this boy—Charles H. Best—to grow up, like Galen, in the country and I am glad to note that it was in the United States: Pembroke, Maine. From his father, a country doctor, he gained self-respect and confidence at the age of twelve, by giving the anaesthetic during operations as Will and Charles Mayo did for their father.

How dependent Sir Frederick Banting was upon him and how outspoken in proclaiming it! When Dr. Best was telling the story of insulin in the packed amphitheatre of our Vanderbilt Dormitory (incidentally, a replica of its Toronto counterpart) I was annoyed to receive a telegram. Having read it, I passed it over to President Eliot who had come from Cambridge for the lecture. When Dr. Best finished, President Eliot rose and read:

At any meeting or dinner please read following. I ascribe to Best equal share in discovery. Hurt that he is not so acknowledged by Nobel Trustees. Will share with him.

BANTING

A fitting sequel to this incident is the beautiful obituary Dr. Best wrote for Dr. Banting.

Charles Best was as young as Vesalius when he went to Padua in 1536 at the age of 22 and a short time subsequently was made Professor. He had the spark of youth, and by his discovery of insulin with Banting he proved that a medical student was *ipso facto* an investigator and deserved to be regarded as such. From the very beginning Dr. Best realized also that the discovery of insulin was not only a scientific achievement but also a major contribution to the future of mankind. The late John D. Rockefeller, Jr., sensed this and with the advice of Dr. Simon Flexner gave funds to several of us to make insulin useful immediately. As a result of insulin the average diabetic's life has been prolonged on the average at least ten years;* thus for the 3,000,000 diabetics in the United States we now have 30,000,000 more life years of diabetes to treat.

This volume contains the early papers describing the discovery of insulin followed by those dealing with its preparation, extraction, and physiologic effects, the limitation of its presence to the pancreas and its absence in the plant kingdom, with an estimate of the insulin content of the pancreas and the influence of diet upon it. Included are papers written with his colleagues on the prevalence of diabetes in Canada and a short paper by Dr. Best discussing its future. One-half of the volume gives results of research by him and his associates on subjects closely related to diabetes. There are also papers on the action of histamine, the group of studies on lipo-tropic agents, especially those related to lecithin and choline, my old friends, to whom I was introduced by R. H. Chittenden of Yale in 1890. Others shed new light on the action of heparin upon the control of coagula-tion in experimental trauma. Fortunately for us all it has been Dr. Best's habit from early 1922 up to the present to review the prevailing knowledge of diabetes and especially of insulin, thereby allowing student and practi-tioner to be *au courant* with diabetes every few years.

The first public recognition of Banting's and Best's work was the Reeves Prize of fifty dollars, awarded to them in 1923 by a committee of professors of Anatomy, Physiology, Biochemistry, Pharmacology, Pathology, and Patho-logical Chemistry for the best scientific research accomplished in any department of the Faculty of Medicine of the University of Toronto by

*This is the average extension of life by insulin irrespective of the age of onset of diabetes. Many diabetics who received their first insulin in the early 1920's are alive and well, i.e., after forty years. AUTHOR'S NOTE

junior members of the staff. Other grants followed and the recent gift of Mr. Garfield Weston, in Best's honour, will allow what he has begun to be perpetuated.

When Imhotep, credited by Sir William Osler as the world's first recognized physician, built the Pyramid in 2980 B.C. he stood alone as its creator and with his flail in his left hand compelled thousands to join in the task. It was very different with the marble Cathedral of Milan. To be sure, there were master minds and architects, and engineers were selected with care, but thousands and thousands of simple folk voluntarily gave their labour for its excavation and construction over four centuries. Dr. Best has succeeded in making diabetics and research workers feel that they all are working with him, and they are proud to be among his willing helpers.

My prized possession is the page recording the experiment which Banting and Best carried out on August 6, 1921. I believe this is the only leaf of their notebook not in Toronto. Day and night to them were alike. The dog was prepared for the experiment at 5 P.M., but the first dose of the material possibly containing insulin (first called in this publication "isletin") was given at 12 midnight when the blood sugar was 430 mg. Subsequently, 8 cc were injected hourly and the blood sugar dropped steadily so that by 4 A.M. it had been demonstrated that an anti-diabetic substance had been extracted from the pancreas and would lower the blood sugar to normal.

I feel so grateful to the University of Toronto for the privilege of writing this introduction that, with the consent of Harvard University, I am returning this page to complete the notebook of Banting and Best, to which, in addition to their signatures, I am adding my own.

January 1962

On January 28, 1962, very soon after he completed this introductory article, Dr. Elliott P. Joslin died. He was in his 93rd year.

1. A Canadian Trail of Medical Research

CHARLES H. BEST

[*This lecture was part of the Proceedings of the Seventy-Fifth (Ordinary) Meeting of the Society for Endocrinology, held at the Royal Society, Burlington House, London, on June 23, 1959. At this meeting the President, Sir Charles E. Dodds, made the first award of the Dale Medal to Dr. Best and presented a second medal to Sir Henry Dale. Dr. Best then delivered the Annual Lecture.*]

The depth of my appreciation of this first award of the Dale Medal will, I trust, be apparent in the course of this lecture, with which your Society for Endocrinology has honoured me.

Sir Henry Dale appears many times on my pathway through or around the obstacles which one meets in nearly forty years of medical research and, indeed, on several occasions he has blazed a trail for me. His great influence on the development of Canadian physiology in this century has been accomplished in large part by his publications and his innumerable discussions with biochemists, physiologists, and pharmacologists who have worked in our country. My close friends, F. C. MacIntosh, from Cape Breton, Nova Scotia, who is now head of Physiology at McGill University, and Charles Code, from Winnipeg, Manitoba, and now head of Physiology at the Mayo Clinic, and I, have passed on to many young physiologists in the New World some of the inspiration and stimulus which Sir Henry Dale gave to us as his junior colleagues here in London.[1] Returning to my Canadian story, I may say that, with the exception of Frederick Grant Banting, no scientist has been so frequently and so happily in my mind as Sir Henry. This statement is incomplete because it leaves unmentioned the innumerable kindnesses which my wife and I have received from Sir Henry and Lady Dale. Without these warm friendships, trails of medical research could be very bleak journeys.

Originally appeared in the *Journal of Endocrinology*, XIX (1959), 1–17.

[1]Since I have mentioned the United States as well as Canada, I should include the inspiration transmitted by a brilliant group of clinicians—Dickinson Richards, Walter Bauer, Oliver Cope, and A. M. Harvey (all physiologists at heart) who were also exposed to the Dale stimulus at a formative period in their careers. I should have mentioned first, perhaps, three more senior figures in pharmacology, biochemistry, and physiology in the United States, all of whom were scientific colleagues and close friends of Sir Henry here in London—A. N. Richards, Henry Dakin, and Herbert Gasser.

In 1953 I received from Henry Hallett Dale a copy of his *Adventures in Physiology*. When I read the introduction and comments and re-read the papers, the wisdom and enthusiasm of my close friend since 1922 stimulated me as they always have. I decided to select a number of my own articles—which I hope will have either historical or contemporary interest—and to publish these with an introduction and comments under the title *A Canadian Trail of Medical Research*. I must admit that no publisher has, as yet, urged me to hurry along with this effort, but perchance a discussion of this matter and the presentation of a lecture such as this, which might even serve as an introduction, may reveal a hidden interest. This will not be a very scientific presentation but an informal and undoubtedly too personal account of the medical research matters which have continuously fascinated me.

The effects of environment and opportunity, which play such dominant roles in the courses which all of us have followed, will be obvious. Another great factor—heredity—seems to have exerted its influence by making me eager to remain in Canada. Two of my ancestors, William Best and John Burbidge, went from the Isle of Wight with Cornwallis to found Halifax, Nova Scotia, in 1749. They were active in the building of the first Protestant church in Canada, St. Paul's in Halifax, in the laying out of the Public Gardens, and in the development of the great orchard industry in the fertile Annapolis and Cornwallis valleys. They both sat in the first Legislative Assembly of Canada in 1758. My father was the sixth generation to be born and brought up in Nova Scotia. We went there for our vacations as children, and my earliest recollection of medical lore came from discussions with him while we watched the loading of thousands of barrels of Nova Scotian apples, destined for England, into the great ships which, at low tide, rested on the mud and listed slightly against the tall wharves. At high tide they floated some forty to fifty feet higher and looked down majestically at their frail connections with the land. My father, aunt, and uncle attended Dalhousie University, which was founded in part by monies collected as customs duty by the British at the Port of Castine in Maine during the War of 1812. My father had intended finishing his medical course at McGill, but he missed his class because of a second attack of typhoid fever. He completed his medicine in New York City and graduated with honours. What was to have been a brief *locum tenens* on the Maine–New Brunswick border turned out to be forty-five years of devoted and expert medical service in a small town and country practice in which my Nova Scotian mother constantly played a vital role. They lived on the United States side of the border and my father took many of his seriously ill patients to a hospital in St. Stephen, New Brunswick, Canada. For two years we lived in the little city of Eastport, Maine, which looks across at the island of Campobello. Eastport was occupied by the British during the War of 1812, with the active help of Admiral Owen, a Cambridge graduate, who received a King's grant of the Island of Campobello and lived there in feudal grandeur. He named his territory by latinizing that of his friend, General Campbell, a comrade in one of the Mediterranean campaigns. This was the summer home of Franklin Roosevelt, who knew well and loved, as I do, the Grand Manan Archipelago and its splendid tide runs. I met him on Campobello and later in Ottawa, where, acting as Public Orator for the University of London, England, I presented the President to Lord Athlone for an honorary degree. Lord Athlone, our Governor General at that time, was Chancellor of the University of London.

My father had a small private hospital in Eastport for two years and his only nurse was his sister, Anna Best who—like many other girls from Nova Scotia—trained at the Massachusetts General Hospital in Boston. She knew Dr. Elliott P. Joslin who was a houseman at that time. In the early years of this century my aunt became diabetic No. 875 in Dr. Joslin's series. When she was living with us she was following the starvation regimen and she died in diabetic coma a few years before insulin became available.

I went to a collegiate in Toronto in 1916 to prepare for my university examinations. I volunteered again and again for military service but a cardiac systolic murmur, and perhaps my age, prevented my acceptance until I found a homeopath who did not listen to my heart and gave me a grading of A 1, which was presumably correct as I represented my unit in several strenuous athletic activities, including horseback wrestling. I came to England for the first time as a Sergeant in the Canadian Army in the summer of 1918. My unit was decimated by influenza during a seventeen-day trip across the North Atlantic. There were no doctors or nurses in the ship and there were many casualties. I never got closer to the front than Southampton, and a skirmish between battalions of young Australian and Canadian soldiers in Rhyl provided my only campaign experience.

I resumed my studies in the University of Toronto at the age of nineteen and soon transferred from a General Arts Course to a specialized one in Physiology and Biochemistry, which was designed to provide a training for medical research. I was intensely interested in medical matters as a young boy, and began giving anaesthetics under my father's direction at the age of twelve. The family interest in diabetes played a part in my selection of a department for postgraduate work in the University of Toronto. In my fifth year at the University, and the final year of that course, I divided my time between the Department of Biochemistry under Professor

Andrew Hunter and Professor Hardolf Wasteneys, where I applied Dakin's butyl alcohol method for the separation of amino acids derived from the protein gliadin, and the Department of Physiology, under Professor J. J. R. Macleod, where my problem with another student was the pathway of Claude Bernard's piqûre impulses from the medulla to the liver. Every practical point which I learned in that year, in the handling of proteins, in distillation techniques, and in the accepted procedures for investigations of carbohydrate metabolism: blood and urine sugars, nitrogen, ketone bodies, respiratory quotients, glycogen estimations, and so on, were utilized to the full in the research which I began with F. G. Banting on the day after I had finished my final examinations in Physiology and Biochemistry. This was May 17, 1921.

I have paid my tribute of admiration and affection to Fred Banting on many occasions. One should look back to the statements made at the time to secure proper and accurate perspective. Copies of memoranda that Professor Macleod, Fred Banting, and I wrote in 1922 in response to an invitation from the Board of Governors of the University of Toronto, will be deposited in London in the Wellcome Historical Medical Library. I was the only graduate student of that year who made arrangements to work throughout the summer of 1921 and the following year in Professor Macleod's department. There was no tossing of coins to decide who would work first with Fred Banting, and no mention of this myth was ever made by Professor Macleod who was entirely responsible for these arrangements and who has recorded: "I assigned one of my recently graduated students, C. H. Best, to work with Dr. Fred Banting." Professor Macleod also stated that "knowledge of physiological and biochemical procedures used in the study of carbohydrate metabolism, was essential if the venture was to have any chance of success." As I worked without any stipend that summer, I have always been under the impression that I volunteered for the job. Fred Banting has recorded in his official account the well-known circumstances leading to his initiation of the research in Toronto. I wrote, at the time, "I assisted Banting in the surgical aspects of the study and he assisted me in the chemical procedures." As you know, we worked as vigorously as we could, and during the eight months of our partnership we established a number of unassailable facts. Our main effort was directed towards proving that a neutral, or preferably an acid, aqueous or alcoholic extract of degenerated, or intact dog pancreas and of foetal or adult beef pancreas always provided us with a potent antidiabetic material. We were overwhelmed by a multitude of ideas which demanded investigation, but we persisted, until on seventy-five occasions, without any failures, we had been able to secure a material potent in lowering blood sugar and which on many occasions produced dramatic clinical improvements in our depancreatized—and sometimes almost moribund—animals. No statistics were needed to establish the fact that we could invariably extract an antidiabetic material from pancreas. We amassed a great volume of data, only a part of which was ever published. Professor Macleod has recorded that he gave Banting and me complete credit for the consistent demonstration of an antidiabetic principle in extracts of degenerated dog's pancreas and in foetal calf pancreas. I think the evidence was equally convincing when we used whole beef pancreas which was available in adequate amounts, but at this phase circumstances prevented us from developing our discovery alone as all explorers would plan and hope to do. There were two great pressures upon us. One was exerted by the diabetic patients who needed insulin. After the announcement of our findings to the medical faculty, November 14, 1921, the forerunners of the thousands of letters from diabetics appeared and soon patients, many from distant places, began to arrive. Parents with diabetic children found their way right into our laboratory and, in spite of anything we could do, came day after day until plans were made to care for them.

The second pressure was exerted by senior and more experienced investigators, who had not invested an hour's work before the discovery but who were now more than anxious to appropriate a share of it. Every experiment which we did to improve the preparation of insulin was successful, but we had no scientific or technical assistance and few facilities, and progress seemed slow. Before the end of 1921 both Banting and I had secured opportunities in other departments. He went to Pharmacology and I to the Connaught Laboratories. This made the continuation of our partnership difficult but we preserved our independence.

I will now present a few figures and graphs to illustrate some of the points I have made. Figure 1 is a page of our notebook, written in late July 1921, which shows the definite but moderate lowering of blood sugar. In Figure 2a a more dramatic record of the sweeping decline in blood-sugar level produced by insulin is illustrated. On August 14, 1921, we produced for the first time a definite hypoglycaemia in a depancreatized dog by giving 30 ml. of the extract intravenously (see Figure 2b). Figure 2c depicts our preliminary finding on August 17 on the efficacy of neutral and acid-cold saline to extract the insulin from the pancreas of a normal dog. The alkaline extract had no effect on blood sugar. In November, while still working alone, we lowered the blood sugar of a dog from a very high level to one at which some of the signs of hypoglycaemia were produced and we demonstrated and recorded the effect of glucose. The extract was made from whole beef pancreas and the test dog at autopsy proved to have been completely depancreatized. The announcement, i.e., our first presenta-

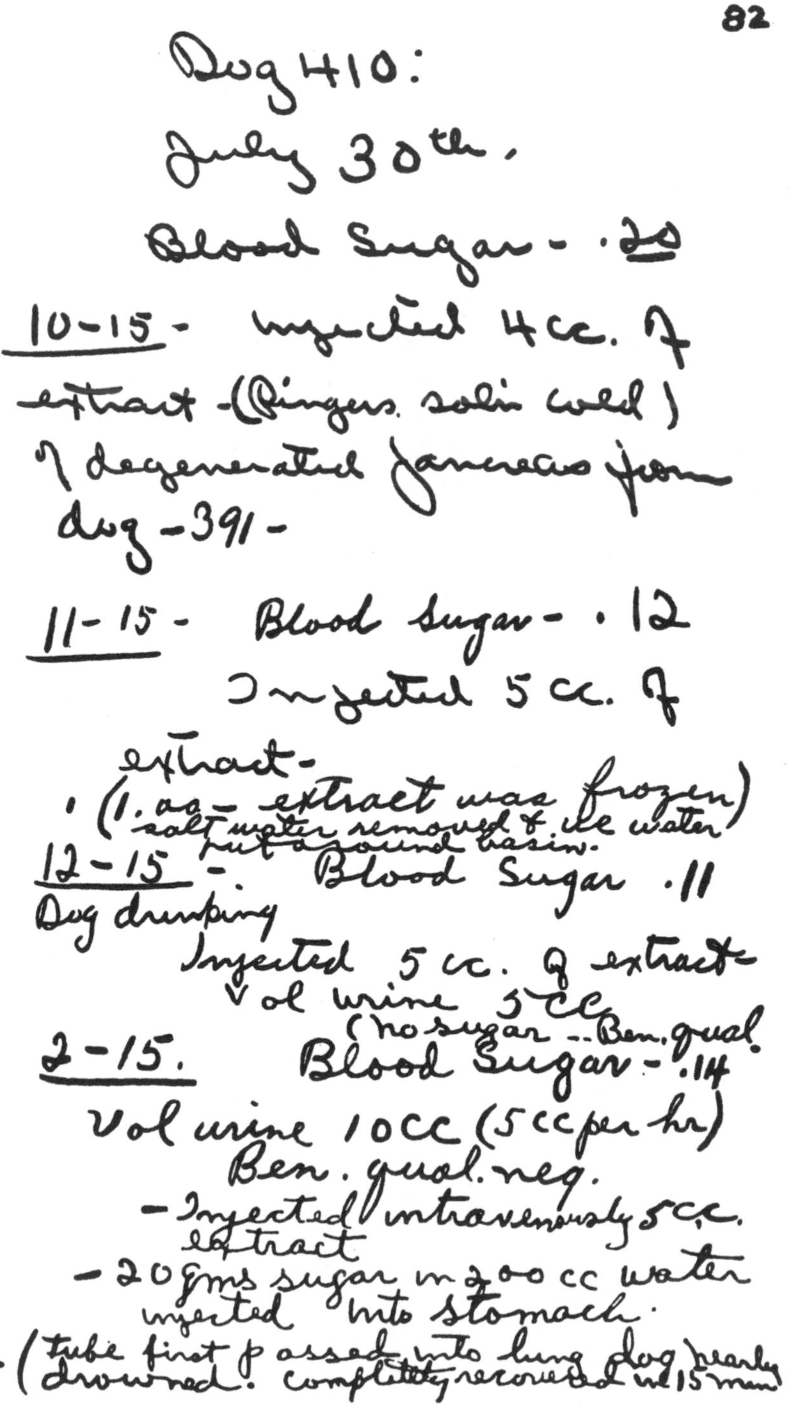

Dog 410:

July 30th.

Blood Sugar - .20

10-15 - injected 4 cc. of extract -(Ringers soln cold) of degenerated pancreas from dog -391-

11-15 - Blood Sugar - .12
Injected 5 cc. of extract-
. (1.oz- extract was frozen)
salt water removed & ice water
put around basin.

12-15 -. Blood Sugar .11
Dog drinking
Injected 5 cc. of extract-
Vol urine 5 cc
(no sugar ...Ben. qual.

2-15. Blood Sugar -.14
Vol urine 10 cc (5 cc per hr)
Ben. qual. neg.
- Injected intravenously 5 cc.
extract
- 20 gms sugar in 200 cc water
injected into stomach.
- (tube first passed into lung dog nearly
drowned. completely recovered in 15 min

FIGURE 1. Page from notebook, July 1921.

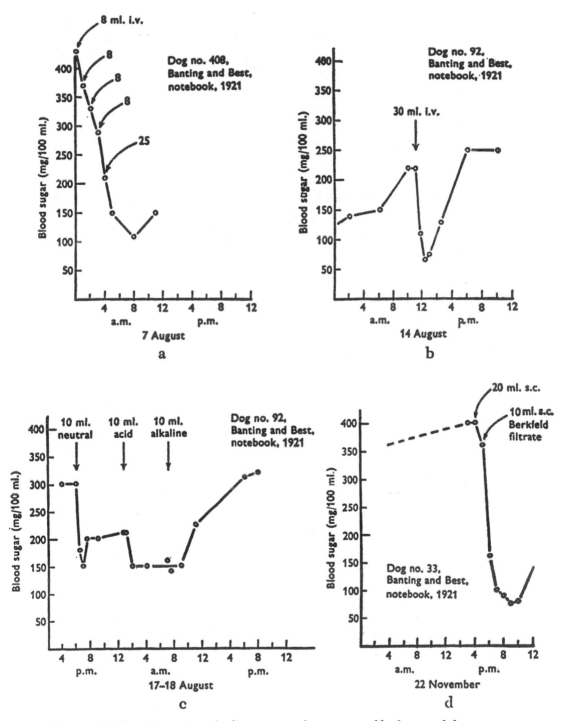

FIGURE 2. Effect of injections of saline extracts of pancreas on blood sugar of depancreatized dogs. (*a, b*) Extract of degenerated pancreas; (*c*) extract of normal pancreas; (*d*) extract of pancreas of foetal calf. (Redrawn, 1958.)

tion was given before the Faculty of Medicine of the University of Toronto, and this was the first paper on insulin [40]. Professor Macleod added his name to a preliminary communication given before the American Physiological Society at Yale, Christmas 1921, and this note [49]—which should, perhaps, not be considered to constitute priority although it has performed this function in several strategic places—actually was published a week or so before the more complete account, which Banting and I had sent in several months before the note was submitted. The preliminary observations on ketone body excretion, on liver fat, and on various other signs of the diabetic state, were not published by Banting and myself alone, but were amplified and developed by the team which was later organized, and the complete evidence for the first demonstration of these effects of insulin will be found in a series of papers published in the *Transactions of the Royal Society of Canada* [43, 44, 45, 46, 47, 207].

When the time came to test our extract on a human diabetic, Banting was intensely anxious that I should make the extract and this actually was the case. I felt very strongly that our potent, sterile, and relatively clean preparation from foetal calf pancreas should be utilized. We knew that it was much more potent than that from whole beef pancreas, but Banting felt that we might be criticized because we had not made the material from a commercially available source. I have always regretted that I allowed myself to be persuaded to make this extract from normal beef pancreas. It was potent but there was a great deal of inert protein present. We injected it into each other. It was life-saving and not toxic when given to a diabetic dog, but a great deal of unnecessary debate and trouble would have been avoided if the potent sterile extract of foetal calf pancreas (Figure 2d) had been used in the first patients. Quite recently my colleagues Dr. J. M. Salter and Dr. O. Sirek have made and tested an extract from foetal calf pancreas, produced by exactly the same procedure which I used in 1921. This gave a sweeping fall of blood sugar in animals and in diabetic children on Professor A. L. Chute's wards, and there were no signs whatever of any local reactions or toxic effects.

I must resist the desire to tell you about some of the dramatic effects on patients of the early lots of insulin. The improvements in production developed by J. B. Collip had been incorporated. We had passed through a stage when Collip had lost the secret of making larger lots of insulin and some of the patients, who had been successfully treated, died from lack of the hormone. Collip went back to his department in Alberta and I was forced to return to the task of producing insulin. I *could* tell you about some of the patients who received the first lots of insulin in Toronto who are still alive; about the insulin which Sir Henry Dale brought back to

England in 1922; about the insulin which I sent to Professor Oskar Minkowski; about the material which was given to Sir Francis Fraser in Toronto and which he used to treat the Captain of his ship who had lapsed into diabetic coma; and about the first insulin sent to the United States to treat a boy who is now alive and well thirty-seven years later.

I remember reading copies of the correspondence between the secretary of our Insulin Committee in Toronto and Sir Walter Fletcher, secretary of the Medical Research Council, and with what excitement I looked forward to the arrival of H. H. Dale and Harold Ward Dudley. The Medical Research Council made no mistake in the selection of that pair, and my life was fuller from the moment that I met them. We had many wonderful talks. I remember explaining the procedures which we were forced to use in the larger-scale production of insulin, the difficulties which we had encountered, and how we had overcome them by the construction of a great wind tunnel where acetone extracts of pancreas were rapidly evaporated under open electric heaters. We used a fan that had been designed to ventilate a whole building, and the gale of wind sucked off the vapour and perhaps blew out the sparks. Before Dale and Dudley arrived, this apparatus had been replaced by a 25 gal. metal vacuum still with a condenser which ravenously consumed the several tons of ice hoisted into its open mouth every 24 hours.

Dudley and I went from Toronto to Chicago, where we spent an interesting day discussing the preparation of insulin with Dr. Robin T. Woodyatt. We met Dale in Indianapolis. This was one of the nine trips which I made to the Eli Lilly and Company during that year to help them get started on the large-scale production of insulin and to learn from their fine staff industrial techniques and scientific facts which I utilized as Director of Insulin Production for Canada in the Connaught Laboratories. We were very fortunate in our choice of a company with which to co-operate, and the development of insulin owes a great deal to members of the Lilly family and to Dr. G. H. A. Clowes, the English-American scientist who was the Scientific Director of the Company.

Dale and I together depancreatized a dog in the Lilly Laboratories, and if I remember correctly it was the first one which survived the intense heat and made its contribution to the preparation of insulin. I have never been sure whether I assisted Dale or he assisted me, but I have a vivid recollection of his taking the needle holder out of my hand, and completing, with dextrous touch, the sewing up of the skin wound. I can hear him laugh as he patted my shoulder and said, "Fingers are really quite adequate for this type of work."

I wrote my M.A. thesis in Physiology in the spring of 1922, on one aspect of the effects of insulin, and I was undecided whether to proceed to a Ph.D. or to qualify in medicine. I decided on the latter, and for three years I superintended the production of insulin, conducted research on the methods of its preparation and studied medicine. My association with D. A. Scott, F.R.S., had already begun and we were intensely interested in all the procedures which gave us better yields of insulin. We found insulin-like activity in tissues [115] where Banting and I had failed to detect any. Somewhat later I had the maturing experience of sorting out a vexatious and somewhat humiliating problem. Our test rabbits had been unreliable and apparently sometimes showed spontaneous hypoglycaemia. We also decided that the dust of the room and invisible traces of previous lots of insulin must be eliminated with scrupulous care from glassware and apparatus. We eventually satisfied ourselves and reported again [99] as Banting and I had originally, that the pancreas contains the only appreciable reserves of insulin in the body. With present-day methods, other tissues can, of course, be shown to contain small amounts. A number of laboratories in Europe, in England, and the United States had fallen into one or more of the same pitfalls, and I remember writing to each of them explaining our difficulties and suggesting that they repeat their work with added precautions. As you all know, David Scott, my close friend for thirty-seven years, was to go on and show that the crystalline insulin prepared by Abel and Geiling was the zinc salt, and with another colleague of mine, Dr. Albert Fisher, to prepare protamine zinc insulin [685].

When Dale was in Toronto in 1922 he had agreed to accept me as a junior colleague in the summer of 1925, and I came to London as soon as I finished my medical course. I was anxious to work on anything except insulin. I had decided to live in Canada, and, as an M.A. in Physiology, I had refused several offers in the United States, which paid more at that time than I have ever received in the University of Toronto. To facilitate my progress in Canada I felt that a D.Sc. degree from the University of London would be helpful. Dale said, "This will not make you a better physiologist," but he went to great trouble to get himself appointed a recognized teacher at the University of London, and I believe that I was his first graduate student. The time in Dale's laboratory in 1925 and 1926, and again in 1928 was a great joy to me. I learned physiological and pharmacological techniques from Dale and chemical procedures from Dudley. P. P. Laidlaw and Percival Hartley were my particularly close friends. With Dale, Dudley and Thorpe I helped to isolate histamine for the first time from tissue which did not have the opportunity to become contaminated bacteriologically. I played a very minor role in this work, but I learned a great deal. I became interested in the effects of choline and

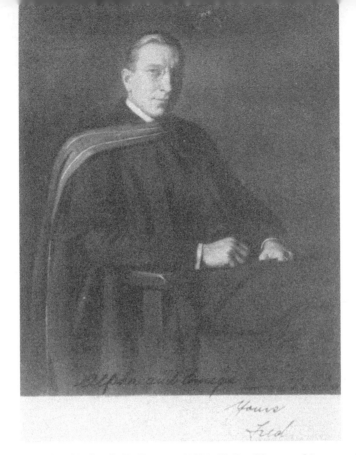

PLATE 1. (a) Dr. Frederick G. Banting (1891–1941). Photographic copy of the painting by Curtis Williamson, sent by Banting to Best with inscription "Alpha and Omega—Charlie, Yours Fred." (b) Dr. Charles H. Best presents citation from the American Diabetes Association to Dr. Elliott P. Joslin on the occasion of his ninetieth birthday (at the annual A.D.A. banquet, Atlantic City, June 1959).

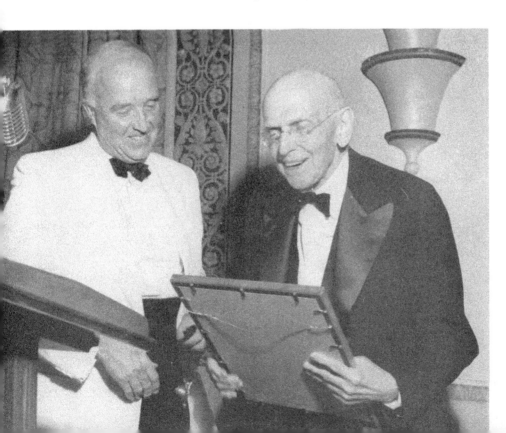

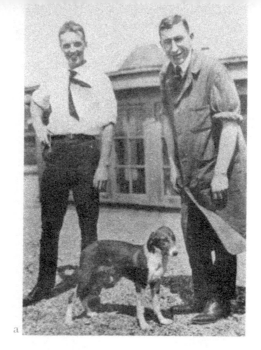

a

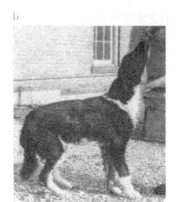

b

PLATE II. (*a*) Banting (*on right*) and Best with the first dog to be kept alive by insulin (Paper 27). (*b*) Dog Marjorie (referred to in Paper 5) nine weeks after pancreatectomy; she received insulin daily. (*c*) Former University Y.M.C.A. building which housed the insulin plant from 1922 to 1927.

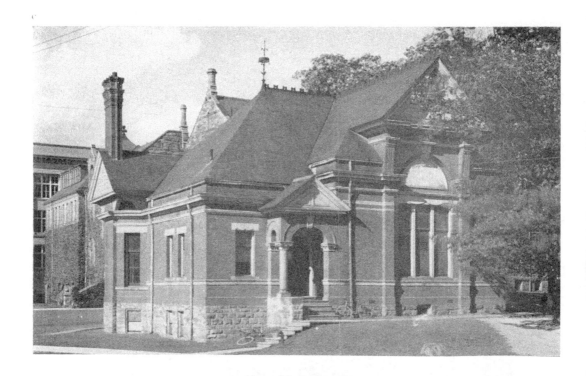

c

histamine together in lowering the blood pressure. Matching doses of histamine and choline were given separately. Half doses of the two together had a greater effect [82]. We had developed a quantitative method for the analysis of histamine in tissues and I thought it would be interesting to study the possibility that histamine was made from histidine, but, to my surprise, the added histamine and that naturally present in lung tissue disappeared rapidly. This did not occur in heated extracts [69]. This subject was further developed with McHenry after my return to Toronto. I suggested the name histaminase for the system which destroyed histamine [107]. The subject of the catabolism of histamine has changed tremendously over the years and Schayer [672] has suggested that there are at least six pathways by which histamine may be broken down *in vivo*. He states, "The controversy over histaminase versus diamine oxidase has not been settled. The matter has become worse since it has been shown that diamine oxidase oxidizes monoamines and monoamine oxidase oxidizes diamines, including histamine." Schayer goes on to say that, "It seems desirable to discontinue use of the term 'histaminase' as soon as a satisfactory system of nomenclature for amine oxidases can be formulated." An *alternative* course would be to retain the name "histaminase" for all of the enzymes which destroy histamine, and to characterize each one individually in accordance with the chemical changes which it produces in the histamine molecule.

When I arrived in Hampstead, Dale, Burn, and Marks were very busy with studies of the effects of insulin in the eviscerated animal. I was truly anxious to gain experience in other lines of research, but the lure of the work on insulin proved irresistible, and, before long, Joseph Hoet, of Louvain, who was to become one of my closest friends, and I were participating in an extension of these studies on the action of insulin. With Sir Henry and Marks, we made a balance sheet of the sugar which disappeared as a result of the effects of insulin, and we came to the conclusion that glycogen formation and oxidation would account for essentially all of it. We assumed that in the presence of an excess of sugar with a respiratory quotient of 1, and in the absence of a functioning liver, all the oxygen utilized was employed in the oxidation of carbohydrate [83]. We based our assumption, also, on the work of several previous investigators who also felt that this was valid under these particular conditions. Of course, direct evidence for the oxidation of sugar had to await the availability of isotopically labelled glucose. There was also the possibility which we *now* know, that appreciable amounts of the sugar may have been transformed into fatty acid. But I would not be surprised if the use of the most modern techniques in an experiment of the type in which we were then interested, would lead to essentially the same conclusions which we then drew. One of my former students and colleagues, Dr. Samuel Soskin, has criticized our old-fashioned experiments, somewhat unjustly. It seems to me that he yielded to the temptation to twist the lion's tail, and those of his pups, somewhat more than the facts and his Canadian background would warrant. In another investigation, which I conducted by myself, I was pleased to find a dramatic effect of insulin on the rate of disappearance of sugar from the isolated perfused hindlegs of the cat [68]. This was, essentially, a muscle preparation and it provided perhaps the earliest direct evidence of the effect of insulin on muscle tissue.

Variations in the amount of insulin extractable from the pancreas under standard conditions have fascinated me ever since 1921. With Dr. (now Professor) R. E. Haist and Dr. Jessie Ridout, extended studies were conducted of the effect of diet on the extractable insulin and the dramatic lowering which is produced by fasting or fat feeding [85]. The reduced level can be lowered even further when insulin is given to the fasted animals. After the demonstration of the production of permanent diabetes in dogs given anterior pituitary extract, by my friend and one-time colleague in Toronto, Professor Frank Young [821], Haist, Campbell, and I showed that the onset of diabetes in these pituitary-treated dogs could be prevented if insulin was given prophylactically. The insulin extractable from the pancreas remained at a much higher level in the insulin-treated dogs. In the transient diabetes produced by pituitary extract, the insulin content of the pancreas fell but returned to normal when the pituitary injections were discontinued (Figure 3).

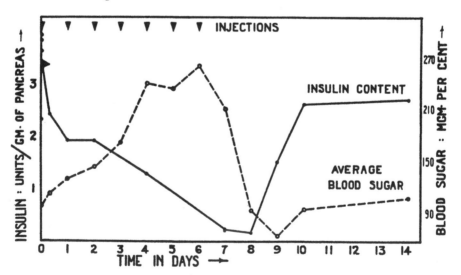

FIGURE 3. Effect of anterior pituitary extract on the insulin content of pancreas and average blood sugar.

When permanent diabetes was produced the insulin content remained at essentially zero [347]. More recently my pupil and colleague, Dr. Gerald Wrenshall, has studied the insulin extractable from the human pancreas. He finds almost no insulin in the pancreas of the so-called growth-onset diabetic, and approximately 40 per cent of the normal value in the pancreas of the maturity-onset diabetic. In dogs permanent diabetes is always accompanied by virtual loss of all insulin from the pancreatic tissues. These findings on human diabetics with the maturity-onset type of disorder have assumed very great significance in the light of the effects of the oral hypoglycaemic agents. One aspect of their action is either to liberate insulin or to stimulate a reaction for which the presence of at least some insulin is necessary.

It was never my good fortune to work with my friend Professor A. V. Hill, C.H., F.R.S., in the beautiful and fundamental studies which have earned him his great and enduring reputation. However, I did work with him for a short time, and was stimulated to carry on for several more years studying the respiratory quotient of the excess metabolism of muscular exercise and the dynamics of sprint running. A. V. Hill derived a lot of pleasure from experiments of this type and so did I. He gave me the apparatus which he had used in some of his experiments at Cornell University at Ithaca, New York, and I explored—with my very competent biophysical colleague, Dr. Ruth Partridge—the dynamics exhibited by the young Canadian sprinter, Percy Williams, who won both the 100 and the 200 metres in the 1928 Olympic Games, and by a famous woman sprinter, Myrtle Cook. We retained Williams for some weeks as a member of our staff (Figure 4). At the same Olympic Games I studied the blood sugar of the marathon runners and found that several of them, at the end of their 26 miles, exhibited signs of hypoglycaemia, and that the level of sugar in their blood showed that this was actually the case [110].

The work on heparin in Toronto was stimulated, in part, by my experiences with Sir Henry Dale. The need for a much purer and more active anticoagulant was obvious, and on my return to Toronto in 1928 I organized a team to explore the sources of heparin and to test the purified products in the prevention of experimental thrombosis. The possibility of clinical application was constantly in our minds. I recently described in some detail [76] at a meeting of the New York Academy of Medicine to honour the late J. McLean, who discovered heparin in Howell's laboratory in 1916 [535], the advances which we made in Toronto. Dr. Scott and Dr. Charles, working in what was then my section of the Connaught Laboratories and in the Department of Physiology, found that beef lung was an excellent source of heparin, and they went on to prepare various

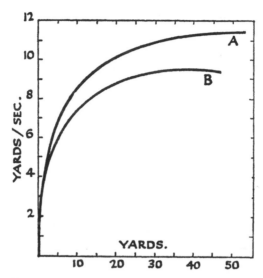

FIGURE 4. Dynamics of sprint running. Change of speed with distance. (A) Percy Williams; (B) Myrtle Cook.

crystalline salts [200]. The purified heparin not only was some twenty-five times as active as that which had been previously available from dog's liver in preventing the clotting of blood, but it also stopped the agglutination of platelets. This property of heparin had not been convincingly demonstrated before. Dr. Gordon Murray collaborated with us in some aspects of the experimental work, and went on to apply these results to surgical practice [589]. In the two years just before the outbreak of the last war, D. Y. Solandt, R. Nassim, and I were very busy in the extension of this work on heparin, and we found that we could prevent the occurrence of experimentally induced coronary thrombosis in dogs, and that we could inhibit, also, the development of the great mural thrombi, which are produced when an irritating substance is injected just under the endocardium. These papers were published in the *Lancet* and stimulated clinical interest in the anticoagulants [722].[2]

The availability of a potent anticoagulant made possible innumerable studies, some of which had clinical application. With Dr. William Thalhimer, Dr. Solandt and I studied exchange transfusion between a nephrectomized animal which became uraemic, and a normal dog [750], and we demonstrated the dramatic lowering of the blood urea of the uraemic animal. The use of a practical artificial kidney or of the artificial heart has, of course, depended on the availability of purified heparin. The

[2]The recent reports of the clinical teams working under the Medical Research Council confirm the favourable effects of the anticoagulants in certain situations.

recognition of a heparinase system [424], the first use of siliconed tubing to minimize clotting [425], and the isolation of heparin in crystalline form from the blood of dogs in anaphylactic shock, were other products of the work of this group of colleagues.

When the war threatened in 1939 we began experiments on traumatic shock and initiated, under the auspices of the Canadian Red Cross Society, a blood donor system which provided over two million contributions of blood serum. This was dried in the Connaught Laboratories and shipped here for use in the Allied Medical Services. I felt that I must set a good example in this wartime venture, so I became the No. 1 donor, but after ten bleedings I felt a bit anaemic and joined the Navy! The Naval Medical Research Unit, formed in 1940, in which my colleagues Solandt, Sellers, Campbell, Parker, Locke, Cowan, and many others, served, made scores of practical contributions to Naval Medicine. The stimulus and some of the basic information for one of our projects was provided by Professor A. V. Hill. After confirmation and extension of this work by Solandt, he and I were able to install for the first time a type of lighting in naval vessels which preserved night vision. The original attempts to test this procedure in the Royal Navy, initiated by the late Dr. Lythgoe, had failed because the sea trials had been conducted in what we later found were conditions which demanded day, rather than night vision. My colleagues and I made frequent trips to sea and studied problems at our bases in Newfoundland, Iceland, and Scotland. A special number of the *Journal of the Canadian Armed Services* [16] has described in detail the results of this Naval Medical Research. The study of seasickness was an extremely difficult matter. We had no landing craft available. We organized trials on liners like the *Queen Elizabeth* with adequate controls. That particular crossing on the *Queen Elizabeth* was exciting but it was so calm that no one was seasick. We made other trials in corvettes and destroyers, when the weather was so severe that even the observers were incapacitated. My colleagues did a lot of excellent work in testing old remedies and investigating new ones. Trustworthy evidence that some of the old compounds were actually effective was obtained. The R.C.N. "seasickness pill," in its various forms, was a boon to the Canadian Navy. An outburst of unwarranted publicity about the pill would have been quenched immediately if I had been in Canada, but I had crossed in a bomber to Greenock, Scotland, to study other problems which our naval personnel were encountering there. I remember a stimulating talk with Sir Henry Tizzard while waiting for our separate bombers on a cold evening in Gander Airport in Newfoundland, and with my friend of longer standing, Sir Edward Mellanby, on various naval medical research matters, when I came to London.

I stayed with Sir Henry and Lady Dale at Mount Vernon House on one of my trips during the war, and at another time I was with them at the Royal Institution on Albemarle Street. Sir Henry was extremely helpful arranging to inform our British colleagues of the results of the red lighting experiments and other advances of a practical nature. He will recall that Solandt and I had some difficulty convincing certain senior medical officers of the Royal Navy of the significance of red lighting. This process was facilitated by the contact which Dale arranged with Lord Hankey and with Admiral Sir Bruce Fraser. Sir Henry will, I think, remember quite vividly the crossing to Canada on the old liner *Bergensfjord*, when he, Adrian, Solandt, and I shared a very small cabin. In the middle of one of the long nights the ship's duty medical officer, Wing-Commander Kidd from Belfast, came into our cabin and awakened us. His question was, "Do any of you chaps know any biochemistry?" Sir Henry, from the lower bunk pondered the matter for a moment and then he replied, "Actually, not much, but you might try Best." He added as an afterthought, "He is younger." The problem was an unconscious American Army boy deep in the bowels of the ship, with the smell of acetone on his breath. Insulin was obtained from the Norwegian skipper of our ship, Captain Colle, who was himself taking 80 units a day. The American boy regained consciousness and made an uneventful recovery.

After Fred Banting's tragic death on February 21, 1941, while carrying scientific information to this country, I was requested to resign my posts in the Connaught Laboratories and the School of Hygiene and to assume responsibility for the Banting and Best Department of Medical Research in addition to that of the Department of Physiology. All of our research problems at that time had some relation to military medicine.

With Professor Phillip Greey and Dr. Colin C. Lucas, a pilot plant for the production of penicillin was organized in the Department of Bacteriology and in the Banting and Best Department of Medical Research, and this later was transferred with some of the key personnel to the Connaught Laboratories where the large-scale production of penicillin in Canada has continued. The contributions of Dr. S. F. MacDonald to the pilot plant studies were invaluable.

At the termination of the war the activities of our departments were reorganized, and many of the old problems on insulin, on heparin, and on choline were attacked by research sections headed by my various colleagues, most of whom had been my students. We have been reinforced from time to time by fine new Canadians, among whom I may mention Dr. Bruno Mendel, Dr. Hermann Fischer, Dr. Erich Baer, Dr. Aaron Rappaport, Dr. Otakar Sirek, and Dr. Anna Sirek.

I need say very little about the work on choline and its precursors, the lipotropic agents, since I have reviewed this field in my Croonian Lecture [74]. I remember remarking to Dale after I had given this lecture that I had attempted to cover too much ground. Sir Henry reassured me by saying: "Almost everyone since 1738 has done the same thing." It would now appear that a great deal of fundamental work on lipid metabolism must probably precede any great advance in our understanding of the mechanism of action of choline.

I may summarize the outstanding developments in this field very rapidly; it was an obvious step to provide minced pancreas in the diet when insulin-treated, completely depancreatized dogs developed signs of liver damage. It has been a long time since Hershey and Soskin [388] reported from my laboratory that some component of crude lecithin could replace the beef pancreas. With Dr. Elinor Huntsman, now Mrs. Colin Mawson, we purified lecithin, and developed a test for the detection of the lipotropic factors, using normal rats given a diet rich in fat [91]. Purified lecithin was lipotropically active and we identified choline as its only active constituent (Figure 5); betaine was also found to be active [94]. The first intimation that protein might contain an active lipotropic agent was reported by Miss Huntsman and myself [95]. Soon methionine was recognized as the main active lipotropic constituent of protein by Tucker and Eckstein [760]. The earliest signs of fibrosis due to choline deficiency were reported

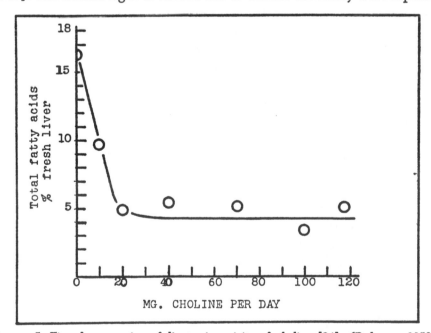

FIGURE 5. First demonstration of lipotropic activity of choline [94]. (Redrawn, 1958.)

in 1934 [532]. The detection of the stages of the development of the huge fatty cysts and their breakdown, with the discharge of fat into the systemic circulation and the eventual laying down of fibrous tissue was due, in large part, to the efforts of my student and colleague, Dr. W. Stanley Hartroft [373]. We found that a few days of choline deficiency in early life resulted in kidney changes, and subsequently in malignant hypertension [372]. The animals were fed an adequate diet throughout the study, except for the five days of choline deficiency. Many years before this Dr. Ridout and I had noted [111] the first effect of choline in decreasing the unsaponifiable fraction of the livers of rats fed cholesterol; this was further explored in collaboration with Dr. Harold Channon [80]. The many recent studies which have been conducted with Professor Colin C. Lucas, Dr. Ridout, and others, cannot be described here.

We should probably have worked more intensely on the factor or factors in the anterior pituitary gland which mobilizes depot fat to the liver. The first clear recognition of this effect was seen in 1936 [78]. Later Dr. Campbell [161] worked out a very useful test for the recognition of this substance or substances. The liver fat of starving or fasted rats or mice increases very rapidly when the pituitary factor is injected. Weil and Stetten [784] repeated and confirmed our findings and suggested the name "adipokinin" for this pituitary material, which may be the same as that which appears in the urine of fasted animals. It is by no means established, as yet, whether this effect is due to pure growth hormone, adrenocorticotrophic hormone, or other components of the anterior pituitary gland. There is still a possibility that the effect may be due to a new substance, but I would suggest, at the moment, that it appears more likely that it is exerted by two or more different pituitary factors.

During the last eight years a number of very promising younger men have joined our group. The most recent, Dr. Geza Hetenyi, formerly Chairman of the Department of Physiology at Szeged, Hungary, is working with our biophysicist, Dr. G. A. Wrenshall, on one approach to the mechanism of the action of insulin. Dr. Ronald Williams, graduate in Biochemistry from Liverpool, and a colleague of Professor Britton Chance of Philadelphia for some years, is attacking the mechanism of the action of choline with the tools of the physical chemist and the enzymologist. Dr. Bruno Rosenfeld, a former colleague of the late Dr. Weizmann in Israel, is also working on the action of choline. Dr. Anna Sirek, Dr. Otakar Sirek, and their colleagues [710, 711] have explored in detail the effects of the oral hypoglycaemic agents in normal and in depancreatized dogs. This species consistently develop signs of liver damage with any of the oral hypoglycaemic agents which we have tested. Dr. Anna Sirek has studied, also, the nature of the material liberated from the splanchnic area when growth hormone is injected. This is not glucagon but may prove to be serotonin or some new substance [709].

I have been keenly interested with my younger colleague, Dr. James Salter, in the action of insulin as a growth hormone. Everyone knows that insulin is a growth hormone, but there is some debate as to the mechanism of this growth effect in hypophysectomized animals. Since a diet containing carbohydrate presumably liberates insulin from the pancreas of the hypophysectomized animal and since somatotrophin probably does the same thing, the only way to explore the effects of known amounts of insulin or somatotrophin alone and the two together, is on depancreatized-hypophysectomized animals. There seems little doubt from the work of Lukens [518] and of Scow[3] [689, 690] in Professor Houssay's laboratory, and of Salter and of Campbell in my department, that insulin alone exerts a definite anabolic effect in Houssay cats, rats, and dogs. It is necessary to provide carbohydrate to demonstrate the anabolic effect of insulin, but it is not surprising that the hormone is ineffective without its fuel [660, 661].

The work on glucagon, in the physiological and biochemical aspects of which Dr. James Salter has been the leading figure, has given us a lot of excitement and pleasure. There is a definite increase in basal metabolic rate when glucagon is administered [247]. When glucagon is given in oil, or when very frequent injections are made over the 24 hours, there is a profound diabetogenic effect in rats, rabbits, and human subjects [662, 295]. Glucagon greatly increases the excretion of the products of protein breakdown, and for this reason its effect on rheumatoid arthritis was explored. Some dramatic improvements were observed by the clinical group of the Department of Medicine, but the production of nausea in the patients precludes, at the moment, further clinical exploration of this interesting situation [295]. We reported last year [663] that the growth of certain tumours in rats could be inhibited when insulin and glucagon were given. This work has been confirmed in two other laboratories, and the growth of some five tumours, some of them naturally occurring, can be inhibited if glucagon and insulin or glucagon alone is administered in the appropriate way. It would seem that this effect of glucagon is on the host rather than on the tumour cell, and, therefore, a thorough investigation of the basic physiological effects of glucagon must be made. In confirmation and extension of the work of Lazarus and Volk [490], Dr. Logothetopoulos and Dr. Salter have obtained a profound effect of glucagon in causing

---

[3]Scow did not study Houssay rats without insulin, since these force-fed animals, under his experimental conditions, died. The fact that they lived with insulin is excellent evidence of an anabolic effect of the hormone.

atrophy of the α-cells of the pancreas in rabbits. This effect is confined to the α-cells and is not exhibited by the argentophil cells of the gastro-intestinal tract.

Recently, Logothetopoulos, Sharma, and Salter have conducted a tedious and exciting experiment in which glucagon was injected into rabbits from shortly after birth until the animal had reached the age of five or six months. Glucagon was administered three or four times during the 24 hours, every day in the week. The animals became intensely diabetic, putting out up to 50 g sugar/day, and they have remained diabetic for prolonged periods after cessation of glucagon administration. The success of this particular aspect of the work is due, in large part, to the perseverance and meticulous experimental techniques of Dr. John Logothetopoulos. These findings mean that metaglucagon diabetes has been established. This will, I think, constitute a new landmark in the study of hormones and the diabetic state.[4]

Thus my particular trail of Canadian medical research has revealed more than enough pleasant and exciting vistas to convince me that few other professions are likely to provide as much satisfaction and pleasure. I sometimes try to exercise a little restraint in discussing these matters at our family gatherings because, as some of you know, neither of my two sons is primarily interested in medical research. Their mother, who has been my perfect helpmate since our engagement, well before the work on insulin started, specialized in botany and history for her university degree. One of our sons is a botanist and the other a historian!

It will be obvious to you how very fortunate I have been in my scientific colleagues. I have reached the stage now when I spend most of my time in planning experiments, in appraising results, and in initiating junior workers into the realm of medical research. I do have the pleasure, however, of knowing that my colleagues who are heads of sections in my departments, are always eager to have me participate more actively in their problems. This I constantly plan to do.

It has been a great privilege to give this annual lecture before the Society for Endocrinology and to receive the first medal struck in honour of one of the great men of our time, Sir Henry Dale.

[4]A hint of some advance made in the field of diabetes in our laboratory has reached the daily press. I hope that none of my colleagues here has been bothered by reporters inquiring about this matter. Many years ago Sir Henry was pestered by a reporter who wanted comments on a new cure developed by Fred Banting in Toronto. The reporter stated that it was a "cure for metabolism."

Part I: INSULIN AND GLUCAGON

I T SO HAPPENS THAT MANY OF OUR *handwritten records and the original manuscript of the first communication concerning insulin are still in existence. I thought it might be of historical interest to reproduce as Paper 2 at least a few pages of the manuscript which Banting and I used at the first presentation of the findings to our colleagues in the Medical Building of the University on November 14, 1921, at a regular meeting of the Physiological Journal Club. Later we revised this slightly to put it in the form in which it appeared in the* Journal of Laboratory and Clinical Medicine *in February 1922 (Paper 4, below). This manuscript thus represents not only the first paper presented but also the first sent for publication.*

Page 1 of the original manuscript, which was in my handwriting, was torn and discoloured and subsequently lost. It had been copied by me after it was damaged and this copy is what now appears as page 1. All the other 26 pages are still intact as they were written in November 1921 except page 16 which has disappeared.

On glancing through the original, one is struck by the fact that the writing of four different hands can be recognized. Three of these are easily identified. The upper portion of page 2 is in my own original handwriting, pages 7 and 8 are in Banting's, the lower half of page 12, page 13, and the top of page 14 are in the writing of Miss Margaret Mahon, who later became my wife, with more of mine on the bottom of the page. We were engaged at the time and I remember dictating this material to her at her parents' home at 370 Brunswick Avenue. The lower portion of page 2 and page 3 are in a handwriting that I have been unable to identify. It is not Professor Macleod's, Professor Henderson's, or that of Dr. or Mrs. Fred Hipwell. Fred Hipwell was Banting's cousin who had come to Toronto with him to attend the University. Someone at Banting's request must have copied this part of the manuscript. I remember looking up some of the material used in this section but, after these many years, I cannot remember who copied these three-and-one-half pages. Pages 25, 26, and 27 present our conclusions in my handwriting on Banting's professional note paper. Banting was reluctant to assume responsibility for describing our results in writing and this fell to my lot. He took great pleasure, however, in drawing the charts from which the lantern slides used in our first presentation, and the illustrations in our original paper, were made.

Some time after this manuscript had been sent off for publication to the Journal of Laboratory and Clinical Medicine, *Professor Macleod suggested that an abstract of this paper should be sent to the American Physiological Society and that we should present a brief account of our work at the Yale meeting in December 1921. Professor Macleod has stated that he did not permit his name to appear on our first two papers to give us clear priority on the demonstration of insulin in dog pancreas and foetal beef pancreas. He did, however, give us the impression that as a member his name was necessary on the preliminary communication to the American Physiological Society. The paper was given by Banting. Professor Macleod was the chairman of the meeting. Banting was nervous but presented our findings clearly. Professor Macleod was in his element and answered a number of questions which Banting had anticipated. He and I, after seven months of intensive work with some seventy-five definite successes, were sure that the results would speak for themselves. Macleod, with greater experience, wished to convince all the sceptics. Professor Anton Carlson raised a question about the length of time dogs would survive after pancreatectomy. He inferred that the survival time might be longer than we thought. I caught the chairman's eye and he asked me to reply to Professor Carlson. I stated that if all the pancreas were removed the animals did not survive under our conditions for more than three weeks, at most. He gave me a sharp look but at the first opportunity came to talk with me in the kindest possible manner and that was the beginning of our long friendship.*

Dr. G. H. A. Clowes, the distinguished English-American scientist, who was the Director of Research of the Eli Lilly and Company, was a very interested spectator at the Yale meeting. As he has related in his Banting Memorial Lecture, he was completely convinced by our presentation and was understandably anxious to place the extensive chemical and engineering experience of his company at our disposal immediately. Banting and I later wished that this had been done. The executives and the scientific staff of this company could not have been fairer or more helpful to us. Professor Macleod was opposed to co-operation with an industrial organization at that time, on the grounds that for a period the future development of all aspects of the work on insulin should be carried out in the University of Toronto.

2. The Internal Secretion of the Pancreas (Selected pages)

By F. G. Banting, M.B. And C.H. Best, B.A.

The hypothesis underlying this series of experiments was first formulated by one of us in November, 1920 (F.G.B) while reading an article dealing with the relation of the islets of Langerhans to diabetes. From the passage in this article, which gives a résumé of degenerative changes in the acini of the pancreas following ligation of the ducts, the idea presented itself that since the acinous, but not the islet tissue, degenerates after this ligation, advantage might be taken of this fact to prepare an active extract of islet tissue. The auxiliary hypothesis was that Trypsinogen or its derivatives was antagonistic to the internal secretion of the gland. The failure of other investigators in this much-worked field were thus accounted for.

The feasibility of the hypothesis having been recognized by Professor J. J. R. Macleod, work was begun, under his direction, in May 1921, in the Physiological

(2)

Laboratory of the University of Toronto. In this paper no attempt will be made to give a complete review of the literature. A short resumé, however, of some of the outstanding articles, which tend to link together the islands of Langerhands with the control of carbohydrate metabolism will be submitted.

Historical.

In 1889 Hering + Minkowski[1] found that total pancreatectomy in dogs resulted in severe + fatal diabetes. Following this, many different observers experimented with other animals + all species examined showed glycosuria + fatal cachexia, thus establishing the fact that the pancreas was responsible for this form of diabetes.

Aronson + Vaillard[2] in 1894 ligated the pancreatic ducts in rabbits + found that within 24 hrs. the ducts became dilated, the epithelial cells began to degenerate + that

There[3] were protoplasmic changes in the acinous cells.   On the 7th. day there was beginning round-celled infiltration. On the 14th. day the parenchyma was mostly replaced by fibrous tissue. Ssobolew in 1902 noted in addition to this that there was gradual atrophy & sclerosis of the pancreas with no glycosuria However, in the later stages, from 30 to 120 days after ligation of the ducts, he found involvement of the islets & accompanying glycosuria.

Laguesse[4], an anatomist, first suggested that the islets might be thought of as pancreatic internal secretion. He showed that there were comparatively more islets in the foetus & the newborn than in the adult animal. Consequently, he concluded that the islets could not be changed acini as thought by Kuwaschew.

Schaefer[5], in 1895, announced it as his belief that the islets produced an internal secretion, the disturbance of which was the basis of diabetes.   Opie & Ssobolew[6] [7] independently furnished the first

¶ We submit the following experiments which we believe give convincing evidence that it is this latter mechanism which is in operation.

The ~~early months~~ of our work ~~were~~ spent in the ligation of the ~~ducts~~ dogs ~~the pancreas~~ and in the attempt to ~~secure~~ secure records of control animals.

~~Our first~~

We first ligated the pancreatic ducts in a number of dogs. Blood Sugar estimations in these animals were recorded from time to time ~~and at various phases of degeneration and~~. We have no record of a hyperglycemia.

In the time ~~which~~ interval which we considered necessary for complete degeneration of the acinous tissue, we secured records of dogs depancreatized by the Hédon method.

.

8

chart no. I contains the record of dog 410. This experiment is not one of the most conclusive of those we submit but is very interesting to us at least since [crossed out] administered to this animal the first dose of the extract of degenerated pancreas.

As will be seen from the chart [crossed out] the pancreas with the exception of the processus uncinatus was removed on July 11th. In the interval between this initial operation & the removal of the pedicle on July 18th the percentage of sugar in the blood remained at the -normal level (.090 average from observation on 30 normal dogs by the Myers-Bar (13) Lewis-Benedict method). The Benedict qualitative tests showed no sugar repeated. Animal decreased in weight from 6.5K to 5.8K. Volume ranged from 250 cc to 300 cc per day. The day following removal of pedicle percentage of bl. sugar rose to .18 and .03 grms sugar were excreted in the urine. On the following two days the % Blood sugar rose slightly;

12

The third operation, because of the gradual development of severe diabetes after the second operation gives infection a much greater opportunity to observe the characteristic symptoms in the than the does a complete pancreatectomy performed at the initial incision. Severe diabetes develops very quickly after this latter operation as is shown in chart No. II. The record in dog 408 shows a normal blood sugar .097. Eighteen hours after the operation the % age of sugar in the blood was .37%. Twenty-two hours after the operation (1 p.m. Aug. 4) the blood-sugar was .267. During the twenty-two hours 3.19 grams of sugar were excreted. The volume of urine was 494 cc. At 1 p.m. we administered 5 cc of extract of degenerated pancreas which had been prepared four days previously. At 2 p.m. the blood-sugar was .167. At 3 p.m. the per cent of sugar in the blood had fallen to .15%. From 1 to 3 p.m. .19 grams of sugar were excreted in a volume of 26 c.c. urine. 3.43 grams of nitrogen were excreted in the twenty-four hours following the operation. From 3 p.m. to 7 p.m. the percentage

3

of sugar in the blood shows a gradual rise from .15 to .20. This latter level was maintained until 9 p.m. The chart shows a slight rise in the sugar excretion following the rise of blood-sugar. At 9 p.m. 5 c.c of extract, which had been exposed to room temperature for one hour, was injected intervenously. The blood-sugar was reduced to a value of .18%. The chart shows a gradual ascent from this value to .27% which is reached at 9 a.m. August 5th.

1.30 gms

At 10 p.m. the percentage of sugar in the blood was .27. At this hour 5 c.c of extract of liver, prepared in precisely the same manner as the pancreatic extract, were administered intervenously. One hour later the blood-sugar was .30. This level was maintained during the following three hours, it was unaffected by an injection of 5 c.c of extract of spleen. The chart shows the rise in total volume of urine and amount of sugar excreted. At 2 p.m. (BS.36%) 5 c.c of extract of degenerated pancreas were injected. A sharp fall in percentage of blood-sugar resulted. At ~~2~~ 3 p.m. and again at 4 p.m. a similar dose of extract was given. The chart records the lasting effect. The 2 p.m. level of .30% was regained twelve hours after the first injection. The hourly excretion of sugar ~~fell~~ ran approximately parallel with the percent of sugar in the blood. Between 1 p.m. and 2 p.m. .52 grams were excreted. Less than .02 grams were excreted between 7 p.m. and 8 p.m. The highest glucose to nitrogen ratio, seemed in the urine, was ~~a~~ a 3.1 value obtained for the 22 hour interval between 2 p.m. the sixth of August and noon the following day. (see) At 12 noon August 6th. the % sugar in the blood was .40%. Five cc. of boiled extract of degenerated pancreas ~~was administered into~~ was injected intravenously. We secured no reduction of blood sugar.

At 12 midnight August 6th. five cc. of extract of degenerated pancreas which had been prepared 48 hrs was administered. The blood sugar fell from .49 at 12ᵐⁿ to .37% at 1 AM. Five cc. doses were given at 1. 2 + 3 Pm

Chart no III is the record of Dog no 92. A complete pancreatectomy was performed on this animal at 4 Pm. August the fourth. The main points in the experiment ~~can be~~ are clearly shown in the chart. The extract used at the beginning of the experiment was freshly prepared from a 10 Kilo. dog whose pancreatic ducts had been ligated for ten weeks. One hundred and ~~and~~ twenty five cc of extract was prepared from the gland. This supply was exhausted at 2 Pm August 13th. — The chart at 10 Am August 14th. records the successful attempt to reduce the 90 sugar in the blood below its normal level. — — — Exceptionally high values for volume of urine and urinary nitrogen for August 15th & 16th may be due to adulteration ~~presence~~ of ~~vomit~~ urine with vomit. — Extract made .19. acid with HCl reduces the blood sugar (August 15th). — — — — Extract made .19 alkaline with NaOH causes a slight reduction. The effect may be due to the alkali per se. — — — (17) ~~Acid extract + .05 grams of tissue powder reduces the blood sugar~~ — — — — A normal pancreas from a ten kilogram animal was divided into three equal parts . one third was

Dr. F. G. Banting
442 Adelaide Street

London, Ontario

Conclusions—

Injection of extract from the dog's pancreas of, removed from seven to ten weeks after ligation of the ducts invariably exercises a reducing influence upon the percentage sugar of the blood and the amount of sugar excreted in the urine. This fact has ~~been~~ conclusively ~~shown~~ by over fifty injections of extract of degenerated gland.

The extent + duration of the reduction varies directly with the amount of extract injected.

~~Fresh~~ Pancreatic juice destroys the active principle of the extract. The original hypothesis is ~~proved~~.

~~That~~ The reducing action is not

Dr. F. G. Banting
442 Adelaide Street

London, Ontario

a dilution phenomena is not indicated by the following facts (1) hemaglobin estimations are are similar following the administration of the extract show a percentage similar with that obtained before the injection (2) injection of large quantities of saline does not appear to effect the blood sugar. The percentage blood sugar one hour after the injection of 100 cc. saline shows no reduction. (3), extracts of other tissues dies not cause a reduction of blood sugar.

Extract made. 1% acid is effectual in lowering the percentage blood sugar.

The presence of the extract enables a diabetic, animal to retain a much greater percentage of injected sugar than it otherwise would. Since this sugar

27

Dr. F. G. Banting
442 Adelaide Street

London, Ontario

The extract prepared in neutral solution retains its potency for at least seven days in cold storage.

Rectal injections are not effective.

Subcutaneous injections are effective The action is delayed, but otherwise the results are similar to intravenous injections.

Page 1 of the original manuscript was torn and discoloured and subsequently lost. It was however copied by me exactly as it was written in my handwriting and thus now appears as page 1. All other pages were written in November 1921 Page 1 and 1/3 of page 2 are in my handwriting. The rest of page 2 and pages 3 and 4 were written by someone who was helping us with the historical aspects or perhaps by someone to whom Banting dictated. I can possibly solve this mystery. Page 5 is in my handwriting. Page 6 is by X. Pages 7 and 8 are in Fred Banting's writing. Pages 9, 10, 11 and 1/2 of 12 are mine. The latter half of 12 and page 13 and half of 14 are in Margaret Mahon's writing. We were engaged and I remember dictating these to her at her friend's home 370 Brunswick Ave. The rest of page 14 and pages 15, 17, 18, 19, 20, 21 22, 23, 24, 25, 26 and the above page 27 are in my handwriting. Page 16 has disappeared. Banting made the charts most of which I have, and I revised this manuscript and put it in the form in which it appeared in Feb 1922. This was thus the first paper presented, the first sent for publication.
— Charles H. Best

*The notes for research in pencil ... are in my handwriting

On THE EVENING OF FEBRUARY 7, 1922, *the Toronto Academy of Medicine met in the south lecture room of the Medical Building. The room was crowded with physicians who had come to hear about the new treatment which had already received some publicity in the daily press. Banting and I presented a paper on "The Internal Secretion of the Pancreas." Banting insisted that I should speak first and review our findings from May 17 to November 14, 1921. For the past four months I had been giving an hour's talk each week to the medical students but this was my first major scientific presentation. I described in some detail the experiments, the results of which were illustrated in a series of lantern slides. The subject headings are given on page 38, below. Banting then discussed our newer findings. We did not have an opportunity to proof-read this paper and a number of minor errors appeared in the report as published in the* Transactions of the Academy of Medicine, Toronto. *It is here printed as Paper 3.*

3. The Internal Secretion of the Pancreas

F. G. BANTING

C. H. BEST

Mr. Best presented lantern slides to illustrate the following points:

1. Intravenous injections of dog's pancreas, removed from seven to ten weeks after ligation of the ducts, invariably exercises a reducing influence on the percentage sugar of the blood and the amount of sugar excreted in the urine.

2. Rectal injections are not effective.

3. The extent and duration of the reduction varies directly with the amount of extract injected.

4. Pancreatic juice destroys the active principle.

5. Extracts made 0.1 per cent acid are effectual in lowering the blood sugar.

6. The presence of the extract enables a diabetic dog to retain a much larger percentage of injected sugar than it otherwise would.

7. Extracts prepared in neutral saline and kept in cold storage retain their potency for at least seven days.

8. Boiled extracts are ineffectual in reducing blood sugar.

9. That the reducing action is not a dilution phenomenon is indicated by the following facts: (1) haemoglobin estimations before and after administration of the extract are identical; (2) injections of large quantities of saline do not affect the blood sugar; (3) similar quantities of extracts of other tissues do not cause a reduction of blood sugar.

Dr. Banting then read the following: The results so far reported occupied our time until the middle of November 1921, when a new era was introduced by the discovery that the foetal calf pancreas of under five months' development did not contain pancreatic juice but did contain internal secretion.

Laguesse found that the islets of Langerhans were comparatively more plentiful in the foetus and newborn than in the adult animal. On November 16, the idea presented itself that by making an extract of the pancreas

Originally appeared in *Transactions of the Academy of Medicine, Toronto,* III (1920–22). The paper was read before the Academy of Medicine, Toronto, February 7, 1922.

of foetal calves, we might be able to obtain large quantities of the internal secretion without the destroying influence of pancreatic juice. This was done and, to our great satisfaction, on the injection of such an extract, the blood sugar of a diabetic dog was reduced from 0.30 per cent to normal and the urine became sugar free. This was repeated both in the same dog and in other depancreatized dogs with a similar result.

Carlson has found that in pregnant bitches depancreatized near term glycosuria did not develop until the pups were born. (Allan was unable to confirm this result.) Ibraham was unable to find proteolytic enzymes in the pancreas of the foetus of under four months' development.

However, this finding gave us access to large quantities of potent extract and abolished the delay and expense of obtaining the extract by ligating the pancreatic ducts of the dog and waiting for degeneration. Furthermore, it offered strong evidence that the active principle was universal in the animal kingdom. (We have since tried the bovine extracts on dogs, rabbits, and the human, and the results confirm this view.)

Foetal calf extract was prepared by macerating the glands in Ringer's solution and filtering until a clear solution was obtained. To get an idea of the potency of the extract so obtained, we placed 50 g of tissue in 250 cc of saline, macerated and filtered; 15 cc of this solution were then diluted to 250 cc with saline. A 15 cc dose of this solution reduced the percentage of blood sugar in a 10 kilogram dog from 0.40 per cent to 0.15 per cent in three hours.

Up to this time the extract had been given intravenously. We found that this extract when given subcutaneously gave a slower and more prolonged, but not less marked, fall in percentage of blood sugar.

In the endeavour to secure a sterile extract, we next tried the effect of preservatives. We found that 0.7 per cent tricresol, which is double the strength used in preserving diphtheria antitoxin, did not interfere with the active principle. It was also found that the extract could be Berkefelded, but much of its potency was lost in this procedure.

Alcohol was then tried in the place of saline as an abstractive, and it was found that the active principle was soluble. This was an important fact for it led us to believe that by the use of alcohol, we could extract the active principle from the whole gland. Consequently, we macerated a whole beef pancreas immediately after the death of the animal in 95 per cent alcohol. After allowing it to stand 12 hours, the liquid was squeezed out and filtered until clear. This solution was then evaporated to dryness in a warm air current. The resin-like residue was redissolved in saline and injected subcutaneously into a diabetic dog. The percentage of blood sugar fell from 0.35 to 0.08 in three hours and the urine became sugar free. This was repeated with similar results. We had thus obtained from the whole gland an extract of the active principle which, when washed with toluol, gave a brownish powder, which could be kept sterile, which was soluble in saline, and which in minute doses (50 mg) gave a pronounced effect on the sugar of the blood.

At this stage of the investigation, we secured the services of Dr. Collip, Professor of Biochemistry at the University of Alberta, on a year's leave of absence. He has worked intensively and has now obtained a very potent, soluble, more nearly protein-free extract which is being tested clinically.

Previous to this we had anaesthetized and connected a diabetic dog to a blood pressure recorder. It was found that the protein-containing extract had a temporary but marked depressor effect. Samples of blood were taken every half-hour during the experiment and it was found incidentally that the percentage of blood sugar fell but slightly following the injection of a known, potent extract. This fact may, in part, account for the failures of some observers to obtain results.

The question now arose as to why the extract acted but slightly under anaesthesia. It seemed reasonable to suspect that the glycogenetic function of the liver was in some way involved as glycogen is not built up during anaesthesia. We cannot state definitely, but some of our results would lead us to believe that the presence of the internal secretion of the pancreas is necessary in order that the liver build up glycogen from sugar.

Dog 19 was our first attempt to keep a depancreatized animal alive with artificially administered internal secretion of the pancreas. This dog lived for 19 days. Our next attempt was on dog 27; this dog lived 21 days and death was caused by an anaphylactic-like reaction following an injection of calf extract. When dog 27 died, we were using dog 33 as a trial dog for the effects of the various forms of extract. This dog has been given almost every variety of extract we had prepared and by every method of administration. We had from time to time given therapeutic doses of extract, and at the end of 20 days, the dog was in excellent condition. We then converted her into a longevity experiment. A dose of extract was given twice per day, and later once per day, and the animal was fed on lean meat, milk and dog biscuits. A slight gain in weight was noted. At the end of 70 days, the dog was becoming thinner and weaker but was still able to walk and wag her tail. The animal was then chloroformed and an autopsy performed by Dr. Robinson. No islet tissue whatever was found. However, in the submucous layer of the intestine, there was a nodule of acinous tissue about 2 mm in diameter (serial section of this failed to reveal islet tissue). Thus, we believe that, under favourable conditions, a totally diabetic dog may be kept alive for a considerable length of time if the internal secretion of the pancreas is administered.

In order to prove that this substance is only found in the pancreas, controls were done with extracts of spleen, liver, thymus, muscle, and thyroid. Thyroid extract alone gave a slight fall in blood sugar.

At the present time, Mr. Best and Dr. Hepburn are conducting experiments on the respiratory quotient. Their results, although not sufficient in number as yet to report, strongly indicate that carbohydrate is not burned in the tissue in totally diabetic dogs, but is burned after pancreatic extracts are given. For example, the respiratory quotients before extract is administered range from 0.68 to 0.74, after extract, from 0.85 to 0.94.

At the present stage of investigation, the results we have to offer are purely experimental, and afford no basis for assuming that the extract could be used in curing diabetes. Before the therapeutic value of the extract can be determined, it would be not only necessary to conduct many more laboratory experiments, but also to investigate the effects of the extract in a diabetic clinic. For this purpose, we have been fortunate in securing the co-operation of Professor Graham and his associates, Dr. Campbell and Dr. Fletcher. This will assure a thorough clinical test because of the efficient organization for the study of metabolic diseases.

Since the preparation of the extract consumes much time and expense, we cannot prepare a sufficient amount at present to take care of more than the needs of the Medical Clinic and of the research on animals. As soon as a thorough clinical test has been made and details regarding dose, method of administration, and indications for use, are worked out, we hope that we may have the opportunity of presenting a further report to the Academy.

We wish to express our sincere thanks to Professor Henderson, Professor Macleod, Professor Fitzgerald, and Professor Graham for their help and co-operation.

Tнis вrings us то тне first publi-
cation on insulin. The last data referred to were obtained on November 9,
1921. It is obvious, as one looks at the paper with more experienced eyes,
that our findings could have been presented much more clearly and forcibly.
The dramatic lowering of blood sugar from 0.40 per cent to 0.10 per cent
in three hours, obtained on November 8, could have been depicted much
more appropriately. But we had only five days to complete the paper, for it
was prepared, as I have mentioned earlier, to present at the meeting of the
University of Toronto Physiological Journal Club on November 14, and
sent for publication soon thereafter.

In retrospect, one of the most satisfactory comments which we made
was the following: "In the course of our experiments we have administered
over seventy-five doses of extract from degenerated pancreatic tissue to ten
different diabetic animals. Since the extract has always produced a reduction of the percentage of sugar of the blood and of the sugar excreted in
the urine, we feel justified in stating that this extract contains the internal
secretion of the pancreas." It seemed to us then and subsequently that this
was the essence of the discovery of insulin.

Banting and I were anxious to publish our first paper in the Journal
of the Canadian Medical Association but Professor Macleod, who was one
of the editors of the Journal of Laboratory and Clinical Medicine, said
that he had been remiss in his duty to direct papers to that journal. He
requested that we submit our effort there. We were disappointed that it
would not be published in Canada first but agreed to this.

4. The Internal Secretion of the Pancreas

F. G. BANTING, M.B.

C. H. BEST, B.A.

The hypothesis underlying this series of experiments was first formulated by one of us in November, 1920 [F. G. B., then Assistant in Physiology at the University of Western Ontario, London, Ontario], while reading an article dealing with the relation of the isles of Langerhans to diabetes [56]. From the passage in this article, which gives a résumé of degenerative changes in the acini of the pancreas following ligation of the ducts, the idea presented itself that since the acinous, but not the islet tissue, degenerates after this operation, advantage might be taken of this fact to prepare an active extract of islet tissue. The subsidiary hypothesis was that trypsinogen or its derivatives was antagonistic to the internal secretion of the gland. The failures of other investigators in this much-worked field were thus accounted for.

The feasibility of the hypothesis having been recognized by Professor J. J. R. Macleod, work was begun, under his direction, in May 1921, in the physiological laboratory of the University of Toronto.

In this paper no attempt is made to give a complete review of the literature. A short résumé, however, of some of the outstanding articles which tend to attribute to the isles of Langerhans the control of carbohydrate metabolism, is submitted.

In 1890 Mering and Minkowski [561] found that total pancreatectomy in dogs resulted in severe and fatal diabetes. Following this, many different observers experimented with animals of various species and found, in all types examined, a glycosuria and fatal cachexia after this operation. The fact was thus established that the pancreas was responsible for this form of diabetes. In 1884, Arnozan and Vaillard [18] had ligated the pancreatic ducts in rabbits and found that within 24 hours the ducts became dilated; the epithelial cells begin to desquamate; and that there are protoplasmic changes in the acinous cells. On the seventh day there is a beginning of round-celled infiltration. On the fourteenth day the parenchyma was mostly

Originally appeared in the *Journal of Laboratory and Clinical Medicine*, VII, 5 (February 1922), 251–66.

replaced by fibrous tissue. Ssobolew [731] in 1902 noted in addition to the above, that there was a gradual atrophy and sclerosis of the pancreas with no glucosuria. However, in the later stages, from 30 to 120 days after ligation of the ducts, he found involvement of the islets and accompanying glucosuria.

Lewaschew [499] believed that the islets were modified acinous cells. Laguesse [479], an anatomist, first suggested that the islets might be the organ of pancreatic internal secretion. He showed that there were comparatively more islets in the foetus and the newborn than in the adult animal. Opie [606] and Ssobolew [731] independently furnished the first clinical foundation for the belief that the islets were involved in pancreatic diabetes.

W. G. MacCallum, in 1909 [524], ligated the ducts draining the tail third of the pancreas. After seven months he excised the remaining two-thirds. This was followed by a mild glucosuria. Three weeks later he removed the degenerated tail third. This second operation resulted in extreme and fatal glucosuria. Kirkbride, in 1912 [458], repeated and corroborated MacCallum's findings and, by the use of Lane's [481] method of staining, proved that the atrophic tissue contained healthy islets.

Kamimura in 1917 [436], working on rabbits, traced the degenerative changes in the parenchymatous tissue of the pancreas after ligation of the ducts, and found that the islets remained normal and that the animal did not develop glucosuria as long as the islets were left intact.

The first attempt to utilize the pancreas in defects of carbohydrate metabolism was made by Minkowski. This worker tried the effect of pancreatic feeding, with no beneficial results. Up to the present time only useless or even harmful effects have been obtained from repeated attempts to use this method.

Knowlton and Starling, in 1912 [460], published experiments which showed a marked decrease in the power of using sugar of a diabetic heart perfused outside the body, as compared with a normal heart under similar conditions. Macleod and Pearce [540], using eviscerated animals were unable to confirm the above results. Patterson and Starling [613] subsequently pointed out that serious error was involved in the early experiments due to (1) excess glycogen present in diabetic hearts, and (2) to the irregular disappearance of glucose from the lungs.

Murlin and Kramer [584] prepared an alkaline extract of pancreatic tissue and, after injection of this solution, secured a reduction in sugar excreted in a diabetic animal. Kleiner [459] has pointed out that the reduction secured by Murlin might be due to the alkali *per se*. Kleiner himself has shown that "unfiltered-water extracts of fresh pancreas diluted with

0.90 per cent NaCl when administered slowly usually resulted in a marked decrease in blood sugar." There was no compensating increase in urine sugar, but rather a decrease, which Kleiner suggests may be partly due to a temporary toxic renal effect. Haemoglobin estimations made during the experiment showed that the reduction in blood sugar was not a dilution phenomenon. Paulesco [614] has recently demonstrated the reducing effect of whole gland extract upon the amounts of sugar, urea, and acetone bodies in the blood and urine of diabetic animals. He states that injections into peripheral veins produce no effect and his experiments show that second injections do not produce such marked effect as the first.

From the work of the above-mentioned observers we may conclude: (1) that the secretion produced by the acinous cells of the pancreas are in no way connected with carbohydrate utilization; (2) that all injections of whole-gland extract have been futile as a therapeutic measure in defects of carbohydrate utilization; (3) that the islands of Langerhans are essential in the control of carbohydrate metabolism. According to Macleod there are two possible mechanisms by which the islets might accomplish this control: (1) the blood might be modified while passing through the islet tissue, i.e., the islands might be detoxicating stations and (2) the islets might produce an internal secretion.

We submit the following experiments which we believe give convincing evidence that it is this latter mechanism which is in operation.

In the ten-week interval which we considered necessary for complete degeneration of the acinous tissue, we secured records of dogs depancreatized by the Hédon method [382].

METHODS

The first chart is a record of an animal depancreatized by the Hédon method. The details of this operation are given in Hédon's article. The remaining records are of animals (females) completely depancreatized at the initial operation. The procedure is as follows: under general anaesthesia an upper right rectus incision is made through the abdominal wall. The duodenum is delivered through the abdominal wound, and the pancreas traced to the tail portion. The mesentery beyond is cut between clamp and ligature. Vessels from spleen are then isolated, ligated and divided. Little dissection is then required until the duodenum is reached. The superior pancreatico-duodenal vessels are located and great care is exercised to avoid damaging them. The pancreas is stripped from the duodenum by dry dissection. The vessels to the uncinate process are ligated and divided, and the process freed from its mesenteric attachments. The larger duct of the pancreas is then ligated close to its entry into the duodenum and the pancreas is removed. Special care must be exercised to preserve the splenic vessels. The superior pancreatico-duodenal vessels must be left intact. Failing this, duodenal ulcer is a frequent development. If this procedure is carried out the whole gland with the exception of the portion in contact with the duodenum is covered with mesentery. The abdominal wound is closed layer by layer with catgut. A collodion dressing is used. The urethral orifice is exposed by a midline incision of the perineum and the edges of the wound drawn together to facilitate healing.

We have found that animals between eight and sixteen months old are the most suitable for this operation. At this age the pancreas is not so firmly fixed as it becomes later.

We first ligated, under general anaesthesia, the pancreatic ducts in a number of dogs. (Blood sugar estimations on these animals were recorded from time to time. We have no record of a hyperglycaemia.)

The extract was prepared as follows: The dog was given a lethal dose of chloroform. The degenerated pancreas was swiftly removed and sliced into a chilled mortar containing Ringer's solution. The mortar was placed in freezing mixture and the contents partially frozen. The half frozen gland was then completely macerated. The solution was filtered through paper and the filtrate, having been raised to body temperature, was injected intravenously.

We have never found it necessary to cut down on a vein under general or local anaesthetic. The skin surface above the vein is shaved and the needle inserted into the vein which is dilated by compression. The dogs make very little resistance to this procedure and after the first few punctures lie quietly during the operation. Sugar injections (100 cc of fluid) as well as the numerous administrations of extract were conducted by this method.

We performed several experiments with the object of exhausting the zymogen granules of the pancreas. Prolonged secretin injections and vagus stimulation below the diaphragm were practised. Fortune favoured us in the first experiment. In subsequent attempts we were never able to exhaust the gland sufficiently to obtain an extract free from the disturbing effects of some constituent of pancreatic juice.

The blood sugar estimations were made by the Myers-Bailey [591] modification of the Lewis-Benedict method. The results of this method were corroborated by the Shaffer-Hartmann [694] method at high and low percentages of blood sugar. The former method gave results which were consistently slightly higher (0.01 per cent) than those obtained by the Shaffer-Hartmann method. We find the average normal blood sugar, from observations on thirty normal dogs, to be 0.090 per cent.

Haemoglobin estimations were made by the carbon-monoxide saturation method, using the du Boscq colorimeter.

RESULTS

Figure 6 contains the record of a 6.5 kilogram dog (410). This experiment is not conclusive but is interesting to us at least, since we administered the first dose of extract of degenerated pancreas to this animal. On July 11, the pancreas, with the exception of the processus uncinatus, was removed. The processus was allowed to remain until July 18. In the interval between the operations there was no hyperglycaemia or glucosuria. The curves on subsequent days show the effect produced by the removal of the pedicle. It will be noted that as the experiment progresses the percentage of blood sugar did not rise to the level usually attained in completely depancreatized animals, and also that there was a marked decrease in the daily amounts of nitrogen and sugar excreted and the volume of urine voided. The animal continued to lose weight and seemed to be entering the cachexial condition characteristic of depancreatized animals which had become infected.

The chart for July 27 shows the effect produced on the percentage of blood sugar and on the sugar excretion by the oral administration of 25g of dextrose in 250 cc of water.

At 10 A.M. July 30, the percentage of blood sugar was 0.20. Four cc of extract of degenerated pancreas were injected intravenously. At 11 A.M. the blood sugar had fallen to 0.12 per cent. The injections of extract are shown in the chart. At 12 A.M. 20 g of sugar in 200 cc of water were given by stomach tube. The chart records the effect.

The obvious criticism of this experiment is that the animal was moribund when the effect of the extract was tried. The interesting features, which gave us great encouragement are (1) the extract caused a sudden fall in the blood sugar and (2) that in the presence of the extract the animal excreted 0.21 g of a 20 g injection in a period of five hours following the injection, in contrast to an excretion of 15.88 g of a 25 g injection in the same interval, when no extract was administered.

Figure 7 is the record of dog 92, weight 11.9 kg. A complete pancreatectomy was performed on this animal at 3 P.M. August 11. The first injection of extract was given six hours after the operation and subsequently an injection every four hours. This extract was freshly prepared from a 10 kg dog whose pancreatic ducts had been ligated for ten weeks. One hundred and twenty-five cc of extract were prepared from the gland residue but this supply was exhausted by 2 P.M., August 13, after which other extracts were used. Blood samples were always taken before the injections of extract.

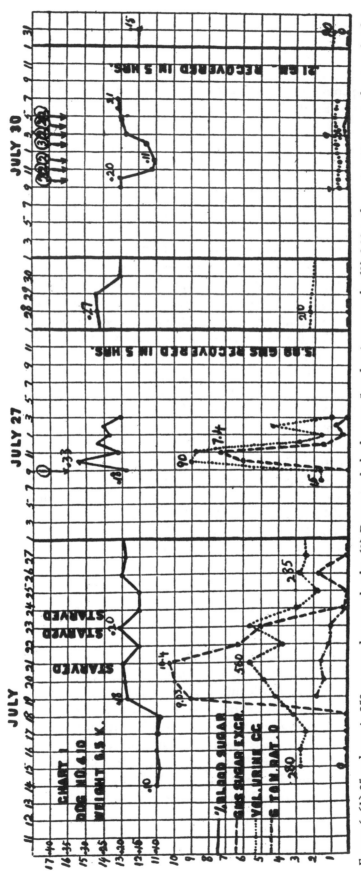

Figure 6. (1) 25 g glucose in 250 cc water by stomach tube. (2) Degenerated gland extract, 5 cc dose intravenously. (3) 0.20 g glucose in 200 cc water by stomach tube. Dog died July 31—cachexia.

On August 12, the blood sugar curve shows that neither 5 nor 8 cc of this extract every four hours were sufficient to counterbalance the upward trend of the percentage of sugar of the blood. A 10 P.M. the dose was increased to 12 cc and a marked fall is noted. The chart at 10 A.M. August 14 records the reduction of the percentage of sugar in the blood below its normal level, as a result of extract from another degenerated gland. (The exceptionally higher values for the volume of urine and the urinary nitrogen for August 15 and 16 may be due to the adulteration of urine with vomit.) On August 15 at 10 A.M. the chart shows the effect produced by 10 cc of the same gland extract made 0.1 per cent acid with HCl. This extract made 0.1 per cent alkaline with NaOH causes a slight reduction (August 15, 8 P.M.). The effect may be due to the alkali.

The extract administered at 10 A.M. August 16 was neutral and made from the same degenerated gland.

On August 16 and 17 effects of extracts from normal glands were tested. A normal pancreas from a 10 kg animal was divided into three equal parts. One-third was extracted with neutral saline, the second portion with 0.1 per cent HCl and the third with 0.1 per cent NaOH. On August 17 at 4 P.M. the neutral whole gland extract was administered. A marked fall in blood sugar resulted. The acid and alkaline extracts were injected at 12 P.M. August 17, and 7 A.M. August 18. The last two injections were perhaps not given a fair opportunity to develop their effects. We do not take colorimeter readings by artificial light and therefore did not have an accurate knowledge of the height of blood sugar at these times.

The conclusion from this experiment is that freshly prepared neutral or acid extracts of the whole pancreas do have a reducing effect on blood sugar, thus confirming Kleiner. It may be stated here that repeated injections of whole gland extracts cause marked thrombosis of the veins where the injections are made and a noticeable interference with kidney function. It is obvious from the chart that the whole gland extract is much weaker than that from the degenerated gland.

On August 20, we attempted to exhaust the pancreas of a 19 kg dog by continued injections of secretin and repeated stimulation of the vagus nerve below the diaphragm. We obtained 85 cc of pancreatic juice and considered the gland exhausted. It was swiftly removed and immediately chilled. The marked effect of injection of this material is shown on the chart at 7 P.M. August 20. On August 21 we incubated 10 cc of the extract and 5 cc of pancreatic juice for two hours at body temperature in alkaline solution. This solution was injected at 6 P.M. August 21. The curve shows the very slight effect produced. As a control on the above, 10 cc of extract and 5 cc of saline were incubated under similar conditions for two hours. The chart at 10 P.M. August 21 records the marked effect of the injection of this second solution. On August 22 at 6 P.M. 8 cc of extract from the normal pancreas of a cat were injected. We obtained a marked anaphylactic-like reaction. The curve shows the effect upon the blood sugar.

No further injections were given to this animal after August 22. The dog died on August 30, nineteen days after the operation. The autopsy showed consolidation and necrosis of a large area in lower lobe of right lung, infection in right pleural sac. The operation wound was well healed. There was no sign of pancreatic tissue. The abdomen was not infected.

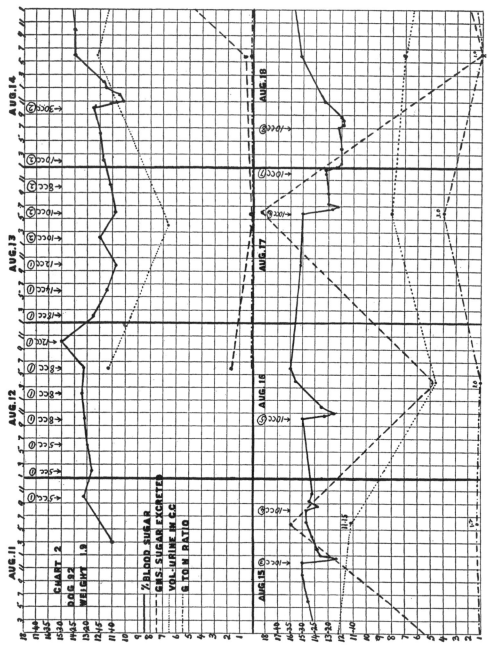

Figure 7. (1) Degenerated pancreas, dog 394. (2) Degenerated pancreas, dog 390. (3) Degenerated pancreas + 0.1 per cent HCl. (4) Degenerated pancreas + 0.10 per cent NaOH. (5) Degenerated pancreas + 0.1 per cent HCl. (6) Whole gland extract, fresh, cold. (7) Whole gland extract + 0.1 per cent HCl. (8) Whole gland extract + 0.1 per cent NaOH.

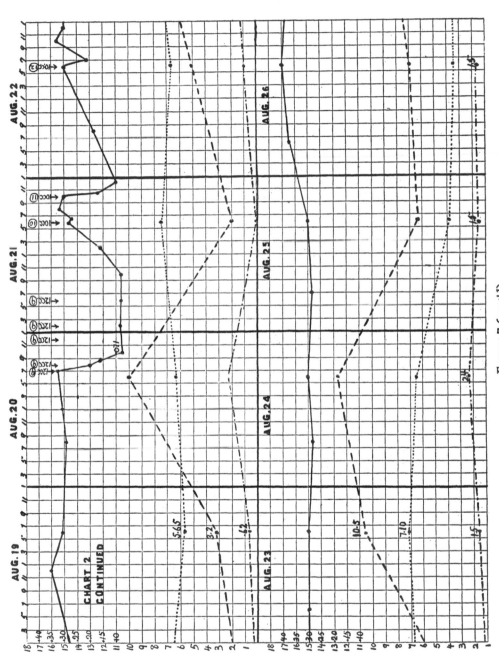

FIGURE 7 (cont'd)

(9) Exhausted gland extract. (10) 10 cc exhausted gland extract + 5 cc pancreatic juice incubated 2 hours. (11) 10 cc exhausted gland extract (— pancreatic juice) incubated 2 hours. (12) Whole gland, cat. Dog died August 30.

Figure 8 is the record of dog 408. The weight of this animal was 9 kg. The details of the experiment will be given rather fully.

The normal blood sugar of dog 408 was 0.090 per cent. Eighteen hours after pancreatectomy the percentage of sugar in the blood was 0.27. Twenty-two hours after the operation, 1 P.M. August 4, the blood sugar was 0.26 per cent. During the twenty-two hours 3.10 g of sugar were excreted. The volume of urine was 494 cc. At 1 P.M. we administered 5 cc of extract of degenerated pancreas which had been prepared four days previously and kept in cold storage. At 2 P.M. the blood sugar was 0.16 per cent. At 3 P.M. the percentage of sugar in the blood had fallen to 0.15. From 1 to 3 P.M. 0.19 g of sugar were excreted in a volume of twenty-six cc of urine. Three and forty-three hundredths g of urinary nitrogen were excreted in the twenty-four hours following the operation. The G. to N. ratio for this period was 1.4:1. From 3 P.M. to 7 P.M. the percentage of sugar in the blood shows a gradual rise from 0.15 to 0.25 per cent. This latter level was maintained until 9 P.M. The chart shows a slight rise in sugar excretion following the rise of blood sugar. At 9 P.M. 5 cc of extract which had been exposed to room temperature for one hour was injected intravenously. The blood sugar was reduced to a value of 0.18 per cent. The chart shows a gradual ascent from this value to 0.27 per cent. At 10 P.M. the percentage of sugar in the blood was 0.27. At this hour 5 cc of extract of liver, prepared in precisely the same manner as the pancreatic extract, were administered intravenously. One hour later the blood sugar was 0.30 per cent. This level was maintained during the following three hours. It was unaffected by an injection of 5 cc of extract of spleen. The chart shows the rise in volume of urine and amount of sugar excreted. At 2 P.M. (blood sugar 0.3 per cent), 5 cc of an extract of degenerated pancreas were injected. A sharp fall in the blood sugar resulted. At 3 P.M. and again at 4 P.M. a similar dose of extract was given. The chart records the lasting effect. The 2 P.M. level of 0.30 per cent was regained twelve hours after the first injection. The hourly excretion of sugar ran approximately parallel with the percentage of sugar in the blood. Between 1 P.M. and 2 P.M. 0.52 g were excreted. Less than 0.02 g were excreted between 7 P.M. and 8 P.M. The highest glucose to nitrogen ratio observed in this experiment was a 3:1 value for the 22-hour interval between 2 P.M. the 6th of August and noon the following day. At 12 noon August 6 the percentage of sugar in the blood was 0.40 per cent. Five cc of boiled extract of degenerated pancreas were injected intravenously at this stage and caused no reduction of blood sugar. At twelve midnight August 6, 5 cc of extract of degenerated pancreas which had been prepared 48 hrs previously were administered. The blood sugar fell from 0.43 per cent at 12 P.M. to 0.37 per cent at 1 A.M. Five cc doses were given at 1, 2, and 3 A.M. and a 25 cc dose at 4 A.M. The chart shows the reduction in blood sugar to a normal level and the beginning of an upward trend five hours after the last injection of extract. The animal died at 12 A.M. August 7.

A brief description of the clinical condition of the animal at various stages of the experiment is necessary for the correct interpretation of the above results. The animal made a good postoperative recovery and was able to retain water and meat after the second day following the operation. On the morning of August 5 we noticed that the condition of the animal was much worse. It appeared

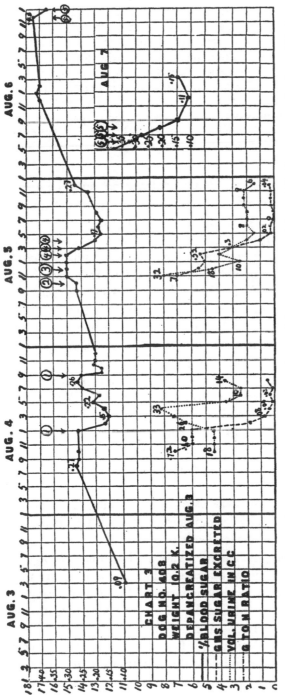

FIGURE 8. (1) 5 cc four-day-old extract of degenerated pancreas. (2) 5 cc extract of liver. (3) 5 cc extract of spleen. (4) 5 cc extract of degenerated pancreas. Dog died August 7—general peritonitis.

excessively tired, did not eat, and vomited after drinking water and also after extract of spleen given intravenously. At 5 P.M. August 5 the animal appeared considerably improved. It retained water and ate meat. On August 6 at 10 P.M. the abdominal wound was moist with exudate, and the animal was not so active as on the preceding day. No marked variation from this condition was observed until 4 A.M. when 25 cc of extract were administered. After this injection the animal had a marked reaction and appeared to be dying. It was revived slightly by intravenous and intraperitoneal injections of warm saline. Considerable improvement was noted at 7 A.M., the dog being able to stand. The improvement was short-lived. The dog died at 12 A.M. August 7. The post-mortem showed a widespread abdominal infection. There was no sign of pancreatic tissue.

The entire degenerated pancreas from one 8 kg dog and approximately one-half the degenerated gland from a 6 kg dog was the substrate of the extract used in this experiment.

Figure 9, dog 9, gives additional evidence on several important points which have been referred to previously. At 6 P.M., September 8, we administered 10 cc of extract of degenerated pancreas *per rectum*. There was no reduction in blood sugar at 7 P.M. when we gave 12 cc of extract of exhausted gland intravenously. The chart records the effect of this and subsequent injections of the same material. At 6 A.M., September 10, we administered 15 cc of extract of exhausted gland *per rectum*. There was no effect. At 8 A.M., September 10, 15 cc of extract of exhausted gland were injected intravenously. The drop in blood sugar was very marked. Twenty cc of exhausted gland extract, made 1 per cent alkaline with NaOH, were incubated three hours at body temperature with 10 cc of active pancreatic juice. This solution was neutralized and injected intravenously at 7 P.M. September 10. No reduction in blood sugar resulted. At 2 P.M. September 11, 20 cc of acid extract incubated for three hours at 37.5° C were injected. The curve shows the drop in blood sugar. On September 13 at 9 A.M. and 2 P.M. the effect of extracts from the partially exhausted gland of a cat is shown. This extract produced a pronounced general reaction.

We observe that extracts prepared from these more or less exhausted glands, while retaining to some extent the reducing effect upon blood and urine sugar, produce many symptoms of toxicity which are absent after injections of extracts from completely degenerated glands.

Figure 10 is the graphic record of an experiment on a 10 kg dog in which we have attempted to prove that the reduction of the percentage sugar in the blood is not a dilution phenomenon. Our plan of campaign was to inject at a given hour on the first day (2 P.M., October 7), 100 cc of isotonic saline (1). On the second day at the same hour the animal received 100 cc of 10 per cent sugar solution (2). Extract (3) (10 and 15 cc doses) was given one hour, and a second dose thirty minutes before the corresponding

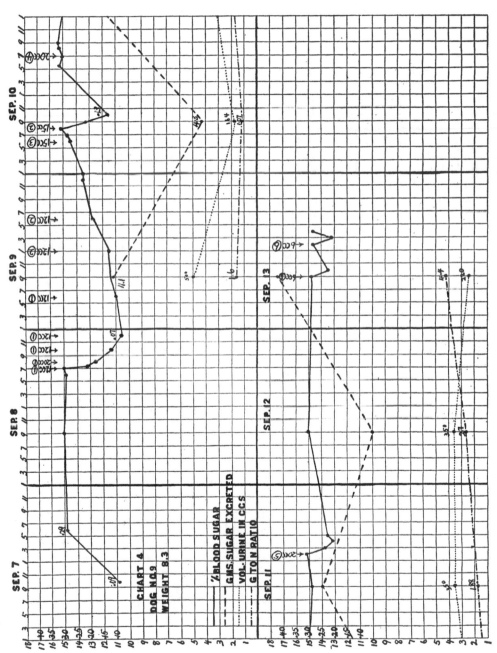

Figure 9. (1) Exhausted gland extract 1 per cent HCl. (2) Exhausted gland extract neutralized. (3) Exhausted gland extract neutralized, per rectum. (4) 20 cc exhausted gland extract and alkali + 10 cc pancreatic juice incubated 3 hours at 37° C then neutralized. (5) 20 cc exhausted gland extract incubated 3 hours at 37° C, 0.1 per cent HCl. (6) Exhausted gland of cat, 0.2 per cent HCl.

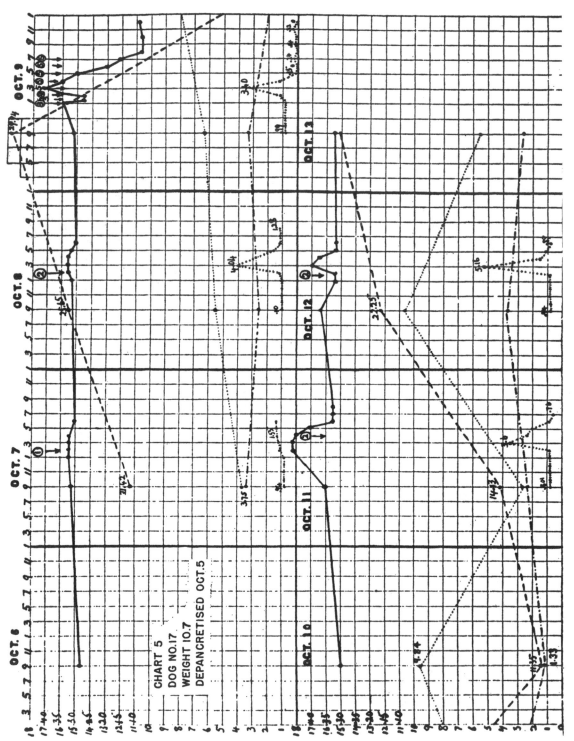

FIGURE 10. (1) 100 cc saline. (2) 10 g sugar + 100 cc water. (3) 10 cc extract A. (4) 10 g sugar, 80 cc water, 20 cc extract A. (5) 20 cc extract B. Note: Extract A was made from uncinate process. Extract B from tail portion of pancreas.

hour on the third day and 70 cc of distilled water containing 10 g of sugar were injected on the hour (4). Extract in 20 cc doses was injected at 3, 4, 5, 6, and 7 P.M. (5). To interpret correctly the curve for this day, a brief description of extracts (3) and (5) is necessary. The pancreas from which these extracts were made was not completely degenerated. The pancreatic ducts of the animal had been tied six weeks. Extract (3) was made from the processus uncinatus. Extract (5) was made from the remainder of the gland. The extract from the uncinate process was much weaker than the latter. In the four hours following the first injection of sugar we recovered 9.94 g in the urine. In the corresponding period on the following day after the injection of sugar plus extract 4.49 g were recovered. Had we used the more powerful extract first, the reducing action might have been even more strikingly demonstrated.

We were surprised that we did not secure a raised blood sugar one hour after the first injection of sugar. The rise after the second injection was very marked. We gave the animal a one-day rest and repeated the consecutive injections with the same results as above. The interpretation of the results of the first of the later injections is complicated by an unexplainably high percentage of sugar present before the injection. This phenomenon cannot be wholly explained by the rate of output of sugar, since, on the fourth injection, the first hour excretion was the maximum of the series and we did obtain a definite rise in blood sugar. An injection of 1 g of sugar per kg given to a normal dog showed a pronounced rise in percentage sugar of the blood after a 15-minute interval. This hyperglycaemia rapidly subsided and at the end of an hour the blood sugar had regained its normal level; 2.29 g of sugar were excreted.

Haemoglobin estimations were made (1) one hour after the first sugar injection, (2) just before the first injection of extract, and (3) at 12 P.M., October 9. The blood sugars at these times were 0.33 per cent, 0.35 per cent, and 0.09 per cent respectively. The haemoglobin was identical at the second and third determinations; a slightly lower value was obtained at the first determination.

Figure 11 is the record of a short, but very interesting experiment which again demonstrates the remarkable effect of the extract of degenerated pancreas upon the power of a diabetic animal to retain sugar. On November 8 at 11 A.M. (blood sugar 0.35 per cent), 10 g of sugar were injected intravenously. The curve shows the rise in blood sugar. In the four hours following the injection, 10.88 g of sugar were excreted. From 3 to 9 P.M. 78 cc

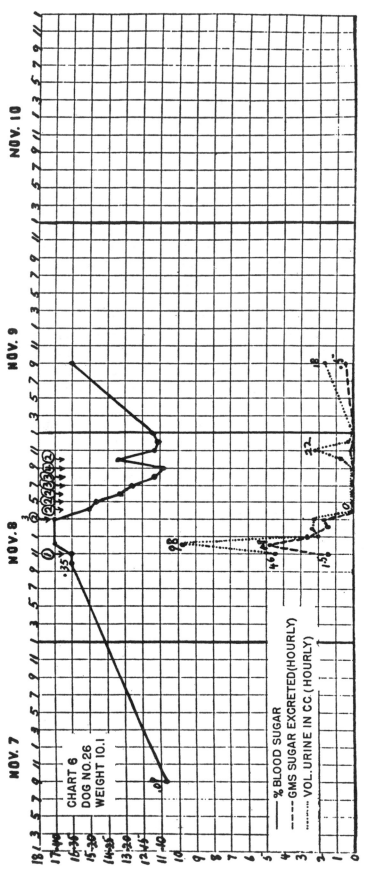

FIGURE 11. (1) 10 g sugar in 100 cc water. (2) 15 cc extract degenerated pancreas (4 weeks after ligation of ducts). (3) 6 cc extract degenerated pancreas (7 weeks after ligation of ducts). (4) 10 g sugar in 100 cc water. Dog died November 10—duodenal ulcer.

of dilute extract were injected in 13 cc doses. At 9 P.M. (blood sugar 0.09 per cent), 10 g of sugar were injected. The curve shows the effect on blood sugar and sugar excretion. The effect of partially degenerated gland extract, five weeks after ligation of the ducts, upon the kidneys is shown here. This extract may produce a raised threshold to sugar or a condition of anuria, as in this experiment. Haemoglobin estimations before and after administration of extract were identical. Duodenal ulcer was the cause of the early termination of the experiment.

A more detailed description of the histological sections obtained during our experiments will be included in a subsequent communication. Suffice it here to note that the pancreatic tissue removed after seven to ten weeks' degeneration shows an abundance of healthy islets, and a complete replacement of the acini with fibrous tissue.

In the course of our experiments we have administered over seventy-five doses of extract from degenerated pancreatic tissue to ten different diabetic animals. Since the extract has always produced a reduction of the percentage sugar of the blood and of the sugar excreted in the urine, we feel justified in stating that this extract contains the internal secretion of the pancreas. Some of our more recent experiments, which are not yet completed, give, in addition to still more conclusive evidence regarding the sugar-retaining power of diabetic animals treated with extract, some interesting facts regarding the chemical nature of the active principle of the internal secretion. These results, together with a study of the respiratory exchange in diabetic animals before and after administration of extract, will be reported in a subsequent communication.

We have always observed a distinct improvement in the clinical condition of diabetic dogs after administration of extract of degenerated pancreas, but it is very obvious that the results of our experimental work, as reported in this paper, do not at present justify the therapeutic administration of degenerated gland extracts to cases of diabetes mellitus in the clinic.

CONCLUSIONS

The results of the experimental work reported in this article may be summarized as follows: (1) Intravenous injections of extract from dog's pancreas, removed from seven to ten weeks after ligation of the ducts, invariably exercises a reducing influence upon the percentage sugar of the blood and the amount of sugar excreted in the urine. (2) Rectal injections are not effective. (3) The extent and duration of the reduction varies directly with the amount of extract injected. (4) Pancreatic juice destroys the active principle of the extract.

That the reducing action is not a dilution phenomenon is indicated by the following facts: (1) Haemoglobin estimations before and after administration of extract are identical. (2) Injections of large quantities of saline do not affect the blood sugar. (3) Similar quantities of extracts of other tissues do not cause a reduction of blood sugar.

Extract made 0.1 per cent acid is effectual in lowering the blood sugar. The presence of extract enables a diabetic animal to retain a much greater percentage of injected sugar than it would otherwise. Extract prepared in neutral saline and kept in cold storage retains its potency for at least seven days. Boiled extract has no effect on the reduction of blood sugar.

We wish to express our gratitude to Professor Macleod for helpful suggestions and laboratory facilities and to Professor V. E. Henderson for his interest and support.

Our SECOND COMPLETE PAPER WAS entitled "Pancreatic Extracts" (Paper 5 below) and several new findings were discussed. By this time we had prepared very active extracts from foetal calf pancreas. We were, of course, looking for a source of pancreas free from digestive enzymes. A search of the literature revealed that granules appeared in the islets before they did in the acinar cells so it seemed probable that at five months insulin was present but digestive enzymes were not. Sweeping falls in the blood sugars of our diabetic dogs were produced by these extracts. As we shall see (Paper 24), after slight purification they provided safe and very potent insulin when, many years later, they were tested clinically.

We also discussed the preparation of highly potent extracts from adult beef pancreas. These contained much more inert protein than those from the foetal pancreas and were apt to cause abscesses localized at the site of subcutaneous injection. They could be given intravenously without difficulty. We described the experiment in which a completely depancreatized dog was kept alive by insulin for seventy days. The animal received extracts made from foetal pancreas and from whole beef pancreas. Again we did not make the most of our data. There were many diversions and we were inundated with requests for insulin.

5. Pancreatic Extracts

F. G. BANTING

C. H. BEST

In a previous paper [40] we have reported experiments which justify the conclusion that some constituent of the pancreas destroys the active principle of the internal secretion of the gland when extracts are made of the gland by the usual methods. To eliminate these digestive substances, extracts were prepared from degenerated pancreatic tissue ten weeks after ligation of the ducts of the pancreas by which time the acinar but not the insular cells are said to have disappeared. From this material we secured small quantities of very active extract. The question of a more rapid and economical method of securing larger quantities of the extract soon became of prime importance.

Ibrahim [413] could obtain no conclusive evidence of the presence of an active proteolytic enzyme in the pancreas of the human foetus till after the fourth month of intrauterine life. Carlson [175] reported that in pregnant bitches near term, complete pancreatectomy was not followed by severe glycosuria in uncomplicated cases till the young were born. Allen [9] was unable to confirm this finding. The most natural interpretation of Carlson's result is that the pancreas of the foetus furnishes to the mother an internal secretion which is necessary for the metabolism of sugar. These facts coupled with the evidence afforded by our previous experiments suggested the possibility that the foetal pancreas might prove a source of an extract rich in internal secretion and yet free from the destructive enzymes of pancreatic juice.

In order to test this hypothesis a quantity of pancreas was obtained from foetal calves of less than five months' development. The tissue was macerated in Ringer's solution, and the liquid filtered off. The filtrate was tested on several different diabetic dogs and found to produce similar effects upon the percentage sugar of the blood and on the sugar excreted in the urine as did the extract prepared from degenerated pancreatic tissue. The extract was not found to contain any proteolytic enzyme.

Originally appeared in the *Journal of Laboratory and Clinical Medicine*, VII, 8 (May 1922), 464–72.

In this paper we are reporting two experiments in which such extracts of foetal calf pancreas were used.

Experiment I

A total pancreatectomy was performed upon dog 27 on November 14; weight of the animal, 5 kg. The effects of injections of the extract are given in Table 5.I.

TABLE 5.I

Dog 27—Pancreatectomy November 14, 1921—Weight 5 Kilograms

Date	Hour		Blood Sugar (%)	Extract	Sugar Excreted	Weight
Nov. 15	10	A.M.	0.11	—	—	5.0 k (Total pancreatectomy)
Nov. 16	3	P.M.	0.28	—	—	—
Nov. 17	8:30	A.M.	0.30	5 cc	12 noon 16 to	4.1 k
	9:15	A.M.	0.20	—	9 A.M. 17—	
	10	A.M.	0.17	5 cc	4 g	
	6	P.M.	0.15	5 cc		
Nov. 18	9	A.M.	0.175	10 cc	Previous 24 hr	4.1 k
	10	A.M.	0.08	—	vol. of urine	
	6	P.M.	—	10 cc	100 cc no sugar	
Nov. 19	9	A.M.	0.21	—	Previous 24 hr	4.2 k
	6	P.M.	—	10 cc	vol. of urine 225 cc sugar free	
Nov. 20	10	A.M.	0.20	10 cc		4.3 k
Nov. 21	10:15	A.M.	0.26	10 cc		
Nov. 22	9	A.M.	0.25	12 cc		
Nov. 23	9	A.M.	—	12 cc		
Nov. 24	9	A.M.	—	10 cc		
Nov. 25	9	A.M.	—	10 cc		
Nov. 28	6	P.M.	—	2 cc (concentrated)		
Nov. 29	6	P.M.	—	5 cc (concentrated)		
Dec. 2	11	A.M.	0.15	—	Previous 24 hr	4.0 k
	12	A.M.	—	6 cc	vol. 320 cc 0.5 g sugar	
Dec. 4	12	A.M.	—	6 cc		

Dog 27 was removed from the metabolism cage on November 20. Sugar excretion was not followed in the interval between November 20 and December 1. On November 20 the animal was in excellent condition which was maintained until December 2. At noon December 2, 6 cc of foetal calf extract prepared 16 days previously was injected subcutaneously. This extract had been prepared under aseptic conditions and immediately after its preparation was found to have a very low bacterial count. The solution was kept in a refrigerator some distance away from the ice. At 3:30 P.M. December 2, the dog showed symptoms of a peculiar nature. Periods of unconsciousness with convulsive twitchings, retraction of the head, salivation, and frothing alternated with periods of semi-consciousness. These symptoms lasted from 3:30 P.M. to 6 P.M.; after 6 P.M. the animal gradually improved and at 8 P.M. was resting quietly. On December 4 at 12 A.M., 6 cc of the same extract was again given. At 1:30 P.M. the animal began to exhibit symptoms similar to but more severe than those noticed on December 2. The dog died during the night of December 4. Postmortem examination showed that all the pancreas had been removed and there was no evidence of infection. Twelve cc of the same extract as was used in the latter part of this experiment injected into a normal dog produced no apparent reaction.

Experiment II

Figure 12 is the graphic record of some interesting experiments performed upon a dog (no. 33) from which the pancreas was removed on November 18, 1921. Daily sugar excretion in grams and 24 hour urine volume are clearly shown in the chart, from which it will be seen that in twenty-four hours after the operation (November 19, 10 A.M.), the percentage of sugar in the blood was 0.33 per cent. Ten cc of filtered foetal calf extract were injected intravenously and one hour later the blood sugar was 0.17 per cent. At 7 P.M. November 19, the blood sugar was 0.37 per cent when 10 cc of extract that had been passed through a Berkefeld filter were injected. At 8 P.M. the blood sugar was 0.26 per cent. At 9 A.M. November 20 the blood sugar was 0.37 per cent when 10 cc of neutral Berkefeld extract which had been kept in a water-bath at 78° C for thirty minutes were injected intravenously without causing any change in blood sugar. From this and other experiments we believe that the active principle of this extract is destroyed by heating it to approximately 65° C. At 4 P.M. November 20, 10 cc of extract which had been boiled twenty minutes in the presence of 2 per cent HCl were injected intravenously. No reduction in the percentage of blood sugar was observed. Similar results were obtained with corresponding concentrations of other acids. At 7 P.M. November 20, when the blood sugar was 0.40, 10 cc of neutral and Berkefeld extract, given intravenously, lowered it to 0.23 per cent in three hours.

On November 21 the blood sugar was lowered from 0.43 per cent at 10:15 A.M. to 0.3 per cent at 2 P.M. by the subcutaneous injection of 20 cc of Berkefeld extract. On November 22, 10 cc of a freshly prepared concentrated extract of foetal calf pancreas were injected subcutaneously with the remarkable result that the sugar of the blood fell from 0.40 per cent at 4 P.M. to the subnormal level of 0.075 per cent at 9 P.M. On November 24 at 10 P.M., 10 cc of a seven-day-old extract containing 0.7 per cent tricresol caused the percentage of blood sugar to fall from 0.43 to 0.22 per cent at 11:15 A.M. On November 28 at 9:30 A.M. the blood sugar was 0.43 per cent and 10 g sugar in 100 cc of water injected intravenously raised it to 0.60 per cent and 8.53 g of sugar were excreted in the urine in the four hours following the injection. We were unable to follow the blood sugar curve as closely as desirable owing to the difficulty of obtaining blood by venepuncture. At 6 P.M. on the same day 6 cc of a more concentrated foetal calf extract were given subcutaneously and next morning (at 9:30 A.M. November 29), the blood sugar was found to be 0.18 per cent when 4 cc of the same extract were again injected. The blood sugar at 2:30 P.M. was 0.048 per cent and the urine collected from 9:30 A.M. to 3 P.M. was sugar free, the volume excreted between 12 noon and 3 P.M. being 68 cc. At 3 P.M., 4 cc extract were administered and at 4 P.M. 10 g of sugar in 100 cc of water were injected intravenously. The blood sugar at 7:30 P.M. was 0.05 per cent and in the two hours following the injection of sugar 0.51 g was recovered in the urine after which the urine was free of sugar. On November 30 the animal was in good condition. On December 1 it excreted 14.84 g of sugar in a volume of 520 cc of urine and on December 2, 320 cc of urine and 10.94 g of sugar.

At 10 A.M. on December 3 after eighteen hours' starvation the blood sugar was 0.28 per cent when 10 cc of concentrated foetal calf extract were given by stomach tube in order to find out whether absorption of the active principle of the extract might occur through the gastric mucosa. At 2 P.M. the blood sugar stood at 0.23 per cent when another 10 cc of extract were given by mouth. The blood sugar rose slightly during the next hour. On the following days, December 4, 5, and 6, the animal excreted 4.95, 8.40, and 15.70 g of sugar, respectively.

Since the animal at this stage was still in fairly good condition, even though there had been considerable irregularity in the administration of extract, it was decided to discontinue using it for the purpose of testing the relative potency of different forms of extract and to administer to it the most efficient of these in regular dosage so as to determine for how long a time the animal could be kept alive. On December 7 the injection was made with foetal calf extract prepared as described above, but on December 8 an extract, prepared by extracting the pancreas with alcohol, evaporating to dryness, and redissolving the residue in distilled water, was used with the result that 4 cc caused the blood sugar to fall from 0.30 to 0.15 per cent in one hour. A second injection of this extract (12 cc) was given at 1 P.M. and at 5 P.M. the blood sugar was 0.12 per cent. It will be seen that the principle upon which the preparation of this latter extract depends is the same as that of E. L. Scott [688] and the favourable results led us to see whether adult pancreas could be used in place of foetal. Six cc of whole gland extract prepared as above were therefore injected daily from December 8 to January 3 inclusive. On January 4 the administration of extract was discontinued and on this day the dog excreted 12.86 g of sugar in a volume of 450 cc of urine. The animal was in good condition and was on a diet of lean meat. On January 5 it was not so hungry or so lively as on previous days and 4 g of sugar in 350 cc of urine were excreted. On the next day (January 6) 3.5 g of sugar and 320 cc of urine were excreted and the animal was in a very poor condition compared with that of a few days previously. On January 6 the diet was changed to one of milk and biscuit along with meat, and the sugar excretion rose to 25 g. At noon on January

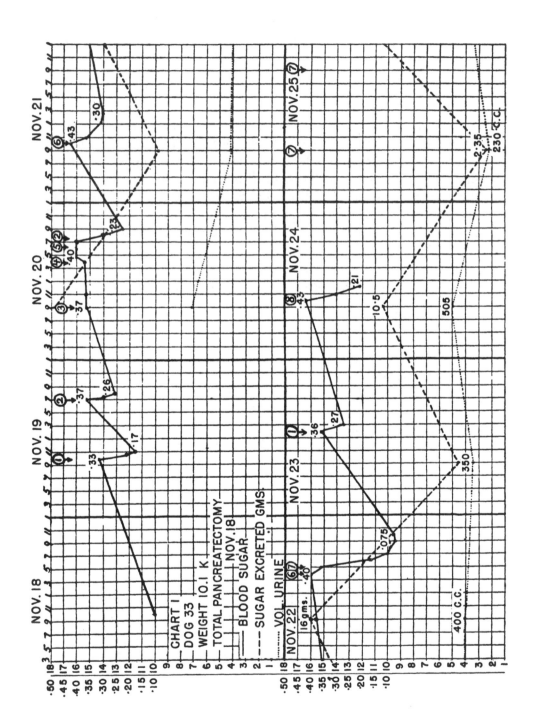

CHART I
DOG 33
WEIGHT 10.1 K
TOTAL PANCREATECTOMY NOV.18
——— BLOOD SUGAR
- - - SUGAR EXCRETED GMS.
VOL. URINE

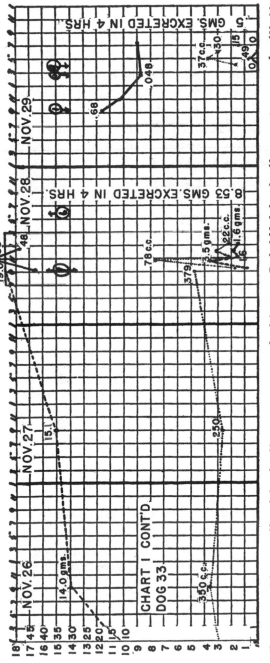

Figure 12. (1) 10 cc filtered foetal calf extract intravenously. (2) 10 cc Berkefelded foetal calf extract intravenously. (3) 10 cc of (2) heated to 78° C for 30 minutes. (4) 10 cc of (2) + ⅛ cc glacial acetic boiled for 30 minutes. (5) 10 cc of (2) + ⅛ cc hydrochloric boiled for 30 minutes. (6) 20 cc Berkefelded foetal calf extract subcutaneously. (7) 10 cc of (1) subcutaneously. (8) 10 cc degenerated pancreas of dog intravenously. (9) 100 cc water. 10 g dextrose. Dog converted to longevity experiment December 5. Chloroformed January 27, 1922.

7, while on the same diet, 8 cc of whole gland extract were injected and the twenty-four hour sugar excretion was found to be 22 g. A further injection of 10 cc of extract at 9 A.M. on January 8 brought the sugar excretion down to 2.0 g.

The original weight of the animal (33) was 10.1 kg, and one week after the pancreatectomy it was 8.1 kg. This was maintained fairly constant throughout the second and third weeks after the operation and then slightly increased. From the fifth to the ninth week (see Plate II (b)), during which time daily injections of 6 cc of whole gland extract were given, the condition remained good and was so on the 63rd day when, to convince ourselves that the extract was necessary to the health of the animal, we discontinued its administration for three days (21, 22, and 23 of January) with the result that the dog became so weak that it was barely able to stand. Extract was again given on January 24 and 25 with decided improvement. On January 27 when the dog weighed 7.9 kg it was killed by an overdose of chloroform and a careful autopsy was immediately made by Dr. W. L. Robinson, Pathologist at the General Hospital, Toronto. His report is as follows:

REPORT OF AUTOPSY FINDINGS ON DOG NO. 33

We made a very careful examination of this dog with the object of determining if any pancreatic tissue had been left from the operation, or if possible, an accessory pancreas were present.

The area formerly occupied by the pancreas showed no gross evidence of pancreatic tissue. There were a number of firm fibrous adhesions about the duodenum. These were sectioned, and on microscopic examination showed no evidence of pancreatic tissue remaining in them.

The duodenum was then examined and nothing abnormal found except for a small nodule about 3 mm. in diameter situated in the wall at the mesenteric attachment and 10 cms. below the pylorus. This on microscopic examination was found to consist of what is apparently a nodule of pancreatic tissue, lying in the submucosa. Serial microscopic sections of this however, failed to show the presence of any Islands of Langerhans.

No other gross or microscopical evidences of pancreatic tissue could be found.

W. L. ROBINSON,
Pathologist,
Toronto General Hospital.

EXPERIMENT III

To study the effect of an intravenous injection of whole gland (normal beef pancreas) extract upon the blood pressure of a diabetic animal, dog 27 was anaesthetized and its blood pressure recorded (see Figure 13). After the intravenous injection of 5 cc of extract, the blood pressure fell approxi-

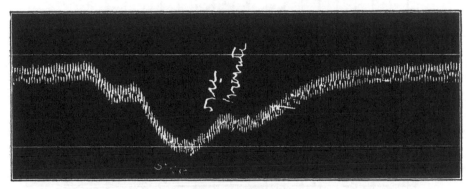

FIGURE 13. Blood pressure tracing following administration of extract.

mately 50 mm, but regained its original level in less than two minutes. The effect of a similar dose of extract upon the blood sugar of an unanaesthetized diabetic animal would have lasted for at least six hours, and the lowest level would have been reached in from one to two hours after the injection. The fact that administration of extract to this animal caused very little fall in the blood sugar indicates that, in anaesthetized diabetic animals, extract of known activity causes only a slight reduction in the blood sugar, a fact which we had observed before. Further details of the interrelationship of the effects of anaesthesia and extract will be reported later.

Experiment IV

The purpose of reporting this experiment is to show the relative effects of extracts prepared in various ways. (No attempt was made to prove the dog totally diabetic, nor was the excretion of sugar followed closely since we wished simply to ascertain by the blood sugar whether a particular extract contained the active principle or not.) On December 8, 1921, dog 35 was completely depancreatized. The animal made a good postoperative recovery. On December 11 we injected 6 cc of an extract (see Figure 14) prepared from the pancreas of this animal in the following way. The entire pancreas immediately after removal was cut into small pieces which were put into 0.2 per cent HCl in 95 per cent alcohol and allowed to stand till December 10. It was then macerated, filtered, and the clear filtrate evaporated to dryness in a warm air current. On December 11 this dry resin-like residue was emulsified in 25 cc Ringer's solution and 6 cc were given intravenously at 10 A.M. The blood sugar dropped from 0.46 to 0.18 per cent in three hours.

On December 12 at 3 P.M., 20 cc of an extract made from the pancreas of a cow, in the same manner as outlined above, were given on an empty

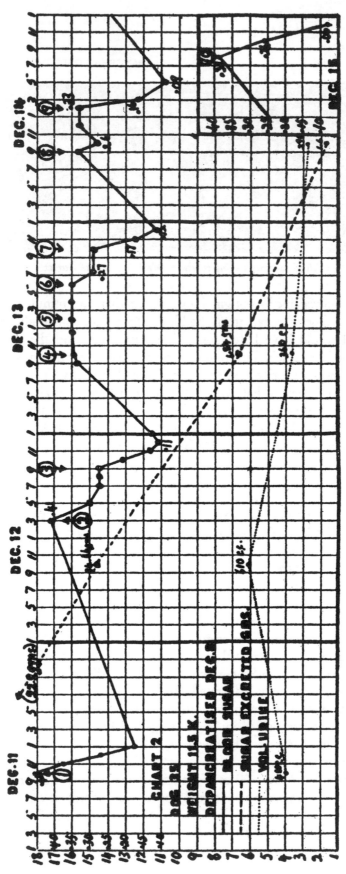

FIGURE 14. (1) 6 cc extract whole dog pancreas intravenously. (2) 10 cc extract whole cow pancreas intravenously. (3) 10 cc extract whole cow pancreas per stomach. (4) 10 cc extract liver intravenously. (5) 10 cc extract spleen intravenously. (6) 10 cc extract thyroid intravenously. (7) 10 cc extract pancreas intravenously. (8) 10 cc extract thymus intravenously. (9) 6 cc extract whole pancreas of cow dialysed. (10) 10 cc dried extract redissolved in saline. Dog chloroformed December 19. Cachexia.

stomach by stomach tube. The blood sugar fell from 0.41 at 3 P.M. to 0.28 at 7 P.M. At 9 P.M., 10 cc of this same extract were given intravenously. The blood sugar fell from 0.28 at 9 P.M. to 0.11 at 12 P.M. On December 13 about 20 g each of liver (4), spleen (5), thyroid (6), and pancreas (7) were extracted in identically the same manner as outlined above. There was no reduction in blood sugar following the intravenous injection of extracts of liver or spleen; a slight fall occurred (from 0.35 to 0.27) following the administration of extract of thyroid and a marked one (from 0.27 to 0.12) following one of pancreas.

On December 14 at 9:30, 10 cc of extract of thymus (8), made in the same way as were the liver, spleen, and thyroid, were injected intravenously. There was a slight temporary fall from 0.33 to 0.26 in one hour. At 2 P.M., 6 cc of an extract, prepared as above from pancreas and which had been placed in a parchment dialyzer in running water for twelve hours, caused the percentage of blood sugar to fall from 0.33 to 0.09 per cent in three hours.

On December 15, 200 mg of the residue of ox pancreas extract were washed twice in toluol and then in 95 per cent alcohol, then dried again and emulsified in saline. At 10 A.M. this was given intravenously. The blood sugar dropped from 0.37 to 0.06 per cent in four hours. On December 16 at 9 A.M., 10 cc of concentrated foetal calf extract were given *per os*. Blood sugar fell very slightly (0.38 to 0.35 per cent). On December 19, the animal, by this time considerably emaciated, was killed by chloroform.

DISCUSSION

The foregoing observations were undertaken partly to determine whether extracts having an antidiabetic power equal to those prepared from the degenerated pancreas could also be prepared from the normal gland, and partly to find out whether frequent injection with active extracts would prolong the life of a depancreated animal far beyond the limit of time which such animals ordinarily survive. In connection with the preparation of the extract it has been found that foetal ox pancreas and, with certain modifications in the method of preparation, adult pancreas as well, furnish highly potent extracts. These extracts are, however, somewhat toxic, and they are apt to cause local abscesses at the point of injection. This method of preparation is being materially improved by various important modifications which are being worked out by Dr. J. B. Collip and which will be reported in the near future. In connection with the effect of the extract on the longevity of the depancreated animal, one of our observations would seem to afford fairly conclusive results. This animal (no. 33) lived for seventy days and at autopsy no pancreatic residues were found by macroscopic examination although by microscopic examination of serial sections of the duodenum a small nodule of pancreatic tissue (containing no islets) was found in the submucosa. It does not seem likely that so small a piece of pancreas could be responsible for the maintenance of life in the animal but, of course, the experiment is not finally conclusive. We are engaged in its repetition and will report the results in due time.

CONCLUSIONS

(1) By intravenous and subcutaneous injections of neutral saline extracts prepared from the pancreas of the bovine foetus at about the fifth month, the percentage of blood sugar and the daily urinary excretion of sugar are markedly reduced in depancreated dogs. (2) Daily injections of extract of pancreas enabled a depancreatized dog to live for seventy days. (3) The active (antidiabetic) principle of such extracts is destroyed by boiling in strongly acid reaction but it is not affected by the presence of tricresol which may therefore be used as a preservative. (4) The depressor action of the extract is short-lived.

AT THE 1922 MAY MEETING (41ST) OF
the Royal Society of Canada, which was held in Ottawa, five papers on
insulin were presented (grouped as Paper 6, below). In the first section of
the first paper are summarized several of the procedures which Banting and
I had used for the preparation of insulin: extracts made with Ringer's
solution, with an equal amount of alcohol, or later with acid alcohol. In
the second section, Collip's extension of our procedure is reported. The
problem was to remove most of the protein and salts and all of the lipoid
material from the extracts without destroying the active principle, to give
a product of sufficient purity for repeated subcutaneous or intravenous
administration in man. Abandonment of the use of acidified alcohol, in the
belief that insulin was too labile to withstand such treatment, was only
temporary as will be described later (page 172). The first published mention
of the use of acid in the extraction medium is to be found in the paper of
Banting and Best read to the Toronto Academy of Medicine on February
7, 1922 (Paper 3, above).

The other four papers by Banting, Best, Collip, Hepburn, Macleod, and
Noble, record some very significant findings. It is quite likely that many
students of diabetes have not had available the Proceedings and Transactions of the Royal Society of Canada where these reports were published.
All of them deal with researches which Banting and I had listed in our
letter of August 1921 to Professor Macleod. We had hoped to secure
assistance and to pursue these problems ourselves. Banting had given the
effect of insulin on liver glycogen his highest priority, and I was most
anxious to determine its effect on the respiratory quotient of the diabetic
organism. We were not happy, I think understandably, after six months of
productive independent work, to become members of a large team. How-

ever, as the results show, the joint attack was effective and new facts, many of which are still receiving widespread scientific attention, were secured. Banting and I had noted that the livers of our untreated diabetic dogs were yellow with fat, as Minkowski had reported thirty-two years previously, and that our insulin-treated animals appeared to have less hepatic fat. We had noted on several occasions, with our qualitative tests, a decrease in urinary ketones after insulin. The quantitative procedures which Professor Collip set up demonstrated these effects clearly. The dramatic decrease in ketone excretion was obtained with the simple alcoholic extract of adult ox pancreas, made by the procedure which Banting and I had first used.

Although the first dramatic fall in blood sugar was seen in a dog on August 7, 1921 (Figure 2(a), Paper 1), the first deliberate attempt to produce hypoglycaemia by overdosage with insulin was made on August 14 (Figure 2(b) of the same paper). Later, with Collip, Macleod, and Noble, Banting and I studied this in more detail. In Paper 5 (foot of Table 5.I) the first description appears of a dog in convulsions following overdosage with insulin; in Paper 6 a detailed description was given of the characteristic signs seen in rabbits when given an overdosage of insulin. The correspondence between the fall in blood sugar and the incidence of convulsions was noted and the causal relationship was recognized. The prompt recovery from convulsions or coma when injections of glucose were given, and the inability of saline solution or pentose sugars to alleviate the condition, proved that the convulsions following injection of excess insulin resulted from the hypoglycaemia. The first clinical study of the effects of an overdose of insulin was made in the Department of Medicine, University of Toronto, by Dr. A. A. Fletcher and Dr. W. R. Campbell in 1922.

The clinician distinguishes between low blood sugars resulting from overdosage with insulin and hypoglycaemia arising from spontaneous liberation of an excessive amount of insulin. Among the early visitors to the Toronto laboratories was Dr. Seale Harris of Birmingham, Alabama. He recognized that the symptom-complex induced by overdosage with insulin resembled that which he had seen occurring spontaneously in certain of his patients and he assumed that these episodes were induced by oversecretion of insulin by the pancreas. Consequently he diagnosed this symptom-complex as hyperinsulinism or dysinsulinism. This diagnosis was unacceptable to some clinicians because the symptoms could result from glandular abnormalities or other changes not involving the pancreas.

In 1927 Wilder, Allan, Power, and Robertson reported the first case in which an excessive secretion of insulin was established. A cancer of the pancreas was revealed at laparotomy with a number of metastases in the liver. *The patient died four weeks later and large amounts of insulin were shown to be present in the hepatic metastases as well as in the primary tumour.*

The first recovery of a patient with an islet cell tumour after surgical removal of the growth was reported from the Toronto General Hospital in 1929 by Drs. Howland, Campbell, Maltby, and Robinson. The tumour was removed by the late Professor Roscoe Graham.

6. Preliminary Studies on the Physiological Effects of Insulin

I. THE PREPARATION OF PANCREATIC EXTRACTS CONTAINING INSULIN

F. G. BANTING, M.C., M.B.

C. H. BEST, M.A.

J. B. COLLIP, PH.D.

J. J. R. MACLEOD, M.B., F.R.S.C.

A. *The Preparation of the Earlier Extracts* (procedures used by F. G. Banting and C. H. Best)

In two previous papers a brief outline of the preparation of pancreatic extracts has been given. Active anti-diabetic extracts of degenerated gland, exhausted gland, foetal gland, and finally adult beef gland, were made. The main problem in the preparation was to get rid of or avoid the presence of proteolytic enzymes.

The first extract used was obtained by ligating the pancreatic ducts of the dog, and waiting from seven to ten weeks for degeneration of the acinar tissue. The remnant, which contained healthy insular tissue, was removed and macerated in ice-cold Ringer's solution. By this procedure a non-toxic extract which markedly reduced the blood sugar and the excretion of sugar in diabetic dogs was obtained in small quantity. Active extract was also prepared from the pancreas of a dog that had been injected with secretin.

The foetal calf extract was at first made by macerating pancreas of foetal calves of under four months development in Ringer's solution and filtering. Later, 95 per cent alcohol was used in place of Ringer's solution.

The alcoholic filtrate was evaporated to dryness in a warm air current and the resin-like residue redissolved in saline. This solution when injected subcutaneously or intravenously into a diabetic dog caused a marked fall in blood sugar and in sugar excreted in the urine. It was further found that

Originally appeared in the *Transactions of the Royal Society of Canada*, Series III, XVI Section V (1922), 27–44. A group of five papers, collectively given the general title "Preliminary Studies on the Physiological Effects of Insulin," are reproduced here as read before Section V at the May meeting.

this extract did not contain trypsin, that it was destroyed by boiling, that the active principle was insoluble in 95 per cent alcohol, and that daily injections enabled a totally depancreatized dog to live a much longer time (70 days) than has hitherto been recorded after such an operation.

Potent extracts of the whole gland of the adult ox were obtained in a similar manner, using equal volumes of 95 per cent alcohol and pancreas, with the exception that the alcohol was made 0.2 per cent acid by the addition of HCl. It was found that the fatty substances in the extract could be removed by washing twice with toluol without deterioration of the potency of the extract. The alcohol could also be removed by distillation *in vacuo* at low temperature and it was found by reducing the volume to one-fifth instead of to dryness that a watery extract of the active principle was obtained. This could be sterilized by passing it through a Berkefeld filter. The extract in this form was given to a human diabetic and results in every way comparable to those obtained on the depancreatized dog were observed. However, owing to the high percentage of protein also present, sterile abscesses formed in few instances at the site of injection.

B. The Preparation of the Extracts Used in the First Clinical Cases (as developed by J. B. Collip)

The demonstration by Banting and Best that extracts of pancreas, prepared with certain precautions, contain a substance having the power to lower the blood sugar and to raise the sugar tolerance in diabetes, both in dogs and man, warranted an attempt to isolate this substance in a sufficiently pure state for repeated subcutaneous or intravenous administration in man. The problem was to remove most of the protein and salts and all of the lipoid material from the extracts without destroying the active principle. In the endeavour to solve this problem various methods were tried and the following was found to be most satisfactory.

To a small volume of 95 per cent ethyl alcohol freshly minced pancreas was added in equal amount. The mixture was allowed to stand for a few hours with occasional shaking. It was then strained through cheesecloth and the liquid portion at once filtered. The filtrate was treated with two volumes of 95 per cent ethyl alcohol. It was found by this treatment that the major part of the protein was removed while the active principle remained in alcoholic solution. After allowing some hours for the protein precipitation to be effected the mixture was filtered and the filtrate concentrated to small bulk by distillation *in vacuo* at a low temperature (18° to 30° C). The lipoid substances were then removed by twice extracting with sulphuric ether in a separating funnel and the watery solution returned to the vacuum still, where it was further concentrated till it was of a pasty consistency. Eighty per cent ethyl alcohol was then added and the mixture centrifuged. After centrifuging, four distinct layers were manifested in the tube. The uppermost was perfectly clear and consisted of alcohol holding all the active principle in solution. Below this, in order, were a flocculent layer of protein, a second clear watery layer saturated with salt, and a lowermost layer consisting of crystals of salt. The alcohol layer was removed by means of a pipette and was at once delivered into several volumes of 95 per cent alcohol, or better, of absolute alcohol. It was found that this final treatment with alcohol of high grade caused the precipitation of the active principle along with adherent substances. Some hours after this final precipitation the precipitate was caught on a Buchner funnel, dissolved in distilled water, and then concentrated to the desired degree by use of the vacuum still. It was then passed through a Berkefeld filter, sterility tests made and the final product delivered to the clinic.

The essential points relating to the extract prepared as outlined above are: (1) It contains only a minimum of protein. (2) It is practically salt free and can readily be made isotonic. (3) It is lipoid free. (4) It is almost free from alcohol soluble constituents. (5) It can be administered subcutaneously without fear of any local reaction.

II. THE EFFECT OF INSULIN ON NORMAL RABBITS AND ON RABBITS RENDERED HYPERGLYCAEMIC IN VARIOUS WAYS

F. G. BANTING, M.C., M.B.

C. H. BEST, M.A.

J. B. COLLIP, PH.D.

J. J. R. MACLEOD, M.B., CH.B., F.R.S.C.

E. C. NOBLE, M.A.

The successful demonstration of the beneficial influence of insulin in the diabetes of depancreated animals raised in our minds the question whether it would also affect the blood sugar of normal animals and of those made diabetic in other ways than by pancreatectomy. If such were the case a ready means would be at hand by which to test the activity of the extracts at various stages in their production. In the present communication we record briefly results bearing on these two questions.

1. *The Effect of Insulin on Normal Rabbits*

In over 150 normal rabbits, fed with oats and sometimes also with sugar, the percentage of sugar in blood from the marginal ear vein was determined, before and at various intervals following subcutaneous injections of insulin. The average percentage of sugar in 90 of these rabbits prior to the injections was 0.133 with a maximum of 0.186 and a minimum of 0.095 (Shaffer-Hartmann method). A marked fall from the initial values was observed to occur within an hour or so of the injection and for purposes of physiological assay we have come to designate as one rabbit dose the amount of insulin (given subcutaneously) which lowers the blood sugar by 50 per cent in 1–3 hours. This method of evaluation of the potency of insulin seems to be fairly satisfactory, for we have found that relatively greater effects in reducing the blood sugar are obtained when the same extract is used on diabetic dogs. Thus, 10 cc of a certain extract injected into a rabbit reduced the blood sugar from 0.135 to 0.071 in 1½ hours, after which it began to rise again, whereas 20 cc of the same extract given to a diabetic dog weighing about five times more than the rabbit caused the blood sugar to fall from 0.375 to 0.030 in 7 hours. The lowest percentage of blood sugar observed in rabbits treated with insulin was 0.01 in 2 hours and 45 minutes after the injection. The purer the preparation of insulin used the more rapid is the fall in blood sugar. The fall seems to be equally rapid in well-fed and starving animals.

Some time after the injection of insulin the rabbits often show characteristic symptoms. A preliminary period of hyperexcitability gives place to a comatose condition in which the animal lies on its side, breathing rapidly (often periodically) with sluggish conjunctival reflex and widely dilated pupils (rectal temperature normal). On the slightest stimulation, as shaking of the floor, violent clonic convulsions supervene in which the animal either throws itself over and over, or lies on its side with head markedly retracted and the limbs moving rapidly as in running. These convulsive seizures usually last 1–2 minutes, and they often come on without any apparent stimulation, when the interval between them is about fifteen minutes. They frequently terminate in death from respiratory failure.

Out of a total of 123 rabbits receiving insulin, convulsions were observed in 26 cases, and the maximum percentage of blood sugar at which they occurred was 0.047 (except in one animal in which 0.067 was found), and the minimum percentage at which there were no convulsions was 0.037.

This close parallelism between the percentage of blood sugar and the incidence of convulsions suggests that a causal relationship exists between the two. This view is supported by the observations of F. C. Mann on dogs rendered hypoglycaemic by removal of the liver from the circulation [548], and by the fact that we have found that subcutaneous injection of dextrose (4 g in 20 per cent solution) restores the animal to the normal condition within a few minutes of the injection. Occasionally recovery may ensue without injections of dextrose, but this is rare. The animals restored by dextrose may subsequently relapse into convulsions which can again be removed by dextrose. Injections of saline solutions or of pentose sugars have no effect.

2. *The Effect of Insulin on Hyperglycaemic Animals*

For these experiments the rabbits were fed on oats and sugar so as to ensure an abundant accumulation of glycogen in the liver. Portions of liver were also removed after death for determination of glycogen.

The methods employed to cause hyperglycaemia were asphyxia, carbon monoxide poisoning, injection of epinephrine (adrenalin), piqûre, and ether. Having satisfied ourselves, by at least four observations in each group,

TABLE 6.I

Piqûre

Time	Uninjected Rabbit	Time	Rabbit Injected with Insulin
10.15	0.137	12.50	0.123
11.00	piqûre	3.30	insulin
11.30	0.305	4.30	0.083
12.05	0.420	4.45	piqûre
12.50	0.457	5.15	0.081
2.20	0.386	5.20	insulin
3.20	0.244	6.00	0.064
4.25	0.187	6.30	0.093
—	—	8.15	0.045

TABLE 6.II

Epinephrine

Time	Uninjected Rabbit	Time	Rabbit Injected with Insulin
9.15	0.154	12.00	0.159
10.20	epinephrine	12.05	insulin
10.55	0.364	2.00	0.040
11.30	0.397	3.05	insulin
12.00	0.440	3.35	epinephrine
1.00	0.440	4.00	0.040
2.05	0.410	4.30	0.057
—	—	5.00	0.065
—	—	5.35	0.060

TABLE 6.III

ASPHYXIA

Time	Uninjected Rabbit	Time	Rabbit Injected with Insulin
9.50	0.140	9.50	0.124
9.55	asphyxia (20 min)	10.00	insulin
10.23	0.383	11.00	0.077
10.55	0.376	2.00	insulin
11.25	0.370	2.20	0.045 (hyperexcitable)
11.55	0.222	2.22	asphyxia (20 min)
12.25	0.200	2.45	0.159
—	—	3.15	0.075
—	—	3.45	0.046

that the above methods cause marked hyperglycaemia in untreated rabbits we then repeated them on rabbits previously injected with insulin. In every case we found in the injected animals either that there was no rise whatsoever in the percentage of blood sugar or that the rise was very markedly less than in untreated animals. Tables 6.I to 6.III give the percentages of blood sugar.

III. THE EFFECT PRODUCED ON THE RESPIRATORY QUOTIENT BY INJECTIONS OF INSULIN

F. G. BANTING, M.B.

C. H. BEST, M.A.

J. B. COLLIP, PH.D.

J. HEPBURN, M.B.

J. J. R. MACLEOD, M.B., CH.B., F.R.S.C.

It is generally recognized that the most satisfactory evidence of the utilization of carbohydrate in the animal body is afforded by the behaviour of the respiratory quotient, i.e., the ratio between the volume of CO_2 expired and of O_2 absorbed. In the normal animal this quotient approaches unity in proportion as carbohydrates replace fats and proteins in the total metabolism; thus, when sugar is given to the animals that are starving or living on a fat and protein diet the quotient promptly rises. In the completely diabetic animal on the other hand, whether this condition be brought about by removal of the pancreas, by administration of phloridzin, or by disease, the quotient remains at the level of about 0.7 (which is characteristic of the metabolism of a mixture of fat and protein) even when large amounts of carbohydrate are ingested.

At an early stage in our work on the influence of insulin on diabetes it became necessary to observe this quotient. This has been done on a case of severe diabetes in man and on several depancreated dogs. The patient (aet. 29) (Dr. G.) has been suffering from diabetes for six years. During the past few months his diet has contained approximately 10 g carbohydrate with total calories of 1200. The total daily excretion of sugar has been 15–30 g, the blood sugar between 0.28 and 0.33 per cent, and acetone bodies always present. On February 17, 1922, while on the above diet, the R.Q. was found to be 0.74 and it remained unchanged in several observations made during the succeeding two hours. Insulin (4 cc) was then injected subcutaneously and 20 g cane sugar was taken by mouth with the result that the quotient rose to 0.90 in two hours. In a second observation of the same type, but in which only 2 cc of insulin was injected, the quotient rose to 0.82 in about three hours. Results of a similar character were obtained by Dr. W. R. Campbell on two other diabetic patients in the medical clinic of the University.

The observations on depancreated dogs were carried out by placing a closely fitting mask over the head and connecting it through two-way valves and wide-bore tubing with a spirometer. There was no great difficulty in training the animal to lie quietly on his side during the observation and great care was taken to see that there were no leaks around the edges of the mask.

The usual procedure was to determine the quotient several times, then to administer cane sugar or pure dextrose either by mouth or subcutaneously, with or without injections of insulin, and then to observe the quotient at frequent intervals. Observations have so far been made on five animals, at periods varying from 48 hours to 154 hours after the pancreatectomy. We are aware that several observers have found that the depancreated animal still retains, for 4–5 days, some power to utilize carbohydrate as shown by a small rise in the quotient when sugar is ingested. This, however, does not detract at all from the value of our results.

Experimental Data

Dog II. Before pancreatectomy, R.Q., after 22–23 hours starvation was 0.85 and 0.86. Thirty g sucrose by mouth caused it to rise to 1.0 in 35 minutes and it remained exactly at this level for two hours. The animal was then depancreated (Jan. 21) and the R.Q., 48 hours later (Jan. 23), was 0.63 rising to 0.76–0.78 in 1½ hours after 20 g sucrose. In 74 hours (10.46 A.M.) after pancreatectomy 25 g sucrose (by mouth) and 10 cc insulin, subcutaneously, caused the quotient to rise to 0.86 in 31 minutes and 0.90 in 1½ hours; it then fell to 0.77 in 3–3½ hours. The animal was again given 20 g sucrose and 8 cc insulin at 3.15 P.M. and the R.Q. rose within 50 minutes to 0.91 then 0.94 (1 hr, 37 min), 0.93 (3 hrs, 17 min), and 0.87 (4 hrs, 1 min). Next morning (Jan. 25) R.Q. stood at 0.68 and 20 g sucrose raised it to 0.82 (3 observations) and 0.85 (1 observation). On Jan. 26, R.Q. was 0.68–0.72; 20 g sucrose raised it to 0.81 in 1 hour, and 10 cc insulin 5 hours later caused it to rise to 0.90 in 40 minutes.

The earlier results of this experiment are not entirely convincing because there was a definite increase in R.Q. with sucrose alone. This may be because sufficient time had not elapsed since the pancreatectomy for the power to utilize carbohydrates (especially laevulose) to disappear. The observations on Jan. 26, five days after the pancreatectomy, are more satisfactory.

Dog III. R.Q. 0.65 (49 hrs after pancreatectomy); after 7 cc insulin subcutaneously (without sucrose) it rose to 0.70 (1 hr, 34 min), 0.68 (1 hr, 51 min), and 0.67 (2 hrs, 7 min). 20 g sucrose, given orally 5 hours after the insulin, caused the quotient to rise 0.89–0.86.

A repetition of this experiment on the next day raised R.Q. to 1.06.

Dog IV. R.Q. 0.63 (48 hrs after pancreatectomy); after 25 g sucrose it rose to 0.70 (in 52 min) returning to 0.65 in 1 hr 35 min. Two days later 5 cc insulin followed in 1½ hours by 30 g sucrose caused the quotient to rise to 0.83 in about 1 hour after the sucrose. On Feb. 20, six days after pancreatectomy, this animal was fed sugar *ad lib.* 10 cc of insulin then caused R.Q. to rise from 0.76 (on the previous day) to 0.95.

Dog V. Sucrose caused a decided rise in R.Q., from 0.67 to 0.81, in 51 hours and a smaller rise (from 0.69 to 0.73) in 107 hours. On the sixth day 8 g dextrose injected subcutaneously along with 10 cc insulin only raised R.Q. from 0.73 to 0.80.

Dog VI. This animal was not depancreated but was starved for three days. It was given 4 cc insulin subcutaneously with the result that R.Q. rose from 0.77 and 0.75 to 0.90 (in 42 minutes after injection) and then fell to 0.85 (1 hr, 6 min) and 0.78 (1 hr, 36 min).

Although the above observations were not as adequately controlled as we should have desired, they show conclusively that insulin given along with sugar to depancreated dogs raises the respiratory quotient to a much higher level than occurs with sugar alone.

IV. THE EFFECT OF INSULIN ON THE PERCENTAGE AMOUNTS OF FAT AND GLYCOGEN IN THE LIVER AND OTHER ORGANS OF DIABETIC ANIMALS

F. G. BANTING, M.B.

C. H. BEST, M.A.

J. B. COLLIP, PH.D.

J. J. R. MACLEOD, M.B., CH.B., F.R.S.C.

E. C. NOBLE, M.A.

1. *Glycogen in the Liver, Heart, and Muscles*

(a) *Liver.* Minkowski found that after total extirpation of the pancreas in dogs, the percentage of glycogen in the liver fell to 0.5 or less even when large quantities of dextrose had been ingested. When laevulose was given (in three cases) considerably larger amounts of glycogen were deposited (0.72 to 8.14). Several investigators have confirmed these observations except that Cruickshank [234] has found that laevulose also does not form glycogen provided the extirpation of the pancreas is complete. He infers that Minkowski's results with laevulose were due to the fact that all pancreatic tissue had not been removed.

In two depancreated dogs which were given large quantities of cane sugar for several days preceding death we found in the livers 0.044–0.047 per cent in the one, and 1.29–1.35 per cent of glycogen in the other.

Very different results were obtained when insulin, as well as sugar, was given to depancreated dogs for a few days before the animal was killed. Thus, in one animal (Jan. 3) 13.27 per cent, in another (Feb. 21) 12.58 per cent, and in a third (March 28) 11.4 per cent of glycogen were found in the liver. These striking differences indicate that one effect of insulin is to stimulate the glycogenetic function of the liver and this fact, coupled with the knowledge that it also raises the respiratory quotient in an hour or two after it is given subcutaneously, lends support to the hypothesis that carbohydrate can be utilized in the body only after it has been converted into glycogen.

In two other cases less striking results were obtained, namely, 2.85 per cent in one (Jan. 14) and 4.9 per cent in another (April 2). In one animal that took sucrose very greedily and to whom large doses of insulin were given during the two days preceding death considerably more than 12 per cent of glycogen was found in the liver.

(b) *Heart and muscles.* Cruickshank found that glycogen in the hearts of six normal dogs averaged 0.5 per cent, the maximum being 0.85. In 16 depancreated dogs the average was 0.7; in one case it was 1.05 per cent. Macleod and Prendergast [542] found in two normal dogs that the glycogen in the ventricle is increased by starvation to 1.00 and 1.05 per cent respectively. In the present investigation, 0.79–0.92 per cent and 0.98 per cent glycogen were found respectively in the hearts of two depancreated dogs fed sugar but receiving no insulin. In four other depancreated animals to whom insulin was given, as well as sugar, the values were 0.725, 0.600, 0.570, and 0.296. These few observations indicate that insulin reduces the glycogen percentage in the heart of diabetic animals to within the normal limits.

With regard to the skeletal muscles, nothing conclusive can as yet be said although there is some indication that insulin causes the percentage of glycogen to increase (cf. table 6.VI).

2. *Total Fatty Acid in Liver, Heart, and Blood*

Fat. This has been determined as fatty acid by Leathes modification of the Kumagawa-Suto method with the following results, the animals in all cases being given large amounts of sugar (see Table 6.IV).

TABLE 6.IV
Dogs Not Receiving Insulin

No.	Liver (%)	Heart (%)	Blood (%)
48	12.25	4.26	—
50	14.10	2.59	1.21
51	9.90	—	1.12

Although much larger percentages of fat than these have been observed to occur in the liver after phosphorus or phloridzin it is nevertheless much above the average for laboratory animals, which is given by Leathes as about 4–6 per cent. With regard to the blood our results compare with those given by Bloor for severe diabetes viz., 1.01 per cent. These values were decidedly altered in animals receiving insulin (see Table 6.V).

TABLE 6.V
Dogs Receiving Insulin

No.	Liver (%)	Heart (%)	Blood (%)
52	7.425	3.00	(1) 0.333
			(2) 0.270
55	2.190	2.08	0.531
56	4.410	—	—

TABLE 6.VI
SOME EFFECTS OF INSULIN IN DIABETIC DOGS

No.	Date Oper.	Date p.m.	Total Fatty Acid (%) Liver	Heart	Blood	Glycogen-dextrose (%) Liver	Muscle	Heart	Sugar	Insulin	R.Q.	Sugar blood (%)	Remarks and evidence of diabetes
41	II/14	II/21	—	—	—	12.58	0.38	0.725	yes	yes 17th–21st	0.63	—	R.Q. rose from 0.63 to 0.70 after sugar. R.Q. rose to 0.78, 0.79 and 0.83 after sugar and insulin. Dog died during night
48	III/3	III/9	12.25	4.26	—	—	—	—	yes	no	0.64	0.3 / 0.35	R.Q. before sugar 0.65, 0.65; after sugar 0.67, 0.67
49	III/3	III/14	—	—	—	0.047 / 0.044	0.58 / 0.48	0.918 / 0.787	yes / yes	no / no	0.65 / 0.67	—	Died during night
50	III/14	III/18	14.10	2.59	1.207	—	—	—	yes / yes	no	0.63 / 0.69	—	R.Q. before sugar 0.63, 0.63; after sugar 0.66, 0.65, 0.67, 0.69
50	III/18	III/25	9.90	—	1.121	1.354 / 1.287	0.034 / 0.034	0.98 / 0.98	yes	no	—	—	took large amounts sugar for 3 days before death. R.Q. before sugar 0.67–0.68; after sugar 0.67, 0.67, 0.67
52	IV/8	IV/14	7.425	3.00	0.333[1] / 0.270[2]	—	—	—	yes	yes on 13th	—	0.31[1] / 0.030[3]	[1]Fat and sugar of blood on IV/12 while on diet of meat and biscuit. [2]Fat in blood on IV/13 after which large dose insulin
54	IV/19	IV/22	26.350 / 26.375	3.00	0.368	0.34	—	—	no	yes on 21st	—	0.305	[3]Sugar in blood when moribund fed meat and biscuit—large dose insulin given on 21st and moribund on 22nd
53	IV/19	IV/22	10.276	—	—	—	—	—	no	yes on 21st	—	0.33	same as 54, only died during night
C₁	I/10	I/14	—	—	—	2.567 / 2.845	0.41	0.600	yes	yes on 14th	—	—	animal in very poor condition at time of death
C₂	—	XII/22	—	—	—	Over 12	0.600	—	yes	yes 20th–22nd	—	—	
55	IV/25	IV/28	2.189	2.08	0.531	11.4	0.764	0.570	yes dextrose	yes 26th–28th	0.62–0.64, 0.67, 0.85[2]	0.30, 0.105[1], 0.111[2]	[1]After dextrose. [2]After dextrose and insulin—dog in good condition at time of death
56	IV/27	V/2	4.410	—	—	4.92 / 4.70 / 4.78	—	0.293 / 0.299	yes dextrose	yes (1st)	—	0.396 / 0.410	dog dead but not cold when liver was removed for glycogen

There were two dogs, however, in which the liver fat was not found to be reduced following insulin. In both of these (53 and 54) excessive doses of insulin were given so that the one animal (53) died during the night and the other (54) in the forenoon following the administration. In the former case 10.276 per cent and in the latter 26.360 per cent of fatty acid were found in the liver.

The results so far obtained on the fat of blood show insulin to have a decided reducing effect.

The observations taken as a whole show that insulin given to sugar-fed diabetic animals causes the fat to become reduced in the liver at the same time as glycogen accumulates. Whether glycogen would also accumulate in this organ without ingestion of sugar, we cannot at present say. It is clear that there must be a stage following the administration of insulin when glycogen and fat both are present in considerable percentage in the liver. This is shown in experiment 56. The protocols of these experiments are given in abbreviated form in Table 6.VI.

V. THE EFFECT OF INSULIN ON THE EXCRETION OF KETONE BODIES BY THE DIABETIC DOG

F. G. BANTING, M.B.

C H. BEST, M.A.

J. B. COLLIP, PH.D.

J. J. R. MACLEOD, M.B., CH.B., F.R.S.C.

As the production and excretion of ketone bodies is one of the cardinal symptoms of the diabetic individual the effect of the administration of extracts of pancreas containing the active principle of the gland (insulin) upon the excretion of these substances by depancreatized dogs was studied. This study was initiated before a purified extract was produced. The extracts used were made by alcoholic extraction of the whole gland of the ox, the alcohol being subsequently removed by vacuum distillation. They had a fair degree of potency but contained considerable protein, lipoid, and salt and were relatively very crude as compared with later products. The results obtained, however, show in a very striking manner the influence upon the excretion of ketone bodies, a fact which has subsequently been confirmed on clinical cases (cf. *Canadian Medical Association Journal*, March 1922 [see Paper 7, below]).

The animals used were depancreated and placed in metabolism cages. The urine was collected over twenty-four hour periods and the total excretion of ketone bodies determined by the method of Van Slyke [765]. When a very definite ketonuria had developed extract was administered by subcutaneous injection.

The results are shown in Table 6.VII.

TABLE 6.VII

EXCRETION OF SUGAR AND KETONE BODIES IN DEPANCREATED DOGS

No.	Date	Whether Insulin Given	Urine Volume (cc)	Total Dextrose Excretion (g)	Total Acetone Bodies (mg)	Remarks
I	Dec. 14	no insulin	1,000	—	75.0	♀ wt. 15 kg
	" 15	"	885	24.0	62.0	
	" 16	"	1,150	36.0	80.0	
	" 17	"	1,000	25.0	60.0	
	" 18	"	750	27.0	—	
	" 19	"	850	29.0	190.0	nitrogen 1.14
	" 20	"	800	28.0	210.0	nitrogen 1.15
						blood sugar 0.309%
						blood sugar ⎧0.217%
						following ⎨0.085%
						insulin ⎩0.051%
	" 21	insulin	600	none	none	
II	Jan. 6	no insulin	1,000	29.7	100.0	
	" 7	"	375	28.4	187.0	Blood sugar 0.351%
	p.m.	insulin	—	—	—	lowered blood sugar to 0.085%
	Jan. 8	no insulin	425	4.25	none	
	" 9	"	325	9.95	none	
	" 10	"	370	9.6	none	
	" 11	"	275	25.2	34.0	
	" 12	"	325	25.4	55.0	
	" 13	"	750	18.0	114.0	
	p.m.	insulin				
	Jan. 14	"	600	8.0	none	
III	Jan. 13	no insulin	750	22.4	206.0	♀ wt. 5 kg
	" 14	"	1,750	63.0	3.141	blood sugar 0.295%
	p.m.	insulin	500	30.0	none	insulin given at 9 a.m. dog killed at 4:30 p.m.

The most convincing of these experiments is number II in which administration of insulin on one day, January 7, caused the acetone bodies to disappear from the urine of the next three days, during which no insulin was given. After this they again gradually appeared to be removed a second time by injection of insulin.

P APER 7 IS THE FORERUNNER OF THE
tens of thousands of reports on the effects of insulin on diabetic patients.
The results of the clinical work which had started on January 11, 1922,
with the administration to Leonard Thompson of the extract from adult
ox pancreas, which Banting and I had made, were now prepared for publication. We had actually given our diabetic friend, Dr. Joe Gilchrist, a large
dose of insulin orally in late December 1921. As we had expected from the
results of our animal studies, this had no effect. Although Banting and I
had found that the best results were achieved in dogs when the extracts
were injected intravenously, the clinicians in charge decided to give the
extract to Leonard Thompson subcutaneously. They were cautious, and
commendably so, because the extract contained protein foreign to the
human species. The dose given to the boy was much less on a body
weight basis than we had used in the dogs. We were disappointed but not
too surprised at the small decrease in blood sugar and lack of clinical
improvement following the first injections. Nearly two weeks elapsed
before heavier dosage with an improved material prepared by Collip was
tried and definite improvement was observed. The data in this first clinical
paper confirmed the experimental findings in a most satisfactory fashion.
Even more dramatic results were soon to be seen on the hospital wards. It is
unfortunate that our very potent sterile extract of foetal calf pancreas was not
used for the first clinical trial, but the source of supply would soon have
been exhausted.

A little later unexpected difficulties developed with tragic consequences.
Pitfalls in the transfer of laboratory procedures to larger scale production
are now well known but at that time they brought the production of insulin
to a halt and two of the original group of patients died. Professor Collip had

returned to his post in Alberta and I was forced to resume responsibility for production. I have described this hectic period elsewhere. Banting refers to it in his Nobel Lecture. During the night and day struggle for six weeks in the basement of the Medical Building, Professor Macleod appeared briefly on two occasions. He tried his best to be helpful but his only suggestion was that we return to the small scale procedure which had invariably given potent lots of insulin. This was what I was trying to do, but the collection and handling of larger amounts of pancreas introduced many new problems.

7. Pancreatic Extracts in the Treatment of Diabetes Mellitus: Preliminary Report

F. G. BANTING

C. H. BEST

J. B. COLLIP*

W. R. CAMPBELL†

A. A. FLETCHER†

Since the year 1890, when von Mering and Minkowski [561] produced severe and fatal diabetes by total removal of the pancreas in dogs, many investigators have endeavoured to obtain some beneficial effect in diabetes mellitus, either by feeding pancreas, or by administration of pancreatic extracts.

Minkowski, Sandmeyer [665], Pflüger [619], and others found that feeding pancreas was followed by negative or even harmful results. More recently, Murlin and Kramer [584], Kleiner [459] and Paulesco [614] have tried the effects of aqueous extracts of the pancreas intravenously, on depancreatized animals and have found transitory reduction in the percentage of blood sugar and in the sugar excreted in the urine.

In 1907, Rennie and Fraser [636], recognizing the possibility that pancreatic enzymes might have harmful effects on the internal secretions, secured islet tissue from teleosteal fishes, where it exists separately from the rest of the pancreas, and fed it to human diabetics. Their studies demonstrated no beneficial influence on the condition of the patient. E. L. Scott [688] in 1912 sought to eliminate the influence of proteolytic enzymes by using alcoholic extracts of the pancreas. He did not find, however, that such extracts caused as marked a reduction in the urinary sugar or in the G/N ratio as when extracts were made with acidulated water. The whole question has been reviewed recently by Allen [7, 10]; by him, and,

Originally appeared in the *Canadian Medical Association Journal*, XII (March 1922), 141–46.

*From the Department of Pathological Chemistry, University of Toronto.

†From the Department of Medicine, University of Toronto, and the Toronto General Hospital.

indeed, by the majority of recent writers, it is usually stated that pancreatic extracts have no clinical value whatsoever. During the past ten months, two of us (F.G.B. and C.H.B.), working in the Department of Physiology of the University of Toronto, have reinvestigated the problem. Certain of the results obtained have already been published [40], others are now in press. These may be briefly reviewed here.

Believing that extracts of the pancreas, as usually prepared, did not satisfactorily demonstrate the presence of an internal secretion acting on carbohydrate metabolism, because the active principle was destroyed by the digestive enzymes also present in such extracts, attempts were made to eliminate these enzymes. In the first experiments, this was done by taking advantage of the fact that the acinous tissue (from which the digestive enzymes are derived) but not the insular tissue of the pancreas degenerates in seven to ten weeks after ligation of the pancreatic ducts. Extracts were therefore made, with ice-cold Ringer's solution, of degenerated pancreatic tissue removed ten weeks after the ligation of the ducts. The extract obtained by this procedure, when injected intravenously or subcutaneously into diabetic dogs, invariably caused a marked reduction in blood sugar and in the amount of sugar excreted in the urine. It also enabled a diabetic dog to retain a much higher percentage of injected sugar than it otherwise would. Extracts of liver or spleen, prepared in the same manner as the extracts of degenerated pancreas, were found to have neither of these effects. The active principle of the extract of degenerated pancreas was destroyed by boiling in neutral or acid solution or by incubating for two hours at body temperature with pancreatic juice.

In later experiments, it was found that the pancreas of foetal calves of under five months' development did not contain proteolytic enzymes, thus confirming the observations of Ibrahim [413]. By extracting such foetal pancreatic tissue, a highly potent and readily procurable preparation was obtained. Besides affording a much more practicable method for securing larger quantities of extracts, this result demonstrated that the active principle is essentially the same from whatever animal it is prepared. A method was finally evolved by which an active extract, which would retain its potency for at least one month, could be obtained from normal adult ox pancreas. Daily injections of pancreatic extract (foetal calf or adult beef pancreas) prolonged life of a completely diabetic dog to seventy days, at the end of which time the animal was chloroformed. Allen states that in his experience completely diabetic dogs do not live more than fourteen days. The first results of a study of the respiratory exchange in completely diabetic dogs, before and after administration of extract, showed that the extract confers on the diabetic animal the power to burn carbohydrates.

Thus, in a diabetic dog, on starvation or lean meat diet, the respiratory quotient was found to be in the neighbourhood of 0.7. The ingestion of carbohydrate caused no rise in the CO_2/O_2 ratio, but when preceded by an injection of extract gave a value which approached 1.0, indicating that carbohydrate was being burned. Besides the above, it should be recorded that the administration of extract very quickly caused striking improvement in the various symptoms known to be characteristic of complete pancreatectomy.

As the results obtained by Banting and Best led us to expect that potent extracts, suitable for administration to the human diabetic subject, could be prepared, one of us (J. B. C.) took up the problem of the isolation of the active principle of the gland. As a result of this latter investigation, an extract has been prepared from the whole gland, which is sterile and highly potent, and which can be administered subcutaneously to the human subject. The preparation of such an extract made possible at once the study of its effects upon the human diabetic, the preliminary results of which study are herein reported. The extract containing the active principle is being further purified and concentrated. A detailed report of the method of extraction, purification, and concentration will be published at an early date.

For the investigation of the clinical application of these extracts in the treatment of human diabetes, Professor Graham has placed at the disposal of two of us (W. R. C. and A. A. F.) the cases of diabetes mellitus in the wards of the Medical Service of the Toronto General Hospital.

Patients were placed on a constant diet, varying with the severity of each individual case, and their reaction to such treatment studied for a period of a week, after which various samples of extract were administered and the effects observed. The ordinary routine clinical examinations were carried through. Blood sugar was estimated at intervals by the revised Folin-Wu method, urinary sugar by Benedict's methods, the acetone bodies by Van Slyke's methods, and the respiratory quotient by the Tissot-Haldane and Douglas-Haldane methods.

Up to the present time, February 22, 1922, the effects of these preparations have been observed in seven cases of diabetes mellitus and it is now evident that certain definite results can be obtained by their administration. The effects observed in depancreatized animals have been paralleled in man. The fall in blood sugar occurs and in two cases, repeatedly examined, a rise in the respiratory quotient, indicating carbohydrate utilization, occurs more or less coincidentally with the attainment of a normal blood sugar level. Patients report a complete relief from the subjective symptoms of the disease. The sugar excretion shows marked decrease or, if dosage be ade-

quate, disappears. Ketonuria is abolished, thus confirming a similar observation by Collip in diabetic animals (results as yet unpublished). These
results taken together have been such as to leave no doubt that in these
extracts we have a therapeutic measure of unquestionable value in the
treatment of certain phases of the disease in man. In agreement with observations of other investigators in laboratory animals, it has been found that
without careful control severe toxic reactions may be encountered and this
will undoubtedly be a factor in the evaluation of the ultimate therapeutic
utility of the method.

The following case report illustrates these observations:

Name: L. T. (Boy). Aged 14.
Admitted to the Medical Wards, Toronto General Hospital, December 2,
1921.
Present Illness. About December 1919, he was taken to his family physician
because he had been wetting the bed at nights, and also because his ankles
became swollen occasionally. One month later, sugar was found in the urine.
He states that at this time he was in good health, his appetite was somewhat
excessive, but no increased thirst was complained of. Careful dietetic regulation
was prescribed and he states that he adhered to this diet fairly well. This his
family physician will not confirm. Fasting was also tried apparently without
success. The glycosuria persisted, he began to lose weight, frequency of micturition, both day and night, increased up to the time when his physician recommended admission to hospital.
Past Illness. Always healthy up until two-and-one-half years ago, with the
exception of an attack of chicken-pox at the age of ten and of discharging ear
for two years as a baby.
Personal History. Born in Canada, went regularly to school, able to work well
up to time of onset of present illness. Has always been fond of sweet food
and previous to the onset of this condition ate freely of candy.
Family History. Mother and father, one brother and two sisters, all in good
health. No diabetes or other familial diseases known.
Examination. On admission he was poorly nourished, pale, weight 65 pounds,
hair falling out, odour of acetone on the breath, tonsils and teeth in good
condition, abdomen large and tympanitic. Blood pressure 100–70. He appeared
dull, talked rather slowly, quite willing to lie about all day. Hands show marked
xanthochromia. No findings of note in examination of cardio-vascular, respiratory, abdominal systems or of the blood. The urine at the time of admission
was strongly acid, specific gravity 1.030 to 1.040. The test for sugar strongly
positive. Rothera and ferric chloride tests for ketones strongly positive. 24
hour amount of urine, 3–5 litres. Blood sugar 5.8 mg per cc.
Treatment. He was put to bed and was quite content to remain there most
of the time. However, when he wished to do so, he was allowed to get up and
wander about the ward, which he did very little during the first month. His diet
was as follows:
Dec. 2. 5, 10, and 15 per cent vegetables as much as desired.
Dec. 11. 60 g lean meat daily added to diet.

Dec. 15. 4 bran cakes daily added to diet.

Jan. 4. Daily ration to consist of 50 g lean meat, 5 and 10 per cent vegetables, and fruits and bran cakes to make up exactly 100 g of carbohydrates per day. Clear broth, cocoa, tea, and coffee in moderation. Total intake about 450 calories.

No further change in diet was made.

This case was one of severe juvenile diabetes with ketosis. Previous to admission, he had been starved without evident benefit. During the first month of his stay in hospital, careful dietetic regulation failed to influence the course of the disease and by January 11 his clinical condition made it evident that he was becoming definitely worse.

The extracts given on January 11 were not as concentrated as those used at a later date, and, other than a slightly lowered sugar excretion and a 25 per cent fall in the blood sugar level, no clinical benefit was evidenced.

Daily injections of the extract were made from January 23 to February 4 (excepting January 25 and 26). This resulted in immediate improvement. The excretion of sugar as shown in Figure 15 became much less. On days of treatment, this varied from 7.5 g to 45.1 g compared with a previous amount well over 100 g daily. The acetone bodies disappeared from the urine. The boy became brighter, more active, looked better and said he felt stronger. No extract was given from February 5 to February 15. During this time sugar again appeared in the urine in large amounts along with traces of acetone. Administration of extract in smaller doses after February 16 again resulted in lowered sugar excretion and disappearance of acetone from the urine. Figure 16 shows the fall in the total acetone bodies of the urine during the periods of treatment after January 23. Figure 17 gives a four-hour record of the blood sugar following the administration of a single dose of 6 cc extract on February 17. Figure 18 shows the influence of extract on the amount of glucose excreted in each two hourly period when extract was being used. Table 7.I records the volume of urine and amount of sugar excreted each day and blood sugar determinations. The qualitative test for the daily excretion of acetone bodies in the urine and the amount of extract given is also tabulated.

Although the other six patients treated by these extracts were all favourably influenced by its administration, particular reference might be made to one—a severe case who had been excreting 20 g of glucose on a diet containing 10 g carbohydrate and 2400 calories per day. Following injection of the extract his urine became sugar free, and he obtained complete relief from severe depression and extreme lassitude. Respiratory quotients in this same case showed a definite rise after injection of the extract, confirming the increased utilization of carbohydrate.

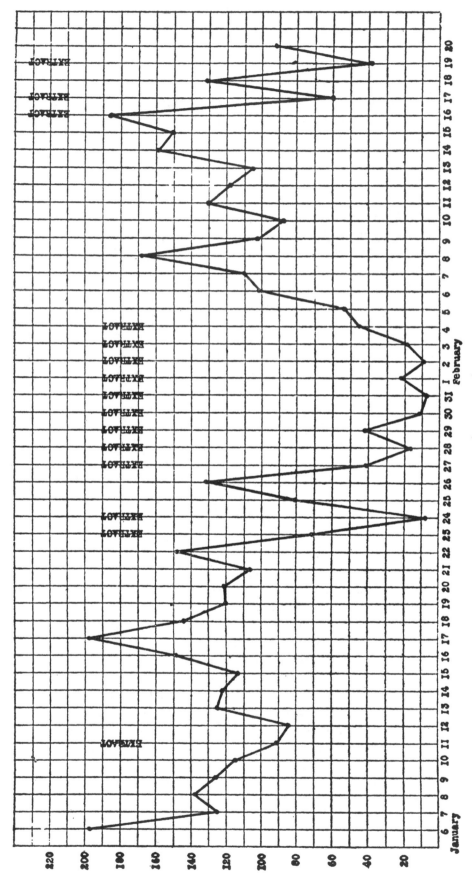

Figure 15. Effect of extract on glycosuria

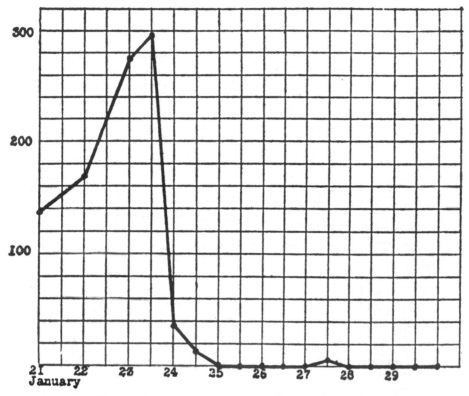

FIGURE 16. Showing the cessation of ketonuria following administration of extract.

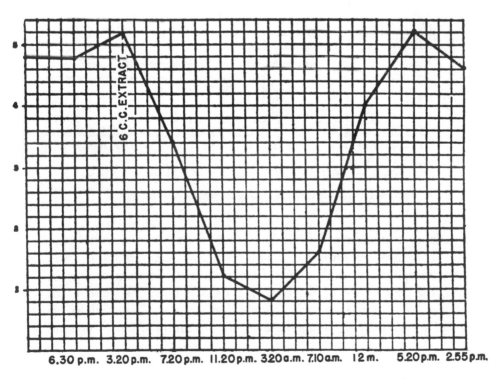

FIGURE 17. Effect of one injection of extract on blood sugar (mg per cc = tenth per cent).

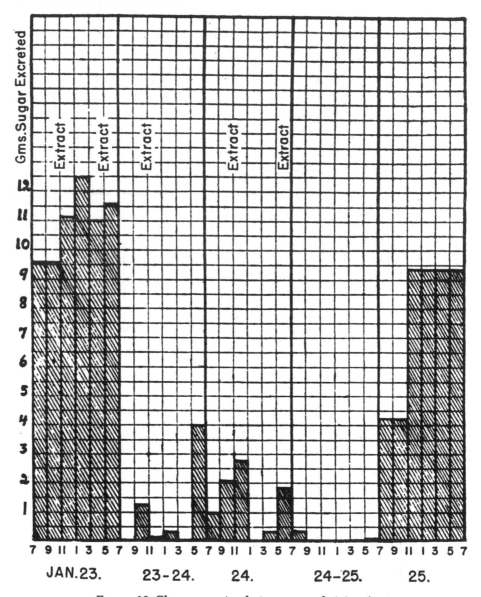

FIGURE 18. Glucose excretion during extract administration.

All patients were improved clinically. It is difficult to put in words what is meant by clinical improvement. Those who have been treating diabetes will have recognized as early signs of improvement a certain change in the skin, the appearance of the eyes, the behaviour of the patient, his mental and psychic activity, and the physical evidences, as well as his testimony, of increased vigour and desire to use his muscles. Under present-

TABLE 7.I

CLINICAL PROTOCOLS (L.T.)

Date	24 hr Amount of Urine in cc	24 hr Excretion of Glucose in g	Blood Sugar in mg per cc	Rothera Test		Total Acetone Bodies in mg per litre	Subcutaneous Injection of Pancreatic Extract in cc a.m.	p.m.
Dec. 12	—	—	5.8	plus	plus	—	—	
20	—	—	4.5	plus	plus	—	—	
29	—	—	5.2	plus	plus	—	—	
Jan. 3	—	—	5.2	plus	plus	—	—	
6	4500	187.8	—	plus	plus	—	—	
7	4020	126.2	—	plus	plus	—	—	
8	3650	137.2	—	plus	plus	72	—	
9	3690	126.7	6.2	plus		540	—	
10	6870	114.0	—	plus	plus	—	—	
11	3625	91.5	3.2–4.4	plus	plus	188		15
12	4060	84.0	4.9	plus	plus	69	—	
13	3950	125.5	—	plus		—	—	
14	3780	123.5	—	plus	plus	—	—	
15	3900	114.7	—	plus	plus	—	—	
16	3910	148.0	—	plus	plus	—	—	
17	3960	197.3	6.7	plus	plus	—	—	
18	4300	144.6	—	plus	plus	—	—	
19	3770	120.6	—	plus	plus	—	—	
20	3840	121.9	—	plus	plus	—	—	
21	4580	107.3	—	plus	plus	137	—	
22	4540	148.5	—	plus	plus	167	—	
23	4210	71.1	5.2	plus	plus	282	5	20
24	4120	8.7	1.2–3.0	plus		30	10	10
25	3880	80.5	—		0	0	—	
26	5070	130.3	—		0	0	—	
27	3040	42.2	—	plus		4	4	4
28	5125	16.7	—	trace		0	2	4
29	3275	42.5	—		0	0	4	
30	2715	11.5	—	trace		0	4	4
31	4415	7.5	—		0	0	4	4
Feb. 1	3145	21.8	—		0	0	4½	4
2	2700	9.1	—		0	0	5	4
3	4150	18.2	—		0	0	5	4
4	3740	45.1	—		0	0	5	4
5	3475	53.3	—		0	0	—	
6	3900	101.5	—		0	0	—	
7	3700	110.1	—		0	0	—	
8	4910	167.1	—	trace		0	—	
9	4940	101.7	—		0	0	—	
10	4710	86.9	—	trace		0	—	
11	4510	129.9	—	trace		0	—	
12	3170	117.7	4.87	trace		0	—	
13	2595	106.7	4.9	trace		0	—	
14	4670	158.5	—	trace		0	—	
15	3275	151.4	—	trace		0	—	
16	4611	185.0	4.73	neg.		0		5
17	3930	60.4	0.85–5.2	neg.		0		6
18	4790	132.3	2.0–4.5	neg.		0	—	
19	3105	39.6	—	neg.		0		4
20	3985	92.0	—	neg.		0	—	

day treatment, such improvement occurs in diabetics free from acetone but is undoubtedly more striking in patients recovering from a ketosis. This is the nature of the improvement seen clinically as a result of the administration of these extracts, and, while it is of a temporary nature, we believe that it justifies the hope of more permanent results following more adequate and carefully regulated dosage.

Summary

Following the production of what appears to be a concentrated internal secretion of the pancreas and the demonstration of its physiological activity in animals, and, under careful control, its relatively low toxicity, we are presenting a preliminary report on the pharmacological activity of this extract in human diabetes mellitus. Clinical observations at this juncture would appear to justify the following conclusions: (1) Blood sugar can be markedly reduced even to the normal values. (2) Glycosuria can be abolished. (3) The acetone bodies can be made to disappear from the urine. (4) The respiratory quotient shows evidence of increased utilization of carbohydrates. (5) A definite improvement is observed in the general condition of these patients and in addition the patients themselves report a subjective sense of well-being and increased vigour for a period following the administration of these preparations.

Acknowledgments

For their hearty co-operation and kindly assistance and advice, we have great pleasure in presenting our best thanks to Professor J. J. R. Macleod of the Department of Physiology, to Professor V. E. Henderson of the Department of Pharmacology, to Professor J. G. Fitzgerald of the Department of Hygiene, and to Professor Duncan Graham of the Department of Medicine of the University of Toronto.

D URING AUGUST, SEPTEMBER, AND
October 1921, in the intervals between our appointments with our diabetic
dogs, Fred Banting and I occupied ourselves planning the experiments
which we hoped to do with insulin. In our August letter to Professor
Macleod, we had placed the study of the effects on normal animals in a
prominent position and we were anxious to start the investigation. A very
large part of my own time during the spring of 1922 had to be devoted to
making insulin for the clinical and the experimental studies. Fred Banting
was dividing his time between the clinic and the laboratory. Thus a major
part of the first demonstration that insulin counteracts the hyperglycaemia
produced by piqûre, epinephrine, asphyxia, and ether, was contributed by
other members of the team.

Another paper was presented at this time under the names of Banting,
Best, Collip, Campbell, Fletcher, Macleod, and Noble. Professor Macleod
read this communication at the May 1922 meeting of the American Association of Physicians. Since neither Banting nor I had been consulted about the
plan to give the paper and since we had no part in its preparation, it will not
be included here.

Paper 8 describes the effects of insulin on some types of experimental
hyperglycaemia in rabbits.

8. The Effects of Insulin on Experimental Hyperglycaemia in Rabbits

F. G. BANTING

C. H. BEST

J. B. COLLIP

J. J. R. MACLEOD

E. C. NOBLE

In a previous paper it was shown that a marked fall occurs in the percentage of blood sugar in normal rabbits when they are injected subcutaneously with insulin. Taken in conjunction with the fact that insulin also reduces often to the normal level, or even below it, the high percentages of sugar found in the blood of depancreated dogs and of diabetic patients, it would appear that its action must be a fundamental one in the control of the blood sugar level [48]. The present investigation was undertaken to obtain further evidence of the scope of the action of insulin by studying its effect on the various experimental conditions that are known to cause marked hyperglycaemia in rabbits.

It is unnecessary to review here the extensive literature which bears on the methods used to cause these various forms of hyperglycaemia. We will only refer to those investigations which have a direct bearing on our own results, in connection with each of the varieties which we have investigated.

METHODS

The rabbits used were as uniform in size and breed as possible and they were fed for some days preceding the experiments an abundance of oats and hay, sometimes with sugar added. The blood was collected at frequent intervals in 1 cc quantities from the ear veins and the percentage of sugar determined in the samples by the Shaffer-Hartmann method. At the termination of the experiments, whenever possible, the percentage of glycogen

Originally appeared in the *American Journal of Physiology*, LXII (November 1922), 559–80.

was determined in the liver by Pflüger's method, using the Shaffer-Hart-mann method for measurement of the reducing power of the hydrolysed solutions. The insulin used was not always of uniform potency since during the progress of this research we were also engaged in working out the most suitable method for its preparation. As a preliminary to each experiment it was therefore the practice to inject the preparation of insulin into normal rabbits. Provided the preparation was found to be active, either the same rabbit or another (normal) rabbit was subjected to one or other of the procedures for the production of hyperglycaemia. These were piqûre, injection of epinephrine, mechanical asphyxia, carbon monoxide poisoning, and ether.

RESULTS

Piqûre

In order to be certain that hyperglycaemia will result in this experiment it is necessary to make sure that the liver contains adequate amounts of glycogen and that the puncture is not too far above the calamus of the medulla and is near the midline.

With regard to the latter condition it is our opinion that certainty of correct puncture can best be assured by reflecting the skin from the occipital bone under local (ethyl chloride) anaesthesia and then, with the head bent as far forward as possible, puncturing at the occipital tubercle in the direction of the outer canthi of the eyes until the point of the instrument is felt to come against the basilar process. We have found that an ordinary trochar is a suitable instrument to use. This operation necessarily wounds the cerebellum with the result that after it the animal shows forced movements. Usually also there is a certain amount of haemorrhage into the 4th ventricle. Stewart and Rogoff [740] recommend actual exposure of the 4th ventricle by Eckhard's method, which involves separating the muscles lying over the occipito-atlantoid ligament, which is then incised. We believe, however, that this is unnecessary and that it is an advantage to avoid it because of the danger of haemorrhage. At the termination of each experiment the exact position of the puncture was determined by post-mortem examination.

The results of piqûre on three normal well-fed rabbits are given in Figure 19 along with two of Stewart and Rogoff's. It will be seen that the rise in blood sugar follows the piqûre very rapidly indeed, the maximum being reached in about one hour, and that the return to normal is much slower, occupying from 5 to 8 hours. The glycogen content of the rabbit showing the steepest curve (no. 2) was found to be 2 per cent on the day following the experiment. It was lower, 0.6 per cent, in another (no. 3) animal in which the curve was somewhat lower. The considerable variability in the position of the punctures in these three definitely positive cases of hyperglycaemia shows that some latitude is permissible.

Turning now to the experiments in which the piqûre was performed on animals under the influence of insulin very different results are evident.

TYPICAL PROTOCOLS*

Piqûre, no insulin. Rabbit III, 3

Normal blood at 10:15 A.M.—0.137 per cent sugar.
Piqûre at 11:00.
Blood at 11:30—0.305 per cent sugar.
Blood at 12:05—0.420 per cent sugar.
Blood at 12:50—0.457 per cent sugar.
Blood at 2:20—0.386 per cent sugar.
Blood at 3:20—0.244 per cent sugar.
Blood at 4:25—0.187 per cent sugar.
Blood at 12:30—0.170 per cent sugar (next day).
Animal killed at 12:30 next day.

The liver at this time showed a glycogen content of 2.0 per cent. Post-mortem showed a puncture through the vermis of the cerebellum in the midline, and through the medulla 1 mm to the left of the midline, 11 mm above the calamus.

Piqûre plus insulin. Rabbit IV, 2

Normal blood at 12:50—0.123 per cent sugar.
At 3:30, 5 cc of insulin.
Blood at 4:30—0.083 per cent sugar.
Piqûre at 4:45.
Blood at 5:15—0.081 per cent sugar.
At 5:20, 4 cc of insulin.
Blood at 6:00—0.064 per cent sugar.
Blood at 6:30—0.093 per cent sugar.
Blood at 8:13—0.045 per cent sugar.
Blood at 3:00—0.124 per cent sugar (next day).

At 8:15 the rabbit was in convulsions as described in the previous paper and dextrose solution was injected subcutaneously, resulting in rapid recovery. The rabbit was killed at 3:30 the next day, and the liver showed only 0.27 per cent glycogen. The medulla showed two punctures, one on the right cerebral penduncle, 6 mm above the calamus, and the other 10 mm above in the midline.

Piqûre plus insulin. Rabbit VI; weight, 2.4 kilos

Normal blood at 9:50—0.117 per cent sugar.
At 10:00—7 cc of insulin.
Blood at 11:00—0.075 per cent sugar.

*Three protocols in the original and a diagram showing the position of puncture in the floor of the 4th ventricle have been omitted.

Blood at 11:45—0.056 per cent sugar.
Piqûre 11:50 (2 punctures) about 5 cc of blood lost.
Blood at 12:35—0.068 per cent sugar.
Blood at 1:10—0.062 per cent sugar.
Blood at 2:40—0.052 per cent sugar.
At 3:00—3 cc of insulin.
Blood at 3:45—0.042 per cent sugar, mild convulsions.
Blood at 4:55—0.035 per cent sugar, mild convulsions.
Animal killed at 5:00. Liver contained 2.64 per cent glycogen. Puncture through vermis in midline, two in floor of 4th ventricle.

The punctures of the medulla in these cases were such as to ensure hyperglycaemia. The amounts of glycogen found present in the livers were entirely adequate in two cases (5 and 6) but rather small in one (4). In this case the animal was not killed until twenty-two hours after the operation, during which time a considerable amount of glycogen may have been hydrolysed. In experiment 4 the blood sugar during the first four hours following piqûre did not rise above 0.093 per cent, a figure considerably under the normal level. In no. 5, the sugar was not reduced to the same extent as in no. 6, before piqûre was performed; in thirty minutes it had risen to 0.177 per cent slightly above normal, and then, following another dose of extract, fell off gradually to 0.063 per cent. (These results are shown in graphic form in Figure 19.)

From these experiments, we may conclude that the severe hyperglycaemia which occurs in rabbits whose livers are rich in glycogen, following piqûre, may be markedly reduced, if not entirely inhibited, if the operation is performed subsequent to the injection of suitable doses of insulin. The experiment (no. IV, 2), in which 0.27 per cent of glycogen was found in the liver, is the only one in which there can be any doubt as to the inhibiting action of insulin. It is somewhat similar to one described by Stewart and Rogoff [740] in which no hyperglycaemia occurred in a piqûred rabbit with 0.34 per cent of glycogen in the liver. In this case the blood sugar rose only from 0.124 per cent to 0.143 per cent following piqûre and to 0.151 per cent following asphyxia. In our case, as a result of insulin, the blood sugar fell to 0.045 per cent and then recovered to 0.124 per cent by next day. This recovery probably indicates that the glycogen had been drawn on to restore the blood sugar to its normal level. In light of the corroborative nature of the results of other experiments on piqûre we do not consider it necessary at the present to add further observations.

Epinephrine Hyperglycaemia

Bang [39] found that the subcutaneous injection of 1 mg epinephrine in rabbits caused the blood sugar to rise to a maximum in 2 to 3 hours returning to the normal in 7 to 9 hours. The curve was similar in starved and well-fed animals except that it did not begin to rise quite so quickly in the former. Reference to other investigations are given by Bang, the most sig-

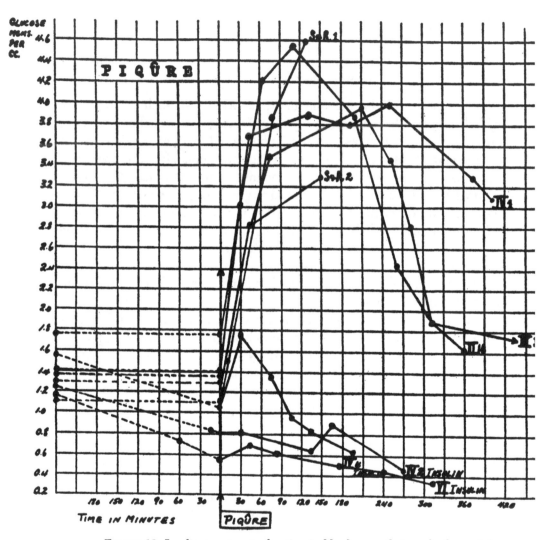

FIGURE 19. Insulin counteracts elevation in blood sugar that results from piqûre.

nificant point being that injection intravenously of the above amount of epinephrine causes only a transient and slight increase in blood sugar.

In order to satisfy ourselves that marked hyperglycaemia invariably follows subcutaneous injection of epinephrine in rabbits, the following experiments were done using solutions of adrenalin chloride.

Rabbit IV, 3; weight 1.45 kilos; well-fed

Normal blood at 9:15—0.154 per cent sugar.
At 10:20, 2 cc adrenalin chloride solution 1—1000 injected subcutaneously.
Blood at 10:55—0.364 per cent sugar.
Blood at 11:30—0.397 per cent sugar.
Blood at 12:00—0.440 per cent sugar.
Blood at 1:00—0.440 per cent sugar.
Blood at 2:05—0.410 per cent sugar.

Rabbit II, 6; well-fed

Normal blood at 10:50—0.141 per cent sugar.
At 2:35, 2 cc adrenalin chloride solution 1—1000 injected subcutaneously.
Blood at 3:10—0.34 per cent sugar.
Blood at 4:55—0.36 per cent sugar.
This is the same adrenalin solution as used in the insulin experiment (III, 6) (below).

To study the influence of insulin on this form of hyperglycaemia, two methods were used. In the following two experiments 2 cc adrenalin and 5 cc of insulin were injected at the same time.

Rabbit III, 6; well-fed

Normal blood at 12:00—0.122 per cent sugar.
At 2:45, 5 cc of insulin and 2.0 cc adrenalin chloride 1—1000 were injected subcutaneously.
Blood at 3:30—0.090 per cent sugar.
Blood at 4:15—0.132 per cent sugar.
Animal died at 5:40 P.M. No glycogen determination made.

Rabbit X

Normal blood at 9:50—0.138 per cent sugar.
At 9:56, 4.0 cc insulin + 2 cc adrenalin chloride 1—1000.
Blood at 10:30—0.232 per cent sugar.
Blood at 11:00—0.303 per cent sugar.
Blood at 11:30—0.347 per cent sugar.
Blood at 12:10—0.365 per cent sugar.
Blood at 1:10—0.388 per cent sugar.
Blood at 2:10—0.325 per cent sugar.
Blood at 3:10—0.233 per cent sugar.
Blood at 4:10—0.165 per cent sugar.
This insulin caused convulsions in a control animal.

In the following experiment 2 cc adrenalin were injected after the hypo-glycaemic effect of insulin had become evident.

Rabbit VII, weight, 4.25 kilos

Normal blood at 10:15—0.127 per cent sugar.
At 10:17, 4 cc insulin.
Blood at 11:15—0.106 per cent sugar.

2 cc adrenalin chloride 1—1000, subcutaneously.
Blood at 11:45—0.183 per cent sugar.
Blood at 12:15—0.227 per cent sugar.
Blood at 12:45—0.240 per cent sugar.
Blood at 1:15—0.244 per cent sugar.
Blood at 1:45—0.307 per cent sugar.
Blood at 2:15—0.324 per cent sugar.
Blood at 2:45—0.304 per cent sugar.
Blood at 3:45—0.235 per cent sugar.
Blood at 4:45—0.147 per cent sugar.
Blood at 6:30—0.115 per cent sugar.

In the following experiments 1 cc adrenalin was injected after the hypo-glycaemic effect of insulin had become evident.

Rabbit XII

Normal blood at 9:05—0.105 per cent sugar.
At 9:10, 2.0 cc insulin.
Blood at 11:15—0.083 per cent sugar.
Blood at 12:15—0.050 per cent sugar.
1.0 cc adrenalin chloride 1—1000.
Blood at 1:15—0.054 per cent sugar.
Blood at 2:15—0.090 per cent sugar.
Blood at 3:20—0.090 per cent sugar.
Blood at 4:15—0.090 per cent sugar.
Glycogen = 2.26 per cent.

Rabbit XIII

Normal blood at 9:25—0.100 per cent sugar.
At 9:30, 2.0 cc insulin.
Blood at 11:25—0.066 per cent sugar.
Blood at 1:10—0.074 per cent sugar.
1.0 cc adrenalin chloride 1—1000.
Blood at 2:10—0.120 per cent sugar.
Blood at 3:15—0.131 per cent sugar.
Blood at 4:10—0.127 per cent sugar.
Glycogen = 1.80 per cent.

It is clear that insulin is capable of greatly reducing the hyperglycaemia caused by epinephrine, provided the latter be not given in massive doses. Out of a total of five experiments in which 1 cc adrenalin chloride was injected after the hypoglycaemic effect of insulin had become evident, the blood sugar did not rise above 0.130 per cent in three, in one it rose to 0.190 and in another to 0.265. In the two last-mentioned cases, however, the insulin used was evidently extremely weak, the blood sugar being only reduced to about 0.09 per cent prior to the injection of adrenalin, thus contrasting with the marked reduction in the other cases. In the three experiments in which 2 cc adrenalin were injected following insulin a decided hypoglycaemic effect remained in one, but distinct increase in blood sugar occurred in the other two. In two experiments in which 2 cc adrenalin were injected at the same time as insulin, a marked hyperglycaemia developed in the one but not in the other. Taking these results as a whole it is plain that much more work must be done before it can be told to what extent insulin can antidote the adrenalin effect. We are hopeful that it may be possible to determine the dosage of insulin in terms of the amount capable of antidoting the effect of a standard dose of adrenalin. [Protocols of eight experiments and two figures dealing with the antidotal effects of insulin and adrenalin have been omitted.]

Asphyxial Hyperglycaemia

There is no more certain means for causing a marked degree of hyperglycaemia than asphyxia brought about by constriction of the upper air passages. In rabbits the most practical way for doing this is by placing a piece of waterproof material over the snout and holding it there until the heart rate becomes definitely slowed. The animal is then allowed to breathe freely for a few breaths when it is again asphyxiated. This procedure is kept up for twenty minutes. With so many observations of this type on record (cf. Stewart and Rogoff, and Macleod) it was not considered necessary to perform more than one control experiment of which the following is the result.

Rabbit IV, 3; weight 2.3 kilos; well-fed
  Normal blood at 9:50—0.140 per cent sugar.
  Mechanical asphyxia from 9:55–10:20.
  Blood at 10:23—0.383 per cent sugar.
  Blood at 10:55—0.376 per cent sugar.
  Blood at 11:25—0.370 per cent sugar.
  Blood at 11:55—0.222 per cent sugar.
  Blood at 12:25—0.200 per cent sugar.

Three experiments were then performed on well-fed rabbits which were asphyxiated for twenty minutes following the injection of insulin.

Rabbit IV, 4; weight 2.05 kilos
  Normal blood at 9:50—0.124 per cent sugar.
  At 10:00, 3 cc insulin injected subcutaneously.
  Blood at 11:00—0.077 per cent sugar.
  At 2:00, 3.0 cc insulin (same) subcutaneously.
  Blood at 2:20—0.045 per cent sugar (animal hyperexcitable).
  Mechanical asphyxia from 2:22–2:40.
  Blood at 2:45—0.159 per cent sugar.
  Blood at 3:15—0.075 per cent sugar.

Blood at 3:45—0.046 per cent sugar.
Animal was asphyxiated again, and died during the operation.
Blood at 4:15—0.144 per cent sugar obtained from the heart after death.
Liver contained 2.04 per cent glycogen.

Insulin had the effect either of preventing entirely any asphyxial rise in blood sugar or of greatly reducing the rise which usually occurs. [The protocols of two experiments and one figure dealing with the experiments on insulin and asphyxia have been omitted.] In Experiment IV, 4, the sugar rose from 0.045 to 0.159 per cent during a twenty-minute asphyxial period, an increase of 0.114 per cent as compared with 0.243 per cent in the control experiment (no. IV, 3) but it will be observed this rise was of a very temporary nature, the percentage returning to its pre-asphyxial level in one hour. A similar sharp return to the pre-asphyxial level is also to be observed in the second period of asphyxia in experiment IV, 9.

Carbon Monoxide Poisoning

In order to study the effect of a less acute form of asphyxia than the foregoing we have also investigated carbon monoxide poisoning. The method was to place the animal in an air-tight box just large enough to contain it comfortably, and provided with an observation window. A mixture of air and illuminating gas was then allowed to circulate slowly through the box at the rate of 0.6 litre per minute. This mixture contained 0.8 per cent carbon monoxide by calculation. In the 0.8 per cent atmosphere hyperpnea developed early and in forty-five minutes the animal was in a semi-conscious condition and was removed from the box. It was then unable for several minutes to stand on its feet and some time elapsed before the hyperpnea disappeared. Four of the five experiments performed were carried out on two well-fed rabbits, each of which was first subjected to forty-five minutes' gassing, and then in a week's time, underwent a second period of gassing, after being given insulin. The fifth experiment is an additional control performed on a normal rabbit. The results of one experiment follow. [One chart and protocols for two rabbits have been omitted.]

(a) *Rabbit III, 10; weight 2.2 kilos; well-fed*
  Normal blood at 2:30—0.149 per cent sugar.
  Gassed from 2:30–3:18, 0.8 per cent CO (by calculation).
  Blood at 3:19—0.245 per cent sugar.
  Blood at 3:49—0.334 per cent sugar.
  Blood at 4:19—0.347 per cent sugar.
  Blood at 4:49—0.320 per cent sugar.
  Respirations at 3:20—240 per minute.
  Respirations at 3:45—250 per minute.
  Respirations at 4:30—190 per minute.

(b) Same animal seven days later
    Normal blood at 10:00—0.125 per cent sugar.
    At 10:05, 3.0 cc of insulin, subcutaneously.
    Blood at 10:40—0.089 per cent sugar.
    At 10:45, 5.0 cc insulin, subcutaneously.
    Gassed from 10:52–11:37, 0.8 per cent CO.
    Blood at 11:40—0.081 per cent sugar.
    Blood at 12:10—0.083 per cent sugar.
    At 12:15, 2.5 cc insulin subcutaneously.
    Blood at 12:40—0.070 per cent sugar.
    Blood at 1:10—0.060 per cent sugar.
    Blood at 2:30—0.070 per cent sugar.
    Blood at 3:30—0.062 per cent sugar.
    Animal was in very weak condition when removed from the chamber.

In experiment I(b) the results are very striking; the blood sugar immediately after the animal was removed from the chamber, was slightly lower than when the animal was inserted forty-five minutes before. The same rabbit seven days previously had responded to the same period of gassing, without the injection of insulin, by a rise in blood sugar to as high as 0.347 per cent.

No glycogen determinations were made on the livers of these animals, but it is evident, from the initial hyperglycaemia following carbon monoxide, that an ample amount of this material was present, and the animals were fed, until the second experiment, on the same carbohydrate-rich diet.

These results indicate that insulin prevents, or at least greatly depresses, the hyperglycaemia which follows the administration of carbon monoxide to well-fed rabbits.

Ether Hyperglycaemia

It is well known that the percentage of blood sugar rises during ether anaesthesia. In rabbits the degree of this hyperglycaemia, according to Fujii, is proportional to the intensity of the etherization. Of course it is impossible to be certain that the animals used in a series of experiments such as this are all etherized to the same degree, but nevertheless, even under very light anaesthesia, a certain degree of hyperglycaemia always develops, provided of course the liver contains an ample supply of glycogen. The changes in blood sugar following ether administrations to normal well-fed rabbits are shown in Figure 20.

Ether. Rabbit IV, 7; weight, 1.75 kilos
    Normal blood at 12:00—0.147 per cent sugar.
    Ether commenced at 12:15.
    Blood at 12:50—0.45 per cent sugar.
    Blood at 1:25—0.50 per cent sugar.

The rise in blood sugar is rapid, and it persists as long as the etherization: in each case until the death of the animal.

When ether was administered after injecting the animal with insulin, the following results were obtained:

Ether after insulin. Rabbit IV, 10; weight, 2.7 kilos; sugar-fed
  Normal blood at 9:50—0.095 per cent sugar.
  At 10:00, 7.0 cc of insulin, subcutaneously.
  Blood at 10:45—0.073 per cent sugar.
  At 11:45, 5.0 cc of insulin, subcutaneously.
  Blood at 1:25—0.057 per cent sugar.
  Blood at 2:30—0.052 per cent sugar.
  At 2:35, 5.0 cc of insulin, subcutaneously.
  At 2:40 ether commenced, continuous to 4:25.
  Blood at 3:10—0.065 per cent sugar.
  Blood at 3:40—0.060 per cent sugar.
  Blood at 4:10—0.071 per cent sugar.
  Animal died at 4:25. Liver contained 3.91 per cent glycogen.

The results in Figure 20 show that even with considerable amounts of glycogen in the liver there was only a slight and transient increase in the percentage of blood sugar while the animal was under ether. [Three protocols dealing with the effects of ether and insulin have been omitted.]

In another case, insulin was not given until some time after the animal had been lightly under ether, with the following results:

Ether before insulin. Rabbit IV, 6; weight, 1.85 kilos; sugar-fed
  Normal blood at 1:30—0.114 per cent sugar.
  Ether commenced at 1:45 P.M., continuous to 5:15 P.M.
  Blood at 2:15—0.142 per cent sugar.
  Blood at 2:45—0.150 per cent sugar.
  At 2:50, 10.0 cc of insulin, subcutaneously.
  Blood at 3:20—0.120 per cent sugar.
  Blood at 3:50—0.082 per cent sugar.
  Blood at 4:40—0.060 per cent sugar.
  Blood at 5:10—0.047 per cent sugar.
  Animal killed at 5:15. Liver contained 0.77 per cent glycogen.

The degree of hyperglycaemia in this experiment is somewhat less striking possibly because of the relatively low glycogen content of the liver. The effect of insulin is, however, quite definite.

The effect of insulin in inhibiting the hyperglycaemia of ether anaesthesia is of importance from both experimental and clinical standpoints, from the former because it offers greater opportunities for the experimental investigation of the exact mechanism of the physiological action of insulin, and from

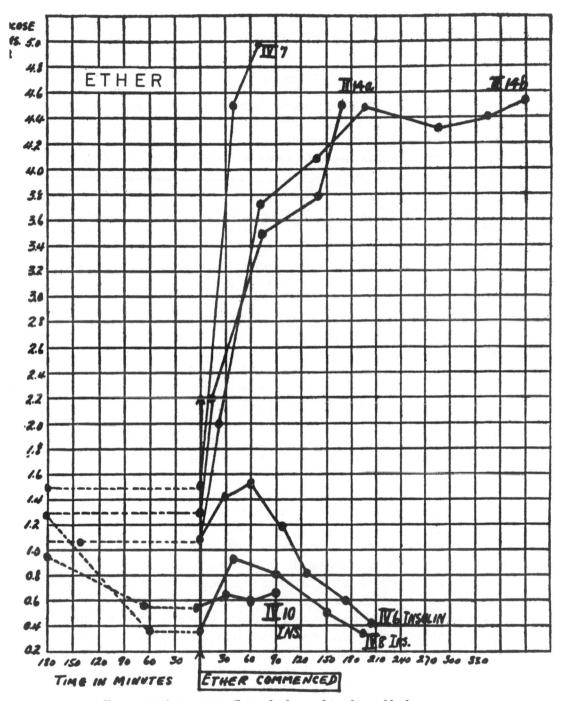

FIGURE 20. Antagonistic effects of ether and insulin on blood sugar.

the latter because it offers a means by which hyperglycaemia may be controlled when surgical anaesthesia is necessary in diabetic patients.

DISCUSSION

Considering these results as a whole there can be no doubt that insulin in suitable dosage more or less inhibits the development of hyperglycaemia in rabbits subjected to various conditions which otherwise cause it. The degree of this inhibition is usually sufficient entirely to mask any rise in blood sugar but sometimes a rise occurs to a certain extent. This rise may be quite marked when the insulin is injected at the same time as the application of the stimulus used to cause hyperglycaemia, as is especially evident when this is epinephrine. In the latter case, indeed, the degree of hyperglycaemia may be as great as the usual when the injections of epinephrine and insulin are made simultaneously. This would seem to indicate that there is a considerable latent period before insulin unfolds its full action, a conclusion which is borne out by the preliminary observations which we have made on the behaviour of the respiratory quotient following insulin. During this preliminary stage a powerful hyperglycaemia-producing stimulus like epinephrine can apparently almost annul the effect of insulin. Further work on this aspect of the problem is in progress.

That insulin acts not only in the experimental forms of hyperglycaemia discussed in this paper but also in that following pancreatectomy and in diabetes in man indicates that its action on carbohydrate metabolism is fundamental. Its effect on blood sugar is just as striking in a pancreatic diabetic animal with only a trace of glycogen in the liver as on a normal one whose liver is loaded with this material. In the former case insulin also influences the excretion of ketone bodies, the mobilization of fat and the respiratory quotient, which must be interpreted as meaning that it is essential in the regulation of the series of intermediary metabolic changes that culminate in the complete utilization of both fat and carbohydrate. By more intensive investigations of the metabolism of pancreatic diabetic animals treated with insulin it is therefore to be hoped that some light may be thrown on the problem of ketogenesis.

Concerning the *modus operandi* of insulin in preventing the purely experimental form of hyperglycaemia, we have no hypothesis to offer. Before any such is attempted it will be necessary to obtain precise data on the amounts of glycogen in the liver and muscles before and during and after insulin action. Only then can it be known whether insulin actually stimulates glycogenesis to the extent that it takes glucose away from the systemic blood.

Conclusions

1. When the fall in blood sugar due to subcutaneous injection of insulin is thoroughly established, piqûre, epinephrine, mechanical and carbon monoxide asphyxia, and ether do not cause the usual degree of hyperglycaemia. There may be a distinct increase in the percentage of blood sugar but very seldom is this sufficient to raise it to the normal level existing before insulin was given.

2. Even when the insulin is given at the same time as the animal is subjected to the experimental condition used to cause hyperglycaemia the latter may be either entirely absent or greatly diminished.

IN THE SPRING OF 1922, DAVID A. SCOTT, Ph.D., F.R.S., *because of his chemical experience and proven ability, was appointed by the Connaught Laboratories to help me with the preparation of insulin. Fred Banting and I were devoted to "Scotty" and fervently wished that he could have joined us earlier. Before long he was carrying a great deal of the responsibility for insulin production in Canada. His subsequent outstanding work on the preparation of insulin, the significance of zinc in crystalline insulin, the preparation (with Dr. A. M. Fisher) of protamine zinc insulin, the distribution, purification, and crystallization of heparin (with Dr. Arthur Charles) is very widely known and appreciated. In 1922 Scott and I prepared several bulletins on the preparation of insulin, which were sent to interested pharmaceutical companies in many countries. Paper 9, published in 1923, is a review of the situation at that time.*

This is not the place to review the history of the purification of insulin, but I would like here to pay particular tribute to the valuable contributions of Harold Ward Dudley, of Doisy, Somogyi, and Shaffer, and of Moloney and Findlay, although many others deserve mention.

9. The Preparation of Insulin

C. H. BEST

D. A. SCOTT

When the Insulin Committee suggested that we should report on the recent progress in the preparation of insulin an extensive review of the history of pancreatic extracts was at first contemplated. Macleod [538], Dale [237], and others, however, have recently reviewed certain parts of the literature, and since a study of that portion of this literature which describes the preparation of the extracts shows that many of them are of minor significance in the present connection, we have decided to refer only to those investigators whose work, in our opinion, led them very near to the solution of the problem.

Zuelzer [827], a German investigator, was one of the early workers in this field. He prepared extracts from pancreas in several ways, one of which is as follows. The pancreas was minced and sufficient sodium bicarbonate was added to produce a weak alkaline reaction. The mixture was then left to autolyse for several days. (This procedure in our experience results in a great loss of potency of the material. Zuelzer stated, however, that this step might be omitted.) The liquid was then pressed out and alcohol added until no more albuminous substances were precipitated. When the solution was free from albumin, it was filtered and concentrated in a vacuum still. The final product obtained, Zuelzer says, was a fine, dry, grey powder. This powder, he states, was easily soluble in water or dilute alkali; was free from ferments; and gave none of the known protein reactions. Insulin, as we know it at present, is less stable in alkaline than in acid solution. The purest preparation we have as yet obtained from mammalian pancreas gives a positive biuret reaction.

Zuelzer tested his preparation by determining to what extent it antidoted the hyperglycaemia and glucosuria caused by administration of epinephrine. Von Fürth and Schwarz [315] and others have reported that many other substances counteract the effect of epinephrine.

Zuelzer's extract was administered to several diabetic patients, and in

Originally appeared in the *Journal of Biological Chemistry*, LVII, 3 (October 1923), 709–23. From the Insulin Division of the Connaught Antitoxin Laboratories, University of Toronto.

certain of these cases was partially successful, in his own hands, in alleviating the symptoms of diabetes. In the hands of others (Forschbach [306]), however, the toxic effects overshadowed the beneficial action to such an extent that further treatment was abandoned.

Although Zuelzer nearly discovered in 1908 the active pancreatic principle which we call insulin, his work in the light of subsequent events must be considered an abandoned research.

E. L. Scott [688], working on the hypothesis that later was independently formulated by Banting, narrowly missed demonstrating in 1912 the internal secretion of the pancreas. He was unable to secure complete atrophy of the acinous cells of the pancreas in dogs, after attempting to ligate the pancreatic ducts. He did not report the effect of administration of extract of this partially atrophied gland. Scott also tried to extract the internal secretion by means of alcohol, but in his endeavour to inhibit the action of the external secretion, he raised the concentration of alcohol to such a height that a large proportion of the active principle was undoubtedly never extracted from the gland. The alcoholic extract obtained from the gland was concentrated *in vacuo* and the residue extracted with ether. The ether extract was discarded. The residue was dissolved in 95 per cent alcohol. Since insulin from mammalian pancreas is only slightly soluble in alcohol of this concentration, Scott could have had very little of the active substance in his final extract. In the preparation of watery extracts Scott used a preliminary alcoholic extraction. The concentration of alcohol was approximately 85 per cent for the first extraction of the glands. At this concentration a part of the insulin would go into solution. This was evidently discarded. A large part of the active substance would be left behind, however, and should have been present in the second extract which was obtained by treating the glands with water. Possibly one reason why better effects were not obtained with this material was that an inhibiting substance which is at least partially precipitated by 80 per cent alcohol, must have been present in large amounts in the watery extracts.

Rennie and Fraser [636] in 1907 studied the effects on diabetic patients of the oral administration of the principal islets of certain bony fishes. In one case these investigators administered a saline extract of islet tissue by subcutaneous injection. No beneficial influence on the symptoms of diabetes was observed. Since insulin in a purified form has not as yet been administered successfully by mouth, we have not far to look for the cause of failure of those experiments in which the crude islet tissue was orally administered. The subcutaneous injection of the extract of the islet tissue produced very profound symptoms of toxicity.

Knowlton and Starling [460] hazarded the opinion that the pancreatic hormone "would be a body diffusible, soluble in water, unstable in alkaline solution, but more stable in slightly acid solution, and not destroyed immediately at the temperature of boiling water." It is interesting to note that these speculations (with the exception of that one relating to the diffusibility of the substance) are correct. We have not as yet obtained a preparation which dialyses through parchment. The diffusibility of the active principle is a property which has to be retested every time a purer preparation is obtained. We have carried out the procedure used by these investigators in the preparation of their extract, and have demonstrated the presence of insulin in the resulting mixture. The tests are much more conclusive, however, if the crude extract so obtained is purified in any one of the several ways which we will attempt to outline in the body of this paper. The work of Knowlton and Starling [460] and of Patterson and Starling [613] has been reviewed in several communications by the Toronto group [40]. We merely wish to point out here that had these investigators used criteria other than the change in sugar consumption of the perfused mammalian heart to determine the potency of their material, more encouraging results might have been obtained.

Murlin and Kramer [584], in 1913, prepared alkaline extracts of pancreas. The administration of this extract reduced the degree of glycosuria in diabetic dogs. It was discovered, however, that this effect was produced by the administration of alkali alone. With the exception of experiments in which the respiratory quotients of several diabetic animals were studied, no further work was reported by Murlin and his collaborators until after the publication of the initial experiments of the Toronto investigators.

Kleiner [459] showed that the administration to diabetic dogs of unfiltered watery extracts of fresh pancreas which had been diluted with 0.90 per cent sodium chloride, usually resulted in a marked decrease in blood sugar. A decrease in the amount of sugar excreted in the urine accompanied the reduction of the blood sugar level. Kleiner suggested that the diminished excretion of sugar might be partly due to the toxic renal effects. Kleiner's experiment was repeated and confirmed by Banting and Best [40]. Anuria was observed, however, in the experimental animal.

Very significant results have been obtained by a group of workers who have attempted to demonstrate in blood or in pancreatic perfusates a substance necessary for the proper combustion of carbohydrates in the body. The most important of these contributions are those of A. H. Clark [203], Lépine [492], Drennan [263], Hédon [382; 383; 384], Forschbach [305], and Murlin and Kramer [584]. Since we contemplate reporting on the demonstration of insulin in blood, a review of the work of these investigators will perhaps be more advantageously included in that communication.

PREPARATION OF EARLIER EXTRACTS

In July 1921 [40], extracts were prepared in the Department of Physiology of the University of Toronto, which were shown to contain the internal secretion of the pancreas. In the preparation of this extract the degenerated pancreas was removed from dogs ten weeks after ligation of the pancreatic ducts. The gland was obtained as soon as possible after the death of the animal and was sliced into a chilled mortar containing Ringer's solution. The mortar was placed in a freezing mixture and the contents were partially frozen. Sand was added and the tissue was completely pulverized. The temperature of the contents of the mortar was then raised and the resulting liquid filtered through paper. The filtrate was administered intravenously to diabetic dogs. The results of the injection of this material have been published [40]. Extracts were prepared by this simple procedure from the normal pancreas of the dog and from foetal calf pancreas. The normal pancreas did not yield as much of the active principle per gram of tissue as did the degenerated gland. The pancreas of the foetal calf, however, provided comparatively large quantities of the substance. It would be interesting to compare the amounts of active material obtainable from these sources, if the tissues were treated with a high acid extractive, as in our present procedure. This causes the immediate inactivation of proteolytic enzymes and a comparatively efficient extraction of the active principle.

Banting and Best [41] prepared active extracts from the normal pancreas of the ox by extraction of the gland with alcohol, which had been made acid by the addition of 0.2 per cent hydrochloric acid. The concentration of alcohol in the mixture was in some cases as high as 60 per cent. The liquid was removed from the glands by filtration and the filtrate evaporated either in porcelain dishes placed in a warm air current or by means of a laboratory vacuum still. The liquid was usually evaporated so that from 5 to 10 cc contained one dose for a depancreatized dog. This material was administered to several diabetic dogs. One animal, in particular, dog 33, which lived 70 days after pancreatectomy, received many injections of this preparation. Rigid aseptic precautions were not observed in the administration of the extract to this animal. However, so long as daily doses of active material were administered there was little or no suppuration at the sites of injection. Numerous abscesses developed when insulin was omitted. These disappeared, however, when the treatment was resumed. The improvement in the clinical condition of the animals receiving this material was very marked. The respiratory quotients of completely diabetic dogs were definitely raised and large amounts of glycogen [47] were deposited in the livers of the animals when glucose and insulin, which had been prepared by the above procedure, were administered. In some cases the filtrate referred to was evaporated to dryness and the residue extracted with toluene to remove the lipoid material. This procedure caused no loss in potency. *These investigators were able to demonstrate that the active principle contained in this residue was practically insoluble in 95 per cent ethyl alcohol.* They treated an aliquot portion of the dried residue with 95 per cent alcohol. The mixture was filtered and the filtrate evaporated. The residue was dissolved in saline solution. Administration of this solution produced no effect upon the blood or urinary sugar of a depancreatized dog. A saline solution of the material which did not dissolve in 95 per cent alcohol, however, definitely lowered the blood sugar and diminished the sugar excretion of the same animal. A watery solution of this material was passed through a Berkefeld filter, but a considerable loss of potency was observed. Tricresol in excess of that amount used as a preservative in biological products, such as diphtheria antitoxin, did not injure the active substance. Material prepared by these investigators from beef pancreas was administered to several diabetic patients in the clinic of the Toronto General Hospital. A decrease in blood sugar and a lowered sugar excretion resulted. A certain degree of local irritation was observed in some of the cases. This was probably due to the high percentage of protein present in the extract. The results of these experiments showed that insulin could be derived from a readily available source—beef pancreas; that a preparation could be secured from this source which was efficient in completely removing the symptoms of diabetes from depancreatized animals; and that these results, as far as the effects on hyperglycaemia and glucosuria were concerned, could be duplicated in the clinic. The practical application of the results was very evident.

A method for the further purification of insulin was evolved principally by J. B. Collip who joined forces with the discoverers of insulin in December 1921. This method has been reported [44; 207]. The details are briefly as follows: 95 per cent alcohol was added to freshly minced pancreas so that the volumes of extractive and glands were approximately equal. After an interval of a few hours, during which the mixture was stirred, the liquid was filtered off. 95 per cent alcohol was added to the filtrate to secure a concentration of approximately 80 per cent alcohol. The mixture was then filtered and the filtrate concentrated *in vacuo*. The vacuum was secured by the use of a laboratory water pump. When the liquid had been concentrated to a small volume the lipoid substances were removed by extraction with ether. The watery solution was then further concentrated to a pasty consistency. This material was treated with 80 per cent alcohol and the mixture centrifuged. The active principle was found to be contained entirely in the alcohol which formed the uppermost layer in the centrifuge tube. The alcoholic solution was removed and was added to several volumes of 95 per cent or absolute alcohol. The active principle, as mentioned above, was practically insoluble in alcohol of this concentration. The precipitate obtained by the above procedure was removed by a Buchner filtration, dissolved in distilled water, and concentrated to remove traces of alcohol and to secure the desired concentration of active substance. The preliminary clinical effects of this preparation have been reported [42]. This method of purification worked out satisfactorily for a short time, on a small scale. Larger scale experiments were not successful and subsequently it was found impossible to duplicate consistently the earlier results on any scale. For a period of 2 months scarcely any insulin was available. A method was then evolved, however, in this laboratory, with the assistance of various members of the Toronto group, which utilized the facts reported by Banting and Best and many of the details of Collip's procedure. The method gave consistent results, and furnished all the insulin used in Toronto for clinical and experimental work for a period of 3 months prior to the beginning of collaboration with Eli Lilly and Company. This method was as follows: Minced pancreas was extracted with an equal volume of 95 per cent acetone. A small amount of formic or acetic acid was added. Collip had previously found formic acid advantageous. The concentration never exceeded 0.1 per cent. (Higher acid was first used in this laboratory as a result of a conversation with H. H. Dale, in which the acidity of the extractive was discussed.) The pancreas acetone mixture was allowed to stand for several hours and was then filtered. The filtrate was placed in enamel lined trays (500 cc to each tray measuring $18 \times 18 \times 2.5$ inches). The trays were placed in a tunnel through which a current of hot air was rapidly drawn. The 500 cc were evaporated to approximately 50 cc in about 1 hour. The temperature of the liquid never exceeded $35°$ C. The residue was removed from the trays, chilled to $0°$ C, and filtered. Lipoid material was largely eliminated in this manner. The filtrate thus obtained was treated with 95 per cent ethyl alcohol to secure a concentration of approximately 80 per cent alcohol. The mixture was then filtered and the filtrate added to 5 or more volumes of 95 per cent alcohol as in the previous method. The precipitate which formed was allowed to settle to the bottom of the alcoholic solution. From 24 to 48 hours were allowed for the precipitate to settle. The alcohol was then decanted off and the precipitate dissolved in distilled water. Traces of alcohol were removed by vacuum distillation. This was the method originally adopted and applied to larger scale production by Eli Lilly and Company when information regarding the production of insulin was communicated to them by the Toronto Committee.

One of the first contributions made by the scientific staff of Eli Lilly and Company was the employment of rotary high vacuum pumps which immediately made possible the efficient concentration of the original acetone or alcoholic filtrate and also of the filtrate after the 80 per cent alcoholic precipitation.

Benzoic Acid Method

This method of preparing and purifying insulin was evolved in these laboratories by Moloney and Findlay [575]. The principle of this process is based on the fact that certain substances readily adsorb insulin. The particular adsorbing substance used by these investigators was benzoic acid. The method briefly is as follows:

Minced pancreatic glands were extracted with alcohol and the filtrate was concentrated in an efficient vacuum still. To each litre of the crude aqueous concentrate 50 cc of a 25 per cent sodium benzoate and 12.5 cc of concentrated hydrochloric acid were used. These amounts were usually sufficient to saturate the solution with benzoic acid. However, these quantities can be increased or decreased proportionately depending on the amount necessary to cause a first lasting precipitate. Then to this saturated benzoic acid solution 40 cc of 25 per cent sodium benzoate and 10 cc of concentrated hydrochloric acid were added. The precipitate thus formed was allowed to settle and the solution filtered. This precipitate usually contained about two-thirds of the potent material. The filtrate was again treated with 40 cc of sodium benzoate and 10 cc of hydrochloric acid to secure a second precipitate. This precipitate was filtered off and the filtrate again treated if this was considered necessary. The benzoic acid precipitates were mixed and added to a small volume of 80 per cent ethyl alcohol which dissolved both the insulin and benzoic acid. Certain inert materials, however, settled out and the alcoholic solution was filtered. The filtrate was concentrated to dryness *in vacuo* and the benzoic acid dissolved by treatment with ether. This solution was transferred to a separatory funnel and a small volume of water was added. The insulin was contained in the aqueous layer.

The introduction of the benzoic acid method of purification marked a distinct advance in the production of insulin. By this process the large amounts of alcohol necessary for the fractional precipitation of the proteins and the final precipitation of the insulin in the previous methods were avoided. Chemically, it gave a product which was much freer from protein material, as determined by the nitrogen content, than anything we had hitherto been able to obtain. Clinically, the toxic and indurating effects which characterized all the earlier extracts were greatly reduced. The main disadvantage which this process possessed was that the separation of the benzoic acid precipitates often required long and tedious filtration. However, the benzoic acid method has been a very important factor in the production of insulin over a considerable period of time. This is shown by the fact that approximately 250,000 units of insulin made by that method under our direction in this laboratory were used clincally in Toronto in the autumn of 1922, with very satisfactory results.

WATER EXTRACTS

In the past many attempts have been made to obtain the substance necessary for the utilization of carbohydrates in the body by watery extraction of the pancreas. Knowlton and Starling, as previously stated, prepared an extract from the pancreas by extracting the gland with acidulated cold water. Shortly after the original publication by the Toronto group, Sansum (personal communication) was able to obtain a small quantity of insulin by hot water extraction of beef pancreas. Because of the possible economic significance of a watery extraction of the pancreas in the manufacture of insulin, this method has been investigated in our laboratories. Some 150 experiments using different modifications in the extraction, such as varying the time, the temperature, the acidity, etc., have been carried out. While all these experiments are of interest, we will report only a few which have given the most promising results.

Two pounds of minced beef pancreas were added to 300 cc of distilled water which had been acidified with 4 cc of concentrated sulphuric acid. After 20 minutes, 1 litre of boiling water was added to the mixture, and the temperature raised to 80° C by a jet of live steam. This temperature was maintained for a period of 2 minutes. The mixture was then poured into a flask and cooled quickly by connecting the flask to a high vacuum pump. The cooled contents were filtered. An almost colourless filtrate was obtained. After the completion of the filtration which usually took about ½ hour, the glands were re-extracted with 1 litre of acidified water at room temperature for a period of 3 hours. The liquid was filtered off as in the first extraction. The insulin in the combined filtrates was purified either by the method elaborated by Banting, Best, Collip, and Macleod, or by the present method of purification used in our laboratories.

We were able to obtain equally satisfactory results by cold water extraction of the pancreatic glands. The method was as follows: 2 pounds of minced pancreas were added to 1,500 cc of distilled water which was acidified with 3.5 cc of concentrated sulphuric acid. The mixture, after extraction for 2 hours, was filtered through fluted filter paper. The filtrate was quite clear and had a pH of approximately 3.5. It is very essential that this pH be very close to the above value for two reasons. The acidity is outside the isoelectric range of many of the proteins in the pancreas, and at this hydrogen ion concentration there is obtained a mixture which filters readily and gives a clear filtrate. The glands were re-extracted with acidified water, as above, for 2 hours and the liquid filtered off as in the first extraction. The insulin in the combined filtrates may be purified by any of the methods described in this paper.

Under conditions as described above we were able to obtain fairly satisfactory yields of insulin (see p. 128). The results, however, though very encouraging, have not as yet shown nearly as great a unitage per pound of pancreas as that obtained by the alcohol or acetone method of extraction under the best experimental conditions.

THE METHOD OF DOISY, SOMOGYI, AND SHAFFER [259]

The investigators have described a method of purification of insulin, the salient new features of which were the precipitation of insulin from watery solution with half saturation of ammonium sulphate and the so-called isoelectric precipitation. Ammonium sulphate in one-half saturation had been previously used in these laboratories by Moloney. Full details of the isoelectric precipitation of insulin from watery solutions containing the active substance were communicated to us by Professor P. A. Shaffer and, almost immediately afterwards, by Dr. Clowes of Eli Lilly and Company. This method was evidently worked out independently in two laboratories at about the same time. We have profited by discussion of this method with Professor Shaffer and Dr. Clowes on several occasions. The experimental work in the research laboratories of Eli Lilly and Company was carried out by G. Walden under the direction of Dr. Clowes. The crude material, to which the "isoelectric" method of purification was applied, was obtained by different procedures by the two groups of investigators. It appears from experiments we have carried out that insulin can be removed from watery solution at various hydrogen ion concentrations by procedures which cause a precipitate to settle out. For example, the addition of copper sulphate to obtain a concentration of 1 per cent, in a solution of insulin at pH 3.7 causes separation of a precipitate which may contain much of the potent material. Similarly, if insulin is added to a solution of edestin and the hydrogen ion concentration adjusted to 6.89, the isoelectric point of this protein, a precipitate forms which may contain all the potency of the original solution.

THE PRESENT METHOD

In our present process we have employed various steps of many of these methods. The precipitation of insulin from alcoholic solution by the addition of ether was suggested to us by an experiment performed by H. W.

Dudley, in this laboratory. In this experiment Dudley demonstrated that the addition of an equal volume of ether to the alcohol used in the final precipitation of insulin in the procedure of Banting, Best, Collip, and Macleod, resulted in a much more efficient precipitation of the active principle than that obtained by the use of alcohol alone.

Fresh pancreatic glands from the ox are obtained from the abattoirs. After separating as much of the fat and connective tissue as possible the glands are placed in large containers which are collected every 3 hours and taken to the laboratory.

The glands are weighed. They are then run through a power meat chopper in which they are finely minced. This minced material is poured into large earthenware crocks which contain a weight of 95 per cent denatured alcohol (10 per cent methyl and the remainder ethyl), equal to that of the glands. The alcohol is acidified to 1.3 per cent with acetic acid. It is important that a high hydrogen ion concentration be secured at this stage. It inhibits the action of proteolytic enzymes and affects the proteins in such a way as to facilitate separation of the solid and liquid materials at a later stage of the process. Sulphuric acid may be used in place of acetic acid, but, if so, a more highly coloured filtrate is obtained. This colour is difficult to remove at a later stage. The minced glands are extracted for 3 hours in this acid alcohol solution. During this time they are slowly agitated in order to facilitate extraction. At the end of 3 hours this alcoholic mixture is poured into a rotary centrifuge to separate the alcoholic extract from solid materials. After the completion of the centrifuging the solid material remaining in the centrifuge is re-extracted for 3 hours with a volume of 60 per cent alcohol equal to that of the liquid removed after the first extraction. The alcoholic extract, after 3 hours, is separated by means of the centrifuge. The extracts from the first and second extractions are mixed, neutralized to litmus with sodium hydroxide, and chilled in a brine tank to 0° C (the chilling may be omitted). During the chilling the filtrate becomes turbid due to the separation of lipoid and protein materials. The mixture is filtered through large glass funnels which have been fitted with fluted filter papers. The alcoholic extract thus obtained is almost colourless. The filtrate which contains the active principle is concentrated to about one-twentieth of its original volume in an efficient vacuum still. During the distillation the temperature is not allowed to rise above 30° C. The reasons for this are as follows: excessive heat will coagulate much of the protein material. This is undesirable at this stage because some of the insulin would be adsorbed on the precipitated proteins. Excessive heat over the period required for the concentration produces highly coloured decomposition products which greatly increase the difficulty of purification of insulin. After the completion of the distillation the concentrate is quickly heated to 55° C. At this temperature lipoid and other materials rise to the surface and are readily skimmed off. This fatty mass which contains about one-quarter of the total potency of the concentrate is treated with sufficient ether to dissolve the lipoid material and is allowed to stand overnight. The ether is then removed and the residue made up to 80 per cent with denatured alcohol. This mixture is filtered through paper.

Ammonium sulphate is added to the liquid portion of the concentrate to secure half saturation (37 g per 100 cc). This mixture is stirred well and almost immediately protein material separates out and readily rises to the top of the liquid. After standing ½ hour the protein precipitate is skimmed off and allowed to drain on hardened filter paper for 3 to 6 hours. It is then added to sufficient 95 per cent alcohol to secure a final concentration of 75 to 80 per cent alcohol. The amount of alcohol added is usually very small, but varies with the amount of moisture held in the protein precipitate. Much of the protein material is precipitated by this concentration of alcohol and is removed by filtration. This filtrate is mixed with that obtained when the residue from the fatty mass (which was extracted with ether), is treated with 80 per cent alcohol, as described above. The active principle in these combined filtrates is precipitated by adding to them an equal volume of sulphuric ether. On standing overnight this precipitate settles to the bottom of the flask and the ether-alcohol solution is decanted. The precipitate is brought to dryness *in vacuo* and is then treated with dilute ammonium hydroxide of such a concentration that the pH of the resulting solution is approximately 8. At this pH the insulin is completely soluble. The hydrogen ion concentration is then adjusted to a pH of 3.5. At this hydrogen ion concentration a precipitate containing dark coloured material usually separates out. This is removed by filtration. The filtrate which is an aqueous extract containing the active principle may be pure enough for clinical use. However, it is advisable to purify it further either by the so called isoelectric precipitation [259], by Dudley's picrate method, or by the use of charcoal. This latter method of purification has been worked out by J. P. Moloney and D. M. Findlay in this laboratory and has been found very satisfactory [The details were not published until a year later [576].] The purified product is diluted with acidified water (pH 2.5) to the desired potency as estimated by the rabbit test.

After determining the strength of the insulin, 0.1 per cent tricresol is added, and the solution is passed through a Mandler filter. The insulin, after passing through the filter and before the vials are filled, is retested carefully to determine its potency. It is then diluted with sterile distilled water, pH 2.5, so that it contains 10 or 20 units per cubic centimetre. The method of standardizing insulin has been described elsewhere [275]. The tested insulin is poured into sterile glass vials with aseptic precautions, and the sterility of the final product thoroughly tested by approved methods.

YIELDS OF INSULIN

The unit of insulin has recently been defined in several communications. It is one-third the amount of material required to lower the blood sugar of a 2 kilo rabbit, which has been fasted 24 hours, from the normal level (0.118 per cent) to 0.045 per cent over a period of 5 hours.

The earlier extracts obtained from the degenerated pancreas of the dog, normal dog's pancreas, or the pancreatic tissue of foetal calves, were tested upon diabetic dogs. It is difficult, therefore, since the relative susceptibility of depancreatized dogs and normal rabbits to insulin has not been accurately determined, to quote definite figures in rabbit units for the yield of insulin originally obtained per gram of these tissues.

Pork pancreas has consistently given us somewhat larger yields in experimental lots than has beef pancreas. Beef glands are, however, somewhat easier to process, because they have adherent a smaller amount of fat. They have been used exclusively in this laboratory for the production of larger quantities of material.

During the early part of April 1922 the yield of insulin suitable for clinical use was approximately 15 units per kilo of pancreas. Later in the same month we were able to obtain about 40 units of purified material per kilo. Experimental lots at that time showed as high as 90 units of crude insulin per kilo. Our present procedure, as previously described, gives a yield of approximately 400 units of purified material per kilo. *The increase in acidity of the extractive has been the greatest single factor in improving the yields.*

The yields secured by watery extraction of the glands are extremely promising. The extraction with boiling water under the most favourable conditions gives a consistent yield of approximately 225 units per kilo. The results of extraction by cold, highly acidified water are even more interesting, at the present time, than those with hot water. Extracts obtained by these procedures are at present more difficult to purify than those obtained by alcoholic extraction.

The highest yields we have as yet obtained were secured from beef pancreas by alcoholic extraction. In several experiments (15 pounds of pancreas were used in each experiment) we have been able to obtain approximately 900 units of purified insulin per kilo of pancreas. In the preliminary experiments of this series, however, large volumes of extractive were used, and we are not certain as yet that the procedure will be practical. The material was purified in some cases by the benzoic acid method, and in others by the ammonium sulphate and isoelectric method. Recent results tend to show that the volume of the extractive may be greatly diminished without lowering the yield if certain precautions are observed. These experiments have been carried out with the assistance of W. J. Grant.

DISCUSSION

During the year 1922, those of us who were responsible for the preparation of insulin for clinical use had insufficient opportunities for the systematic investigation of the chemical properties of the material we were struggling to prepare for patients who were being treated by our clinical collaborators. Changes in the method of production were rapidly introduced, and in many cases were discarded after a brief trial. As our knowledge of the properties of the material has increased, improvements in the method have been introduced.

Alcohol was the extractive used by the original investigators in the University of Toronto in the preparation of insulin from beef pancreas. At many times in the past and especially very recently it has appeared that water would be a more economical solvent. To increase the number of units of insulin obtainable per kilo of pancreas or to introduce a cheaper extractive and thus to assist in lowering the cost of insulin is very desirable, but the question of yields must always be subsidiary to that of the purity of the product. In consideration of this latter point, we believe at the present time that alcohol is the most preferable extractive we have yet investigated.

The active interest of the members of the Department of Physiology, Biochemistry, and Pharmacology, in our work has been a very important factor in our progress. We have benefited by the suggestions of the representatives of the British Medical Research Council, who visited our laboratory. An ingenious method of purification evolved by Dudley [268] which has been extensively used in England, promises to be of use in the preparation of a dry powder. Insulin in this form seems to be very stable. The collaboration of the investigators mentioned in the body of this communication has been greatly appreciated. The research staff of Eli Lilly and Company has played a prominent part in the rapid development of efficient methods for large scale production.

It has been our intention to review the methods used in Toronto for the preparation of insulin, and not to discuss in detail the properties of this substance. However, certain obvious characteristics of the material are discernible from a study of the various procedures used in the preparation.

The stability of insulin is of particular interest and suggests that further research may result in a more highly purified product being obtained.

We regret that we have not had the opportunity to test thoroughly various procedures for the preparation and purification of insulin which have been developed by Professor T. Brailsford Robertson, and Professor A. B. Anderson of the University of Adelaide, Australia, and by Professor August Krogh of Copenhagen University, Denmark. The details of these procedures were communicated to Professor J. J. R. Macleod, and we are indebted to him for very promptly making them available to us.

ACKNOWLEDGMENTS

We wish to express our thanks to Dr. J. G. FitzGerald and Dr. R. D. Defries for their helpful criticism and energetic support.

It is a pleasure to acknowledge our indebtedness to Mr. A. S. Wall and Miss Jessie H. Ridout for their efficient assistance in our work.

AN ARTICLE BY BANTING AND MYSELF, "*The Discovery and Preparation of Insulin,*" *which was published in the University of Toronto Medical Journal in February 1924, was the last of our joint publications.*

After obtaining my M.A. in Physiology in 1922, I was busy with my medical course and my duties in the Connaught Laboratories. Fred Banting and I had many long talks during which we relived the wonderful, happy, and exhilarating times of that summer of 1921. I struggled, as I have ever since, to keep up with the literature on insulin. Banting submerged himself completely in other problems. He was anxious that I should become an Associate Professor in the Banting and Best Department of Medical Research immediately after obtaining my medical degree. This was a new department which came into being in the University of Toronto in 1923, and Banting was appointed the first professor. For several years it was housed temporarily on the ground floor of the old Pathology Building on University Avenue until more permanent quarters became available in the Banting Institute at 100 College Street. Professor V. E. Henderson offered me a comparable position in the Department of Pharmacology. These were attractive opportunities but I felt that H. H. Dale's laboratory in London would provide stimulation and broader training.

In the first Paper of this volume I have described the fortunate circumstances which gave me the opportunity in 1925 to work with Dr. Dale in the National Institute for Medical Research at Hampstead in London. I was most anxious to learn the physiological and biochemical techniques utilized in his investigations involving histamine and choline and I did work exclusively in these fields for the first few months. The opportunity to test the action of insulin in perfused isolated limbs and to help remove some of the confusion which then obscured this field was too tempting. Paper 10 describes the dramatic effect of the hormone on what was essentially a skeletal muscle preparation. The subsequent attempt with Dale, Hoet, and Marks to account for the complete effect of insulin on the eviscerated spinal preparation, has also been referred to in Paper 1. It would be interesting, using dextrose labelled with radioactive carbon, to determine whether appreciable formation of fat would be stimulated by insulin in the preparation which we used in 1926.

10. The Effect of Insulin on the Dextrose Consumption of Perfused Skeletal Muscle

CHARLES H. BEST*

The experiments of Hepburn and Latchford [385], which have been confirmed by Burn and Dale [157], show that insulin accelerates the rate of disappearance of dextrose from the fluid used to perfuse the isolated mammalian heart. Burn and Dale also demonstrated that insulin greatly increases the rate of disappearance of dextrose from the circulating blood of the decapitated and eviscerated cat. Cori, Cori, and Goltz [226], working on rabbits, and Lawrence [485] and Pemberton and Cunningham [615], from clinical studies, have reported that insulin increases the loss of sugar from the blood during its passage through a limb. Frank, Nothmann, and Wagner [308] have obtained similar results by analysis of blood samples drawn simultaneously from the femoral artery and vein, after the injection of insulin into the femoral artery. Macleod [539] states that, in experiments in his laboratory, no increased discrepancy between the dextrose content of the arterial and venous blood was observed after the administration of insulin in normal or diabetic animals.

Attempts to prove that insulin causes an increased disappearance of sugar from the fluid perfused through the isolated limbs of laboratory animals have been made by Macleod and his collaborators [539] and Staub [734]. Macleod states that his experiments were unsatisfactory because of oedema of the muscles or the development of marked resistance to the perfusion. Staub has reported experiments in which the rate of sugar disappearance, before and after the addition of insulin, from the defibrinated blood used to perfuse the hind limbs of the dog, are recorded. In some of Staub's experiments insulin appeared definitely to accelerate the sugar disappearance. Because of the very rapid disappearance of sugar from the blood before the addition of insulin, however, it is difficult to demonstrate

Originally appeared in the *Proceedings of the Royal Society*, B, XCIX (1926), 375–82. Communicated by Dr. H. H. Dale, Secretary, Royal Society. From the National Institute for Medical Research, London.
*Fellow of the International Health Board of the Rockefeller Foundation.

convincingly, by this type of experiment, that the rate of disappearance is really accelerated by insulin.

Since an efficient perfusion apparatus by which the perfusion fluid is circulated continuously was available in this laboratory, it was thought worth while to attempt to obtain more convincing evidence of the effect of insulin on the disappearance of sugar from fluid perfused through a skeletal muscle preparation. In the experiments reported in this paper defibrinated blood was perfused through the vessels of the hind limbs of the cat.

Methods

The sugar concentration of the blood was prevented from falling rapidly in the preliminary period by the addition of dextrose at a known rate. When insulin was added to the blood, the rate of this artificial addition of dextrose was usually increased, so as to mitigate the fall produced by insulin. Full particulars of the perfusion apparatus used in these experiments are given in a recent publication by Burn and Dale [157]. The following procedure by which the tissue was set up for perfusion is similar to that described by these investigators. The anaesthetized cat was bled from the aorta. About 40 cc of saline were run in through the jugular vein during the bleeding. After the death of the animal mass ligatures were applied at the level of the upper lumbar vertebrae. The hindquarters were then separated from the rest of the body by a transection just above the mass ligatures, and the spinal canal was firmly plugged with plasticine. Cannulae were placed in the aorta and the vena cava, and connections with the arterial and venous blood tubes of the perfusion apparatus were made.

In many of the experiments it was necessary to use the blood from two cats, since the perfusion apparatus was constructed for a volume of 225 cc. The blood was defibrinated by whipping and was then filtered through cotton wool. The blood flow through the limbs was kept as nearly constant as possible throughout the experiment. The burette of the slow infusion apparatus described by Burn and Dale [157] was connected by rubber tubing with a small glass tube, which was fitted in a hole bored in the top of the oxygenating chamber, so that 4 per cent dextrose was added at a known rate to the blood and completely mixed with it during oxygenation. In all the experiments the infusion of dextrose was started as soon as the perfusion was properly under way. Blood samples were taken every 20 minutes from the reservoir which receives the blood from the pump. As much blood as possible was kept in the reservoir during the experiment, so that these samples should be fairly representative of the whole volume of blood in circulation. The dextrose determinations were made by the

Shaffer-Hartmann method. Insulin was added to the blood by delivering the required quantity, dissolved in 0.25 to 0.5 cc of saline, into the funnel which received the blood from the venous cannula.

The values for the sugar disappearance were calculated from the sugar-infusion figures and the change in sugar concentration of the blood. In the calculations the volume was assumed to be the same as the volume of blood originally placed in the apparatus. During the experiment the blood was concentrated somewhat by evaporation of water during oxygenation and was diluted slightly by the fluid in which the sugar was added. The discrepancy between the volume of blood recovered from the apparatus, *plus* the amount used for analysis, *plus* or *minus* the gain or loss of weight of the perfused tissue on the one hand, and the amount of blood originally taken *plus* the volume of sugar solution added on the other hand, is accounted for by evaporation. This was tested in some experiments by haemoglobin estimations made at the beginning and end of the experiment, the loss of water calculated from these accounting satisfactorily for the missing volume.

EXPERIMENTAL RESULTS

The essential details of the experiments are recorded on the graphs. Only very brief protocols are therefore submitted.

Experiment 1 (Figure 21). Weight of tissue perfused was 1248 g. Volume of blood used in perfusion was 220 cc. Blood samples were taken every 20 minutes. The blood-sugar values were 0.210 per cent, 0.212 per cent, 0.223 per cent, 0.223 per cent (insulin 10 units), 0.220 per cent, 0.188 per cent, 0.168 per cent, 0.161 per cent, 0.146 per cent, 0.132 per cent, 0.119 per cent. The sugar infusion, as shown in Figure 21, was increased when insulin was added. At the end of the experiment 125 cc of blood were recovered from the apparatus. The perfused tissue increased in weight by 52 g. 34 cc of blood had been taken during the experiment for analysis. 41 cc of 4 per cent sugar solution were added to the blood during the experiment. Rate of blood flow before insulin, 2080 cc per hour; rate of blood flow in first hour after insulin, 2307 cc per hour. Temperature was 37–38° C.

Calculation shows that in the hour before insulin 376 milligrams of sugar disappeared, while in the first hour after insulin the disappearance was 643 milligrams.

Experiment 2 (Figure 22). Weight of tissue perfused was 652 g. The volume of the blood used was 270 cc. The sugar in the blood was estimated every 20 minutes. The values were as follows: at the beginning, 0.178 per cent, 0.174 per cent, 0.183 per cent, 0.178 per cent (insulin 15 units), 0.178 per cent, 0.196 per cent, 0.221 per cent, 0.219 per cent, 0.229 per cent, 0.224 per cent, 0.197 per cent, 0.210 per cent. Volume of blood recovered at the end of the experiment was 230 cc. Samples accounted for 26 cc. Weight of tissue at end of

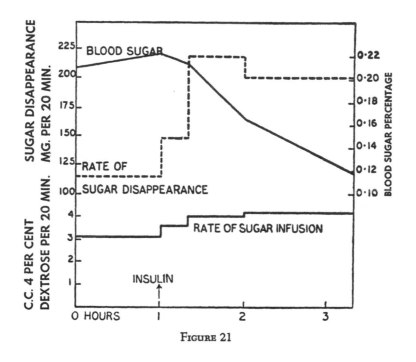

FIGURE 21

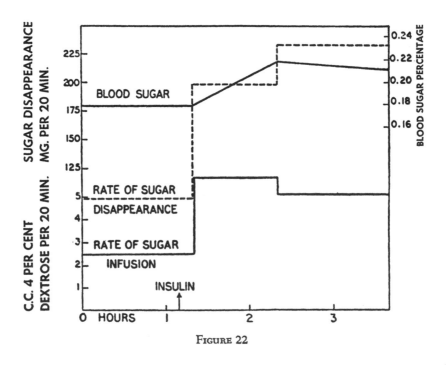

FIGURE 22

experiment was 642 g. 47.6 cc of sugar solution were added. Rate of blood flow before insulin, 2352 cc per hour; rate of blood flow in first hour after insulin, 2122 cc per hour. Temperature, 37–38° C.

In the hour before insulin was added to the blood 324 mg of sugar disappeared. After insulin 620 mg per hour disappeared.

Experiment 3 (Figure 23). Weight of tissue perfused was 782 g. 260 cc of defibrinated blood were used in the perfusion. The sugar values, determined at 20-minute intervals throughout the experiment, were 0.221 per cent, 0.238 per cent, 0.224 per cent, 0.232 per cent, 0.215 per cent (insulin 15 units), 0.210

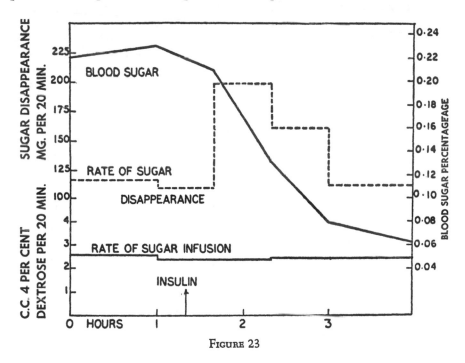

FIGURE 23

per cent, 0.173 per cent, 0.133 per cent, 0.118 per cent, 0.080 per cent, 0.070 per cent, 0.060 per cent, 0.062 per cent. 150 cc of blood were recovered from the apparatus (samples accounted for 36 cc). 29 cc of 4 per cent sugar solution were infused. Weight of tissue at end of experiment was 835 g. Rate of blood flow before insulin, 2396 cc per hour; rate of blood flow in the first hour after insulin, 2374 cc per hour.

Sugar disappearance before insulin was 325.6 mg per hour. In the first hour after insulin the disappearance was 530 mg.

Experiment 4. Weight of tissue perfused was 906 g. Volume of blood used in the perfusion was 250 cc. Sugar was infused at the rate of 4.8 mg per minute. The sugar concentration of the blood remained steady at 0.20 per cent for the first three 20-minute intervals. The sugar infusion was then stopped and the tissue was eliminated from the circulation. The sugar determinations for the next four 20-minute periods were 0.20 per cent, 0.20 per cent, 0.20 per cent,

0.19 per cent. Fifteen units of insulin were then added to the circulating blood. The next three sugar values were 0.19 per cent, 0.18 per cent, 0.18 per cent. Blood recovered from the apparatus was 160 cc. Weight of tissue at end of experiment was 932 g. 8.5 cc of sugar solution were infused. 28 cc of blood were used for sampling.

This experiment shows that there is little or no disappearance of sugar from the blood, either before or after the addition of insulin, when the tissue is eliminated from the circulation.

Experiment 5 (Figure 24). Weight of tissue perfused was 1212 g. Volume of blood was 220 cc. The blood sugar was determined at twenty-minute intervals. The first three values were 0.220 per cent, 0.210 per cent, 0.204 per cent. 15 units of insulin were then added. The next three sugar values were 0.169 per cent, 0.124 per cent, 0.083 per cent. The sugar infusion was then stopped, and the tissue was eliminated from the circulation. The next four sugar values were 0.092 per cent, 0.087 per cent, 0.080 per cent, 0.076 per cent. The slight

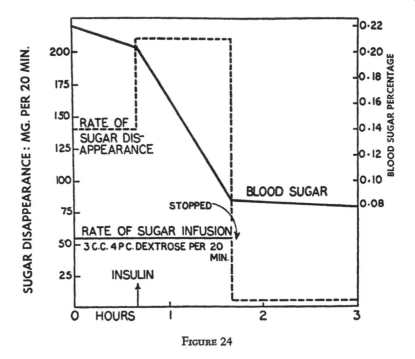

FIGURE 24

rise in sugar concentration was probably due to the fact that the last bit of infused sugar was not mixed with the blood at the time the 0.083 per cent sample was taken. Rate of blood flow before insulin 2280 cc per hour. Rate of blood flow after insulin 2800 cc per hour. One hour and 40 minutes after the beginning of the experiment the perfusion through the limbs and addition of sugar were stopped. The warm blood was pumped through the apparatus during the remainder of the experiment. Temperature throughout experiment was 37–38° C.

This experiment is the same as the preceding, except that insulin was added before the tissue was excluded from the circulation. The results are the same as in Experiment 4.

DISCUSSION

Burn and Dale used a preparation consisting of heart, lungs, skeleton, skin, and muscles. They showed that removal of the skin did not affect the result. In the experiments here described, the heart and lungs have been replaced by a mechanical system, so that it is safe to attribute the effects observed chiefly, if not entirely, to the metabolic activity of the skeletal muscles. Under these conditions, the rate of sugar disappearance from the blood is very rapid, even before the addition of insulin. It is much more rapid, per gram of muscle, than that from the blood of the decapitated and eviscerated cat before insulin is administered. The extent to which the liver, although cut off from direct circulation, contributes sugar by diffusion to the eviscerated preparation is not known. Slightly more sugar, therefore, than would appear from the determinations may disappear from the blood of Burn's and Dale's preparation. On the other hand, the sugar disappearance before insulin in the experiments reported in this paper might be slower if loss of CO_2 from the blood were prevented. Glycolysis by the blood itself, however, is insignificant in the defibrinated blood which has passed through cotton wool, and plays no appreciable part in the observed disappearance of the sugar. In all the experiments carried out in this investigation, the acceleration of sugar disappearance after the addition of insulin was perfectly definite.

SUMMARY

Insulin greatly accelerates the rate of sugar disappearance from defibrinated blood used to perfuse the isolated limbs of the cat. The action is attributable to an effect on the metabolism of the skeletal muscles.

ACKNOWLEDGMENT

The author gratefully acknowledges the kindly criticism and help of Dr. H. H. Dale in the planning and execution of the experiments reported in this paper.

11. The Fate of the Sugar Disappearing under the Action of Insulin

C. H. BEST*

J. P. HOET*

H. P. MARKS

The apparent disappearance of sugar injected into normal animals has for a long time puzzled physiological investigators (Bang, Meltzer and Kleiner, Palmer, Woodyatt). When insulin was discovered it was apparent that an agent was available by which the normal processes could be exaggerated, and therefore more easily studied. It was soon shown that the administration of sugar and insulin to the diabetic animal resulted in an increased combustion of carbohydrate and the accumulation of glycogen in the depôts. When, however, attempts were made to trace the fate of the sugar which disappears from the blood of the normal animal under the influence of an injection of insulin, difficulties were encountered.

McCormick and Macleod [526] studied the effect of insulin on the glycogen reserves of rabbits which had been starved and treated with epinephrine. In some of the experiments glucose was administered subcutaneously during the period of action of insulin. No significant difference between the glycogen content of the muscles of the control animals and of those which received insulin was observed. The glycogen of the livers of the insulin-treated animals was slightly less than that of the control animals. Campbell and Macleod [169] concluded from these experiments "that less glycogen is deposited both in the muscles and the liver when insulin is given along with sugar to previously starved animals than when the same amounts of sugar are given alone." In the experiments of Dudley and Marrian [270], in which the effect of insulin on the liver glycogen of mice was studied, a much smaller amount of glycogen was found in the livers of the animals which received insulin than in those which served for controls. In another series of experiments in which insulin was administered

Originally appeared in the *Proceedings of the Royal Society*, B, C (1926), 32–54. Communicated by Dr. H. H. Dale, Secretary, Royal Society. From the National Institute for Medical Research, Hampstead, London.
*Fellow of the Rockefeller Foundation.

to rabbits which had been previously fed on a carbohydrate-rich diet, the glycogen content of the liver and skeletal muscles of the insulin-treated animals was again much less than that of the control animals. In both series of experiments the animals were killed after convulsions had supervened. The experiments of Babkin [31] are similar to those of McCormick and Macleod. In some of his experiments Babkin kept the blood sugar of the rabbits at a high level by the administration of sugar. He found no increase in glycogen after insulin. Kuhn and Baur [475], in a study of the effect of insulin on the glycogen content of the skeletal muscles of rabbits and guinea-pigs, found that, after insulin convulsions, the glycogen had practically disappeared from the muscles of these animals. They are undecided as to whether the depletion of glycogen is a primary effect of insulin or is to be attributed to the convulsions.

Other investigators believe that the glycogen content of the animal body is increased under the action of insulin. Bickel and Collazo [123] found that the glycogen content of the livers of pigeons, fed on a diet deficient in vitamin B, was increased in those which received insulin. They obtained similar [206], but not very conclusive, results in normal guinea-pigs. Convulsions were carefully avoided in these experiments. Bissinger, Lesser, and Zipf [126], in a study of the effect of insulin on the carbohydrate balance of mice, determined the glycogen content of starved mice, of mice injected with dextrose only, and of mice which received dextrose and insulin. They found that approximately one-third of the sugar which disappeared could be recovered as glycogen. In a more recent paper Bissinger and Lesser [125] have shown that one-half hour after the injection of insulin about one-fifth of the sugar is deposited as glycogen. Cori, Cori, and Pucher [227] have reported that insulin causes an increase in the liver glycogen of normal rabbits when the free sugar of the liver is as low as in a starving animal. Ringer [645], using phloridzinized dogs, found that 40 per cent of the sugar which was metabolized by these animals as the result of an injection of insulin was burned. He assumed that the remainder was laid down as glycogen. Cori [221] has shown that there is an increase in the glycogen of the liver of phloridzinized rabbits and cats when insulin is administered. He has found [222], however, that the liver glycogen of mice is decreased by insulin, even when convulsions are avoided.

The conclusion, that the sugar which disappears from normal animals under the action of insulin is not laid down as glycogen, has been accepted by many investigators, and numerous theories have been advanced to explain this disappearance. One of the most interesting hypotheses is that there is an increase in lactacidogen (Embden) sufficient to account for a large part of the sugar. [Lactacidogen is an obsolete term for an unidentified precursor of lactic acid. At various times it was suspected that it was one of the hexose phosphoric esters, creatine phosphate, or the phosphoric ester of enol-pyruvic acid.] Harrop and Benedict [363], using unanaesthetized animals, compared the lactacidogen content of a muscle removed before insulin with that of the corresponding muscle of the opposite side removed some time after insulin. They believe that they have demonstrated an increase in lactacidogen after insulin. (See also Audova and Wagner [30].) Kay and Robison [442], who have reviewed the literature which deals with the relation of phosphorus to carbohydrate metabolism, also obtained results which convinced them that the lactacidogen of the muscle is increased under the action of insulin. Eadie, Macleod, and Noble [276] have been unable to confirm these findings. Many of the other theories which have been advanced to explain the rapid disappearance of the sugar from the blood have been disproved, while others, which might account for a stage in this process, could not be expected, nor were some of them intended, to explain the ultimate fate of the sugar.

The experiments of Burn and Dale [157] on the eviscerated spinal cat show that the increase in oxygen consumption after the administration of insulin is usually insufficient to account for more than a small part of the sugar which disappears from the blood of this preparation. Our experiments, which may be regarded as an extension of the work of these investigators, are designed to investigate the fate of this sugar which is not burned. Attention was first concentrated on lactacidogen. The change in muscle glycogen attributable to insulin was then investigated.

METHODS

Choice of a Preparation

In many of the experiments which have been mentioned above a series of animals have been used as controls for a second series to which insulin has been administered. The glycogen content of the tissues of the control animals, however, varies within such wide limits that an almost prohibitive number of animals must be used before valid conclusions as to the effect of insulin can be drawn. In studies in which normal rabbits or mice have been used convulsions have frequently occurred in spite of the administration of dextrose. Furthermore, in many experiments in which the intact animal is used, it is not certain that sufficient sugar disappears from the blood, in excess of what may be burned or excreted, to give a detectable increase in glycogen, if this substance were formed. Variations in the interval between the cessation of circulation with the death of the animal and the fixation of the tissues for estimation of this glycogen are difficult to eliminate in experiments on the intact animal. The eviscerated spinal preparation (Burn and Dale) is particularly well adapted to an investigation of this kind. Dextrose is infused at any desired rate into the jugular vein by means of the slow infusion apparatus of these authors. The blood sugar can be kept approximately at any desired level. Convulsions are avoided. The glycogen content of an individual muscle of one leg has been shown to be practically the same as the content of the corresponding muscle of the opposite leg [618]. We have taken advantage of this fact to determine the effect of insulin on the glycogen content of the muscles of this preparation. To obtain the muscles, the skin is removed and each muscle in turn is dissected free from its sheath. Ligatures are placed around the extremities of the muscle. When everything is ready the ligatures are tied; the muscle is removed and immediately dropped into hot alkali.

Methods Used in the Analysis of Tissues

The blood sugar was estimated in the early experiments by the Shaffer-Hartmann method. In the later experiments the Hagedorn-Jensen technique was used. The latter method is much the more suitable for use with the eviscerated spinal preparation, since the small samples of blood required (0.2 to 0.3 cc) can be taken frequently without affecting the blood pressure. Inorganic phosphorus was estimated by the Briggs modification of the Bell-Doisy method. Glycogen was estimated by Pflüger's method. The sugar formed by the acid hydrolysis of the glycogen was determined by a modification of the Bertrand method. Five cc amounts of the sugar solution, copper reagent, and alkali were used, instead of 20 cc as recommended in Bertrand's paper. The solutions were heated together for ten minutes in the boiling water-bath, instead of being boiled for three minutes over the flame. Bertrand's permanganate solution was diluted five times. The use of smaller quantities of sugar solutions made duplicate determinations possible. Embden's technique, except that trichloracetic acid was used instead of Schenck's reagent to precipitate the proteins, was followed in the lactacidogen determinations.

EXPERIMENTAL RESULTS

I. Phosphate Metabolism

Inorganic phosphorus. The decrease produced by insulin in the inorganic phosphorus of the blood of normal animals has been observed by many investigators. In the first series of experiments reported in this paper the effect of insulin on the inorganic phosphorus of the blood of the eviscerated spinal preparation has been studied.

Three control experiments showed that the inorganic phosphorus of the blood of the eviscerated spinal preparation remains fairly steady when the blood sugar level is kept constant by the infusion of sugar. [The protocols of these experiments have been omitted.]

Insulin experiments

Experiment 4. Cat, 3.7 kg. Eviscerated spinal preparation. Sugar infused at the rate of 150 mg per hour.

Time	0	45 min.	55 min.	1 hr. 20 min.	2 hrs. 50 min.	3 hrs. 10 min.
Blood sugar percentage	0.237	0.242	Insulin 5 units	0.166	0.063	0.053
Inorganic phosphorus of whole blood	6.3	6.4		5.3	4.2	3.9

Experiment 5. The details of this experiment are shown in Figure 25. The rate of sugar infusion was increased slightly after the administration of insulin so as to diminish the rate and extent of fall of the blood sugar.

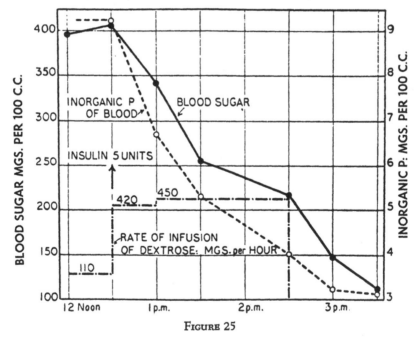

FIGURE 25

Experiment 6 (Figure 26). In this experiment the rate of sugar infusion was increased when insulin was given and there was no fall in blood sugar.

These experiments show that insulin produces a decrease in the inorganic phosphorus of the blood of the eviscerated spinal preparation, and that when the blood sugar is prevented from falling by accelerating the infusion of dextrose, the fall in blood phosphate persists. The change in blood phosphate is, therefore, related to the disappearance of sugar and not to the fall in sugar concentration in the blood. In this preparation it is improbable that the blood receives phosphorus from any source, and we may assume that the phosphorus disappearing from the blood goes to the muscles. The effect of this additional inorganic phosphorus on the concentration of this substance in the muscles may be seen from the following calculation. The muscles of a cat weighing 3.0 kg weigh about 1.5 kg. The active volume

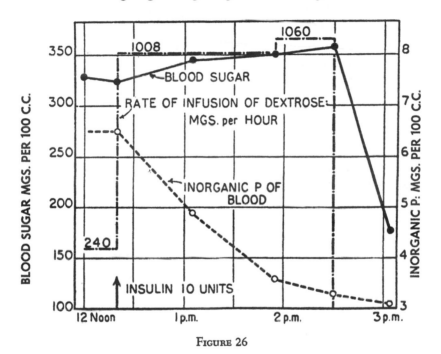

FIGURE 26

of the body fluids of the eviscerated spinal preparation made from this animal may be estimated as 500 cc (Burn and Dale). This "active volume" has been used in calculations throughout this paper. If the inorganic phosphorus of the blood decreases by 6 mg per 100 cc, 30 mg of phosphorus have been distributed to the muscles, if our assumptions are correct. Thirty mg of phosphorus spread over 1,500 g of muscle would give an increase of inorganic phosphorus of approximately 2 mg per 100 g of muscle. The change would be within the range of error of the methods used in the estimation of the phosphorus. This calculation takes no account of the effect which variations in the other forms of phosphorus of the blood might have on the inorganic portion. There appears, however, to be very little change in these other compounds (Kay and Robison). [Two paragraphs of text and a large table dealing with the effect of insulin on the lactacidogen content of skeletal muscle have been eliminated. The figures appear to indicate that there is a slight increase in that part of the combined phosphoric acid which is referred to as the lactacidogen of Embden. The differences, however, are so small that even their reality is doubtful.]

We can safely conclude that no significant proportion of the sugar which disappeared from the muscles is stored as a phosphoric ester. It had been shown that the removal of sugar from the circulation of the eviscerated spinal preparation is associated with a disappearance of free phosphate, and thus it appeared that phosphoric esters play a part in the phenomenon. It seemed clear, therefore, that they could only function as a stage on the way to the true storage form.

II. *Glycogen*

The second part of our investigation consists in a study of the variation in the glycogen content of the skeletal muscles when insulin and sugar are administered to the eviscerated spinal preparation. A series of control experiments are recorded first. The great variation in the glycogen content of the different muscles of the same animal, and in similar muscles of different animals, is well demonstrated. The contents of the corresponding muscles of the two hind limbs, however, agree rather closely under the conditions of these control experiments. Although in some cases there is a difference of 20 per cent between the glycogen contents of two corresponding muscles, the difference between the average values for several corresponding muscles of the two sides is small. The small differences between the glycogen figures for corresponding muscles are probably due, in part, to the unavoidable variations in the technique of removal.

1. *Control experiments.* [Protocols of one control experiment have been omitted.]

TABLE 11.I
GLYCOGEN IN SKELETAL MUSCLE

	Right (%)	Left (%)
Gastrocnemius	0.337	0.385
Tibialis	0.338	0.421
Sartorius	0.433	0.401
Biceps	0.302	0.325
Rectus femoris	0.479	0.440
	Av. 0.378	Av. 0.394

Experiment 8 (II). Cat, 3 kg. Eviscerated spinal preparation. Muscles of right side taken first, left side 20 min later. (See Table 11.I.)

In Experiments 9, 10, and 11 muscles were taken in the same way from eviscerated spinal cats subjected to constant intravenous infusion of dextrose, at rates of 400–500 mg per hour. The muscles of the right leg were taken early in each experiment, those of the left leg after 1 hr, 15 min, 2 hrs, 30 min, and 5 hrs respectively in the three experiments. The percentage of dextrose in the blood rose from 0.276 to 0.302 in Experiment 9, from 0.354 to 0.398 in Experiment 10, and from 0.294 to 0.430 in Experiment 11, during these periods. The muscles were therefore exposed to progressive hyperglycaemia of 0.3 to 0.4 per cent for these different periods, and furnish good controls for those from the later experiments, in which sugar was given with insulin. The averages of their glycogen contents were as given in Table 11.II. It will be seen that the maximum difference, 0.031 per cent,

TABLE 11.II

GLYCOGEN IN SKELETAL MUSCLE AFTER INTRAVENOUS INFUSION OF DEXTROSE

	Right	Left	Difference
Experiment 9	0.257	0.261	0.004
" 10	0.589	0.598	0.009
" 11	0.388	0.419	0.031

is so small as to have doubtful significance. The maximum difference between individual muscles was 0.086 per cent. These experiments confirm the statements of Külz [618], of Hatcher and Wolf [378], and of others, that isolated mammalian muscles do not form glycogen when perfused with blood rich in dextrose.

[Three-and-one-half pages of the original paper have been omitted; these give protocols of Experiments 12 to 17 and five tables of data.]

2. *Insulin experiments.* In Experiments 12–17 insulin was administered and the rate of sugar infusion was increased in an attempt to maintain a hyperglycaemia comparable to that which was present in the control experiments. The initial dose of insulin in these experiments was 12 units. This dose was repeated at the end of each 90 minutes during the "insulin period."

The results of the foregoing insulin experiments are summarized in Table 11.III. The results show that, in the preparation used in these experiments, when plenty of dextrose is supplied, insulin will cause the deposition of a large proportion, about 45 per cent on an average, as glycogen in the skeletal muscles.

The conditions of the experiments hitherto described practically limited the action of insulin to the muscles, as the only tissues remaining which

TABLE 11.III

INSULIN EXPERIMENTS

No. of Experiment	Duration hrs min		Sugar Disappearing (g)	Glycogen Found (g)	Sugar Not Recovered as Glycogen (g)
12	2	40	4.5	1.9	2.6
13	5	30	8.3	4.7	3.6
14	3	40	5.3	2.9	2.4
15	5	45	9.2	2.8	6.4
16	3	30	5.7	4.3	1.4
				(one muscle)	
Average (without Expt. 16)			6.8	3.1	3.7

In our more recent experiments we have found that several important sources of carbohydrate are not considered in these estimates. It has been found that, although the vessels carrying blood to the liver are tied, an appreciable quantity of dextrose enters the blood from this source during the experiment. Therefore more sugar is used than our calculations indicate, and the figure for sugar disappearance is too low.

In some more recent experiments the oxygen consumption has also been measured. The figures show that the sugar which disappears, and is not deposited as glycogen, is fully accounted for by the oxygen consumption, as will be shown in a forthcoming paper.

had an important carbohydrate metabolism. It was thought desirable to make further experiments, using the intact animal, and securing immobilization by chemical anaesthesia in place of destruction of the brain. Among anaesthetics available for this purpose, that known as "Amytal" appeared, from the experience of others, to be the most desirable. We made a few experiments with "Amytal" (kindly placed at our disposal by Messrs. Eli Lilly and Company), but we found that even this anaesthetic introduced complications which rendered it unsuitable for our purpose. Under "Amytal" alone the muscles lost glycogen, and a dose of insulin, which reduced the blood sugar to 0.07 per cent, did not prevent this loss. In order, therefore, to include the liver in the range of observation, but to leave the conditions otherwise as in the previous experiments, we made a few experiments on the animal with the brain destroyed, but the abdominal viscera left intact (Experiments 18, 19, and 20).

In Experiment 18 no analysis of the liver was made. During the 4 hrs and 15 min of the insulin period, in which 30 units in all were given, 4.42 g of dextrose were infused, and the blood sugar fell from 0.387 to 0.282 per cent. The average percentage of muscle glycogen increased in the same period from 0.856 to 1.120, i.e., by 0.264 per cent.

In Experiment 19, samples of liver as well as of the muscles were taken just before insulin was first administered, and again at the end of the experiment. In the 4 hours of insulin action 4.57 g of dextrose were infused, and the blood sugar fell from 0.440 to 0.220 per cent. The muscle glycogen increased from 0.930 to 1.142, i.e., by 0.212 per cent, and the liver glycogen from 2.245 to 2.83, i.e., by 0.585 per cent. Such an increase in the liver glycogen would contribute but little to the total gain of glycogen by the preparation, since the weight of the liver was probably not more than 1/15 of that of the muscles.

In Experiment 20, with the idea that the liver might take a greater part in the glycogen formation if the insulin reached it first, both dextrose and insulin were administered, in mixed solution, by infusion into the splenic vein, so that both passed through the liver before reaching the general circulation. The urine excreted in the insulin period was also collected and analysed. The action of insulin lasted for 3 hours, during which 3.036 g of dextrose and 25 units of insulin were infused. Two samples of liver were taken before insulin, and two at the end of the experiment. The blood sugar fell from 0.500 to 0.375 per cent. The urine secreted during the period contained 0.636 g of dextrose. The muscle glycogen increased from 0.935 to 1.297, i.e., by 0.362 g of dextrose. The liver glycogen, however, fell from 6.86 to 2.63 per cent, i.e., by 4.23 per cent, giving extra dextrose to be accounted for, instead of an addition to the glycogen yield.

Weight of cat	3 kg
Weight of liver	100 g
	g
Dextrose from liver	4.23
Dextrose infused	3.036
Blood sugar fell 0.125 per cent, 0.125 $\times$ 5	0.625
	7.891
Dextrose excreted in urine	0.636
Dextrose to be accounted for	7.255
Glycogen increase in muscles, 0.362 $\times$ 15	5.43
	g
Sugar to be accounted for	7.891
Sugar excreted	0.636
Sugar disappearing	7.255
Sugar found as glycogen in the muscles, 0.362 $\times$ 14.8 =	5.36

It will be seen that the increase in liver glycogen in Experiment 19 was relatively very small, and that in Experiment 20, made with the intention of concentrating the insulin effect on the liver as far as possible, there was actually a large loss of glycogen from that organ. It may be doubted, however, whether the conditions of the experiment entitle us to conclude that the liver, under completely physiological conditions, does not participate in the immediate formation of glycogen from glucose under insulin. The experiments are useful, however, as showing that the deposition in the muscles is not an artificial result of the exclusion of other organs. With the abdominal viscera intact, it occurs at least as rapidly as when they have been removed. As we were interested in the fate of the sugar, rather than the effect attributable to natural as distinguished from artificially injected insulin, experiments with infusion of dextrose alone, with intact viscera, were not made.

The effect of hypoglycaemia upon muscle glycogen. It has been suggested by several investigators that when insulin is administered to an animal which has only a small amount of available carbohydrate, the glycogen of the muscle is given up to form some unknown sugar compound. Bollman, Mann, and Magath [137] have recently shown, however, that in hepatectomized dogs the muscle glycogen is not drawn upon to maintain the normal blood sugar level. To investigate the effect of simple hypoglycaemia upon the muscle glycogen of the eviscerated spinal preparation, experiments were performed in which a small amount of sugar, or no sugar at all, was infused. [Two pages of the original paper, describing Experiments 20 to 25, have been omitted.]

The figures for muscle glycogen show a decrease so small as to be of doubtful significance. Practically it may be said that the muscle glycogen is unchanged. The results of the earlier experiments make it probable that, in the preliminary stages of these, when sugar was disappearing rapidly under insulin, there may have been a corresponding small deposition of glycogen, and that this may have been followed by a secondary return to slightly below the original value, to meet the metabolic need of the tissues, raised by the occurrence of some convulsions. However that may be, it is clear that, under these conditions, doses of insulin greatly excessive in relation to the sugar available, and maintaining a severe hypoglycaemia for several hours, do not cause a significant depletion of the glycogen store, or a large conversion of carbohydrate into unidentified forms.

The effect of convulsions on the glycogen content of the skeletal muscles. In many of the investigations from which the conclusion has been drawn that the glycogen of the skeletal muscles is depleted by the administration of insulin, the possible effect of the hypoglycaemic convulsions has not been eliminated. We therefore made a series of experiments in which lethal doses of insulin were administered to rabbits in which one sciatic nerve had been cut, under ether anaesthesia, a few days previously. (These operations were performed for us by Dr. Dale.) The animals died after periods of varying length, in which violent convulsions alternated with intervals of, at first, partial recovery, and later coma. Immediately after death the tibialis and gastrocnemius muscles of the denervated and normal sides were removed and analysed for glycogen. The muscles of the normal side were removed first. The results are shown in Table 11.IV.

TABLE 11.IV
MUSCLE GLYCOGEN AFTER VIOLENT CONTRACTIONS OF INSULIN CONVULSIONS

Rabbit	Amount of Insulin	Interval between Injection of Insulin and Time of Death	Glycogen Percentage			
			Normal side		Denervated side	
			tibialis	gastroc.	tibialis	gastroc.
No. 1	20 units	7 hrs	<0.01	0.025	0.732	0.392
" 2	20 "	11 "	0.161	0.274	0.445	0.457
" 3	10 "	3 "	<0.01	0.180	0.755	0.640
" 4	10 "	6½ "	<0.01	0.025	0.305	0.355
" 5	10 "	8 "†	0.171	0.040	0.760	0.563

†Animal killed.

To show that denervation of itself will not produce any corresponding contrast, one sciatic was cut under ether in each of two rabbits, which were kept for 3 days under the same conditions as the insulin rabbits, and then killed, no. 1 by a blow on the neck, no. 2 by coal gas. The glycogen analyses are shown in Table 11.V.

TABLE 11.V
CONTROL RABBITS

Rabbit No.	Muscle	Normal	Denervated
1	gastrocnemius	0.477	0.473
2	gastrocnemius	0.445	0.466
	Tibialis anterior	0.497	0.491
	Av.	0.473	0.476

These results demonstrate very convincingly that insulin convulsions play a very important role in the depletion of the muscle glycogen. In the denervated muscles, which participated only passively in the convulsions, the glycogen content was within normal limits in spite of the prolonged hypoglycaemia.

DISCUSSION

The puzzle presented by the action of insulin has been of the following kind. In the diabetic animal insulin revives the missing function of storing carbohydrate in the form of glycogen; in the normal animal, on the other hand, most of the available evidence seemed to indicate that, so far from promoting such storage, insulin caused the disappearance from the body of glycogen already present. With the exceptions mentioned in the introduction, no observer had been able to detect storage of glycogen, even as a preliminary phase in the effect of a large dose of insulin on the normal animal. The prevalent view, accordingly, was that the carbohydrate, disappearing from the circulation and from the glycogen stores of the normal animal treated with excess of insulin, must be deposited in the body in some other form, in which it was temporarily withdrawn from oxidative metabolism. On that view it would be necessary to suppose either that the deposition of glycogen in the diabetic under insulin is a relatively late result of the action, and does not represent the immediate effect of insulin on the carbohydrate metabolism, or else that the action of insulin in the diabetic organism, where the sugar available is large in proportion to the insulin, is qualitatively different from its action on the normal animal, where insulin is in excess in relation to the available sugar.

The first of these two possibilities our experiments may be said to have settled. The accelerated combustion of dextrose and synthesis of a further quantity to glycogen, seen in the diabetic subject, represent its immediate effects. The changes in blood phosphate suggest that the sugar becomes a phosphoric ester in a stage in the synthesis, but there is no significant storage in that form, and the sugar lost from circulation, and not oxidized, can apparently be found as glycogen in the muscles. The evidence for the oxidation of what is not stored as glycogen will be presented in a later paper. The demonstration of glycogen formation has been made possible by the nature of our experiments. The use of the spinal preparation has eliminated the complications due to convulsions, and when the preparation has also been eviscerated the problem has been reduced to its simplest terms, since the dextrose to be accounted for has been, in addition to that originally present in the body, the accurately measured amount infused. The observation that, while the muscles of different animals and even different muscles of the same animal vary widely in their glycogen load, that of corresponding muscles from the two sides of the same animal is always practically identical, gave us an accuracy of control which no method of observation can afford, in which one animal, or one set of animals, is used as control for another.

Lest it should be supposed that, by using eviscerated preparations, we were dealing only with the conditions presented by the diabetic animal, and that our results are therefore not applicable to the normal one, it should be noted that in spinal preparations not eviscerated we have obtained essentially the same results. The one point which our experiments do not make clear is the part played by the liver, under normal conditions, in the immediate storage of dextrose as glycogen in response to insulin. Our experiments, at their face value, would seem to indicate that the liver takes little part in this primary effect; indeed, in the one case in which an attempt was made to concentrate the action on the liver, by allowing the dextrose and insulin to pass through this organ on their way to the general circulation, the net result was a loss of a large amount of glycogen from the liver, and its deposition as glycogen in the muscles. We think it may fairly be argued, however, that the conditions of our experiment are unphysiological, in exposing the liver to persistent splanchnic stimulation, and that the results are no more indicative of its true function than the many failures to demonstrate storage of glycogen under insulin action in livers artificially perfused. It is still an open possibility that the storage of glycogen in the liver of the diabetic animal under insulin is a later and indirect effect; but our experiments cannot be held to prove the point. The one point which they appear definitely to establish is the immediate storage in the muscles, as glycogen, of sugar removed from the circulation by the action of insulin, either in the eviscerated preparation, or in that which is still normal to the extent that the pancreas and liver are intact. We agree with Lesser and his co-workers, therefore, whose results on whole mice have led them also to the conclusion that the removal of circulating dextrose by insulin in the normal, as in the diabetic organism, is produced by the oxidation of some and the synthesis to glycogen of the remainder.

In order to obtain a clearly recognizable increase of glycogen in the muscles, it was necessary to infuse abundance of dextrose to meet the insulin, and thereby to prevent any serious depression of the blood sugar below the normal level. But our experiments were not all of this kind. Even when the blood sugar was allowed to fall, under insulin, to a very low level, and to remain there for a long period, the glycogen of the muscles was not perceptibly depleted. When the sugar available was insufficient to produce a definite increase, the glycogen remained practically unaltered. Under the conditions of our experiments, therefore, with the animal immobilised by destruction of the brain, insulin even in large excess does not cause glycogen to be removed from the muscles and stored in another form. It must be supposed, therefore, that the disappearance in the normal animal is not due to a direct action of insulin, but to a call on the carbohydrate reserves by the metabolic requirements of the normally active organism, greatly intensified, as we have shown, by convulsions when they occur. The full discussion, however, of the relation of the effects here recorded to those observed in the normal, intact animal, may be deferred to a later paper, for which more complete data will be available.

SUMMARY AND CONCLUSIONS

(1) The disappearance under insulin of inorganic phosphate from the blood of the eviscerated spinal preparation is related to the disappearance

of sugar, and not to the fall in sugar concentration in the blood. (2) No significant portion of the sugar which disappears from the blood of this preparation, under the influence of insulin, is stored in the muscles as a phosphoric ester. (3) When an abundance of sugar is available, a large proportion of the sugar which disappears from the blood of the spinal cat is deposited as glycogen in the skeletal muscles of the animal. (4) Insulin hypoglycaemia, lasting for from one to three hours, does not appreciably lower the glycogen content of the resting skeletal muscles of the spinal cat. (5) The decrease or complete disappearance of the muscle glycogen of normal rabbits, produced by large doses of insulin, is chiefly due to the convulsions.

ACKNOWLEDGMENT

It is a pleasure to acknowledge the active direction and kindly criticism of Dr. H. H. Dale throughout this investigation.

12. Oxidation and Storage of Glucose under the Action of Insulin

C. H. BEST

H. H. DALE*

J. P. HOET

H. P. MARKS

Experiments published by three of us (B., H., and M.) [92] have demonstrated that, in a spinal animal with the muscles at rest, a large part of the glucose disappearing from the circulation under the action of insulin is deposited as glycogen in the muscles. The view that the remainder, which was in most cases the larger, and in some cases the much larger part, had been oxidized, was quite compatible with the observations of Burn and Dale [157], who had measured the oxygen consumption, but not the glycogen increase, under similar conditions. It was important, however, to put this possibility to a quantitative test by simultaneous measurement of the consumption of oxygen and the accumulation of glycogen in the same preparation. The experiments here described represent such an attempt to make a complete experimental balance sheet, representing the fate of the whole of the glucose.

METHODS

The methods of making the preparation, infusing glucose, and taking samples for analysis were identical with those described in earlier papers [92; 157], the eviscerated spinal cat being used in all cases.

For measurement of the oxygen consumption we had the advantage of using a circulating respirometer, recently designed and constructed for the purpose by our colleague, Dr. E. H. J. Schuster. In principle it is quite similar to that which he previously designed [681], and which was used by Burn and Dale, but the details of construction have been so altered

Originally appeared in the *Proceedings of the Royal Society*, B, C (1926), 55–71.
From the National Institute for Medical Research, Hampstead.
*Secretary, Royal Society.

that the whole apparatus can be easily accommodated at the end of the operating table. The double-barrelled piston-pump of the earlier design is replaced by a two-chambered diaphragm-pump, with mechanically operated and synchronized valves. The pistons of both chambers are operated by a common crank-shaft, and the throw can be altered, if necessary, without stopping the pump, by turning a micrometer screw, which alters the position of the fulcrum. The wedge-shaped gasometer, previously used, is replaced by a counterpoised, cylindrical gasometer, into which, as before, the expired air is driven through a tower filled with soda-lime. When the gasometer, through absorption of oxygen, and consequent reduction of volume of the whole system, has fallen to a certain level, the counterpoise lifts a light trigger, bringing into play a clutch, and producing one stroke of a small accessory pump. This delivers a definite volume (4.016 cc) of oxygen into the gasometer, and the resulting fall of the counterpoise throws the clutch out of action, until shrinkage to the same volume again brings it into play. The strokes of the accessory oxygen-pump are registered by a mechanical counter, and the number occurring in each five-minute period was recorded in the notes. At the end of the experiment the total volume in cubic centimetres introduced in any period, representing the volume of oxygen absorbed in that period, could be calculated by multiplying the total number of strokes by 4.016, and then reducing to 0° and 760 mm.

In most experiments two doses, each 10 units, of insulin were injected by the saphena vein, the second being given 1½ hours after the first. In the later experiments, for reasons which will become clear, we found it necessary to determine the free glucose in the muscles, before and after insulin, as well as the glycogen. It was decided also to analyse samples from the liver, though the afferent vessels to it had been tied, in order to control the slow leakage of glucose from this source into the circulation during the experiment. For the determination of muscle-sugar some of the samples of muscle taken were divided into two, one being dropped immediately into hot potassium-hydrate solution, for determination of the glycogen, and the other, weighing about 5 g, into 20 cc of cold alcohol in a centrifuge-tube in which the alcohol had been cooled below 0° C in a freezing mixture. The weight of the sample of muscle was determined by weighing the tube of cold alcohol before and after its addition. The muscle was minced finely, under the alcohol, with scissors, these being finally washed into the tube with a further 20 cc of cold 70 per cent alcohol. The mixture was allowed to stand for about one hour, and then thoroughly centrifuged. The total volume was taken to be 40 cc + the number of cc corresponding to the weight of the muscle sample, reckoned as water. It was assumed that the free sugar was distributed equally between the solid and liquid constituents of this total volume. The clear alcoholic extract was decanted off from the compacted solid layer, and 35 cc were taken. This was evaporated to dryness on the water bath and taken up in about 15 cc of distilled water. Five cc of 0.5 per cent dialysed iron was then added, in order to remove proteins and other colloidal constituents, and the mixture was diluted to 25 cc and filtered. In the water-clear filtrate, suitably diluted, glucose was determined by the Hagedorn-Jensen ferricyanide method, which seems to be less sensitive to other reducing or inhibiting substances than any of the methods depending on reduction of cupric oxide. From the figure so obtained the "free sugar" per gram of muscle was calculated. It may be doubted whether the attribution of the whole of the observed reduction to glucose is strictly justifiable; but the object of the determinations being essentially comparative, and the glucose being the only muscle constituent likely to vary significantly under the conditions of the experiment, the difference between the values obtained from corresponding muscles, before and after insulin, probably represented the change in the content of free glucose with an accuracy comparable to that of comparative blood sugar determinations.

The liver samples were treated in the same way, except that, in this case, separate samples were not taken directly into hot potash for determining the glycogen, but the solid residue, after removal of the cold alcoholic extract, was dried to remove alcohol and then worked up by Pflüger's method for glycogen. The glycogen being determined as glucose, the figure obtained was added to that for the free glucose in the alcoholic extract, and the total carbohydrate remaining in the liver, when the sample was taken, was thus calculated. Again the difference between two successive such estimates gave a reasonable figure for the glucose escaping into the blood from the *cul de sac* of the liver vessels in the interim.

Results

In the first two experiments the analyses made and the calculation of results from them followed the same lines as those adopted in the earlier paper. In the period before the injection of insulin we observed in each case, as Burn and Dale had observed in similar experiments, a consumption of oxygen much in excess of that required to account for the apparent use of glucose, as calculated from the quantity infused and the change in the blood sugar. The meaning of this discrepancy will become clear later, and there is no need to record the figures so obtained. A similar discrepancy, though much smaller in proportion to the total quantities concerned, appeared in the insulin period, when the calculated total glucose disappearing was compared with the sum of the glycogen accumulated in the muscles and the glucose equivalent of the oxygen used, as may be seen from the following experimental details.

Experiment 1. Weight of cat = 2,450 g. Total period of insulin action, 3 hrs 10 min 6 per cent glucose infused at an average rate of 3.6 cc in each 10 minutes; 68.4 cc in all = 4.104 g glucose.

Blood sugar fell from 0.410 to 0.360 per cent. "Active volume" of body
  fluids calculated as 408 cc, so that additional glucose loss

	= 4.08 × 0.05	= 0.204 g
Total calculated loss of glucose	= 4.104 + 0.204	= 4.31 g

Glycogen percentage in muscles—Before insulin	= 0.804
Final	= 1.102
Gain	= 0.298

Weight of muscles = 1,225 g. Total gain of glycogen = 12.25 × 0.298   = 3.65 g
Oxygen used, at 0° and 760° = 1,969 cc
0.75 L oxygen is equivalent to 1 g glucose
Glucose equivalent to oxygen used = 1.969 × 4/3   = 2.63 g

Total glucose accounted for   = 6.28 g

Glucose accounted for, in excess of calculated loss   = 1.97 g

In a second similar experiment:

Glucose accounted for, in excess of calculated loss   = 1.46 g

The fact that the glucose accounted for was regularly and materially in excess of that which had been calculated as disappearing clearly indicated a defect in some part of the calculation. [Two pages of the original paper have been omitted which discussed possible sources of error in the calculations and included protocols of Experiment 2.]

We decided, therefore, on a new method of estimation, in which the blood sugar changes were taken to apply only to the calculated volume of the blood itself, and the free glucose in the muscles was determined separately, by the method indicated in an earlier section. The total loss of glucose entailed by an observed fall in the percentage of muscle sugar could then be calculated by use of the same factor as that employed in calculating the total gain of muscle glycogen.

Some preliminary experiments were made to determine the regularity of the distribution of free glucose among the muscles, and the degree to which it changed with changes in the blood sugar, whether produced by insulin or otherwise.

Experiment 3. A spinal preparation was taken and eviscerated, and left to itself under artificial respiration on the warmed table for 5½ hours, without the supply of glucose from without or administration of insulin, so that the disappearance of glucose was only what was produced by the metabolic needs of the tissues of this preparation. The blood sugar fell from the initial level of 0.300 per cent to 0.132 per cent in 3½ hours, and to 0.068 per cent in 5½ hours. Samples of four muscles were taken in the usual manner at the beginning, and of the corresponding four muscles at the end of the experiment. Their average glycogen content remained practically constant, that of the initial samples being 0.736 and that of the final samples 0.777 per cent—a difference within the errors of sampling and analysis. The figures obtained for free glucose percentages in the muscles were as given in Table 12.I.

TABLE 12.I
FREE GLUCOSE PERCENTAGES IN THE MUSCLES

	Initial	Final
Gastrocnemius	0.215	0.210
Tibialis anterior	0.225	0.242
Rectus femoris	0.227	0.237
Vastus internus	Lost	0.217
Average (omitting last)	0.222	0.229

It will be noted that the value is very constant over the different muscles, and that it remains practically unchanged during the period in which the blood sugar sinks from 0.3 to 0.068.

Experiment 4. This experiment figures already in the paper by Best, Hoet, and Marks as Experiment 23. It was there pointed out that the accumulation of glycogen, produced in the muscles by the action of insulin, was in this case more than sufficient to account for the glucose infused and that which disappeared from the blood, on the basis of calculation then in use. The full figures for glycogen and free sugar in the muscles analysed were as shown in Table 12.II.

TABLE 12.II
GLYCOGEN AND FREE GLUCOSE IN THE MUSCLES

	Before Insulin		Final	
	Glycogen (%)	Free glucose (%)	Glycogen (%)	Free glucose (%)
Gastrocnemius	1.090	0.236	1.127	0.173
Rectus femoris	0.953	0.332	1.059	0.191
Vastus internus	0.522	0.258	0.758	0.181
Tibialis anterior	Lost	0.220		0.181
Average	0.855	0.262	0.981	0.182

Average increase in glycogen = 0.126 per cent.
Average decrease in free glucose = 0.080 per cent.

It will be clear that two-thirds of the glycogen increase can be accounted for by the loss of free glucose from the muscles themselves; the absence, however, of data as to oxygen consumption and as to the contribution of extra glucose by the liver made it impossible to produce a full reckoning of the carbohydrate balance in this experiment. The values for free glucose in different muscles taken at the same stage are much more uniform than those for glycogen in the same muscles, the only really aberrant figure being that for one muscle (Rect. fem.) before insulin. Calculation of the total change from that in the sample can, therefore, be made with at least as much confidence for free glucose as for glycogen. Though the free muscle glucose in this experiment showed a substantial fall under insulin, it by no means kept pace with that of the blood sugar, which fell in the same period from 0.27 per cent to 0.088 per cent. Nevertheless, the smaller fall in the percentage of muscle sugar makes a much larger contribution to the total of glucose lost than does the larger fall in the blood sugar percentage. The cat weighed 3.725 kilos; we may reckon that the blood volume was about 230 cc, and that the muscles weighed about 1,800 g.

| Lost from blood | $0.182 \times 2.3 = 0.42$ g |
| " muscles | $0.08 \times 18 = 1.44$ g |

Having thus a more satisfactory method for estimating the total amount of glucose disappearing, we proceeded to compare this total with that required by the observed use of oxygen and deposition of glycogen. We may consider first the light thrown, by the analyses of liver samples, on the discrepancy observed by Burn and Dale between the volume of oxygen absorbed by this preparation and the amount of glucose infused, to maintain the blood sugar at a constant level, without insulin. They found that oxygen was consumed in substantially greater amount than was needed to oxidize this glucose, though the respiratory quotient proved that nothing but carbohydrate was being oxidized. We have seen that, in the absence of insulin, the muscle sugar remains remarkably steady, so that the supply of extra glucose from the liver seems the only explanation for the discrepancy. The results of the first stage of Experiment 5 show that it is adequate.

Experiment 5. Weight of cat = 3.2 kilos.

A. *First stage—before insulin.* The period of observation was 50 minutes. Samples of liver were taken for analysis at the beginning and end of the period. The blood sugar remained practically unchanged (0.24 per cent), while 5.6 cc of 4 per cent dextrose were given by slow infusion.

Weight of liver (less that of initial samples) = 70 g

	per cent
Average of 1st samples—glycogen 3.24 per cent + glucose 1.61 per cent	= 4.85
Average of 2nd samples—glycogen 1.26 per cent + glucose 2.35 per cent	= 3.61
Loss of carbohydrate	1.24

Total loss of carbohydrate from liver	= 1.24 × 0.7	= 0.868 g
Glucose infused	5.6 × 0.04	= 0.224 g
Total glucose lost		1.092 g

Oxygen absorbed—784 cc at N.T.P.
Glucose equivalent to oxygen used   0.784 × 4/3 = 1.045 g

It is obvious that the oxygen consumption shows as close a correspondence with the observed loss of glucose as could be expected with the methods of measurement available. The excess consumption of oxygen, observed by Burn and Dale, can be entirely accounted for by the contribution to the blood from the carbohydrates of the liver, which is nearly four times as great as the amount of glucose infused. The total loss of glucose, so calculated, appears, indeed, to be very slightly in excess of that oxidized. Even if the difference were a real one, however, the deposition of 47 mg as glycogen in some 1,600 g of muscle would be altogether beyond the possibility of detection by analysis.

B. Insulin period. After the second liver samples and first muscle samples had been taken, 10 units of insulin were injected intravenously, and the rate of glucose infusion increased. Another 10 units were injected 1½ hours later, and the total period of insulin action was 2½ hours. The third liver and second muscle samples were then taken.

Weight of liver (less that of 1st and 2nd samples) = 58 g

	Per cent		Per cent
Av. liver glycogen just before insulin = 1.26		Av. liver glycogen at end	= 0.70
" free sugar " " = 2.35		" free sugar "	= 1.30
" carbohydrate " = 3.61		" carbohydrate "	= 2.00

Difference = 1.61 per cent
= 1.61 × 0.58 = 0.934 g

Loss of carbohydrate from liver	
Av. muscle glucose before insulin	= 0.25
" " at end	= 0.19
Loss	= 0.06

Total loss of glucose from muscle	= 0.06 × 16 = 0.960 g
Blood sugar fall from 0.240 to 0.130 per cent	= 0.110 per cent
Loss of glucose from blood	= 0.110 × 2 = 0.220 g
Total glucose infused	= 3.250 g
Calculated total loss of glucose	5.364 g

Average muscle glycogen before insulin = 0.654 per cent
"   "   at end   = 0.830   "

Gain   = 0.176   "

Total calculated gain of muscle glycogen $= 0.176 \times 16 = 2.82$ g

Oxygen used = 2,230 cc at N.T.P.

Glucose equivalent of oxygen used $= 2.23 \times 4/3 = \underline{2.97}$ g

          Total glucose accounted for $= \mathbf{5.79}$ g

On this calculation the glucose accounted for by glycogen formation and oxidation, 5.79 g, is slightly in excess of the detected loss, 5.364 g. The difference cannot, however, be regarded as having any true significance. The calculations of the total loss of muscle sugar and gain of glycogen, in particular, have not a high degree of accuracy. They depend on the multiplication of the figures obtained from sample analyses by the large factor 16. If we divide 0.426, the difference between the totals for glucose lost and accounted for, by 16, the result is 0.028 per cent, so that an under-estimate of the muscle sugar loss by 0.014 per cent, and an overestimate of the glycogen gain by the same percentage, would account for the whole difference in the final totals. The comparison of one set of muscles with the corresponding ones of the opposite leg, either for free sugar or glycogen, is liable to inaccuracy at least as great as this. We cannot, therefore, regard the difference between the totals on the two sides of the final account as a real one; but we are entitled to conclude that *the glucose disappearing under the action of insulin is, in this experiment, fully accounted for by the sum of what is oxidized and what is deposited as glycogen.*

Experiment 6. Weight of cat = 2,600 g. In this experiment no sample of the liver was taken until just before insulin was given, so that no balance can be made between glucose lost and oxidized in the pre-insulin period. As in all the other experiments, the oxygen absorbed in this period was much in excess of that required to oxidize the glucose infused.

Insulin period. Four muscles and samples of liver were taken just before the first injection of 10 units of insulin, a second similar injection was given about 1 hour later, and a third after a further 1½ hours. The final samples were taken 3½ hours after the first insulin injection, the preparation being, therefore, under the action of insulin for this total period, and receiving 30 units in all. The infusion of glucose was in this case so greatly accelerated after insulin was given that the blood sugar did not fall, but rose somewhat, being over 0.44 per cent during the whole period.

Weight of liver (less that of first samples) = 70 g

	Per cent			Per cent
Av. liver glycogen just before insulin	= 0.81	Av. liver glycogen at end		= 0.71
" free glucose " "	= 1.4	" free glucose "		= 1.04
	2.21			1.75

                                            Difference = 0.46 per cent

Total loss of carbohydrate from liver $= 0.46 \times 0.7 = 0.312$ g

Av. muscle glucose before insulin = 0.22
"   "   after   "   = 0.20

Loss   = 0.02

Total calculated loss of glucose from muscle   = 0.02 × 13 = 0.260 g
    Glucose infused   = 4.80 g
                                                                5.372 g

Blood sugar rose from 0.44 to 0.51 = 0.07 per cent

$$\frac{0.07 \times 167}{100} = 0.117 \text{ g}$$

Total *gain* of glucose in blood

Calculated total loss of glucose   = 5.255 g

                              Per cent
Av. muscle glycogen before insulin = 0.661
    "   "   at end   = 0.851

Gain   = 0.190

Total calculated gain of muscle glycogen   = 0.190 × 13 = 2.470 g
Oxygen used = 1,946 cc at N.T.P. = 1.946 × 4/3 g glucose   = 2.595 g

    Total glucose accounted for   5.065 g

In this case the apparent difference between the two sides of the account is in the other direction, since we account for 190 mg less glucose than the estimated loss; but again the difference has no significance in relation to the accuracy of the method of calculation. The recorded fall in free muscle sugar—0.22 to 0.20 per cent—cannot be regarded as a certain difference; yet it contributes 0.260 g to the balance sheet as presented, and its absence would change the apparent discrepancy to the other side of the account.

In the two complete experiments thus far recorded, the infusion of glucose was raised to such a rate, after insulin was first injected, that the blood sugar percentage, falling in Experiment 5 and rising in Experiment 6, remained in both well above the normal level throughout the period of observation. It was important to know whether the balance would still hold good when the supply of glucose was so small in relation to the insulin given that the blood sugar would fall rapidly to a minimal value. These conditions were realized in Experiment 7.

Experiment 7. Weight of cat = 2,800 g. Glucose was infused throughout the experiment at the rate of 40 to 48 mg in each 10-minute period, except for an hour in the middle of the insulin period, when the rate of infusion was gradually raised, in order to test its effect on the rapid decline in the rate of oxygen absorption, which had appeared about 40 minutes after the first insulin injection. The effect on oxygen usage being small, the rate of glucose infusion was dropped again, and continued at the original slow rate for a further 2½ hours. 25 units of insulin in all were administered, 10 units at the first injection, 5 units 40 minutes later, when the rate of glucose infusion was increased, and another 10 units 1½ hours after the second injection. The blood sugar percentage fell from 0.360 per cent at the time of the first dose of insulin to 0.034 per cent at the end of the experiment, 4 hours 10 minutes later. The first samples of liver and four muscles of one leg were removed shortly before insulin was first injected, and the rest of the liver and the four corresponding muscles at the end of the experiment.

Weight of liver (less that of first sample) = 102.6 g

	Per cent		Per cent
Av. liver glycogen just before insulin =	1.285	Av. liver glycogen at end =	0.625
„ free glucose „ „ =	1.760	„ free glucose „ =	1.570
	3.045		2.195

Difference = 0.850 per cent
= 1.026 × 0.850 = 0.872 g

Total loss of carbohydrate from liver

Av. muscle glucose before insulin = 0.320 per cent
„ „ at end = 0.240 „

Loss = 0.080 „

Total calculated loss of free glucose from muscle = 0.080 × 14 = 1.120 g
Total glucose infused = 1.680 g
Blood sugar fell from 0.360 to 0.034 = 0.326 per cent
Total loss of glucose from blood = 0.326 × 1.75 = 0.570 g

Calculated total loss of glucose = 4.242 g

Av. muscle glycogen before insulin = 0.727 per cent
„ „ at end = 0.799 „

Gain = 0.072 „

Total calculated gain of muscle glycogen = 0.072 × 14 = 1.008 g
Oxygen used = 2,309 cc at N.T.P. = 2.309 × 4/3 g glucose = 3.079 g

Calculated total glucose accounted for = 4.087 g

Again the two totals, of glucose lost and of glucose found as glycogen or oxidized, show as near an identity as it is reasonable to expect with the method, so that we can safely draw the conclusion that *even when insulin is present in such excess, in relation to the supply of glucose, that a severe hypoglycaemia is produced, all the glucose which disappears is either oxidized or stored as glycogen, no significant part of it being deposited in an unrecognized form.*

It is, of course, possible, and even probable, that a very small part of the disappearing glucose forms an addition to the floating balance of hexose phosphate, on its way to storage as glycogen. Our experiments show definitely, however, that no significant proportion is held at any one moment in this form. A point deserving mention is the curious lack of parallelism between the percentages of blood sugar, on the one hand, and "free glucose" in the muscles on the other, seen in every experiment in which the latter was determined. It would clearly be unprofitable to discuss the meaning of the disparity, without fuller evidence as to whether other substances, and if so what substances and in what proportions, contribute to the reduction on which this figure is based. The point is one worth further investigation. For our present purpose it seemed quite justifiable to assume that a fall in the value is due to loss of glucose, just as it is assumed that a fall in the reducing power of a blood-filtrate is due to loss of glucose, though it is known that a small proportion of other reducing substances is present.

DISCUSSION

The results of the experiments are so definite that they need no discussion of themselves. Under the conditions chosen, with a preparation consisting essentially of naturally perfused quiescent skeletal muscle, all the glucose disappearing under insulin is either oxidized or stored in the muscles as glycogen.

The important question remains, Does this action of insulin, thus artificially isolated in our experiments, cover the whole of its effects as seen in the normal animal? It is quite certain that it does not. Failure to detect glycogen storage could easily be explained; but the fact calling for explanation is the very obvious decrease, often the complete disappearance, of glycogen from the normal animal receiving an excessive dose of insulin. That the convulsions consequent on hypoglycaemia greatly accelerate this depletion of the muscle glycogen, and thus help to annul the effect of any initial storage action, has been clearly demonstrated in a former paper (Best, Hoet, and Marks [92]). But the fundamental difficulty remains, namely, that, if this exhaustion of the carbohydrates is attributed to oxidation, additional to that of the normal resting metabolism, the total respiratory exchange must increase, and the body temperature would be expected to rise. In fact this exhaustion is accompanied by a fall in the respiratory exchange, even to as little as one-third of its normal resting value, and by a corresponding fall in the body temperature. These effects can be well seen in the experiments recorded by Dudley with Laidlaw, Trevan and Boock [269], and with Marrian [270], and also in those experiments of Lesser [493], in which he used doses of insulin sufficient to produce "symptoms."

There are two possible explanations for this paradox of accelerated loss of recoverable carbohydrate with concurrent depression of oxidative metabolism. The one which has apparently been found acceptable by most workers on the subject is the supposition that, when insulin is present in excess, the synthesis of dextrose to glycogen is not completed, but stopped at some intermediate stage, or diverted along some other path, so that the carbohydrate is deposited in some unidentified form, in which it is withdrawn from oxidative metabolism, and is either destroyed or not extracted by the methods ordinarily used in analysis. This is the conception provisionally adopted by Macleod [539] and Campbell and Macleod [169] in their exhaustive reviews of the subject. It must be admitted that such temporary immobilization of the carbohydrate, if there were direct evidence of its occurrence, would account for some of the effects observed. The supposition, however, is directly against the evidence of the experiments here presented. Under conditions which should have been ideal for its detection, since relatively large quantities of glucose were made to disappear under the action of insulin, we observed no trace of this conversion into unrecognized forms; all that was not oxidized was recovered as glycogen. The supposition further involves the difficult assumption that insulin, when present in excess, in relation to the carbohydrate available, has an action *qualitatively* different from that which it produces in the presence of abundant carbohydrate.

The second possible explanation seems to us to have a much clearer relation to the known facts. It is suggested by a consideration of the abnormalities of metabolism which the organism presents when insulin is defective or absent—i.e., in natural or artificial diabetes. Under such conditions the body presents two functional defects—defective use and storage of carbohydrate on the one hand, and excessive, wasteful formation of carbohydrate from proteins (and possibly also from fats) on the other. We have no certain knowledge as to the relation of these two effects to one another, such as would entitle us to regard one as a secondary consequence of the other. But we do know that both these defects are removed by insulin in appropriate dosage; and it has been shown to act in both these directions not only in the diabetic patient and in the depancreatized animal, but also in the dog poisoned by phloridzin (Ringer [645], Nash [592]). It is reasonable to suppose that insulin in excessive doses will produce both these, its normal effects, to an abnormal degree.

(1) We should expect it to accelerate the combustion of carbohydrate, and particularly the associated storage as glycogen, to a rate much above the normal. That it has this effect we believe that our experiments, in addition to those of Lesser and his co-workers [125; 126], have sufficiently demonstrated.

(2) We should expect it to depress the new formation of carbohydrate from other substances in the liver to a rate much below the normal. We believe that this effect is clearly evident in a large number of published experimental results, which have shown a depression of total respiratory metabolism, associated with a large rise in the respiratory quotient. The clearest examples, perhaps, are those given by Laufberger [482; 483]. So

much was he impressed by their significance that he made at first the suggestion that this stoppage or restriction of the new formation of carbohydrate was the sole effect of insulin. This suggestion obviously would not fit the facts any better than the suggestion that the sole effect is to promote combustion and synthesis.

It is probably not realized by those who have not examined the figures how small a ration of total carbohydrate, in relation to the metabolic need, is present at any one moment in the body of such an animal as a fasting mouse. Bissinger and Lesser's analyses show that it amounts to about 170 mg per 100 g of body weight. On the other hand, if the mouse were using carbohydrate alone for its metabolism, it would require about 560 mg per 100 g per hour to maintain its normal rate of expenditure. It is obvious, then, that the normal metabolism can only be maintained by the rapid new formation of carbohydrate in the liver. If this new supply is stopped, the existing supply will be exhausted in about 20 minutes, unless the rate of metabolism is rapidly reduced. The effects which follow the injection into such a mouse of an excessive dose of insulin are exactly what, under such conditions, we should expect. There is an initial sharp rise of the respiratory quotient, indicating that, owing to depression of new formation, the oxidative metabolism has been concentrated on the pre-existing carbohydrate. Other carbohydrate is probably, during a very brief period, being removed from circulation to be deposited as glycogen. But the needs even of the rapidly falling metabolism soon begin to call on all the carbohydrate reserves, and the onset of hypoglycaemic convulsions increases the rate of their exhaustion. If the dose has been large enough, and the fall of metabolism is delayed by putting the animal into a thermostat at 37°, it may be expected that the mouse will die in about half an hour, with its initial stores of carbohydrate completely exhausted; and this is what, in fact, occurs.

In the fasting normal mouse or rat, with their rapid metabolism, it is obviously the depression of new carbohydrate formation which will form the most obvious feature in the action of an excess of insulin, and the only one, indeed, which experiment may succeed in detecting. In the diabetic subject both the effects are equally in evidence. In the eviscerated spinal preparation, as used in our experiments, we have artificially eliminated, from the outset, the new formation of carbohydrate, and the preparation is carrying out its metabolism wholly at the expense of carbohydrate originally present in the body as such, or supplied from outside by infusion, so that the oxidation and synthesis are seen isolated from the other effect, which so often complicates their demonstration in the normal animal.

Our experiments can give no indication of the extent to which the liver participates in the storage of glycogen under insulin. Von Issekutz [417], alone among those who have made such experiments, appears to have obtained evidence, on the perfused frog's liver, of a direct inhibition by insulin of the conversion of glycogen to glucose. This is in accord with the demonstrated reappearance of glycogen in the liver of the diabetic animal treated with insulin. Insulin has also been shown to cause storage of glycogen in the liver of an animal under phloridzin (Cori [223]), and, when given in small doses, of a normal fasting animal (Frank, Hartmann, and Nothmann [307]). The fact, which we and others have observed, that rabbits dying of insulin convulsions often have a substantial remainder of glycogen in the liver, though that of the muscles is exhausted, may possibly point in the same direction. Since the liver-glycogen, however, is the primary carbohydrate reserve of the body, there must always be a conflict, when insulin is present in excess, between a direct promotion of storage by insulin in that organ, and the promotion of glycogenolysis by the hypo-glycaemia, acting either directly or through the suprarenal glands. When to this conflict there is added the effect of depressed new formation of carbohydrate, it is not surprising to find that the end-result of the action of insulin on smaller animals, such as mice, with their rapid metabolism, is often a complete exhaustion of the glycogen from the liver as well as from other organs.

On these lines, attributing to insulin when present in excess no other action than the production of its known physiological effects with more than physiological intensity, and without any assumption of unknown and unrecognizable forms of carbohydrate, we believe that it will prove possible to account for all its effects, in any dosage, and on any species. This view, in essence, was put forward some years ago by one of us (H. H. D. [237]) and in greater detail by Lesser [494]. Each in turn [493; 238] later expressed doubt of its adequacy. In the light of more recent evidence Lesser [125] has returned to it, and we regard the evidence here presented as definitely confirming it.

SUMMARY

(1) The glucose which disappears from an eviscerated spinal preparation under the action of insulin is equal to the sum of the glycogen deposited in the muscles and the glucose-equivalent of the oxygen absorbed. (2) This balance is preserved, whether the blood sugar is maintained at a high level by rapid infusion of glucose, or allowed to sink to a very low level by restricting the supply. (3) The view is advocated that the effects of insulin in excess represent an intensification of its physiological effects.

IN THE INTRODUCTION TO PAPER 13 *the distribution of insulin is discussed in the light of the information available in 1932. By 1932 we had finally become aware of many pitfalls in the assay of insulin. In the Connaught Laboratories it was particularly important to avoid the contamination of glassware and filter paper by insulin-containing dust. Insulin is strongly adsorbed on laboratory glassware, but once this was recognized it was easy to remove the last traces. Much more sensitive and specific methods are now available for assaying the insulin content of tissue extracts. Insulin can now be demonstrated in blood, muscle, and other tissues but these small amounts could not have been detected thirty years ago.*

The presence in plants of as yet imperfectly studied saponins, glucosides, alkaloids, and other compounds with an action on the liver, kidneys, or muscles may alter the concentration of sugar in the blood. Only an experienced investigator can distinguish between the different mechanisms by which the blood sugar may be decreased.

The persistence of insulin in the blood of untreated diabetic animals and the indications that it may be present in a bound, inert form do, however, leave us with fascinating problems regarding the distribution of small but physiologically very significant amounts of the anti-diabetic substance.

13. Insulin in Tissues other than the Pancreas

C. H. BEST

C. M. JEPHCOTT

D. A. SCOTT

A review of the literature, in which the distribution of insulin or insulin-like substances has been discussed, reveals the fact that numerous investigators have reported the presence of these active materials in a great variety of animal and vegetable tissues. With the procedure originally used to obtain insulin from the pancreas, insulin was not obtained from other tissues (Banting and Best [41]). It was perhaps not surprising that the improved methods of extracting pancreatic insulin when applied to other animal tissues should apparently yield definite amounts of active material (Collip [211; 212; 213]; Best and Scott [114; 115]; Best, Scott, and Banting [117]; Ashby [25]; Baker, Dickens, and Dodds [37]; Best, Smith, and Scott [118; 119]; Ivy and Fisher [418]; Lundberg [520]; Brugsch and Horsters [153; 154]; Nothmann [599; 600]; Cori [228; 229]; Vincent, Dodds, and Dickens [774]; Penau and Simonnet [616]; Hoshi [398]; Cramer, Dickens, and Dodds [232]; Redenbaugh, Ivy, and Koppanyi [631]; Shikinami [696]. Certain points in these reports on the distribution of insulin stand out very prominently. It is surprising that insulin should be reported to be present in diabetic tissues (Best, Smith, and Scott [118; 119]; Baker, Dickens, and Dodds [37]; Nothmann [599; 600]; Pollak [623]) and in relatively large amounts in the zymogenous tissue of teleosteal fishes (Vincent, Dodds, and Dickens [774]) and in spleens of normal rats (Cramer, Dickens, and Dodds [232]). Furthermore, the urinary secretion of very large amounts of active material after the intravenous or oral administration of insulin, or after its introduction through an intestinal fistula (Fisher and Noble [300]) and the peculiar behaviour of "endogenous" and "exogenous" insulin (Brugsch and Horsters [153; 154]) are very odd phenomena.

Originally appeared in the *American Journal of Physiology*, C (1932), 285–94. From the Department of Physiology and the School of Hygiene, University of Toronto.

The apparently wide distribution of insulin-like material in the animal kingdom led Collip to suggest that this material might be present wherever glycogen was formed. The active material was, however, later thought to be present in extracts of plants, in the tissues of which no glycogen can be detected (Collip [208; 209; 210; 214; 215; 216]). Collip also encountered a strange phenomenon of "animal passage" of the hypoglycaemia-producing principle. Later he suggested (Collip [217]) that the passage phenomenon was probably attributable to a "living agent." It is obviously impossible to decide from the evidence at present available how much of the delayed hypoglycaemia observed after the injection of extracts from vegetable sources was due to a chemical substance, and how much to the effects of the "living agent" which might have been present in the extracts. The evidence suggests that most of the changes observed by Collip were due to a contaminating "living agent." It must be borne in mind, however, that large doses of pancreatic insulin may produce a prolonged hypoglycaemia after a preliminary period in which the blood sugar is not lowered. It is perhaps significant that some of the workers with plant extracts secured prompt hypoglycaemia (Dubin and Corbitt [266]; Best and Scott [116]; Fisher and McKinley [299]; and others). Collip [214; 215] secured only delayed effects from yeast extracts, while Hutchinson, Smith, and Winter [412] secured more rapid effects comparable to those produced by pancreatic insulin. In Collip's work on extract from clams, hypoglycaemic convulsions were observed in rabbits within six hours. The possible role of pancreatic insulin in the production of some of these results will be clearer when the results we have recently obtained have been discussed.

There are a number of reasons why the results of the early work on the distribution of insulin and insulin-like substances are of no significance from the quantitative point of view. It was not then fully appreciated that some rabbits may show a definite fall in blood sugar over the experimental period, and for this reason the results based on one animal are not satisfactory. A standard of comparison was not used in the assaying of insulin in most of the early work. In a number of the papers which have appeared on the subject of the distribution of insulin, no convincing evidence is to be found that any hypoglycaemia-producing substance was present in the extracts which were reported to yield positive results. When we add to these factors the possibility of the presence of a living agent which may cause hypoglycaemia, the possibility that non-specific toxic materials, which may produce liver damage and delayed hypoglycaemia, may have been present, and the possibility of contamination of solutions by pancreatic insulin, it becomes apparent that the whole question of the distribution of insulin and insulin-like substances must be reopened, and that many, if not all, of the results obtained up to the present time be discarded.

In the previous work several investigators have stated that they were able quantitatively to recover insulin added to pancreas or other tissues. Few, if any, of these results will, in the light of the present knowledge, stand critical analysis. In most cases one of the well-known methods for making pancreatic insulin was used. In work of this kind it would be preferable to have available a method that would yield optimal results when applied to pancreatic tissue. With this point in mind, one of us (Jephcott [428]) has thoroughly explored the conditions under which maximal yields of insulin in a form in which it can be accurately assayed are obtainable from pancreatic tissue. The details of the procedure finally adopted are as follows: perfectly fresh glands are finely minced, and after thorough stirring 25-g samples are quickly weighed and transferred to a flask containing 75 cc of 95 per cent ethyl alcohol, 25 cc of water, and 1.5 cc of concentrated hydrochloric acid. Extraction is carried out in a mechanical shaker immersed in a water bath which is kept at a temperature of 36° C. After two hours the mixture is filtered through a double thickness of gauze and the residue is pressed as dry as possible. A second extraction, similar to the first, is then made. The two filtrates are combined, made just alkaline to litmus with ammonia, filtered through a Buchner funnel and re-acidified to pH2 with hydrochloric acid. The alcohol is distilled off under vacuum at about 35° C. The residue is transferred to a 250 cc measuring flask and made up to volume with water. When desirable the active material may be salted out with ammonium sulphate or sodium chloride without appreciable loss. The assay on white mice and rabbits is conducted as soon as possible after the extract has been prepared. The assays are made by comparison of the effect of the unknown solution with that of standard insulin. After the potency of the solution is determined approximately, from thirty to sixty white mice and several rabbits are used for each test. When the procedure outlined above is used to extract insulin from beef pancreas, average yields of approximately 3000 units per kilogram may be consistently obtained. We believe that yields of 3500–4000 units per kilogram represent the maximal amounts of active material which can be secured by the methods available at present from beef pancreas collected in Toronto during the summer months. Higher yields reported by other workers are open to question since the methods of assay then used cannot now be considered adequate. The yields of insulin from the pancreas of various species have been determined by one of us (C. M. J.) and will shortly be reported.

It might be expected that no difficulty would be encountered in recovering added insulin with a method such as we have outlined. Such, however, is not the case. Purified insulin or the crystalline product cannot consistently be recovered quantitatively when the hydrochloric acid procedure outlined above is used. The results of numerous experiments demonstrate that an average recovery of more than 60 per cent of the added material is not usually secured. When sulphuric acid is used instead of hydrochloric the recovery is not significantly improved. Lower yields of insulin from pancreas are always obtained when sulphuric acid is used.

It can be shown, however, that crude insulin withstands this treatment much better than the purer material (Jephcott [428]). One of the factors affecting the destruction of the purified insulin may be the length of time it is exposed to the alcohol and acid. Even when the tissue is extracted rapidly, however, a great deal of the added material may be lost. Insulin prepared by different procedures varies considerably in its stability under these circumstances.

The situation is, therefore, that the method which gives the best yield of insulin from pancreas does not consistently permit more than a partial recovery of purified insulin added to pancreas or to other tissues. When the hydrochloric acid procedure is used to investigate the insulin content of tissues other than the pancreas, negative results might conceivably mean that small amounts of insulin were present but were destroyed by the treatment. If, however, the hydrochloric and sulphuric acid extractions and various methods of purification are carefully applied and negative results are consistently obtained, the suggestion that demonstrable amounts of insulin or insulin-like materials are not obtainable from other tissues would be supported.

The results of the application of these procedures to vegetable tissues, normal beef and dog tissues, to urine, and to diabetic dog tissues will be briefly reported and discussed.

TABLE 13.I

INABILITY TO DETECT INSULIN IN PLANT TISSUES

Tissue	Weight (g)	Method	Mouse Test	Rabbit Test
Onions	1,100	alcoholic HCl	negative	negative
Beet roots	1,400	alcoholic HCl	negative	negative
Beet roots	1,100	alcoholic H_2SO_4	negative	negative
Beet roots	1,800	alcoholic HCl	negative	negative

Vegetable Tissues

It is unnecessary to review in detail the numerous reports on the presence of insulin-like substances in plant tissues (Collip [208, 209, 210, 214, 215, 216]; Funk and Corbitt [314]; Dubin and Corbitt [266]; Winter and Smith

[809]; Hutchinson, Smith, and Winter [412]; Best and Scott [116]; Gottschalk [329]; Eisler and Portheim [280]; Glaser and Wittner [321]; Fisher and McKinley [299]; Simola [705]; Shikinami [696]; Kaufmann [440; 441], etc.). The results of these studies may be divided into three groups: (a) in which there is no convincing evidence of the presence of any active principle; (b) in which there is proof that a delayed hypoglycaemia occurs; and (c) in which the hypoglycaemia appears more promptly. If we make the obvious inference from Collip's suggestion that a living agent may be responsible for the "animal passage" phenomenon, that it might also account for the delayed hypoglycaemia observed after the subcutaneous

TABLE 13.II

INABILITY TO DETECT INSULIN IN OTHER TISSUES

Tissue	Amount	Method of Extraction	Method of Assay	Result*
Arterial blood (dog); no general anaesthetic	160 cc serum	alcoholic H_2SO_4	mouse and rabbit	negative
	205 cc cells	alcoholic H_2SO_4	mouse and rabbit	negative
Arterial blood (dog); no general anaesthetic	540 cc defibrinated blood	benzoic acid	mouse and rabbit	negative
Splenic vein blood (dog); amytal anaesthesia	57 cc	benzoic acid	mouse	negative
Dog's liver	230 g	alcoholic HCl	mouse	negative (toxic effects)
Dog's liver	100 g	benzoic acid	mouse and rabbit	negative
Dog's liver	150 g	picric acid	mouse and rabbit	negative
Dog's liver	75 g	Fisher's method	mouse and rabbit	negative
Sheep liver	60 g	alcoholic HCl	mouse and rabbit	negative (toxic effects)
Sheep liver	100 g	picric acid	mouse and rabbit	negative
Beef liver	10 g	alcoholic HCl	mouse	negative
Dog's muscle	100 g	benzoic acid	mouse and rabbit	negative
Beef salivary glands	100 g	alcoholic HCl	mouse and rabbit	negative
Beef salivary glands	500 g	picric acid	mouse and rabbit	negative
Dog's heart	50 g	picric acid	mouse and rabbit	negative
Dog's heart	38 g	Fisher's method	mouse	negative
Dog's kidney	47 g	alcoholic HCl	mouse	negative
Dog's spleen	35 g	alcoholic HCl	mouse	negative
Beef thymus	800 g	benzoic acid	mouse and rabbit	negative

*The possibility that the very potent but labile form of insulin reported by Dingemanse [255] and more recently observed by Dirscherl [256] may have been responsible for any of the positive results previously obtained can, in our opinion, be regarded as extremely faint.

injection of vegetable extracts, and admit the possibility that contamination of the plant extracts by pancreatic insulin may be responsible for the more rapid effects, there would be no evidence suggesting an insulin-like substance (glucokinin) in vegetable tissues. Collip [217] apparently does not consider that the initial hypoglycaemia produced by the vegetable extract is attributable to the same factors which cause the "animal passage" hypoglycaemia.

When vegetable tissues were extracted by the procedure most successfully used to obtain pancreatic insulin, negative results were secured.

The extracts made from beet roots produced very toxic effects in several of the rabbits.

While sufficient experiments have not been performed to justify the conclusion that an insulin-like substance (glucokinin) is not present in plant tissues, it may be stated that in light of the recent findings the previous reports cannot be accepted at their face value. (The substances which may be extracted from members of the myrtle family, and which are reported to produce an anti-diabetic effect when given by mouth, are not considered in this discussion.)

Normal Animal Tissues

A great many experiments have been conducted in this part of our work. A limited number of typical results will be reported. In addition to the methods we have discussed above, the exact procedures advocated by Fisher and by Baker, Dickens, and Dodds and by others have been used.

Diabetic Tissues

The failure to demonstrate insulin in normal tissues other than the pancreas made it extremely unlikely that any anti-diabetic principle would be found in diabetic organs. We have taken advantage of an opportunity to secure diabetic tissues, however, and these have been analysed by two methods (sulphuric and hydrochloric acid extraction) in an attempt to secure insulin. Liver, skeletal muscle, and heart muscle were removed from a completely depancreatized dog which had received no insulin for 5 days. The results of the assay of the extracts prepared were completely negative. It does not follow from these results that the pancreas of a patient dying in diabetic coma contains no insulin, but a reinvestigation of this subject is perhaps necessary.

Insulin in Urine

A hypoglycaemia-producing substance has been reported to be present in urine by several groups of workers (Best, Smith, and Scott [118; 119];

Kozuka [471]; Partos [611]; Brugsch and Horsters [154]). This aspect of the subject of the distribution of insulin has been particularly developed by Partos and by Brugsch and Horsters. Recently Lawrence, Madders, and Millar [488] have reported that they are unable to confirm the results obtained by these investigators.

We have reinvestigated this field and have been unable to secure demonstrable amounts of insulin from normal dog or human urine.

Recovery of Injected Insulin

The urinary excretion of injected insulin (Fisher and Noble [300]) needs further comment. These investigators reported that large amounts of insulin could be recovered from the urine of normal dogs after the oral or intravenous administration of the active material. Soon after this work was published R. G. Smith in our laboratory attempted to repeat it. In his first experiments he was apparently successful but later in numerous experiments was unable to detect more than traces in the urine even after the oral or intravenous administration of enormous doses to dogs. So many possible variables were uncontrolled in these experiments that the results were not reported at the time. Quite recently we have repeated certain of these experiments with the following results. When an insulin solution is administered intravenously to a dog under amytal anaesthesia at such a rate that 200 units are given in the first two hours it is found that less than 10 per cent of the injected insulin can be recovered from the urine voided during the four-hour experiment. Saline was given during the last two hours of the experiment. The urine was acidified and immediately tested for insulin by injection directly into mice and rabbits. No insulin could be recovered by the benzoic acid method from liver, kidney, muscle, or heart tissues which were removed at the end of the experiment. These results demonstrate that, although most of the injected insulin was lost, a small but definite amount can be recovered from the urine under the conditions of these experiments. In a few experiments in which large amounts of insulin were administered by mouth to normal dogs, none was recovered in the urine.

DISCUSSION

It is necessary to define what is meant by negative result in the assay of solutions for their insulin content by the mouse and rabbit methods. As it is not advisable to administer more than 0.5 cc of solution to a mouse, the volume of all extracts was kept as small as possible. From 0.25 to 0.50 cc was injected. When no symptoms attributable to the presence of insulin are observed in any of the injected animals it is safe to conclude that less than 1/100 unit of insulin is present. As approximately 25 cc of solution were obtained from 100 g of tissue a negative result indicates that less than ½ unit was present in the extract from this amount of material. Mice may occasionally exhibit convulsions which resemble those produced by insulin when tissue extracts which do not contain demonstrable amounts of this active material are injected. It is sometimes difficult to decide whether or not the administration of dextrose solution improves their condition. Repetition of tests, the results of which are difficult to interpret, and comparison with the results of the rabbit assay, however, always enable an investigator to make a correct interpretation of these doubtful results. Rabbits are injected subcutaneously with from 10 to 15 cc of solution. A blood sugar lowering of from 30 to 40 mgm per cent when the normal value is high (0.13 to 0.15 per cent) is not proof of the presence of insulin. It is inadvisable to conclude that insulin is present if very large doses of the extract under test do not lower the blood sugar of some of the test rabbits fairly rapidly to the convulsive level.

One investigator (F. A. Calderone, who was working under the direction of Professor G. B. Wallace) has informed us that he has been unable to confirm the results of the workers who reported the presence of insulin in blood (Best, Scott, and Banting; Nothmann; Hoshi) but as far as we know there have been no published reports to this effect. Until we had secured the negative results reported above, we were inclined to attribute these apparent difficulties to the same factors which, in the early stages of the work on insulin, made it impossible consistently to obtain active material from pancreatic tissue. The demonstration of insulin in blood by physiological methods (La Barre [476; 477]; Zunz and La Barre [828; 829]) seems to be convincing. The real situation very likely is that suggested by the observations of Képinov and Ledebt-Petit Dutaillis [447; 448] and of Heymans [389]. Insulin added to blood kept at body temperature was found to disappear very rapidly. In the light of our recent observations we believe that there is no evidence that any tissue other than pancreatic either produces or stores insulin. It is, of course, possible that methods will be developed which will permit the recognition of the minute amounts of insulin that one would expect to be present. Although we have not attempted to repeat in detail the extensive work of Brugsch and Horsters, from the results of which they conclude that injected insulin liberates endogenous insulin, etc., etc., we suggest that their results may be different if the experiments are repeated, using the precautions suggested by our experimental results.

A great deal of space might be utilized in the further discussion of the results which we have been unable to confirm. Many of these considered to be positive are obviously attributable to what we now know to be faulty interpretations of the results of the assays. The possibility exists that a contaminating living agent may have been responsible for the positive results in some cases. There is no doubt, however, that the active material found to be present in extracts of these various tissues by several groups of workers was insulin. It is perhaps significant that in Toronto, and in Collip's laboratory, large amounts of insulin were being prepared from pancreas. In Dodds' and Dickens' laboratory, work on the preparation of insulin was also in progress. In the laboratories where Fisher and Ashby, and Lundberg were studying, interest in the preparation and purification of insulin was being taken at the time the work referred to above was done. Although insulin clings tenaciously to laboratory glassware, etc., the usual cleaning procedures carefully applied are sufficient to remove the last traces. If contamination of solutions did occur, it is obviously impossible to make any rational suggestion concerning the mechanism.

It is regrettable that a great deal of what appears to be useless work has been done in this field. The results reported in this paper, in our opinion, serve to remove from serious consideration many reports which made it difficult to accept the pancreas as the only source and the only important storehouse of insulin in the animal body.

Summary

Using a method of extraction which yields maximal amounts of insulin from pancreas, we have been unable to demonstrate the presence of an anti-diabetic substance in other normal tissues from the dog or ox or in the tissues of diabetic dogs. Positive results previously reported we believe can be attributed to one or more of several factors, each of which is discussed in this communication. Certain experimental results which have indicated a wide distribution of an insulin-like substance in the plant kingdom have not been confirmed.

We have had the opportunity of discussing these results with Professor E. C. Dodds and Professor A. C. Ivy. These investigators have repeated certain of the experiments performed in their laboratories, the results of which suggested that insulin or an insulin-like substance could be obtained from mammalian tissues other than pancreas. The results of these recent experiments confirm the negative findings reported in this paper.

Many MIDDLE-AGED DIABETICS ARE overweight when their condition is first recognized. Further, the clinical improvement that follows even mild control of their dietary habits is well known. Whether the improvement is entirely due to altered caloric intake, or whether the composition of the diet can in some way affect the availability of insulin, is a question that has intrigued some clinicians. There are, of course, many other mechanisms by which this effect may be mediated. Paper 14 is a preliminary account of studies of the effect of diet on the insulin content of the pancreas of rats.

As I remember the initiation of the experimental work on the influence of diet and hormones on the amounts of insulin extractable from pancreas, our one-time colleague, E. T. Waters (now at the Institute of Physiology, Cardiff, Wales) was very interested in this problem and we had several discussions about it. Professor R. E. Haist has been the most active contributor to this field and his productive interest has been sustained for more than twenty years—ever since, after graduation from the Faculty of Medicine, he began work for his Ph.D. degree in the Department of Physiology. This is not the place to discuss Professor Haist's scientific contributions but it does give me an opportunity to record that his ability and devotion in the teaching of Physiology and our firm friendship have been important factors in permitting me to devote a large proportion of my time to problems of research.

14. Diet and the Insulin Content of Pancreas

C. H. BEST

R. E. HAIST

JESSIE H. RIDOUT

It is well known that fasting, or feeding diets rich in fat and poor in carbohydrate, leads to a change in the metabolism of sugar as judged by (1) the glucosuria following glucose administration, (2) the diabetic type of sugar tolerance curve when glucose is given, and (3) the absence of the normal rise in respiratory quotient after glucose administration. There is evidence that the administration of insulin at least partially restores the normal metabolism of carbohydrate. An excellent review of the relevant literature has recently been published by W. H. Chambers [185].

We have reported in a preliminary communication [349] that a very definite change in the insulin content of pancreas may be produced by alterations in diet. In order to investigate this subject it is necessary to have available (1) an experimental animal which will ingest the diets provided and one from which all the pancreatic tissue can be removed without undue difficulty; (2) an extraction procedure which consistently gives optimal yields of insulin from pancreatic tissue; and (3) a method of testing which gives accurate results when relatively small amounts of insulin are available. The first requirements are satisfied when the Wistar rat is used as the test animal. A suitable method for the extraction of insulin is that outlined by Jephcott [428] and by Scott and Fisher [686]. Satisfactory assays of the insulin content of the extracts are obtained by the mouse method of testing.

The results of these investigations which will now be described demonstrate, among other points, that a very definite decrease in the insulin content of pancreas is brought about by fasting or by the ingestion of diets rich in fat.

METHODS

In most of the experiments male rats weighing from 200 to 300 g were used. They were from 100 to 200 days old. In any one experiment the rats

Originally appeared in the *Journal of Physiology*, XCVII (1939), 107–19. From the Department of Physiology and the School of Hygiene, University of Toronto.

were from the same age group and the initial weights of each group of ten animals were equal. The rats were kept in individual cages. The diet for each animal was weighed and the uneaten residue was recovered and weighed daily. Unless otherwise stated, the food was removed 14 hrs before pancreatectomy. Each test solution was made from the pancreatic tissue of ten animals. The rats were usually anaesthetized by the intraperitoneal injection of a solution of "sodium amytal." All the pancreatic tissue was carefully dissected from the anaesthetized animals and added to the extraction fluid immediately after its removal. The extraction fluid was made by mixing 750 cc absolute alcohol, 250 cc distilled water, and 15 cc conc. HCl. Approximately 5–6 cc of this solution per gram of pancreas were used. The actual procedure for the preparation of the insulin-containing extract was as follows. The container with the required amount of extraction fluid was weighed before and after the addition of the pancreatic tissue. After the second weighing, the pancreas was thoroughly minced with scissors. The mixture was shaken at frequent intervals, allowed to stand overnight in the refrigerator, and was then filtered through cheesecloth. The solid material was pressed until nearly dry and re-extracted with the same volume of the acid solution. The mixture was allowed to stand for 2 hrs and was again filtered through cheesecloth. The two filtrates were combined, made just alkaline to litmus by addition of ammonium hydroxide and the total volume of the extract was measured. After filtering through Whatman no. 1 filter paper, five 9 cc aliquots were placed in 50 cc centrifuge thimbles. Fifteen cc of absolute alcohol and 25 cc of ether were then added to each thimble. These were placed in the refrigerator overnight. The next day the mixtures were centrifuged, the supernatant fluid discarded and the tubes drained. The precipitate in each tube was dissolved in isotonic saline (pH 2.5) and the solutions were combined and made up to a definite volume.

The potency of these solutions was estimated by the mouse method of assay. The procedure which we have followed was essentially the same as that described by Trevan and Boock [757] and by Trevan [756]. This test depends upon the relative number of mice convulsing when the standard and unknown solutions are administered under comparable conditions. The ratio of the potencies of the two solutions is obtained by reference to a standard curve. The characteristic dose-response curve for our mouse colony was obtained by injecting some 6000 mice with various dilutions of the standard solution. From 200 to 300 mice were used in assaying the potency of each extract. The animals were given dextrose as soon as convulsions appeared and those which recovered were used again after one week. For the most part, the insulin content of the pancreas is expressed in terms of units per group of ten rats and also as units per kg initial body weight of rats. Since the amount of pancreatic fat is so variable, it was thought that any expression based on pancreatic weight would be less reliable. However, where portions of a homogeneous mixture of pancreatic tissue are compared, as in the test of the method, results are expressed as units of insulin per gram of pancreatic tissue.

Assay of Pancreatic Tissue

It will be appreciated that the method of preparation of insulin used in these experiments provides us with a relatively crude material. Nevertheless, it is perfectly adequate for determinations of activity and further purification would probably involve a loss of potency. Jephcott [428] has shown that crude insulin added to minced pancreatic tissue can be recovered quantitatively by the extraction procedure we have used. This has been confirmed repeatedly by D. A. Scott in the Connaught Laboratories and by E. T. Waters in the Department of Physiology. It was decided that the best way to test our methods was to secure a homogeneous preparation of pancreatic tissue and conduct extractions and assays on weighed portions of this material. Two such preparations were used. Each was obtained by removing the pancreatic tissue from fifty rats. The first group consisted of normal animals, fasted overnight, while the second had been maintained for seven days on a diet consisting only of beef fat, agar, and vitamins A, B_1, and D. As each pancreas was removed it was dropped into liquid air and, when fifty had been collected, the tissue was ground to a very fine powder in a cooled mortar. The powder was thoroughly mixed and five aliquots were taken for extraction and assay. The results of these experiments, which are collected in Table 14.I, demonstrate the consistency of the findings under these conditions. No further comment is required here except that it may be stated that *the variations on which we have placed significance are*

TABLE 14.I

TEST OF THE METHOD

Control Diet			Fat Diet, 7 Days		
Aliquot No.	Weight of Aliquot of Pancreatic Tissue (g)	Units of Insulin per g of Pancreas	Aliquot No.	Weight of Aliquot of Pancreatic Tissue (g)	Units of Insulin per g of Pancreas
1	14.6	2.08	1	11.8	1.25
2	12.3	1.83	2	10.2	1.12
3	14.6	2.20	3	11.7	1.22
4	14.0	2.21	4	10.8	1.24
5	13.5	2.18	5	12.0	1.20
Average		2.10			1.21

far greater than any which could be expected to result from the errors inherent in the method of extraction and testing.

In practically all cases the solutions were tested on mice within a week after preparation. They were kept in the refrigerator during this interval. Tests have shown, moreover, that under these conditions the change in potency of the solution is barely appreciable when two weeks are allowed to elapse between extraction and test.

Effect of Anaesthesia

In order to determine the effect of certain anaesthetics upon the insulin content of pancreas, three groups of animals were studied. One group was anaesthetized with urethane, one with "sodium amytal," and the third was stunned. In each group half the rats were fasted overnight, and the other half were fasted for seven days. The length of time under anaesthesia was the same for the urethane and "sodium amytal" groups. In the stunned animals, the pancreas was removed immediately. The results in Table 14.II show that no significant difference exists between the insulin contents of the

TABLE 14.II

EFFECT OF ANAESTHESIA ON THE INSULIN CONTENT OF PANCREAS

		No. of Rats	Units of Insulin per Group of 10 Rats	Units of Insulin per kg of Initial Body Weight
Urethane	control	10	31.4	8.4
	fasted 7 days	10	16.6	4.4
Sodium amytal	control	10	28.8	7.7
	fasted 7 days	10	15.2	4.1
Stunned	control	10	31.4	8.4
	fasted 7 days	10	14.5	3.9

pancreatic tissue of the three groups of animals. Blood sugars were determined upon the groups receiving urethane and "sodium amytal" by the Shaffer-Somogyi method [695]. While the sugar content of the blood was definitely higher in the group which received urethane, this apparently produced no effect upon the insulin content of the pancreatic tissue. In most of the subsequent experiments "sodium amytal" was used as the anaesthetic.

Effect of Fasting

The effect of fasting on the insulin content of pancreas is shown in Table 14.III. The total number of fasted rats was 130, and 110 control animals were used. All the animals had previously received a well-balanced diet. The average loss in weight of the fasted animals was 23 per cent of the initial value. Since there was considerable variation in the initial weights

TABLE 14.III

EFFECT OF FASTING ON THE INSULIN CONTENT OF PANCREAS

	Units of Insulin per Group of 10 Rats		Units of Insulin per kg of Initial Body Weight	
No. of Rats	Fasted 7 days	Control	Fasted 7 days	Control
20	11.1	20.0	3.9	6.9
20	11.0	19.0	3.8	6.6
20	13.5	28.4	4.0	7.9
20	16.6	28.8	5.0	8.1
10	16.2	—	4.9	—
20	11.9	20.5	3.3	5.8
20	16.0	23.9	4.5	6.8
10	17.1	—	4.8	—
20	16.6	31.4	4.4	8.4
20	15.2	28.8	4.1	7.7
20	11.1	29.7	3.0	8.1
20	12.2	29.7	3.3	8.1
20	14.5	31.4	3.9	8.4
Average	14.1	26.5	4.1	7.5

of the different groups, it is best to compare the values for the starved and control animals in each individual experiment. It is evident from these figures that fasting produces a definite decrease in the insulin content of the pancreas.

Effect of Feeding Fat or Sugar

The results of an experiment designed to study this point are collected in Table 14.IV. In the first experiment one group of fifty rats ate the balanced diet and a similar group consumed the fat diet *ad libitum*. The definite fall in the insulin content of the pancreas of animals receiving a diet rich in fat is evident. In the second experiment a paired feeding test was conducted on two groups of thirty rats each. The value for the sugar-

TABLE 14.IV

EFFECT ON THE INSULIN CONTENT OF PANCREAS OF DIETS CONTAINING ONLY FAT OR SUGAR*

No. of Rats	Duration of Exp. Days	Loss in Weight (%)	Diet	Units of Insulin per Group of 10 Rats	Units of Insulin per kg of Initial Body Weight
50	7	3	balanced†	28.9	8.8
50	7	13	fat†	13.7	4.2
30	14	17	sugar‡	18.8	6.5
30	14	20	fat‡	10.9	3.8

*Fat or sugar actually constituted 90 per cent of the material given. Agar, salt mixture, and vitamins A, B₁, and D made up the remainder.
†Rats ate *ad lib*.
‡These two groups had the same caloric intake.

fed animals, 18.8 units of insulin per group of ten rats, is below the average value for normal animals, but the insulin content of fat-fed animals receiving the same caloric intake as those which received sugar is much lower than that of the sugar-fed group. A very important point emerges from a consideration of the latter results. The weight loss in the group which received sugar only was 17 per cent of the initial value, while that of the group receiving the same caloric intake in the form of fat was 20 per cent of the initial value. The initial weights of the two groups were the same at the start of the experiment. *These figures show that weight loss alone is not the factor which is responsible for the change in the insulin content of the pancreatic tissue.*

It may be remarked here that when animals are placed on diets composed only of sugar, protein, or fat, the insulin content of pancreas falls in all cases. However, the caloric intake in these groups is not normal. The animals which are provided with protein eat so little that undernutrition plays a large part in the results obtained. Even when this is involved, results of some preliminary experiments indicate quite definitely that the fall in insulin content is not as great in the group receiving protein as in the group where fat only is ingested. For example, in one series the control value was 31 units of insulin per group of ten animals, while the group which received sugar only gave a value of 22 units. In the protein-fed animals 18 units were present in the pancreatic tissue of ten rats, whereas those animals which received fat showed approximately 9 units per group.

In the first experiment described in Table 14.IV the animals on the diet rich in fat ate as much as they desired. The weight loss in this group was 13 per cent of the initial value after seven days. It will be noticed that the decrease in the insulin content was as great as in the group which had been starved for the same period (Table 14.III) although the loss of weight was not nearly so extensive.

In the second experiment described in Table 14.IV the animals receiving sugar and those ingesting fat were fed in pairs so that each group had an equivalent caloric intake. The sugar-fed group ingested 11.6 g per day which provided 41.8 Cal. The group receiving the fat diet ate 4.8 g per day which was equivalent to 38.9 Cal. The loss of weight in the two groups is comparable but, as noted above, the insulin content of the pancreas of the two groups is quite different. These results, in addition to showing the fall in insulin content which occurs when diets rich in fat are used, demonstrate that carbohydrate tends to prevent the decrease.

Effect of Various Diets in Fasted Animals

In this experiment all the animals were starved for 7 days. They were then divided into various groups and placed on different diets. Three

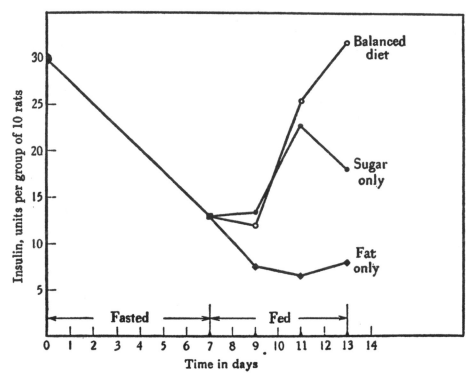

FIGURE 27. Diet and the insulin content of pancreas.

groups received sugar only, three fat only, and three were given a balanced diet. All the rations provided approximately the same caloric intake and this was based on the food consumption of the carbohydrate-fed group. Groups were killed on the 2nd, 4th, and 6th days. The insulin content of the pancreas was determined and the results are shown in Figure 27. It will be quite evident that feeding fat alone does not lead to a restoration of the insulin content. On the contrary, there appears to be a significant further drop. Sugar alone leads to a return towards the normal value, while the adequate diet results in a complete restoration of the normal value within 6 days. At the end of 2 days, however, there was no indication of recovery. The results of this experiment furnish further evidence that loss of body weight may not be an important factor in the decrease in the insulin content of pancreatic tissue. Several sets of figures which illustrate this point are given in Figure 28.

Effect of Diets Moderately Rich in Carbohydrate and Fat

In order to determine whether or not a diet *moderately* rich in fat would exert an effect on the insulin content of pancreas over longer periods of

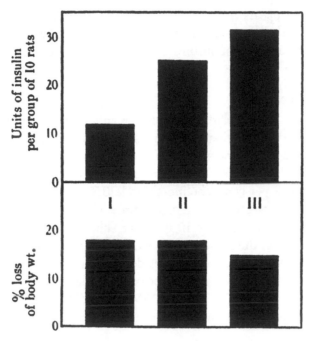

FIGURE 28. Following a fast of 7 days, a balanced diet
was fed for: I, 2 days; II, 4 days; III, 6 days.

time, a diet containing 28 per cent carbohydrate, 15 per cent protein, and
46 per cent fat by weight was provided. The diet high in carbohydrate
contained 69 per cent carbohydrate, 15 per cent protein, and 5 per cent fat.
The control diet consisted of 50 per cent carbohydrate, 18 per cent protein,
and 16 per cent fat. These diets contained a salt mixture, yeast, and cod-
liver oil. The results of these experiments are summarized in Table 14.V.

TABLE 14.V

EFFECT OF MODERATELY HIGH FAT AND CARBOHYDRATE DIETS
ON THE INSULIN CONTENT OF PANCREAS

No. of Rats	Diet	Duration of Exp. Months	Average Weight per Group of 10 Rats		Units of Insulin per Group of 10 Rats
			Initial g	Final g	
30	control	2	1043	2345	26.7
30	fat	2	1033	2373	20.1
60	control	6	955	2661	29.9
59	fat	6	959	2618	23.3
30	control	3	737	2525	25.3
30	carbohydrate	3	655	2246	23.9
18	control	7	691	3337	25.0
67	carbohydrate	7	613	2347	24.9

While there appears to be a decrease in the insulin content when the animals are fed the diet moderately rich in fat, the findings do not suggest that extensive depletion of insulin could be rapidly produced by diets of this type.

Vitamin B₁ Deficiency

While we are contemplating a thorough investigation of the effects of deficiency of the various vitamins, our results thus far are confined entirely to a study of the lack of vitamin B_1. The diet was made up of beef muscle powder 10 per cent, beef fat 20 per cent, sucrose 62.7 per cent, salt mixture 5 per cent, agar 2 per cent, choline chloride 0.3 per cent, and vitamins A and D in the form of cod-liver oil concentrate. One group received 16μg of crystalline vitamin B_1 for every 10 g of diet. The rats in the first group ate freely while those in the second group were given the same amount of food as the animals which received the diet deficient in vitamin B_1 During the first 2 weeks 16.5 μg of vitamin B_1 per rat per day were ingested, in the third week 10.9 μg, and in the fourth week 7.5 μg were ingested. The results of the insulin determinations are given in Table 14.VI and show

TABLE 14.VI

VITAMIN B₁ DEFICIENCY AND THE INSULIN CONTENT OF PANCREAS

No. of Rats	Diet	Units of Insulin per Group of 10 Rats	Units of Insulin per kg of Initial Body Weight
29	B₁ deficient	12.0	9.4
29	B₁ added	13.4	10.5

that, while in both the control and the test group there is a very definite decrease in the insulin content as compared with normal animals, the addition of vitamin B_1 had no effect. Presumably the decrease was due, in large part, to deficient caloric intake. These results are being extended.

Liver Fat and the Insulin Content of Pancreas

In some of the experiments in which diets rich in fat were fed, the rats developed fatty livers. It was therefore considered advisable to determine whether or not fatty changes in the liver might be associated with a change in the insulin content of pancreas. We had the opportunity to conduct tests on the pancreatic tissue from (1) rats poisoned with carbon tetrachloride, (2) rats poisoned with carbon tetrachloride and given choline, and (3) control rats receiving the same diet as those in the first group and a similar caloric intake. The results in Figure 29 show clearly that the insulin content of the pancreas is not affected under these conditions

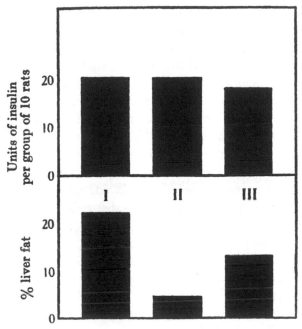

FIGURE 29. I, Animals poisoned with carbon tetrachloride; II, animals poisoned with carbon tetrachloride but receiving choline; III, control animals receiving same caloric intake as group I.

when extensive changes in liver fat have occurred. Further details of these experiments are given in a paper by Barrett, Best, MacLean and Ridout [52].

GENERAL DISCUSSION

It is obvious that the altered carbohydrate metabolism observed in starvation or as a result of feeding diets rich in fat might be produced by factors affecting the production of sugar, the rate of utilization, or both. Factors affecting the production of sugar in the liver or the rate of utilization in the tissues might act directly on these structures, or might exert their effects through one or more of the endocrine glands. At present there are very few facts available which enable one to decide which of these mechanisms are in operation. Our results show conclusively that in rats one definite finding is present under these conditions, namely, that there is a decrease in the insulin content of pancreatic tissue.

In many of the experiments reported the loss of body weight was considerable. In all the experiments, however, the change in insulin content of the pancreas was definitely greater than that which might be expected merely from loss of weight if one makes the unjustifiable assumption that the insulin-producing tissue shares equally with the other tissues in this loss. The exact weight of the pancreatic tissue in rats is difficult to determine since the amount of fat closely associated with the pancreas may vary. *In the experiments where food was administered after fasting, the weight loss still remained extensive even in those animals whose pancreas showed a recovery of the normal insulin content* (Figure 28).

The insulin content of the pancreas represents a balance between the rates of production and liberation of the hormone. A lowered insulin content such as we have observed after fasting or fat feeding may therefore be due to either diminished production or increased liberation or both.

Although no work has yet been done in our laboratory on the glucose tolerance of starved rats, or of rats fed on a diet rich in fat, it would appear from the results of other investigators on other species that the impaired carbohydrate tolerance occurs at a time when, in the light of our experiments, a decrease in the insulin content of the pancreas would be expected. As stated previously, the normal carbohydrate metabolism is partially restored by the administration of insulin (Cori and Cori [224; 230]; Dann and Chambers [246]; Ellis [281]). Since the diminished carbohydrate tolerance in starvation and after feeding fat may be explained, in part at least, on the basis of decreased liberation of insulin, it would seem logical to assume that the low insulin content of pancreas which we have observed is caused by decreased formation rather than by increased liberation of insulin.

While no general relationship between the insulin content of the pancreas and the rate of insulin liberation has been established, there are experimental results which indicate that the liberation is related to the insulin content under certain conditions. It has been shown, for example, that in the permanent diabetes produced in dogs by the administration of anterior pituitary extracts, the insulin content of the pancreas is reduced to extremely low values (Campbell and Best [163]). Furthermore, in many diabetic patients the results obtained by Scott and Fisher [687] show very clearly that the insulin content of the pancreas is reduced well below the normal value. In these cases in which the insulin content of the pancreas is low the organism suffers from severe diabetes and is favourably affected by small doses of insulin. Under these circumstances it is reasonable to suppose that the low insulin content leads to a reduced rate of liberation. There is certainly no evidence at present that there is an increased rate of liberation and that the effect of this is overbalanced by opposing factors. On the other hand, in those clinical cases suffering from liberation of excessive amounts of insulin, i.e. hyperinsulinism, it has been established that the tumours of islet tissue may contain abnormally large amounts of the hormone. For example, in one of the recent cases reported by Campbell, Graham, and Robinson [165] in which D. A. Scott estimated the insulin content of the tumour, the concentration of insulin was 8 units per gram. The patient suffered from a very definite hyperinsulinism which was alleviated by removal of the tumour.

We have merely cited evidence which suggests that under certain conditions there is a relationship between the insulin content of pancreas and the rate of insulin liberation. It is quite possible that under other conditions this relationship may not hold or may be completely obscured by compensatory physiological adjustments. We are postponing a full discussion of the significance of our findings until further studies on the insulin content of pancreas have been made. It may be mentioned here, however, that research along this line will certainly throw further light on such problems as the mechanism of the effect of the undernutrition treatment of diabetes (Allen, Stillman, and Fitz [10]), the role of dietary substances in the aetiology of diabetes (Himsworth [391]), the influence of obesity on the diabetic state (Newburgh, Conn, Johnston, and Conn [597]), and the use of diets very rich in fat in the treatment of hyperinsulinism.

SUMMARY AND CONCLUSIONS

(1) Fasting or the feeding of diets rich in fat produces a very definite decrease in the insulin content of the pancreas. (2) While an abnormally low caloric intake may be one of the factors producing this result in the animals given the diet rich in fat, it is not the only one, since those receiving a certain caloric intake as fat show a much greater decrease in insulin content than those provided with the same caloric intake in the form of carbohydrate. (3) The insulin content of the pancreas, depleted by fasting, is restored within 6 days to a normal value by feeding a well-balanced diet. Carbohydrate alone effects a partial restoration but fat produces no rise in insulin content. (4) The results of preliminary studies on the effect of (a) short periods of anaesthesia and (b) vitamin B₁ deficiency do not suggest that these conditions affect the insulin content of the pancreas in a specific manner. (5) The possible relationship between the low insulin content of the pancreas and the altered carbohydrate metabolism of animals which have been fasted or fed diets rich in fat is discussed.

ANOTHER OF MY PH.D. STUDENTS IN *Physiology, Gerald A. Wrenshall, came to us with a Ph.D. in Atomic Physics. He has a personal interest in insulin which he has repaid by contributing extensively to our knowledge of the hormone. Professor W. Stanley Hartroft, certainly one of my most successful students and colleagues, will be mentioned frequently in the reports describing the choline work, but he also has an abiding and very productive interest in insulin. In Paper 15 the results of Wrenshall's and Hartroft's study of certain aspects of spontaneous diabetes in dogs and in man, are presented. In Paper 16 Professor Wrenshall and I review another problem in which a knowledge of extractable insulin in human pancreas enabled certain predictions to be made about the type of case in which the sulphonylureas would be useful.*

15. Insulin Extractable from the Pancreas and Islet Cell Histology

COMPARATIVE STUDIES IN SPONTANEOUS DIABETES IN DOGS AND HUMAN SUBJECTS

GERALD A. WRENSHALL, PH.D.

W. STANLEY HARTROFT, M.D., PH.D.

CHARLES H. BEST, M.D., D.SC.

The characteristics of diabetes mellitus in man have long been compared, either directly or by inference, with those of diabetes produced in animals by experimental means. From the earliest studies in this field by von Mering and Minkowski [561], in the work leading to the discovery of insulin [40] (1921), and in many later investigations, the dog has occupied a prominent and productive place among experimental animals. In recent years, special aspects of the spontaneous diabetes of dogs have come under study of this laboratory and in that of Professor Henry Ricketts in Chicago.

It is the purpose of this paper to examine the available data to determine the degree to which the spontaneous and the experimentally induced diabetes mellitus of dogs correspond with each other and with the spontaneous diabetes mellitus of man, in terms of the insulin extractable from the pancreas and the histological state of the islands of Langerhans. The relationship of these factors to the diabetic state with which they are associated will also be considered.

MATERIALS AND METHODS

To the best of our knowledge, measurement of the insulin of the pancreas from dogs with spontaneous diabetes is currently limited to eleven cases. Four pancreases from such diabetic dogs were extracted and assayed by us for Dr. Ricketts, while the remaining seven represent subjects from our

Originally appeared in *Diabetes*, III (1954), 444–52. Presented in part at the Nineteenth International Physiological Congress, Montreal, August 30, 1953.

Nine figures showing histological material have been omitted.

own series which have come to autopsy. These were obtained through interested veterinarians and medical men during the past seven years. In four cases the owners did not wish to retain the diabetic dogs as pets. These were killed by intravenous nembutal at the owners' request following periods of laboratory study of eight, ten, twenty-one, and thirty-eight days, respectively.

In another four cases the dogs were returned to their owners with typed instruction sheets following initial two-week periods of adjustment to a measured diet and protamine-zinc insulin. Arrangements were made to readjust diet and insulin dosage for these animals every three months, with autopsy to be held at the laboratory in case of death. While this course of events entails certain experimental hazards, it was adopted since it approximates that to which many diabetic subjects are exposed, and thus establishes a closer parallel between the courses of the spontaneous diabetes of dogs and of man. Data on the insulin of the human pancreas, with which corresponding values for diabetic dogs are compared, have been collected concurrently with those for the diabetic dogs.

The acid alcohol method of Scott and Fisher [686] was used for the extraction of insulin from the pancreas for both human and canine subjects. Estimations of the insulin concentration in such extracts were made, using a mouse convulsion method of assay, meeting the requirements recommended by Bliss [130] for this type of assay.

Sections from the body of each pancreas were taken for histology. These were placed in Bouin's fixative for twelve to sixteen hours. A variety of staining procedures was applied, but those of greatest importance in the present study were Gomori's [326] hematoxylin and phloxine, and Wilson's [807] modification of his aldehyde and fuchsin, which stains beta cell granules a deep purple against a pale green background.

Complete autopsies were performed on all animals, and blocks both for paraffin and frozen sectioning were taken from kidneys, livers, and hearts, and only for paraffin sections from the thyroid, adrenal, pituitary, gonads, and spleen. Frozen sections were stained by Wilson's modification of Lillie's supersaturated Isopropanol Oil Red O technique. Paraffin sections were stained with hematoxylin and eosin and by a variety of methods to demonstrate selected tissues.

Results

Characteristics of the eight dogs of the present series with spontaneous diabetes mellitus are included in Table 15.I. Of these only two were male. One female and one male dog were spayed as pups. The seven of these eight dogs which have come to autopsy varied in age at death between

TABLE 15.I

CHARACTERISTICS OF DOGS WITH SPONTANEOUS DIABETES MELLITUS

General	D-WA	D-CO	D-JU	D-SU	D-LA	D-BO	D-MI	D-DA
Sex	M (spayed)	M	F	F (spayed)	F	F	F	F
Breed	Spitz-Pomeranian	Spaniel	Mongrel	Wire-haired Terrier	Irish Setter	Wire-haired Terrier	Mongrel	Greyhound
Nose to rump distance (cm)	65	74	60	63	103	63	69	96
At admission								
Blood sugar (mg per 100 cc)	300	—	183	340	130	175	192	238
Urine sugar	(positive)	5%	1%	2%	4%	0.2%	5%	5%
Ketonuria	(positive)	—	4+	3+	trace	0	4+	4+
During diabetes therapy								
P.Z. insulin (u/day/kg)	1.3	1.5	2.1	2.0	0.5 later 1.3	2.9	2.7	1.1
Duration (months)	3	18	1.3	1.7	4.8	13	0.8	1.2
At death								
Bilateral cataracts	0	4+	2+	0	1+	0	2+	4+
Condition at death	diabetic coma	intussusception	killed	killed	vaginal infection, pneumonia	living	killed	killed
Age (years)	6.5	8.5	(9)	5.2	8.3	3.3	7	9.6
Body wt. (kg)	8.8	13.6	6.7	10.8	22.5	6.8	10.4	22.9
Pancreas wt. (g)	25 (fatty)	20	27	4.8	47	( )	10	88.3
Extractable insulin Units/kg. body wt.	0.14	0.16*	0.35	0.09	0.16	living	under 0.06	0.25
% of nondiabetic av.	2.9	3.4	7.3	1.9	3.4	—	under 1.3	5.2

*Biopsy.

5.2 and 9.6 years (average 7.7 years). The surviving dog, while mature, is by far the youngest member of the series (3.1 years).

The development of diabetes was preceded by overweight in at least four out of eight of the cases, and was followed by marked weight loss in all cases. In two of the obese dogs, the pancreatic duct was blocked at autopsy and the pancreas had become reduced to a fibrotic remnant. In the other four, the pancreases did not appear abnormal in size or texture, except that in one dog (D-WA) there was fatty degeneration. An active thyroid tumour weighing 86 g was removed surgically from the neck of one of the two male dogs of the series (D-CO); following its removal, the severity of the diabetes was decreased. The relationship, if any, of these factors to the etiology of the diabetes remains inferential at the present time.

Fasting blood sugar concentrations before start of diet and insulin therapy varied between 130 and 346 mg per 100 cc. The lowest of these values was observed in a bitch (D-LA) which showed a negative test for urinary ketone bodies on admission, and which later required nearly three times as much insulin to control the diabetes. At autopsy, no islet cells could be found in the histologic sections of pancreas from this animal. Except for the negative tests obtained for this dog shortly after diagnosis of the diabetes, urine samples from all of the spontaneously diabetic dogs were positive for ketone bodies when insulin therapy was discontinued for two days. Bornstein and Lawrence [140] have reported that ketosis in diabetic human subjects occurs in association with low levels of blood insulin.

Observations on the insulin extractable from pancreas and the abundance and granulation in the beta cells of the islets of Langerhans from the spontaneously diabetic dogs are shown in Table 15.II, together with the histologic observations on four dogs reported by Ricketts and his associates [640].

With the exception of three dogs which were autopsied within one month of the diagnosis of diabetes, few or no beta cells were found in the histologic section of the pancreas and, where found, the abundance of beta cell granulation was very low. Correspondingly, all values for the extractable insulin of the pancreas in dogs autopsied after the one-month interval were extremely low, as indeed were the values in most of those which were autopsied before this time.

A comparable situation was found to exist when a similar chart of extractable insulin and beta cell histology was drawn up for fourteen human subjects whose diabetes had been diagnosed during the normal period of body growth (roughly the first two decades of life). Here again the islets of Langerhans of some of the subjects with newly diagnosed diabetes

TABLE 15.II

SPONTANEOUS DIABETES IN MATURE DOGS

Extractable Insulin of Pancreas and Islet Beta Cell Frequency and
Granulation Compared with Duration of Treated Spontaneous
Diabetes Mellitus in Mature Dogs

Known Duration of Diabetes (months)	Insulin Extractable from Pancreas % of Control	Abundance of Beta Cells	Abundance of Granulation
		(++++ normal)	
0 to 1	<3	++	0
	7	+++	+
	<1	++++	+
	>25	++	+
	2	++	+
	>4	++++	+
1 to 2	3	++	+
	0.3		
4	1	0	0
6	3	++	+
8	0	++	+
18	3	++	

TABLE 15.III

TREATED GROWTH-ONSET DIABETES IN MAN

Extractable Insulin of Pancreas and Islet Beta Cell Frequency and
Granulation Compared with Duration of Treated Growth-Onset
Diabetes Mellitus in Man

Known Duration of Diabetes (months)	Insulin Extractable from Pancreas % of Control	Abundance of Beta Cells	Abundance of Granulation
		(++++ normal)	
0 to 1	<4	++++	++
	88	++++	++
	2	++	0
	1	++	++
	2	++	+
	2	++	+
3	5	+	++
11	6	0	0
13	0.7	+	+
15 to 16	5	++	+
	5	++	0
	1	0	0
17	0.8	++	++
20	0.5	+	+
22	2	+	+

mellitus were found to have appreciable numbers of beta cells but with
scant and poorly granulated cytoplasm. In none of those subjects whose
diabetes had been diagnosed for more than a year were the extractable
insulin, number of beta cells, or abundance of beta cell granulation found
to be above trace levels (Table 15.III).

In human subjects with diabetes of the growth-onset type, as well as in the spontaneously diabetic dogs of our series, depletion of beta cells appears to precede loss of alpha cells to some degree, but eventually both types of cells may become so scarce that it is difficult to locate and identify any islet cells in histologic sections of pancreas from such long-term diabetic subjects.

Lesions in organs other than the pancreas encountered at autopsy are summarized for all seven dogs in Table 15.IV. Only brief mention of findings of special interest will be made here. In dog ju, frozen sections of the kidneys presented a striking picture. The glomerular capsules, as well as the spaces of Bowman within the glomeruli, were filled with masses of stainable fat. In a few glomeruli fat could be seen within the lumina of the glomerular capillaries. The basement membranes of the proximal convoluted tubules in this dog's kidneys were coated with intensely sudanophilic fat. The fat had precipitated on the fibrils of the tubular basement membrane.

The kidneys of dog su were perhaps of even more interest than were the kidneys of the preceding animal. The glomeruli of these kidneys exhibited lesions which closely simulated those of intercapillary diabetic glomerulosclerosis in an early stage. Focal lesions were observed in a small percentage of the glomeruli. In frozen sections of this kidney, lipid plugs could be demonstrated within the glomerular capillaries in the regions of these lesions.

Stainable fat was present in the tubules of nearly all kidneys examined in the series with the exception of dog DAV and dog MI. The fat was confined in most instances to the cells in the walls of the descending portions of the cortical tubules. In two animals, however, D-CO and D-LA, stainable fat was present not only in these portions of the tubules, but also in the convoluted portions of the proximal loops. Abnormal deposits of glycogen were not encountered in tubules of any of the kidneys of the dogs.

In four of the six animals abundant amounts of fat had accumulated in their livers, and in one of the remaining two animals there was a slight trace of liver fat. In every instance in which stainable fat was present in the animals' livers, the distribution of the lipid was centrolobular or nonportal. In one animal only, D-CO, early fibrosis, as well as fat in nonportal regions of the liver, was encountered. Hearts that were examined in this series were not remarkable, with the exception of dogs D-LA and D-DAV. In dog D-LA, fatty degeneration, necrosis, and calcification of heart muscle constituted prominent features. Nearly every cardiac muscle fibre in this animal was swollen with stainable fat droplets. Scattered throughout were focal areas of cardiac necrosis in which inflammatory cell infiltration had occurred with lysis of muscle and calcification of the necrotic debris. The

TABLE 15.IV

SUMMARY OF HISTOLOGIC FINDINGS IN THE TISSUES OF SPONTANEOUSLY DIABETIC DOGS

	D-CO	D-JU	D-SU	D-LA	D-DAV	D-MI
Pancreas						
No. of islets	very scarce	not scarce	very scarce	none found	scarce	very scarce, hyalinized
Beta cell granulation	almost none	almost none	almost none	none	almost none	none
Beta and duct cell hydropic (glycogen) vacuolation	present	present	present	—	present	—
Fat	fatty	normal	normal	normal	normal	fibrosis++
Kidneys						
Glomerular	many fat droplets	capsular and capillary loop fat	capsular and capillary loop fat, glomerulosclerosis	normal except for fat	capsule thickening; fat in capsular space	fat emboli, early glomerulosclerosis
Tubular fat	present in both loops	present in distal loop only	present in distal loop	normal except for fat	little	normal
Liver						
Fat	marked fat vacuolation, early non-portal fibrosis	severe centrolobular fatty change	slight to moderate centrolobular liver fat	uniformly distributed fat, centrolobular congestion	normal (little fat)	centrolobular fat, fatty cysts
Glycogen	abundant	normal	normal	normal	—	normal
Heart	normal	normal	normal	fatty degeneration and necrosis	fat infiltration, coronary artery thickening	coronary artery narrowing
Thyroid	absent	normal	normal	normal	normal	normal
Adrenals	normal	normal	normal	normal	normal	normal
Pituitary body	normal	eosinophils prominent	eosinophils prominent	normal	eosinophils prominent	normal (calcification)
Arteries	normal	normal	normal	normal	normal	aortic, coronary, pancreatic, and renal arteriosclerosis
Spleen	normal	normal	normal	normal	normal	normal

heart of dog D-DAV contained a small amount of stainable fat and a few focal areas of fibrosis, but lesions were not nearly so advanced or widespread as in dog D-LA.

In only one animal, D-MI, were degenerative arterial lesions demonstrated. In this dog, lesions identical with those seen in human atheroma were encountered in the aorta, in the coronary arteries, in the renal vessels, and in the pancreatic arteries. These lesions consisted of subintimal and intimal thickening with deposits of fat and cholesterol in the affected portions. The underlying media had frequently undergone degeneration, fibrosis, and focal areas of calcification. In every site, these changes were indistinguishable from those of atheromatous degeneration in comparable arteries of man.

Although this series of animals does not include examination of a comparable number of control dogs that had experienced environmental conditions similar to those of the diabetic animals, nevertheless the occurrence of lesions in the kidney of one animal that resembled diabetic glomerulosclerosis in man and the presence of advanced atheromatous change in the arteries of another dog are of considerable interest. Similar glomerular lesions were seen in one of the four dogs studied by Ricketts and his associates [640], but these authors did not encounter true atheroma. Stainable fat plugs obstructing flow of blood through glomerular capillaries in dog SU suggests that the pathogenesis of this type of lesion may be the same as we have observed in choline-deficient rats and diabetic man (Hartroft [370]). We have described the stages through which glomeruli pass in choline-deficient rats in the development of lesions that closely simulate glomerulosclerosis in diabetic man. The lesions in the rat were initiated by lipid plugs in the glomerular vessels. Lipid plugs of a similar nature were found in 75 per cent of diabetic patients with Kimmelstiel-Wilson lesions. The evidence provided by the sections of kidney of dog SU suggests that the focal glomerular changes in this animal may have a similar pathogenesis.

The most consistent finding throughout the entire series in organs other than the pancreas was deposition of stainable fat in a variety of organs including the liver, heart, and kidney. It may be significant that deposition of abnormal amounts of fat in these organs and their sequelae (hepatic fibrosis, cardiac necrosis and fibrosis, intercapillary glomerulosclerosis) are all seen in varying degree in choline-deficient rats, spontaneously diabetic dogs, and diabetic man. Although choline deficiency in itself undoubtedly plays little role in either spontaneous canine or human diabetics, it is perhaps more than coincidence that similar lesions are seen in all three conditions. There is undoubtedly, common to all, a disturbance in the metabolism and transport of fat.

Discussion

The early progressive and profound loss of insulin-producing cells from the pancreas in the spontaneous diabetes of mature dogs and of human subjects with growth-onset diabetes reported here corresponds with other available published observations. Schlotthauer and Millar [673] and Ricketts and his associates [640] have surveyed the literature in English on the spontaneous diabetes of dogs, while Hjärre [394] has done so for German publications. In all papers, the close association between the presence of diabetes and degenerative changes in the islets of Langerhans is emphasized. In two of the cases reviewed, diabetic dogs were kept alive for a time before necropsy with diet and insulin. In one case islets were reported to be scarce and very small; in the other, none could be found.

The observed pattern of change with time in the extractable insulin of the pancreas and islet beta cell histology of the spontaneously diabetic dog parallels closely that described by Haist, Campbell, and Best [347] following injection of a diabetogenic anterior pituitary extract in dogs. During the first few days of injection a reversible type of diabetes mellitus associated with degranulation of the islet beta cells and a profound fall in the extractable insulin of pancreas was observed. This condition was followed within a month or so by the disappearance of most or all of the beta cells, and the extractable insulin of the pancreas was then associated with a permanent or metadiabetic state. Since the islet beta cells regularly associated with insulin production are found to be absent from the pancreas in the permanent phases of experimental diabetes in the dog, it is reasonable to conclude, as the above authors did, that the very low levels of extractable insulin of the pancreas regularly associated with them reflect a correspondingly low rate of production of endogenous insulin.

The validity of this interpretation is borne out by the experiments of Houssay and his associates, who demonstrated that the pancreases from dogs with either permanent pituitary diabetes (seven out of seven tested) or permanent alloxan diabetes (six of six tested) had lost most or all of their normal functional capacity to lower the blood sugar of the twenty- to forty-eight-hour depancreatized dog. The islets of Langerhans of such metadiabetic dogs were found to have effectively lost all beta cells when examined histologically 22–144 days after precipitation of the diabetic state (Houssay, Foglia, Smyth, Rietti and Houssay [402]; Houssay, Brignone, and Mazzocco [401]).

One of the most convincing pieces of evidence concerning the nature of growth-onset diabetes in human subjects was presented by Rao and Jackson

[628]. Not only did they find that all of their series of forty-eight subjects required insulin to control their diabetes, but they found also that, within a year of its diagnosis, the amount of insulin required per day to maintain control and normal growth fell into a regular pattern, which increased with the age of the subject until the growth period was passed. This phenomenon would be observed if the endogenous supply of insulin in such subjects were negligible compared with their insulin requirement; that is, if they were "near-total" diabetics in so far as endogenous insulin supply is concerned. It also indicates that no pronounced dispersion in insulin requirement is caused in such subjects by endocrine factors other than insulin.

While the course of spontaneous and experimental diabetes in dogs appears comparable with that in the growth-onset type of diabetes of man in so far as the insulin and beta cells of the pancreas are concerned, it should be emphasized that the spontaneous canine diabetes occurred in *grown* animals in all but one of the seventy-one published cases of which we know.

In a majority of human subjects in whom diabetes mellitus was diagnosed following completion of skeletal growth (maturity-onset diabetes), the situation is quite different. Although the extractable insulin of the pancreas was found to be very low in some of these subjects, it amounts *on the average* to nearly 50 per cent of that found in the nondiabetic controls (Wrenshall, Bogoch, and Ritchie [815]). This is more than twenty times as high as the average found in human subjects with growth-onset diabetes of more than one year's duration. The abundance of islet beta cell granulation, estimated from histologic sections independent of insulin assay values, is found to be correspondingly elevated in the maturity-onset diabetic subjects (Hartroft and Wrenshall [376; 377]). In sharp contrast to the disappearance, within one year of diagnosis, of almost all beta cells and extractable insulin from the pancreas of the human subject with growth-onset diabetes and the dog with spontaneous maturity-onset diabetes, little tendency for these factors to change with duration of diabetes was seen in the human subject with maturity-onset diabetes (Wrenshall, Bogoch, and Ritchie [815]).

The insulin of the pancreas and islet histology in the obese-hyperglycaemic syndrome of mice (Mayer, Bates, and Dickie [559]) is currently being investigated in relation to this group of diabetic human subjects.

SUMMARY

In terms of the insulin of pancreas and the histology of the islet beta cells, the spontaneous diabetes mellitus of mature dogs and the diabetes of the growth-onset type in human subjects run parallel courses which correspond with that seen in the dog following the initiation of experimental diabetes by anterior pituitary extracts or by partial pancreatectomy.

This course is observed to be one of progressive and profound loss of beta cells and of the extractable insulin of the pancreas within relatively short times after onset of diabetes. It is in sharp contrast with the situation found in a majority of human subjects with maturity-onset diabetes, where pancreatic insulin and beta cell granulation are much more abundant and show little tendency to change with duration of the diabetes.

Lesions in organs other than the pancreas are briefly described and discussed, with emphasis on the kidney, heart and liver in the spontaneously diabetic dog.

ACKNOWLEDGMENTS

The authors are grateful to those owners and veterinary doctors whose understanding and co-operation have made this study possible. They wish to acknowledge the co-operation of Dr. A. L. Chute, Dr. W. L. Donohue, and their associates of the Hospital for Sick Children, Toronto, in the collection of the clinical and pathological data relating to diabetes mellitus arising in children.

It is a pleasure to acknowledge the technical aid and skill of Mr. W. D. Wilson, both at autopsies and in the subsequent histochemical treatment of tissues, and of Misses Isabell Jasper and Patricia Dolan.

16. Extractable Insulin of the Pancreas and Effectiveness of Oral Hypoglycaemic Sulphonylureas in the Treatment of Diabetes in Man—A Comparison

G. A. WRENSHALL, M.A., M.SC., PH.D.

C. H. BEST, M.D., D.SC., F.R.S.

The effectiveness of 1-butyl-3-p-aminobenzene-sulphonylurea (BZ-55, U-6987, carbutamide) and 1-butyl-3-p-tolylsulphonylurea (U-2043, orinase) in lowering the blood glucose level and the excretion of glucose in the urine of some but not all diabetic human subjects has been reported [67; 309] and confirmed [457; 564; 568]. The positive response to these sulphonylureas of some but not all diabetic subjects has been interpreted in terms of the presence or absence of a significant supply of endogenous insulin, the effectiveness of which, if present, is restored or enhanced by the sulphonylurea therapy [67; 309; 570].

The purpose of this paper is twofold: (1) to indicate what patterns of association can be demonstrated between the amount of insulin extractable at autopsy from diabetic human pancreas on the one hand and the factors of age at diagnosis of diabetes, known duration of diabetes, and insulin therapy on the other; (2) to compare the frequency of successes and failures in the reduction of blood and urine sugar levels in diabetic human subjects towards normal levels by oral sulphonylurea therapy with the respective frequencies of occurrence of appreciable or negligible reserves of insulin in the pancreas of other diabetic human subjects at autopsy.

Such comparisons are made between different groups of subjects rather than within the same subject or subjects. However, since studies of the latter type are not currently available, the present comparisons are of importance in evaluating an unproven hypothesis, namely, that the effectiveness of the oral sulphonylureas in restoring blood and urine sugar levels

Originally appeared in the *Canadian Medical Association Journal*, LXXIV (1956), 968–72.

towards normal in diabetic man not receiving insulin is dependent on an appreciable although limited supply of endogenous insulin. It is apparent that this hypothesis should be evaluated *prior* to the widespread clinical use of oral sulphonylureas or related compounds in the treatment of diabetes mellitus.

MATERIALS AND METHODS

The observations on the insulin extractable from the pancreas are based on totals of 72 male and 86 female diabetic human subjects, studied individually. Results on 69 of these subjects have been reported elsewhere [815; 817]. The standardized procedures used in the extraction and assay of the insulin obtained from the subjects of the full series have been described [814; 815]. All values for the amount of insulin extractable from the pancreas are expressed as units of insulin per kg body weight at autopsy, while comparisons with levels of extractable insulin in non-diabetic subjects are made using average values for unselected groups of non-diabetic male and female subjects in whom the pancreas was extracted and assayed in the same survey [815].

To facilitate comparisons, measurements on the extractable insulin of diabetic human pancreas at autopsy are illustrated in forms similar to those used by others in reporting the responses of living diabetic human subjects to oral sulphonylurea therapy.

RESULTS AND DISCUSSION

Using a graphic system introduced by Mirsky (personal communication), the individual amounts of insulin extractable from the pancreas in diabetic human subjects are plotted vertically as functions of the age at diagnosis of diabetes, and of its duration until death, in Figure 30. Where the extractable insulin amounted to less than 0.2 unit per kg body weight (that is, to less than about 6 per cent of the average for non-diabetic adult human subjects), the values are shown as empty circles.

The pattern of consistently low levels reported previously [817] for the insulin extractable from the pancreas in subjects surviving more than a year after diagnosis of diabetes during the normal period of growth can be easily seen in Figure 30. The previously reported presence of appreciable amounts of extractable insulin in the pancreases of many subjects with onset of diabetes at maturity, even after many years of treated diabetes, can also be seen.

The least squares plane of best fit correlating age at diagnosis (A) and duration of life thereafter (D), on the one hand, and the amount of

EXTRACTABLE INSULIN OF THE PANCREAS IN MALE AND FEMALE DIABETIC HUMAN SUBJECTS

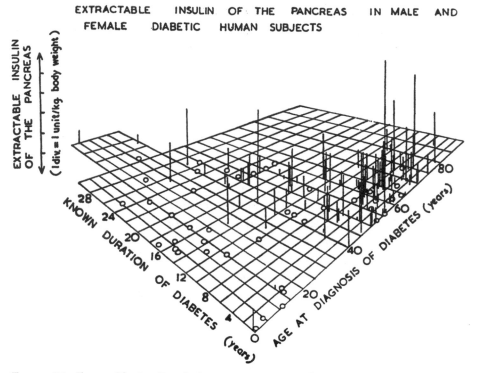

FIGURE 30. Extractable insulin of the pancreas, measured at autopsy in 154 diabetic human subjects, with age at diagnosis and known duration of diabetes. Open circles represent subjects having less than 0.2 unit of extractable insulin per kg body weight.

insulin (I) extractable from the pancreas, on the other, has been calculated by a standard procedure [715] for the 61 male and 78 female maturity-onset diabetic subjects of both sexes. The equation of this plane is:

$$I = (1.49) - (0.0023) A - (0.0231) D \text{ for the 139 male plus female subjects.} \tag{1}$$
$$I = (2.26) - (0.0094) A - (0.0582) D \text{ for the 61 male subjects.} \tag{2}$$
$$I = (1.01) + (0.00079) A + (0.00258) D \text{ for the 78 female subjects.} \tag{3}$$

A and D are measured in years and I in units of insulin extracted from the pancreas per kg body weight at autopsy. In comparison, the average levels of the extractable insulin of pancreas at autopsy in 35 adult non-diabetic male and 23 non-diabetic female subjects were 3.50 ± 0.23 and 3.37 ± 0.31 units of insulin per kg body weight, respectively.

It is seen from equation (1) that, while there is little decrease in I with age at diagnosis of diabetes, there is a more important and progressive fall-off in I with known duration of diabetes in these maturity-onset subjects which appears to occur only in the males (equation 2). The cause and significance of this apparent sex difference are currently under investigation.

Since Bertram, Bendfeldt, and Otto [67] have correlated frequencies of successes and failures in treating diabetic human subjects with BZ-55 following the abrupt withdrawal of insulin therapy with known duration of diabetes, daily dosage of exogenous insulin and duration of insulin therapy, all maturity-onset diabetic subjects of our series were subdivided for comparison into three categories. These categories are: those subjects having less than 10 per cent, those having between 10 per cent and 20 per cent, and those with more than 20 per cent of the extractable insulin of pancreas found on the average in non-diabetic subjects of the same sex.[1] The percentage distribution of maturity-onset diabetic subjects subclassified in the above way is shown in Figure 31a as a function of insulin dosage and in Figure 31b as a function of known duration of diabetes.

Let us consider the *effectiveness* of oral sulphonylureas in the treatment of diabetes in terms of their ability to lower the blood sugar level and the excretion of glucose in the urine towards normal in the absence of injected insulin. To be effective under these conditions these compounds appear to require the presence of endogenous insulin in the diabetic organism [4; 569; 570]. If this premise is correct, it follows that the oral sulphonylureas would not prove effective by themselves in diabetic subjects having no endogenous supply or having very little.

On this basis, it would be predicted from the findings on the extractable insulin of diabetic human pancreas that the chances of effective diabetes therapy with oral sulphonylureas would be minimal in all growth-onset diabetic human subjects surviving more than a year after diagnosis. This interpretation has been supported [67; 568]. In some *newly* diagnosed growth-onset subjects and in two others whose diabetes was diagnosed during the nineteenth year of life, oral sulphonylurea therapy is proving effective in short-term tests [568]. Paralleling this finding, it is interesting in this regard that the only growth-onset diabetic subject from whose pancreas appreciable insulin was extracted was diagnosed as diabetic during his terminal illness (Figure 30).

The observed frequency of occurrence of initial successes with BZ-55 therapy of diabetes in elderly human subjects amounted to 74 per cent in the 38 subjects of Bertram *et al.* [67], and to 72 per cent in the series of 100 subjects of Banse. Franke and Fuchs [309] report successful treatment with BZ-55 in approximately 80 per cent of their series of over 50 treated cases of unspecified ages.

[1]The levels of 10 per cent and 20 per cent were chosen since pancreatic diabetes became evident in the partially depancreatized dog [8] and the alloxan-treated rat [816] when the amount of insulin remaining in the pancreas amounted to between 10 per cent and 20 per cent of that found in normal controls.

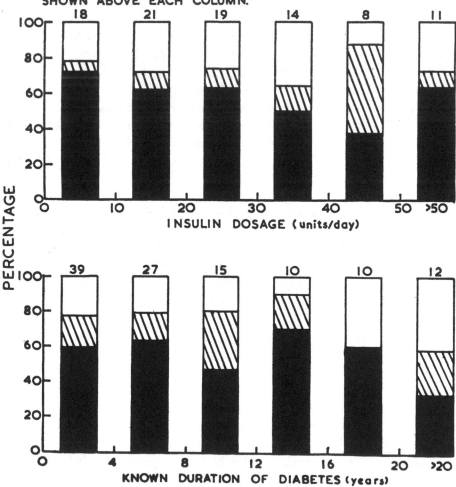

FIGURE 31. Percentage distribution of diabetic subjects with various amounts of extractable insulin expressed as a function of: (a) exogenous insulin dosage taken; (b) known duration of diabetes.

It is, therefore, of some interest to note from Figure 31 that between 60 per cent and 90 per cent of maturity-onset diabetic human subjects had pancreatic reserves of insulin amounting to more than 10 per cent of that found in adult non-diabetic subjects at autopsy. This similarity in range of percentages would indicate that the diabetic subjects who did not show an initial response to the BZ-55 therapy represent those without an appreciable supply of endogenous insulin, and they have been described in this way by the German workers (*Insulinmangeldiabetes*). A similar inference has been based on the absence of a blood sugar lowering effect of U-2043 in alloxan-diabetic rats, which was present in non-diabetic controls [570], and this inference is supported in the finding that the extractable insulin of the pancreas in the alloxan-diabetic rat is very low as a result of beta cell destruction [816].

The age of 45 years has been indicated by Bertram *et al.* [67] and by Banse as a dividing line between the older diabetic subjects who frequently respond favourably to BZ-55 and the younger ones who frequently do not. However, the authors do not make it clear whether they mean age at diagnosis of diabetes or age at time of BZ-55 therapy. It is presumed that they mean the latter, and, if this is the case, a rough parallel exists between their data and average levels of extractable insulin of diabetic human pancreas plotted against age *at death*. In a study by Mirsky *et al.*, the age of 20 years *at diagnosis* of diabetes is taken as the one where a statistically significant change in response to oral sulphonylurea therapy occurs [568].

The parallel existing between the pattern shown in Figure 30 for the extractable insulin of the pancreas and that found by Mirsky and his associates for the blood sugar responses of diabetic subjects to U-2043 [568], is striking. It is apparent in both studies that diabetes diagnosed before the end of the normal period of growth differs from that diagnosed thereafter both in the amount of insulin extractable from the pancreas and in the effectiveness of oral sulphonylurea therapy.

It has been reported that the frequency of occurrence of successful oral sulphonylurea therapy decreases progressively with increasing years of known duration of the diabetes [67; 568]. Based on an analysis made with 38 subjects, Bertram *et al.* [67] have concluded that the effectiveness of diabetes therapy with BZ-55 is mainly limited to subjects in whom the diabetes has lasted for less than 5 to 10 years. While a slow falling-off in the effectiveness of U-2043 with increasing duration of maturity-onset diabetes has been reported for 37 subjects by Mirsky *et al.* [568], inspection of the data in his enlarged series of such subjects indicates clearly that effective responses to U-2043 are still found at least up to 25 years after diagnosis of the diabetes.

Our findings (equation 1, Figure 31b) correlating amount of extractable insulin with known duration of maturity-onset diabetes are in qualitative accord with those of Mirsky. They indicate that a progressive decrease occurs in the endogenous supply of insulin, but one that is so slow in maturity-onset diabetics of both sexes that *on the average* it would require between 30 and 40 years of diabetes for the amount of extractable insulin of the pancreas to fall to 15 per cent of the level in non-diabetic subjects (equation 1). If only male subjects are considered, the 15 per cent level would have been reached after about 20 years of diabetes.

Bertram *et al.* [67] have concluded that, in their series, diabetic subjects treated with insulin for longer than a year or two did not respond well to BZ-55 therapy. We have not gathered sufficient clinical information for a statistical evaluation of the effect of duration of insulin therapy on the extractable insulin of diabetic pancreas. However, in five of seven selected diabetic subjects of the series on whom detailed clinical studies were made, appreciable amounts of insulin were extracted from the pancreas after from 5 to 17 years of insulin therapy. A more extensive study of the above discrepancy in findings is obviously needed.

Our finding of little change with insulin dosage in the distribution of subjects with low levels of extractable insulin of the pancreas (Figure 31a) correlates well with the clinical findings that frequency of success with oral sulphonamide therapy of diabetes is not closely related to prior insulin dosage [67].

The parallelisms drawn in this paper are subject to certain fundamental limitations which should be recognized. Comparisons are made between different national groups of subjects whose patterns of diabetes therapy and levels of control may have differed appreciably. The matching of findings in living with dead diabetic subjects might be considered to represent a comparison of "successful" with "unsuccessful" cases, respectively.

It is tempting to assume that the amount of insulin extractable from the diabetic human pancreas is a measure of the ability of the pancreas to produce insulin. This assumption would lead to a direct functional interpretation of the similarities in pattern which have been found to exist between the amount of extractable insulin in the diabetic human pancreas and the effectiveness of oral sulphonylureas. However, only to the extent that the lowering of the amount of insulin extractable from diabetic pancreas is caused by destruction of functional beta cells can one justify the use of this index as a measure of the ability of the pancreas to produce insulin. Histological evidence indicates that gross destruction of the beta cells has occurred in growth-onset diabetic human subjects [817; 536], and that beta cell destruction is an important factor in many but not all maturity-onset diabetics found to have small amounts of extractable insulin [377].

CONCLUSIONS

Basic similarities in pattern between the presence or absence of appreciable amounts of extractable insulin at autopsy and the effectiveness or ineffectiveness, respectively, of either of two oral sulphonylureas in returning the blood sugar level and urine sugar excretion towards normal have been found to exist for diabetic human subjects. The general ineffectiveness of oral sulphonamide therapy in growth-onset diabetic subjects is paralleled by the absence of appreciable amounts of extractable insulin in the pancreas of such subjects, with selected recently diagnosed cases representing exceptions on each side of the comparison. A progressively decreasing frequency of effectiveness of the oral therapy in maturity-onset subjects of both sexes with increasing years of survival after diabetes diagnosis is matched by a slow decrease in the average amount of insulin extractable from the pancreas, also averaged for both sexes, but mainly assignable to the male subjects.

The comparisons drawn in this paper provide some positive support for the hypothesis that the oral sulphonylureas, administered by themselves, are effective in returning blood and urine sugar levels towards normal only in those diabetic human subjects who possess a source of appreciable amounts of endogenous insulin.

ACKNOWLEDGMENTS

The authors are indebted to Professor J. Hamilton and his associates in the Department of Pathology, University of Toronto, for their friendly support throughout the collection of the data on extractable insulin used in this paper. They wish to thank Dr. I. A. Mirsky, of the School of Medicine, University of Pittsburgh, for his kindness in permitting them to consult his unpublished data on the response of diabetic subjects to therapy with U-2043. They are grateful to Miss Patricia Dolan, Miss Isabell Jasper, and Mrs. Beverly Schaeffer for their technical support in the extraction and assay of insulin from human pancreas.

BECAUSE OF THE VARIABLE FINDINGS *in the studies which have been made of the prevalence of diabetes in different areas, the careful testing of adequate numbers of people in representative communities of all countries is desirable for a variety of reasons. No country in the world has secured a complete knowledge of the incidence of diabetes. This is not the place to discuss the advantages to the patient of early detection of this disorder. Whenever "detection drives" have been conducted the rewards have been great. The results of the first study of the prevalence of diabetes in a Canadian community are described in Paper 17. My interest in this problem, but certainly not my actual contribution to it, was responsible for the invitation to add my name to the report.*

17. A Study of the Prevalence of Diabetes in an Ontario Community

A. J. KENNY, m.b., b.s.*

A. L. CHUTE, m.d.*

C. H. BEST, m.d.†

Diabetes mellitus is not a reportable disease and an accurate estimate of its prevalence is difficult to obtain. Death rates are available for most countries and for several large cities. These figures have been used to calculate the incidence of diabetes. There are, however, two main sources of error for which allowance must be made in such a calculation. First, because the diagnosis of diabetes is frequently omitted from death certificates in cases dying from another cause, mortality figures may understate the incidence. Joslin [433] showed that this understatement may be as high as 37 per cent. Secondly, the calculation requires an estimate of the average duration of the disease from diagnosis to death. Joslin [434] estimates the average duration at 15 years. Beardwood [57] in a study of death certificates mentioning diabetes found the average duration was 7.5 years. By an analysis of death rates, Joslin [434] estimated that there were one million diabetics in the United States in 1946, an incidence of 0.71 per cent. Marks [553] by a slightly different calculation reaches the figure of 675,000 or 0.48 per cent of the population.

Another approach to the problem has been made by house-to-house enquiries in sample populations. The U.S. National Health Survey [593] covered two-and-one-half million people in 1936–37. The results when adjusted for changes in the U.S. population by 1946 give a figure of 725,000 cases of diabetes in the U.S. population or 0.52 per cent. Beardwood [57] has given the results of interviews covering 34,633 people in Philadelphia. Among this group over 1 per cent were cases of diabetes.

The foregoing estimates include only known cases of diabetes, and therefore give an incomplete picture of the problem. Several case finding

Originally appeared in the *Canadian Medical Association Journal*, LXV (1951), 233–41. This research was carried out under the Ontario Provincial Department of Health with funds made available through the National Health Grants of the Dominion Government.

*From the Hospital for Sick Children, Toronto.

†Banting and Best Department of Medical Research, University of Toronto.

studies have been made with the object of revealing undiagnosed as well as known cases. Large groups of selectees for the U.S. forces have been examined for glycosuria. In Blotner's [133; 134] two groups, the first of 45,650 men between 18 and 45 years, the second of 69,688 men between 17 and 37 years at the Boston Induction Station, 208 and 251 cases of diabetes were found. Over three-quarters of these were previously undiagnosed. These figures are equivalent to incidences of 0.45 and 0.36 per cent and these rates are four times as great as those found in the corresponding age group in the National Health Survey. Spellberg [728] conducted a similar investigation at the New Orleans Induction Station. Examination of 32,033 men mostly between 18 and 35, produced only nine diabetics. The large disparity between Blotner's and Spellberg's figures is difficult to explain, and it has been questioned whether the Boston sample was truly respresentative [15].

A recent case finding study has been reported by Wilkerson and Krall [803] in which 3,516 persons in Oxford, Mass., or 70.6 per cent of the population of 4,983 were examined. In the Oxford survey blood and urine samples were examined from each person seen. Blood samples were mostly venous from adults and mostly capillary from children. Blood sugar estimations were made by the method of Folin and Wu [304]. Blood sugar values consistently above 170 mg per cent (venous) or 200 mg per cent (capillary) associated with glycosuria were taken as evidence of diabetes. In interpretation of glucose tolerance tests the height of the curve was given primary consideration. A value above 170 mg per cent (venous) was considered evidence of diabetes if associated with glycosuria.

On these criteria 30 new cases and 40 previously diagnosed diabetics were found. This corresponds to a total incidence of nearly 2 per cent of the tested population. The incidence of previously undiagnosed diabetes was 0.85 per cent. Over half the new cases were above the age of 55. Seventeen of the new cases were diagnosed by the aid of glucose tolerance tests, the remaining 13 on the post-prandial samples alone.

Tabor and Frankhauser [745] in a study of 550 adults over the age of 40 found a total of 22 diabetics of which 16 were previously undiagnosed. The persons selected for this study were from among 1,000 families invited to participate in a nutrition survey in Ottawa county, Michigan. The prevalence of diabetes among this group appears to be similar to the corresponding age groups in Oxford, Mass.

METHOD

Newmarket is a town of 4,800 people. The main source of employment is provided by seven industries, which together employ about 1,200 men and women. Most of the population are of British origin, the only other group of any size is of Dutch origin.

The survey team tried to test all persons over school age. Only a few pre-school children were examined and these only at the special request of the parents. The first survey clinics were held in the schools, about 1,200 students were tested in 6 schools. Next the clinic was set up in each of the seven larger factories; about 1,000 men and women were tested. The remaining people were tested in conjunction with a canvass of the town.

Most of the blood tests were made in the period immediately after breakfast or lunch. About 250 persons normally working out of town in the day were tested in seven evening sessions of the clinic. As far as possible both blood and urine specimens were obtained about one hour after a meal. Sample bottles for urine were usually distributed the day before the appointment for the blood test, with instructions that the sample should be collected one hour after a meal.

With only a little over two hours available each day for testing, the maximum number tested on any day was about 90 persons. While at the clinic a short history was obtained concerning personal and family history of diabetes. In addition, most adults were asked some questions relating to diabetic symptoms. When known diabetics were seen further information was obtained about insulin dosage, diet, and duration of the diabetes.

When the blood sugar was abnormal, or when glycosuria was found, a letter was sent requesting the individual to attend for a second time, when both blood and urine samples were re-examined. If the diagnosis of diabetes was then confirmed, the patient was informed and advised to consult the family physician. A copy of the results was then sent to the physician together with an offer to perform any further blood sugar estimations while the survey clinic was in operation. When the recheck was inconclusive a letter was sent advising a glucose tolerance test. This letter was usually sent about a week before the test and during this period the patient was asked to eat full meals. When known diabetics were tested a report of the results was sent to the family physician and the patient.

Seven months after the conclusion of the survey a follow-up study was made. All diabetics discovered by the survey and a group of persons whose results were equivocal were invited to be re-examined. Those who had previous glucose tolerance tests were re-examined in the same way.

Laboratory Methods

(a) *Urine.* Urine samples were tested qualitatively for reducing substances by means of "Clinitest" [438]; 0.25 ml of urine was mixed with 0.5 ml of water in a test tube and a clinitest reagent tablet added. The resulting colour was recorded in the symbols suggested by the manufacturers of clinitest as follows: negative, tr, $+$, $++$, $+++$, $++++$. When reducing substance was shown to be present, the sample was rechecked by the same test, and also tested for ketones by the nitro-prusside reaction using "Acetone-Test" (manufactured by Denver Manufacturing Company).

No quantitative estimation of urine sugar was made and no attempt was made to investigate the chemical nature of the reducing substances when present.

(*b*) *Blood.* Capillary blood samples taken from the finger-tip or ear lobe were used throughout this survey. It was considered that a capillary method would be more acceptable to the population to be tested than would venipunctures.

Blood glucose estimations were made by a modification of the Somogyi-Nelson [595; 725] colorimetric method. 0.1 ml of blood was used in each estimation. Protein precipitation was made by the method of Herbert and Bourne [386]. In the method used the blood was pipetted into isotonic sulphate-tungstate solution and the precipitation was brought about by the addition of isotonic sulphate-sulphuric acid solution. Herbert and Bourne have shown that this method is effective in preventing the passage of non-glucose reducing substances (mainly glutathione) into the filtrate. This method estimates true glucose and the values obtained are significantly lower than those obtained by the Folin-Wu method.

As blood glucose estimations were made in Toronto there was a delay of several hours between the time the sample was obtained and the time of the estimation. In the case of samples obtained after breakfast, the interval was up to 8 hours while for samples taken after lunch the delay was 2 to 3 hours. During this period the blood samples were standing unprecipitated in isotonic sulphate-tungstate solution, in corked tubes. Any change in the readings caused by this delay was not considered sufficient to affect the clinical interpretation of the results. This factor has been investigated. It was found that 24 hours' delay produced a loss of true blood sugar of 7.5 per cent. When the red cells were re-suspended before protein precipitation was begun, other reducing substances were liberated, causing an apparent increase of 5 per cent above the original estimation (S. H. Jackson, personal communication).

(*c*) *Glucose tolerance tests.* These tests were performed by the same blood sugar method on capillary blood samples taken in duplicate. Fifty g of glucose were given after fasting blood and urine samples had been collected. Further blood and urine samples were taken at one-half hour intervals up to two hours after the ingestion of glucose. Most subjects had fasted overnight, in some cases the test was performed after a four-hour fasting period following breakfast. Subjects were told to eat full meals for one week prior to the test.

Criteria and Procedure in Screening and Diagnosis

(*a*) *Screening values.* Blood glucose values in excess of 160 mg per 100 ml blood occurring between one-half and one-and-one-half hours after a meal, or values above 150 mg per 100 ml between 1½ and 2 hours, or values over 120 mg per 100 ml occurring 2 hours and over after a meal or in the fasting state were considered abnormal. Such persons were asked to attend for a second time when both blood and urine samples were re-examined. Persons showing glycosuria were also re-examined. Persons without glycosuria and blood glucose values below those mentioned were considered non-diabetic.

TABLE 17.1

A SUMMARY OF THE CRITERIA FOR BLOOD SUGAR VALUES USED FOR SCREENING
AND DIAGNOSIS

Test	Blood Sugar mg %	Time after Meal	Interpretation
Initial test	>160 >150 >120	up to 1½ hrs 1½–2 hrs 2 hrs or fasting	abnormal—recheck made
Initial test + recheck test	both >200	anytime	diagnostic of diabetes
Glucose tolerance test (50 g glucose 2 hour curve)	>120 >200 >120	fasting at peak 2 hrs	diagnostic of diabetes together diagnostic of diabetes

NOTE. 1. Blood sugar values are true glucose (Somogyi-Nelson method). 2. All blood samples are capillary. (> indicates greater than.)

(*b*) *Diabetic values.* A diagnosis of diabetes was made (1) if blood glucose values in excess of 200 mg per 100 ml blood were found on two occasions. (2) On the result of glucose tolerance tests. In the interpretation of these tests most stress was laid on the delayed fall of the curve. Diabetes was diagnosed if both the peak was above 200 mg per 100 ml blood and the two-hour level was above 120 mg per 100 ml. A fasting blood sugar of over 120 mg per 100 ml blood was also considered evidence of diabetes, though this was not seen except in curves which were also abnormal from the above considerations. When the blood glucose was markedly in excess of these values the diagnosis was considered justified even when the presence of glycosuria was not established in the samples examined.

A short medical history obtained from each case was also considered before making the diagnosis and as far as possible, other conditions leading to impairment of glucose tolerance were ruled out.

Glucose tolerance tests were performed (*a*) when blood glucose values were found to be abnormal (i.e., above the screening level) on two occasions but one or both tests were below the diabetic level. (*b*) When there was persistent glycosuria of 1+ or more, although blood glucose values were not above the screening level. (*c*) Where there was a marked discrepancy between the first and second tests. For example, a case in which a "diabetic" blood sugar in the first test was followed by a normal result in the second, was usually investigated by a glucose tolerance test. However, a borderline test followed by a normal one was considered non-diabetic unless some factor, such as glycosuria, indicated further investigation.

RESULTS

4,419 persons were tested in the survey in Newmarket and these figures are summarized in Table 17.II. This total includes 843 non-residents most of whom were encountered in the schools and factories visited. In the further analysis of the results of the survey this non-resident group has been included in the total. Children under school age (six years) were not tested, as a rule, by the survey. Out of approximately 500 pre-school children in Newmarket only 79 or 16 per cent were tested. The authors felt that it was very unlikely that any previously undiagnosed cases of diabetes would be found among children of these ages. Among the remaining age groups present in the Newmarket population 81 per cent of the residents were covered by the survey.

TABLE 17.II

ESTIMATED POPULATION OF NEWMARKET AND THE NUMBERS OF
PERSONS TESTED IN THE COURSE OF THE SURVEY

Population of Newmarket	4,800
Population under six years	500
Population over six years	4,300
Total number tested	4,419
Males	2,206
Females	2,213
Non-residents	843
Residents over six years of age	3,502
Percentage of resident population over six years covered	81

As no recent figures are available for the age and sex distribution of the Newmarket population it has not been possible to estimate the proportion in each age group reached by the survey. However, the age and sex distribution of the population of Ontario in 1947 is shown for comparison with the tested group (Figures 32 and 33). The data on which these graphs were based are to be found in Table 17.III. Compared with that of Ontario, the

TABLE 17.III

Age and Sex Distribution of Ontario Population, Tested Population, and Diabetics

Age in Years	Percentage of Population in each Group				No. of Persons in each Group		No. of Diabetics in each Group					
	Ontario* 1949		Tested population in Newmarket		Tested population in Newmarket		New cases		Known cases		Total cases	
	male	female	male	female	male	female	male	female	male	female	male	female
0–9	9.40	9.00	6.00	5.40	265	237						
10–19	7.40	7.22	12.23	10.00	542	443						
20–29	8.22	8.10	6.60	8.20	292	360						
30–39	7.50	7.35	8.05	8.55	357	378	1		1		2	
40–49	6.40	6.10	6.45	6.75	284	299		4	3	1	3	5
50–59	5.30	5.10	4.69	4.95	207	219		4	1	5	1	9
60–69	3.80	3.75	3.80	3.85	168	172	4	4	6	5	10	9
70–79	1.95	2.00	1.74	1.75	75	76	1	2	4	5	5	7
80–89	0.56	0.70	0.32	0.61	14	27		1	1	1	1	2
90–99	0.06	0.09	0.04	0.02	2	1						
Total	50.59%	49.41%	49.92%	50.08%	2,206	2,213	6	15	16	17	22	32

*Estimated population for Ontario 1949, taken from Vital Statistics—Analytical Report No. 1 (Ottawa: Dominion Bureau of Statistics, 1948).

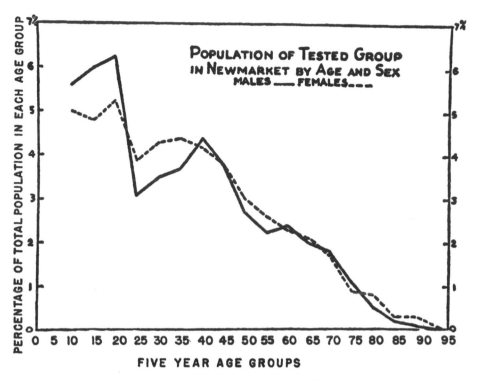

FIGURE 32. Population of tested group in Newmarket.

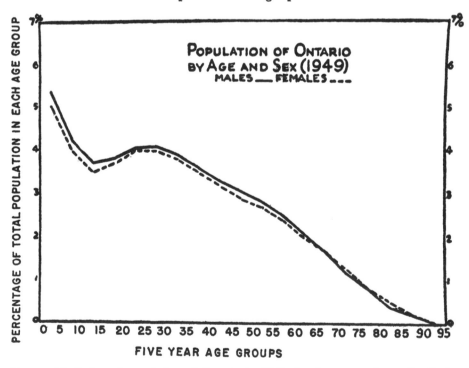

FIGURE 33. Estimated population of Ontario in 1949 showing age and sex distribution of each. Latter data from *Vital Statistics—Analytical Report No. 1*, Dominion Bureau of Statistics, Ottawa, 1948.

tested population shows two main differences: (a) an excess of both males and females between the ages of 5 and 19 years and (b) a deficiency of males between the ages of 20 and 29 years. In the remaining age groups from 30 years upwards, the distribution roughly corresponds with that of Ontario.

The racial origin of the tested population was predominantly Anglo-Saxon; 86.6 per cent of the 3,966 persons for whom a record of the racial origin was obtained were of British descent. Nearly two-thirds of this group were of English origin. The remaining 13.4 per cent were composed of Dutch (5.3 per cent), French (2.8 per cent), German (2.1 per cent) and small numbers of Italians, Slavs, Scandinavians, and Chinese. Those of Jewish origin accounted for only 0.3 per cent of the total.

Diabetics

Among the 4,419 persons seen at the clinic 54 diabetics were encountered; 33 of this number were previously known cases and 21 were new cases diagnosed on the criteria described. The total incidence was 1.2 per cent (known cases, 0.75 per cent; new cases, 0.5 per cent in the tested population).

The non-resident group (842 persons) provided only 5 of the 54 diabetics and the incidence was 0.6 per cent compared with 1.3 per cent in the resident group. The non-residents tested were mostly school children and factory workers. They, therefore, formed a younger group than the residents and contained a predominance of males. These facts presumably account for the lower incidence in this group.

The age and sex distribution of the diabetics is shown in Figure 34. The age range was from 36 to 86 years. The largest single number (19 cases) was found between the ages of 60 and 69. There were 20 cases in three decades from 30 to 59 years and 15 cases in the decades from 70 to 89 years. In the 54 diabetics seen 32 were females and 22 males.

Previously known diabetics. The mean age of this group of 33 cases was 62 years, the range being from 36 to 81 years. 17 were female and 16 male. Nearly half of this group (14 persons) knew of the existence of diabetes in their family histories. The average duration of diabetes in these known cases was 5.6 years, the range from 2 months to 21 years; 8 persons had had diabetes for over ten years. Insulin was taken by 23 persons, the remaining 10 were under treatment by diet alone. On all these cases a report was requested from the family physicians concerned.

Diabetics discovered by the survey. The mean age of this group of 21 cases was 60 years, the range from 37 to 86 years; 15 were female and 6 were males. Four of these persons appeared to be symptom-free at the time of diagnosis, but the remaining 17 had at least one symptom. Tiredness was the most common symptom (12 persons); frequency of micturition, suggested by the fact that such persons rose twice or oftener during the night was present in 9 cases. Unusual thirst was recorded by 5, cramps in the legs by 5, and weight loss by 3 persons. Only 4 gave a family history of diabetes.

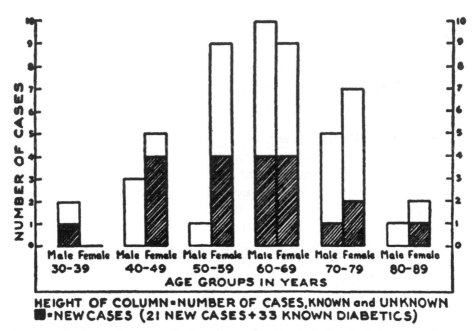

HEIGHT OF COLUMN=NUMBER OF CASES, KNOWN and UNKNOWN
▓=NEW CASES (21 NEW CASES+33 KNOWN DIABETICS)

FIGURE 34. Age and sex distribution of 54 diabetics, including both known and new cases revealed by the survey.

In the initial blood and urine tests of the new diabetics, most (15 persons) showed both hyperglycaemia and glycosuria. One case showed glycosuria as the only abnormality and there were 5 persons who showed hyperglycaemia only. These 5 individuals would have escaped diagnosis in a survey in which urine tests only were used in screening the population.

Seven months after the completion of the survey, 18 of the 21 new cases were interviewed and re-examined. Nine cases diagnosed by the aid of glucose tolerance tests were retested in the same way. Of the remaining 12 diagnosed on the results of post-prandial tests one was untraced, 2 sent reports, and 9 were seen and retested.

The results of this follow-up study were as follows: (1) Treatment: all cases traced had been in the care of physicians since the time of diagnosis. Eight were taking insulin. All had been advised on diet, though the diet followed varied from simple avoidance of sweet foods by some individuals to strict measurement of most foodstuffs by others. (2) Results: most of those who had originally noticed symptoms now claimed to feel much better. Of the 9 tolerance tests, all showed some improvement and 4 were virtually normal curves, following only dietary treatment. Of those retested with single blood sugars all 9 showed improvement over the original tests and 3 gave completely normal results following only dietary treatment. In most cases this improvement was associated with reduction of weight. Four typical pairs of glucose tolerance curves showing the changes that have occurred during treatment are shown in Figure 35 (A-D).

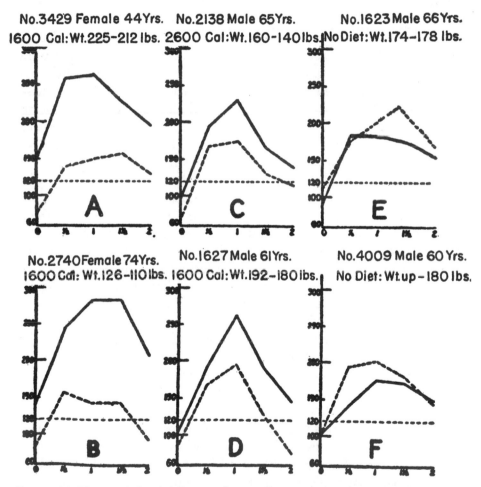

No.3429 Female 44Yrs.   No.2138 Male 65Yrs.   No.1623 Male 66Yrs.
1600 Cal:Wt.225-212 lbs. 2600 Cal:Wt.160-140 lbs. No Diet:Wt.174-178 lbs.

No.2740 Female 74Yrs.   No.1627 Male 61Yrs.   No.4009 Male 60 Yrs.
1600 Cal: Wt.126-110 lbs. 1600 Cal:Wt.192-180 lbs. No Diet: Wt.up-180 lbs.

FIGURE 35. The original and follow-up glucose tolerance curves of six persons. Curve at time of diagnosis in continuous line. Follow-up curve in broken line. Time in hours (abscissæ). Blood sugar in mg per 100 ml (ordinates). A to D: Four previously undiagnosed diabetics showing typical improvement following seven months of dietary treatment. E to F: Two cases previously classified as "doubtful" who showed further impairment of glucose tolerance. Neither was treated in the interval.

DOUBTFUL RESULTS

There are two groups considered under this heading, neither of which was included in either of the foregoing groups of diabetics. First there were 9 persons whose results were abnormal but were not thought to be diagnostic of diabetes. Secondly there were 7 persons who believed that they had or may have had diabetes. No confirmation for their statements could be found, however, either in the results of the survey tests or in reports from their own doctors, when these were obtainable.

The first group contained two persons whose initial tests were suggestive of diabetes but who were unwilling to proceed with any further investigations, either at the survey clinic or, as far as is known, with their own doctor. They were not seen again in the follow-up study. The remaining 7 were persons investigated by glucose tolerance tests. All of these were followed up and the tests repeated after an interval of seven months. Two of these were especially suspicious of diabetes. Post-prandial tests had shown glycosuria accompanied by borderline blood sugars. The glucose tolerance tests showed normal fasting levels, peaks above 180 but below 200 mg per 100 ml blood, and two-hour levels above 150 mg per 100 ml. When the tests were repeated, glucose tolerance had decreased slightly. On the criteria used, these cases would now be classified as diabetic (see Figure 35 E and F). During the interval between the two tests neither of these persons had followed any dietary restriction. Both had gained weight. The other 5 glucose tolerance tests were mostly abnormal in that the height of the curve exceeded 200 mg per cent, the fasting and the two-hour levels being in every case below 120 mg per cent. When these were repeated none showed any increase in the abnormality. Some remained the same, others had returned towards normal.

The second group, comprising 7 persons believing themselves to be diabetic, were all investigated at the survey clinic. Most gave a history extending over several years, all but one covering at least four years. None was taking insulin and none was dieting although three stated that they avoided sugar. None showed any glycosuria and with one exception all post-prandial blood sugars were well below the upper limit of normal. The exception was a known case of cholelithiasis, whose blood sugar 70 minutes after a meal was 165 mg per cent. In all but two cases reports from their physicians were not available concerning the initial blood and urine tests at the time of the supposed diagnosis. In the absence of any definite confirmatory evidence, the authors have not thought it justifiable to include these persons in the list of known diabetics. If they were to be so included the incidence of known diabetes in the tested population would be raised from 0.75 to 0.9 per cent.

Glycosuria. There were 92 persons whose initial sample showed the presence of reducing substances. In addition there were 6, out of the 172 persons who were examined on more than one occasion, who showed glycosuria in subsequent tests although the initial sample gave a negative reaction. Cases showing glycosuria in the initial test are analysed in Table 17.IV.

Of the 92 instances of glycosuria 32 were due to diabetes and of this number 16 occurred in known cases. If these known cases are excluded from the total, 16 out of the remaining 76 cases of glycosuria, or 21 per cent were due to undetected diabetes. Of the remaining 60 non-diabetic glycosurias, 14 cases or 23 per cent appeared to be persistent, in that glycosuria of some degree was present on at least one subsequent occasion. No systematic attempt to classify the non-diabetic glycosurias was possible. There were, however, eight instances in which glycosuria was noticed during glucose tolerance tests which had been judged to be non-diabetic. Of this number three appeared to be related to a lowered renal theshold,

TABLE 17.IV

ANALYSIS OF ALL PERSONS SHOWING GLYCOSURIA IN INITIAL URINE TEST

Result of Test	Total no. of Persons with Positive Results	No. of Diabetics			No. of Non-Diabetics
		Total	Known cases	New cases	
Trace	43	6	4	2	37
+ or ++	18	4	2	2	14
+++ or ++++	31	22	10	12	9
Totals	92	32	16	16	60

and one was associated with a "lag storage" type of curve, or what Lawrence [486] prefers to call the "oxyhyperglycaemic curve." The 60 instances of non-diabetic glycosuria occurred at all ages and in both sexes, but was commoner in males in the ratio of 3 to 2. In females glycosuria most often occurred between 20 and 50 years sometimes associated with pregnancy, while in males most cases occurred after middle age.

DISCUSSION

The diagnosis of diabetes mellitus offers no difficulties in frank cases of the disease. Here symptoms associated with glycosuria and a marked elevation of the blood sugar serve to establish the diagnosis without any doubt. However, in a diabetes survey of a normal population, it is inevitable that a large proportion of the cases discovered should be without symptoms and show only slight elevation of the blood sugar above normal levels. The interpretation of such borderline results raises certain problems.

Glucose tolerance as measured by the standard glucose tolerance test is known to be affected by numerous factors. Previous diet [218; 743; 555; 249] age, physical inactivity [132], absorption rate of ingested glucose, emotional stress, as well as endocrine disorders and hepatic disease are examples of such factors. Mosenthal [578] has focused attention on the necessity for standardizing the conditions of the test and has demonstrated the differences which occur between capillary and venous blood sugar levels and the variable error that arises from the estimation of non-glucose reducing substances in certain techniques.

In interpreting the results of glucose tolerance tests, these factors have been considered. Tests were only performed on ambulant persons. Diet on the days preceding the test was adequate to give a normal response. Mosenthal [578] states that a diet containing 125 g carbohydrate per day is adequate to elicit a normal tolerance curve. Emotional factors were eliminated since patients had already visited the clinic twice before and none was disturbed by the procedure.

The criteria selected are in line with those suggested by several authors. Joslin [434] states that a capillary blood sugar level of over 200 mg per cent after food or 130 mg per cent fasting is indicative of diabetes. Mosenthal [578] suggests that in a normal tolerance test the maximum values for capillary blood should be: fasting, 120 mg per cent; peak, 200 mg per cent; two-hour level, 120 mg per cent. Lawrence [487] also uses substantially the same values. Recently Moyer and Womack [582] have analysed the results of over 100 tolerance tests on non-diabetics and compared them with those from a group of certain diabetics. Venous blood samples were estimated by the Folin-Wu method. They suggest that the upper normal values for fasting, peak, and two-hour level should be 118, 195, and 126 mg per cent respectively. These figures represent in each case the mean normal value plus twice the standard deviation. These authors regard the two-hour level as the most sensitive index for diagnosis.

The improvement of glucose tolerance that many of the new diabetics showed when retested several months after diagnosis might conceivably be interpreted in two ways. First, it might call the original diagnosis into question. It might be argued that the original impairment of glucose tolerance was a transient phenomenon. Against this it may be observed that all these persons had previously shown suspicious blood glucose levels on more than one occasion before the original tolerance test was performed. Secondly, the improvement in tolerance might be regarded as the direct result of the treatment given in the interval between the two tests. There are many reports in the literature of this change occurring following dietary treatment of middle-aged obese diabetics. Simple reduction of calorie intake with no disproportionate reduction of carbohydrate was sufficient in Newburgh's [597] patients to bring about loss of excess weight and return of the glucose tolerance to normal. Himsworth [393] and John [429] have also quoted examples of this effect. Newburgh advances reasons for the view that these cases should not be regarded as true diabetics. John, however, does not accept this reasoning. It is generally agreed that simple weight reduction can bring about cure of both glycosuria and hyperglycaemia in this type of case.

It is of interest that two persons who did not receive any treatment did not show any improvement of glucose tolerance when retested 8 months later. Indeed, there was some tendency towards further impairment. The curves are shown in Figure 35E and F. The original curves just failed to fulfil the criteria for diagnosis—there was a delayed fall, but the peak did not exceed 200 mg per cent. These two individuals would now fall within the diabetic group.

Conclusions

In this survey, as in others reported in the literature, a considerable number of unknown diabetics were found. Most of these cases were in the middle and upper age groups. Their diabetes appeared in most cases to be mild and dietary treatment alone often brought about a marked improvement in glucose tolerance. It seems that there exists a fairly large group of undiagnosed diabetics in the population. It would, therefore, be advantageous for all persons over the age of 40 to have their urine tested at least once a year. This might lead to earlier detection and treatment, with improvement in the sense of well-being and perchance lessen the tendency to complications which may occur as the result of prolonged hyperglycaemia.

Summary

1. Samples of blood and urine from 4,419 persons in Newmarket, Ont., were examined for glucose with the object of estimating the number of diabetics in this community: 81 per cent of the town's population were included in this total. All age groups were covered with the exception of the pre-school group.

2. The literature concerning certain other estimates of the incidence is reviewed briefly.

3. The methods used in the survey are described; capillary blood samples

were estimated by a modified Somogyi-Nelson colorimetric technique. Urine samples were tested with Clinitest.

4. Screening and diagnostic criteria are described.

5. The results of the survey and of a follow-up study seven months later are given. 54 diabetics were seen among 4,419 tested, an incidence of 1.2 per cent. 21 of these were previously undiagnosed. When these cases were re-examined, many showed marked improvement of glucose tolerance. The significance of this effect is discussed.

ACKNOWLEDGMENTS

The authors wish to express their thanks to Dr. Neil E. McKinnon and Mrs. Margaret Richardson of the Department of Hygiene, University of Toronto, for the statistical analysis of the results of this survey.

The authors are also indebted to the following: Dr. K. P. Turner for help in the preliminary organization, Dr. J. G. Cock, the local committee members, the canvassers, and many others who gave voluntary help in the work. Also to the physicians of Newmarket, the Town Council, the *Newmarket Era and Express*, and the many clubs and organizations who gave valuable support.

Thanks are also due to the Ames Company, Elkhart, Ind., for supplies of Clinitest and to the Denver Mfg. Co., Montreal, for supplies of Acetone Test.

THE POSSIBILITY OF PREVENTING DIA-
*betes is very much in our minds. Paper 18 was the first scientific paper in
volume 1 of the* Proceedings of the American Diabetes Association *and for
this reason, and because it contains some interesting discussion by other
students of diabetes, merits inclusion. Some material which had already
been published in other articles has been eliminated.*

18. The Prevention of Diabetes

R. E. HAIST, M.D.

C. H. BEST, M.D.

An article under the title, "The Prevention of Diabetes" was published some eight months ago from our department. The paper was expected to provoke discussion and this expectation has been realized. We are anxious to stimulate interest in the possibility of preventing diabetes, since from the point of view of public health this is the most important aspect of the diabetic problem. Because the discussion of this problem had centred around treatment rather than prevention we brought together certain experimental data which indicated that, in animals, diabetes produced by the only means at present available can be prevented by certain procedures. We therefore made the suggestion that the procedures found to be effective in animals should be tested in man. We are not clinicians—we have made no clinical tests—but this does not relieve us of the responsibility of suggesting that such tests should be made.

Diabetes can be produced in dogs by two methods. The first is by the removal of the pancreas, and the second is by the administration of extracts of anterior pituitary gland. Homans and Allen demonstrated that by leaving a small bit of pancreas in the animal the changes in the islet cells of the pancreas could be observed as the diabetes developed. They found that removal of a large portion of the pancreas in dogs led to diabetes accompanied by degranulation and finally hydropic degeneration of the beta cells of the islets of Langerhans. Allen showed that the intensity of the diabetes paralleled the severity of the islet cell changes. He developed the thesis that the degeneration resulted from exhaustion of the islets through overwork.

Our studies have shown that, in partial pancreatectomy, when enough pancreas is left, the animal does not become diabetic and the islets remain normal in appearance. We have been able to demonstrate that under these conditions the insulin concentration in the pancreatic remnant is within the normal range (Figure 36). If sufficient pancreas is removed, however, the animal does become diabetic. The islet cells show hydropic degenera-

Originally appeared in the *Proceedings of the American Diabetes Association*, I (1941), 31–48.

tion and the insulin concentration in the pancreatic remnant is reduced to very low values. Our findings support Allen's conclusions that the effect of extensive partial pancreatectomy on the islet cells is the result of overwork.

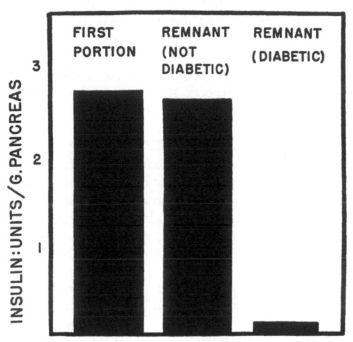

FIGURE 36. Insulin content of the pancreas in dogs following partial pancreatectomy [347].

The second method of producing diabetes in dogs is by administration of anterior pituitary extracts. Houssay, Evans, and others demonstrated that the injection of anterior pituitary extracts gave rise to a diabetic state in dogs. With Dr. J. Campbell, we have shown that the diabetes resulting from the daily injection of certain extracts of the anterior pituitary gland is associated with a progressive reduction in the insulin concentration in the pancreas. With Professor Ham, we have found that there is also a loss of granules in the beta cells of the islets of Langerhans, followed by hydropic degeneration of those cells. The islet picture in these animals is similar to that found in partially depancreatized dogs and is thought to be due to the same cause, namely, overwork of the beta cells of the islets with consequent exhaustion.

We do not wish to imply that the excess stimulation of the islets results from a direct action of the pituitary extract on the pancreas. We know that the extract affects many organs and tissues. It seems probable that at least a large part of the effect on the islets is brought about indirectly by altering the activity of liver and other tissues responsible for the new formation, liberation, storage, and use of sugar.

The diabetes which occurs while the extract is being administered is not permanent if the period of injections is not too prolonged. It is therefore sometimes referred to as "transient diabetes." Recovery of the insulin concentration in the pancreas occurs after the injections of anterior pituitary extract have been discontinued.

Young has shown that a sufficiently long course of injections of anterior pituitary extract leads to a diabetic state, associated with islet changes, which persists indefinitely after the injections are discontinued, i.e., a so-called "permanent diabetes." The exhaustive overwork, if it continues long enough, apparently can lead finally to a permanent reduction in pancreatic insulin content and in functioning beta cells. For long periods (up to 200 days) after the injections of the extract were stopped, the insulin concentration remained at a very low level. In the permanently diabetic dog, diminished islet function appears to be a factor of major importance. Hence this animal resembles the depancreatized dog in many particulars but differs in that it still has available its alpha cells and external pancreatic secretions.

It was thought that a study of the effect of various dietary changes on the insulin content of the pancreas might give some information regarding the factors that influence the activity of the pancreatic islets. One of the first observations was that fasting or the feeding of fat led to a definite reduction in the insulin content of the pancreas in rats. Lately we have found that feeding protein gives much the same degree of restoration as when sugar is given. An attempt is being made to determine quantitatively the relationship between the effect of protein and of carbohydrate, but this study is not yet complete.

While fasting and the feeding of fat led to a reduction in the insulin content of the pancreas of rats, it was not clear whether this was due to a decreased production of insulin and a resting of islet cells or whether it was due, as in the partially depancreatized dogs and the dogs receiving anterior pituitary extract, to an increased activity and exhaustion of islet cells. The resting hypothesis seemed more logical. It was thought that if large doses of protamine zinc insulin were given, some light on this question might be obtained.

The daily injection of adequate amounts of protamine zinc insulin led to a reduction in the insulin content of the pancreas of fed rats (Figure 37). This reduction can hardly be ascribed to overwork and it seems logical to conclude that it results from a decreased production of insulin by the islet cells. When daily injections of protamine zinc insulin were given to fasted and fat-fed rats it was found that the effect of fasting and fat-feeding was enhanced. Figure 38 shows the great reduction in the insulin content of pancreas that resulted when starved rats were given insulin. Figure 39 shows a similar effect obtained when insulin was administered to the animals fed fat. Insulin did not prevent the decrease in insulin

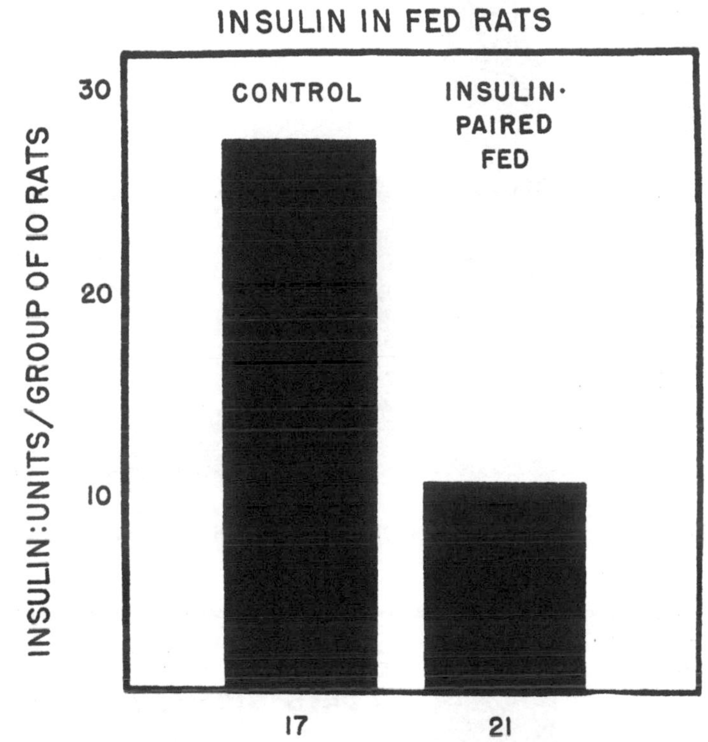

INSULIN IN FED RATS

FIGURE 37. The effect of insulin on the insulin content of the pancreas in normally-fed rats. Numbers under the blocks represent total number of animals [347].

content of the pancreas due to fasting and fat-feeding. On the contrary, it made the reduction still greater. Consequently, it seemed necessary to conclude that insulin administration, fasting, and fat-feeding had similar effects. Since insulin administration probably reduced the need for endogenous insulin and rested islet cells, the other procedures, fasting and the feeding of fat, also probably rested islet cells.

When daily injections of insulin were given at the same time that the animals were starved or fed fat, reduction in the insulin content of the pancreas was very great, to roughly 1/10 of the normal value. This reduction is comparable to that obtained in animals receiving anterior pituitary extract, yet no hydropic degenerative change was evident in the islets. We

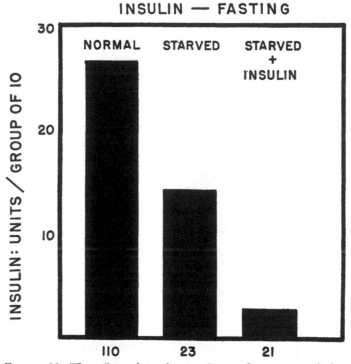

FIGURE 38. The effect of insulin on the insulin content of the pancreas in fasted rats [347].

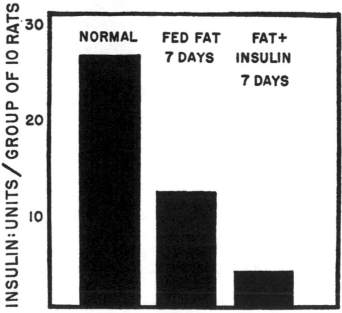

FIGURE 39. The effect of insulin on the insulin content of the pancreas in fat-fed rats [347].

may consider then that the histological picture gives good support to the theory that these procedures rest rather than overstrain the pancreas.

Himsworth and Scott contend that the effects of fat-feeding and fasting on sugar tolerance and insulin sensitivity result from an increased pituitary activity and some may wonder whether an altered pituitary activity might be responsible for the changes in insulin content observed under these conditions. We have found that the effect of fat-feeding on the insulin content of the pancreas can still be obtained in the absence of the pituitary gland (Figure 40). The solid block shows the values for insulin content obtained in the control animals, and the open block the values obtained in

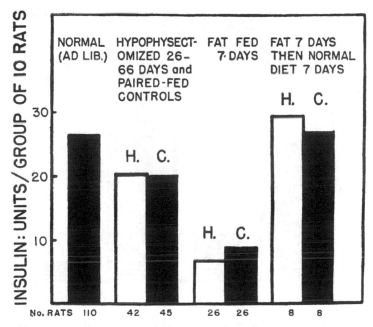

FIGURE 40. The effect of diet on the insulin content of the pancreas in hypophysectomized rats [347].

similarly treated hypophysectomized rats. The reduction in insulin content of the pancreas is evident in the hypophysectomized rats receiving the diet of fat. Moreover, after starvation, feeding a balanced diet will restore the insulin content even in the hypophysectomized rat. These findings show that the pituitary gland is not essential for the reduction in insulin content of the pancreas which occurs as a result of fat-feeding. More recently we have found also that the adrenal glands are not necessary for this effect.

From the work on rats it was concluded that the administration of insulin, fasting, and the feeding of fat tended to rest the beta cells of the islets of Langerhans. If it were true that fasting, fat-feeding and insulin administration rested the islets, then these procedures should prevent overwork of the islet cells and prevent or alleviate experimental diabetes in dogs.

Allen had found that fasting alleviated the diabetes due to partial pancreatectomy and restored the islet cells to a more normal state. Copp and Barclay, and Bowie, found that adequate insulin administration had a similar effect in restoring the islets in partially depancreatized dogs. In some experiments conducted in collaboration with Dr. J. Campbell and Dr. A. W. Ham it was observed that the changes in insulin content and islet picture found in pituitary diabetes could be prevented by the administration of adequate amounts of protamine zinc insulin. Dogs were given

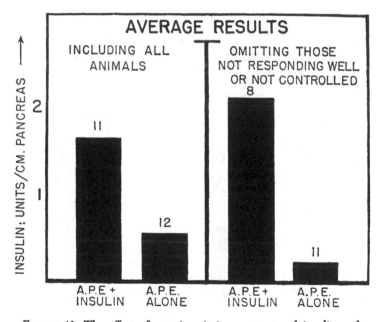

FIGURE 41. The effect of anterior pituitary extract and insulin and of anterior pituitary extract alone on the insulin content of the pancreas in dogs [347].

daily injections of anterior pituitary extract and, in addition, received daily injections of protamine zinc insulin. The administration of the insulin with the extract tended to prevent the reduction in insulin content of the pancreas and degenerative changes in the islet cells (Figure 41). The chart shows clearly that insulin injections tend to prevent the reduction in insulin concentration in the pancreas resulting from anterior pituitary extract administration.

[A figure is omitted showing, on one side, swollen vacuolated cells in an islet of the pancreas of a dog given anterior pituitary extract; on the other side no hydropic degeneration and good granulation of islet cells was evident when insulin injections were given at the same time.]

It seems clear then that, in the dog, the effect of insulin administration, fasting, and fat-feeding act in a manner opposite to the effect of partial pancreatectomy and of pituitary extract administration. This further substantiates the contention that these procedures of fasting, fat-feeding and insulin administration rest the pancreatic islets. The factors that rest the islet cells in the rat tend to prevent the onset of experimental diabetes in the dog. These procedures tend to offset or prevent diabetes in the only types of experimental diabetes as yet available for study.

It may be argued that in certain countries diabetes is a rarity among the poor, whose diet is high in carbohydrate, but is common among the well-to-do whose diet contains a higher proportion of fat. The poor man, however, probably has a low calorie intake, and the rich man a high one. This brings up two points, (1) the effect of undernutrition even though the diet contains a fairly high percentage of carbohydrate, and (2) the effect of diets moderately high in fat.

A reduction in the caloric intake leads to a reduction in the insulin content of the pancreas of rats even though a balanced diet is given (Figure 42). The balanced diet used in this experiment contained 50 per cent carbohydrate. It will be evident from the figure that reducing the caloric intake leads to a decrease in the insulin content of the pancreas. Even when only sugar is given, there is a reduction in the insulin content of the pancreas if the caloric intake is reduced. The second point is that, in normal rats, diets moderately high in fat do not have nearly as dramatic an effect on the insulin content of the pancreas as diets in which fat alone is given, though some effect is evident. In order to increase the depression in pancreatic insulin by a diet moderately rich in fat, the total amount of food ingested should be reduced.

We have pointed out that the procedures that permit the islets to rest prevent or hinder the development of the diabetic state in experimental animals. In animals it would appear that fasting, fat-feeding, and insulin administration tend to rest islet cells, whereas carbohydrate is necessary if these cells are to be stimulated. We are aware that human diabetes may not be entirely comparable to these experimental types and that possibly there may be more than one type of diabetes in man. What we wish to make clear is that the procedures established as beneficial in animals should be tried under as well controlled conditions as possible in human subjects. In the treatment of diabetes in man these procedures have, of course, received consideration. Before the days of insulin it was possible to prolong the lives of diabetics by Allen's undernutrition treatment, and Karl Petren and others used very high fat diets in the treatment of diabetes. We have omitted mention of many clinical studies which might be quoted.

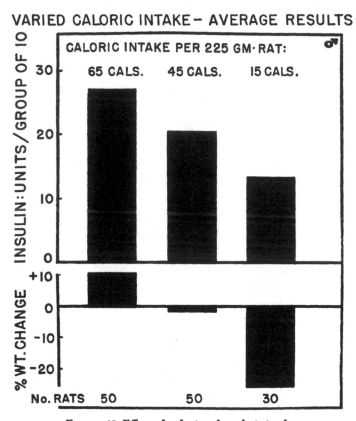

FIGURE 42. Effect of reducing the caloric intake.

We have suggested that the principles derived from the animal experiments might be applied to children with a diabetic family history. The case for the inheritance of diabetes is convincingly stated by White and Pincus in Dr. Joslin's book, *The Treatment of Diabetes Mellitus*. There seems to be general agreement that diabetes runs in families. If it does, then the value of these preventive measures may be tested clinically. Dr. R. D. Lawrence agrees in the main with our interpretation of the animal experiments but does not feel that the suggestions regarding preventive measures in children with a diabetic family history can be taken seriously. As he phrases it, "dogs, yes; children, no." We still feel that the principles derived from the animal experiments can be tested in children without causing them great discomfort, but this is obviously a matter for the clinicians to decide.

DISCUSSION

DR. I. ARTHUR MIRSKY (*Cincinnati, Ohio*): The principles so clearly indicated by the experiments of Dr. Best and Dr. Haist are apparently beyond question. It is concerning their application to the prevention of diabetes that I wish to raise a question in the hope that further discussion of this particular point may be brought out. In this paper, particular emphasis is paid to the fact that the partially depancreatized animal receiving large amounts of sugar develops insulin insufficiency in consequence of an hydropic degeneration of the pancreas. Nevertheless, ever since Allen first proposed the concept that overexhaustion and consequent hydropic degeneration of the pancreas is the cause of the diabetic syndrome in man, attempts to demonstrate this histological phenomenon in man have not been universally successful. Warren, in his studies of the pathology of the pancreas, finds that hydropic degeneration is a rarity in patients dying from diabetes. In fact, he believes that the change is nearly as rare in cases not given insulin as in those receiving insulin. In view of this, I wonder whether in man one is dealing with a situation similar to that in the rat receiving large amounts of pituitary extracts. If hydropic degeneration consequent to exhaustion of the islets is not the cause of the diabetic syndrome in man, then the question as to the efficiency of insulin as a prophylactic measure must be given much careful consideration, for it is possible that instead of resting the islet tissue, one might induce what Selye calls "compensatory atrophy" by the indiscriminate use of exogenous insulin.

DR. WILLIAM D. SANSUM (*Santa Barbara, Cal.*): We clinicians heartily agree with this work. There is plenty of clinical work in support of it. We sort of feel the crux of the whole thing is to keep the blood sugar normal. Now, with protamine zinc insulin we can do that. We couldn't do it before with regular insulin. Now, we can have perfectly normal blood sugars throughout the day and perfectly normal fasting blood sugars.

DR. F. M. ALLEN (*New York, N.Y.*): This paper is exceedingly interesting. One of the questions is about hydropic degeneration. This does occur in human cases, and very marked examples can be shown, but usually it is not discoverable. There is a very simple reason, in the nature of the process itself. It represents an active breakdown of island cells. In partially depancreatized animals, which show this change so strikingly, the beta cells of the islands may be completely lost within a few weeks, and there is necessarily a correspondingly rapid loss of tolerance and aggravation of the diabetes. Human diabetes usually runs a slower course. Granting that the progressive decline of tolerance in uncontrolled cases is due to breakdown of beta cells from functional overstrain, this course is usually so gradual over a number of years that the discovery of an occasional cell in actual degeneration must be uncommon. Microscopic pictures on any scale comparable to those in the dog are seen only in the most intense human cases, for example, in young patients and in some coma cases. With the widespread use of insulin, visible hydropic degeneration becomes naturally a rarity nowadays.

The part of the paper dealing with the insulin content of the pancreas touches on a point which has confused many persons. Some authors have been misled by what was long ago called hunger glycosuria. That is, after several days of fasting or fat diet, the sudden giving of carbohydrate causes exaggerated hyperglycaemia or glycosuria. On the contrary, if carbohydrate or glucose is given repeatedly at short intervals, the usual curve of hyperglycaemia is flattened out by an apparent improvement of assimilation. This has been used as an argument to support claims that high carbohydrate diet stimulates assimilation and increases tolerance in diabetes. As early as 1913 I drew a distinction between real and apparent tolerance. It can be illustrated in a dog which is depancreatized just to the borderline of diabetes. Immediate high carbohydrate feeding will break down the tolerance and make the animal permanently diabetic. But if fasting or only fat diet is given for a few days or a week, and after that the largest possible amounts of carbohydrate or sugar, the result is an immediate heavy glycosuria which is very transitory. After a day or two, no possible amount of carbohydrate feeding will produce continued glycosuria. In other words, the animal was permanently cured by the period of fasting or carbohydrate-free diet which allowed the islands to recuperate by rest. If the undernutrition or carbohydrate deprivation has weakened the true tolerance, the result in such an animal must have been diabetes. The hyperglycaemia or glycosuria after fasting or restricted diet represents only some temporary unpreparedness for the unexpected flood of carbohydrate, whether it be in the pancreas, liver or elsewhere. It has nothing to do with the true tolerance and is not in the slightest conflict with the established fact that fasting or low diet strengthens the island function.

In these and most other respects animals furnish excellent working models of clinical diabetes, and, of course, the pituitary experiments open up wide possibilities which were not available with complete or partial pancreatectomy. There still seems to be one point of mystery, namely, the unknown diabetic element in man. The cure of diabetes in animals is a fascinating development. But if we take a human patient with the mildest possible diabetes, and great obesity along with it, and if we reduce the weight by a hundred or more pounds, we might hope that the great resulting gain of tolerance would eliminate the trivial diabetes and make the patient non-diabetic. In my own experience I have seen great improvements of tolerance but never a cure of diabetes. This sharp unknown demarcation between diabetic and non-diabetic may be the crux of the problem.

DR. BERNARD A. WATSON (*Battle Creek, Mich.*): About ten years ago, in 1931, we became interested in the clinical application of some of the things that have been presented in this paper on the prevention of diabetes. Over a period of ten years all of the entering students of the University of Minnesota who had glycosuria were given a routine glucose tolerance test in an attempt to determine the significance of glycosuria. The type of curves noted were (1) diminished tolerance, (2) diminished assimilation, (3) diminished tolerance and assimilation, (4) chemical diabetes, and (5) clinical diabetes. We found the progression from a diminished tolerance through the various stages to clinical diabetes occurred in many patients and it was possible to check and reverse the process by a restricted fat diet in the first four stages of development of the disease. It was very difficult to reverse the process and obtain a normal tolerance curve in those of the clinical type. The patients were started on a low caloric diet of possibly sixty grams of carbohydrate, sixty of fat and forty-two of protein and as the fasting blood sugar returned to normal and glycosuria disappeared, the carbohydrate and protein were increased very slowly. Glucose tolerance tests were done at periods of six months and very definite evidence of recovery of tolerance was noted. The longest period any of our recovered patients have been followed has been five years. If a recovered patient goes on "a wild spree of eating," the disturbance again becomes evident; but with an average diet, recovery is maintained if weight is not gained. None of these patients were overweight as those Dr. Newburgh reported as recovering a normal tolerance test with weight reduction. Thus the clinical application of the prevention of clinical diabetes is clinically established. We found insulin retarded the recovery of patients, which bears out in part a previous speaker's comments.

DR. C. H. BEST (*Toronto, Canada*): Mr. President, I do not wish to close the discussion and I am not anticipating anything my colleague Dr. Haist may say. I feel, however, I would like to make a point about the early diagnosis of diabetes. This is a clinical problem but certainly there is a great deal to be done. The fact is, as Dr. Allen has emphasized and all the rest of you know, we do not see diabetes until most of the islet cells have been injured. That is not a very satisfactory state of affairs and it would appear to me one of the great problems for clinicians and experimentalists is an attempt, perhaps by entirely new means, to detect the patients who are on the verge of diabetes.

I have no new information about the hereditary factors. As Dr. Haist said, that is not completely settled but certainly there must be some means by which one could detect lesions of the pancreas before so much of the islet tissue is affected.

I was very glad Dr. Allen answered Dr. Mirsky's question. I know that Dr. Mirsky realizes that even the physiologist has seen hydropic degeneration in the human pancreas.

I was sitting next to Dr. Russell Wilder and he urged me to make a point of Dr. Richter's results in diabetic rats which if given a variety of foods, take fats in preference to carbohydrates. I have had no personal experience with that type of experimentation, but it would seem that the depancreatized rat is wise.

I'd like to hear some discussion as to whether it is feasible from the clinical point of view to use insulin prophylactically.

DR. WILLIAM S. COLLENS (*Brooklyn, N.Y.*): Our group have been tremendously impressed and stimulated by the work of Dr. Best and Dr. Haist. I believe one of the most important aspects of their studies is the demonstration of the reversibility of the diabetic state. However, I suspect that the great value of their paper is not so much the prevention of diabetes, as the potentialities of further studies along the path opened by them.

I should like to tell you about some experimental studies that we started in October immediately after the appearance of Best's and Haist's article. We took six patients whose insulin requirements were well over 75 units a day and we thought two methods of approach could be employed as practical therapeutic application of this investigation. We reduced the carbohydrate intake of the diet to less than 20 g and in order to provide a sufficient caloric intake, increased the proteins to 200 g. The fat intake was approximately 150 g. We studied the tolerance and found no evidence of increase in tolerance. The speaker had mentioned the use of high protein diets. I should like to have more specific figures concerning protein feedings.

DR. HAIST: I shall answer the last question first regarding the role of protein. Our results are not yet complete but from those observations that we have made so far, it would seem that protein has an effect very similar to carbohydrate and, in some of our experiments, the effect of the protein was almost as great as that of a carbohydrate diet.

We thought at first that the carbohydrate available from the protein might be the factor involved but the results have been somewhat variable and I can make no statement regarding that point. Fat has no effect in restoring the insulin content after starvation but protein has an effect that is almost though perhaps not as great as carbohydrate. We are not quite sure regarding the role of protein. Certainly there is some evidence that increased protein breakdown will increase the severity of the diabetic state.

It may be interesting to know in connection with the changes in the islets that this reduction in the granulation of the beta cells does not necessarily mean that hydropic degeneration will ensue. We have done some studies using granule stains in the animals that were given fat and those given fat and starved. The preliminary studies indicate there is a granulation in the pancreatic cells.

Now, most of the clinical questions have already been answered by the clinicians. Since the purpose of the paper was to provoke discussion, I think its purpose has been achieved.

IT IS UNNECESSARY TO STATE THAT WE *are enthusiastic about the various actions of insulin and could easily over-estimate its importance. Many investigators including my colleagues and I have studied the intense catabolic effect of pancreatectomy which, in many species, overwhelms all anabolic actions. The reappearance of these ana-bolic processes when insulin is supplied is, of course, thoroughly estab-lished but not completely understood. The exact role of insulin in the action of other hormones merits much more study. In paper 19 Dr. Otakar V. Sirek and I call attention to one of these neglected areas. Dr. O. Sirek and Dr. Anna Sirek, from Czechoslovakia, joined our staff in 1950 and in 1954, respectively. Both have now added a Ph.D. in Physiology to their medical training and have made a number of important contributions to the knowledge of diabetes.*

19. The Protein Anabolic Effect of Testosterone Propionate and its Relationship to Insulin

OTAKAR V. SIREK

CHARLES H. BEST

Since Kochakian and Murlin [461; 462; 463] performed their fundamental experiments on castrate dogs it has been well established that administration of androgenic substances causes a fall in the non-protein nitrogen (NPN) level in blood and at the same time lowers the nitrogen excretion in the urine. It is well known also that insulin has a very similar effect when injected into the diabetic organism (Falkenhausen [297], Chaikoff and Forker [182])—in other words, insulin and the male sex hormone may, under certain circumstances, exert a similar protein anabolic effect. The interrelationship between testosterone propionate and insulin has therefore been investigated and as a first step the behaviour of the NPN and blood sugar levels of normal and depancreatized dogs receiving testosterone has been studied.

EXPERIMENT

This study was carried out on eight well-trained female dogs of a weight between 20–25 kg. Three of them were surgically depancreatized and a standard diet was fed twice a day. Regular (Toronto) insulin was used and administered subcutaneously twice a day in order to keep the urine of the animals sugar-free. Studies were made on (a) normal dogs, (b) totally depancreatized dogs after withdrawal of insulin, and (c) depancreatized dogs receiving various doses of insulin. Each experiment was carried out twice on the same dog, once without testosterone and again after injection of testosterone.

The injections of the male sex hormone (we are grateful to the Ciba Company for supplies of Perandren) were given in the following way: the first morning 50 mg of testosterone propionate dissolved in sesame oil

Originally appeared in *Endocrinology*, LII (1953), 390–5.

were given intramuscularly, the second day 50 mg in the morning and 25 mg in the afternoon. The third day the actual experiment was carried out when 4–7 blood samples were drawn from the animal which was fasted for 24 hours before start of the experiment. A dog treated with testosterone was used again only after an interval of at least 4–5 weeks when it was assumed that all injected testosterone had disappeared from the body.

Blood sugar was determined according to Miller and Van Slyke [565] and for NPN determinations on whole blood Folin and Wu's (Boström [143]) colorimetric method was applied. The precipitation of blood proteins was carried out according to a special modification described by Folin [303]. In this not very common form of protein precipitation blood cells are minimally damaged and haemolysis is prevented. Using this modified precipitation method the results are around 12 mg per cent lower than figures obtained by the original method of Folin and Wu and even small variations in the NPN level can be detected.

RESULTS

The dose of 125 mg of testosterone propionate injected into a normal dog under the standardized conditions of our experiments proved to be highly effective as demonstrated in Figure 43. A similar depression of the

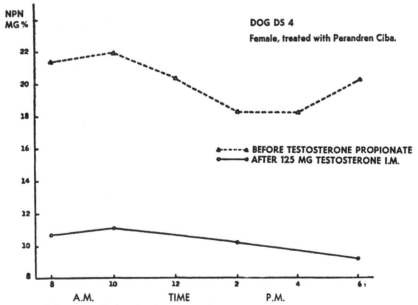

FIGURE 43. The normal female dog responds to testosterone by a remarkable lowering of the non-protein nitrogen level in blood.

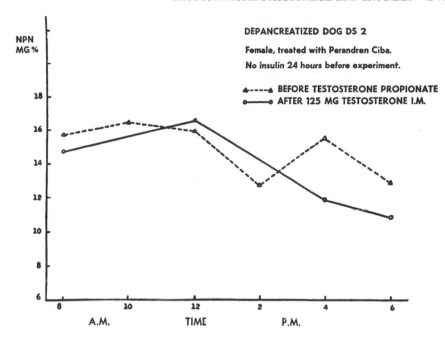

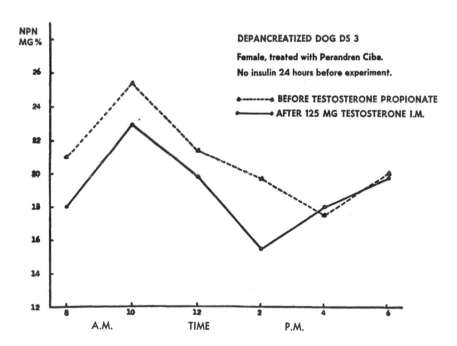

FIGURE 44. (a) The depancreatized dog kept for 24 hours without exogenous insulin exhibits no change of the non-protein nitrogen level after testosterone treatment. Dog DS2. (b) same as (a). Dog DS3.

NPN level in blood was obtained also in the other four intact animals. In contrast to normal dogs, the same dose of testosterone injected into our totally depancreatized dogs did not exert any effect on the NPN level when the exogenous supply of insulin was withheld for 24 hours before the start of experiment. Figures 44a and 44b are good illustrations of the negative response of diabetic dogs when only traces of insulin were present in the body. When under the same conditions an arbitrarily chosen dose of insulin was injected into such a diabetic dog a remarkable lowering of the NPN occurred, as shown in Figure 45, and no further depression of the NPN level could be obtained when the same dose of insulin and testosterone were acting together. The same observation was made after injections of even smaller amounts of insulin, such as 7, 4 or 2 units.

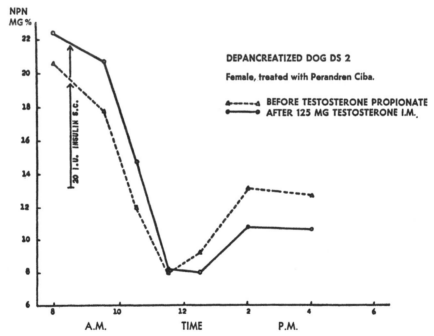

FIGURE 45. The diabetic dog responds to insulin by a prompt lowering of the non-protein nitrogen level. Testosterone neither supplements nor counteracts the NPN-lowering effect of insulin.

As could be expected, however, the decrease in the NPN after smaller doses was not so dramatic as shown in Figure 45. Testosterone had no effect on the NPN in these depancreatized dogs.

The blood sugar level seemed to be entirely unaffected by testosterone treatment under the conditions of this experiment. As shown in Figure 46 testosterone was unable to influence the blood sugar level of the normal

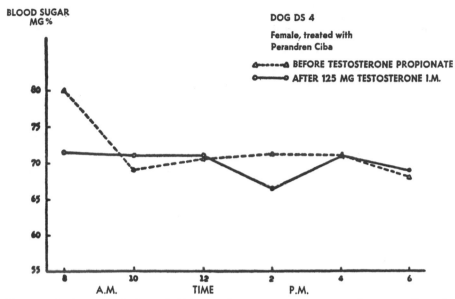

FIGURE 46. A standard dose of 125 mg of testosterone propionate does not affect the blood sugar level of the normal female dog.

female dog. In the depancreatized animal, testosterone did not change the blood sugar level whether insulin was injected or not.

DISCUSSION

The behaviour of the NPN level under the influence of the male sex hormone, testosterone propionate, in the normal and diabetic dog indicates very strongly that the protein anabolic effect of the male sex hormone is intimately associated with the presence of insulin in the body. The fact that testosterone failed to exhibit any influence on the blood sugar of the normal dog does not oppose the evidence indicating that certain physiological amounts of insulin must be available to the body if testosterone is to exhibit any protein anabolic function. There is not, however, any indication from these experiments that testosterone propionate causes a detectable increase in the amount of insulin liberated from the pancreas. Little is as yet known about the mechanism by which testosterone produces the protein anabolic effect for which the presence of insulin appears to be necessary.

SUMMARY AND CONCLUSION

The present paper describes a study of the effect of the male sex hormone, testosterone propionate, on the level of NPN and glucose in blood of normal and totally depancreatized dogs.

In the normal dog following testosterone treatment a significant lowering of the NPN level occurs, while the blood sugar level remains unchanged. In the depancreatized dog after withdrawal of exogenous insulin for 24 hours, testosterone has no effect upon the blood sugar or NPN. When insulin is administered to such a diabetic dog a lowering of both NPN and blood sugar occurs, but no further depression can be obtained when both insulin and testosterone are acting together.

It is therefore concluded that the protein anabolic function of the male sex hormone is intimately associated with the presence of insulin in the body but only a beginning has been made in understanding this relationship.

ACKNOWLEDGMENT

We are greatly indebted to Dr. A. M. Rappaport for performing the pancreatectomies on our experimental dogs.

A CAREFUL LOOK AT OUR FIRST NOTE-books indicates that Banting and I sometimes obtained an initial rise in blood sugar after injections of insulin. We attributed this to liberation of adrenalin. The same explanation was in the minds of other investigators until 1923 when Kimball and Murlin suggested that the initial rise in blood sugar seen after injections of insulin might be due to a new substance, since by the use of acetone and 95 per cent alcohol they were able to separate insulin from a hyperglycaemic substance for which they proposed the name glucagon. Bürger in Germany, Sutherland and Cori in the United States, de Duve in Belgium, and other groups, have greatly extended knowledge of this substance.

Thus it turned out that the methods conventionally used for extracting insulin extract also glucagon, another protein, with some very dissimilar physiological properties. This metabolic hormone remained difficult to separate from insulin preparations for many years but it has now been isolated and its structure determined. Much remains to be learned, however, about its physiological effects.

During the past ten years we have taken an active interest in glucagon. The leading member of our group has been J. M. Salter who, like many of my present colleagues, has passed (to me, very rapidly but to them, all too slowly!) from graduate student to professorial rank. We are primarily interested in glucagon as a physiological substance but useful information can be gained at this stage by administering large amounts. Paper 20 deals with this topic.

20. The Pathologic Effects of Large Amounts of Glucagon

J. M. SALTER, PH.D.

I. W. F. DAVIDSON, B.SC.

CHARLES H. BEST, M.D., D.SC.

The work of Ingle [415] and Cavallero [178] has shown that glucagon will produce a temporary or mild glucosuria in partially depancreatized animals and in animals pretreated with cortisone, but a significant diabetogenic action of glucagon administered alone to intact rats has not previously been shown.

The results of early attempts made in our laboratory to show a diabetogenic action of the pancreatic hyperglycaemic factor were disappointing. We reinvestigated the problem using much larger doses of glucagon attempting, at the same time, to prolong its activity by suspending it in corn oil and administering it subcutaneously at eight-hour intervals. Glucagon administered under these conditions appeared to exert a profound effect.

Figure 47 shows the average changes in weight and food intake of intact male controls injected with corn oil, and of normal male rats injected three times daily with 300 μg of glucagon (Lilly, lot no. 258–234B–33) suspended in corn oil. Weight changes are shown for a second set of controls limited to the amount of food consumed by the glucagon-treated animals.

It is apparent that the glucagon-treated rats consumed much less food than the controls and lost weight rapidly. The weight loss cannot be completely attributed to the reduction in food intake, as the pair-fed controls lost much less weight.

The glucagon-treated animals were not glucosuric but animals similarly treated, and encouraged to eat bread, frequently showed a transient but intense glucosuria. This stimulated us to investigate the effect of glucagon in force-fed rats.

Male Wistar rats weighing 150 to 160 g were fed by stomach-tube at 8:00 A.M., 4:00 P.M., and 12:00 midnight, the high carbohydrate diet

Originally appeared in *Diabetes*, VI (1957), 248–52. Presented at the Symposium on Insulin, Glucagon and the Oral Hypoglycaemic Sulphonylureas sponsored by the Clinical Society of the New York Diabetes Association, Inc., on October 12, 1956.

described by Reinecke, Ball, and Samuels [635]. The volume administered was slowly increased until the tenth day; thereafter each rat received 10 ml of the fluid diet, containing 6 g of solids at each feeding. Five animals served as controls and were injected with corn oil. The remaining five rats

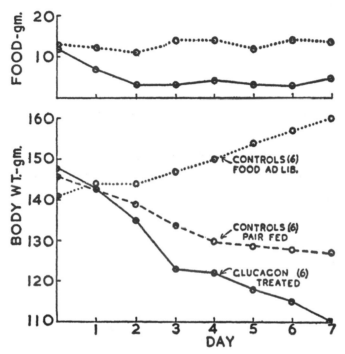

FIGURE 47. Changes in the weight and food intake of male control rats injected with corn oil and of rats injected subcutaneously every eight hours with 300 gamma glucagon in oil.

received subcutaneously at six-hour intervals a total of 1.2 mg of glucagon daily. The glucagon was suspended in corn oil[1] in a concentration of 3 mg per ml.

Figure 48 shows the average daily (a) glucose excretion, (b) urinary nitrogen excretion, and (c) body weight changes in the force-fed controls and in the glucagon-treated animals.

It is evident that the control rats excreted no glucose and gained weight during the experimental period. The glucagon-treated animals excreted approximately 4 g of glucose daily. Their urinary nitrogen excretion was nearly twice that of the controls and they lost weight rapidly. The blood sugar levels of the glucagon-treated animals remained between 350 to 450

[1]We have recently found that it is unnecessary to suspend the glucagon in oil. A neutral saline suspension is equally effective when administered subcutaneously.

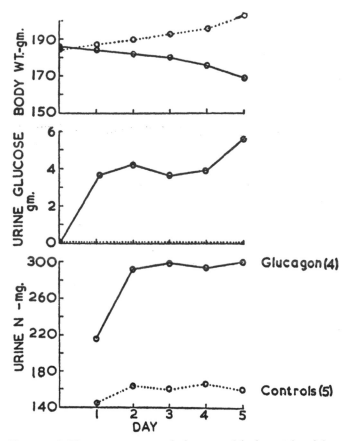

FIGURE 48. Urinary nitrogen and glucose and body weight of force-fed controls and of force-fed rats injected every six hours with 300 gamma of glucagon.

mg per cent throughout the day, while the controls showed only a slight increase in blood sugar concentration after each feeding.

During the experimental period the control rats remained in excellent health while the treated animals became emaciated and ill, with only two of the five rats surviving a seven-day period.

A second experiment was then performed in an attempt to produce permanent diabetes with glucagon. In this experiment twenty force-fed rats were used—ten control rats and ten glucagon-treated. The results substantiated those obtained in the first experiment. Intense glucosuria and hyperglycaemia developed rapidly with some animals excreting as much as 10 g of glucose daily. However, this investigation was difficult to carry out. The force-fed control rats thrived but the glucagon-treated animals became increasingly ill until after a week they required constant attention. The treated rats suffered gastrointestinal disturbances and their stomachs frequently became so distended that it was necessary to aspirate the contents. In other instances the animals would suddenly lapse into a state resembling diabetic coma with blood sugar levels between 800 to 900 mg per cent; this latter condition responded dramatically to insulin therapy. We succeeded in maintaining only two force-fed rats on glucagon for a period of ten days. The animals remained glucosuric and hyperglycaemic for six days following the cessation of all treatment. We feel that if treatment can be maintained for a longer time permanent diabetes may be produced.

In two normal dogs studied with Dr. James Campbell, glucagon in oil produced transient hyperglycaemia and mild glucosuria. Since the supply of glucagon was limited the treatment of these animals was neither intensive nor prolonged. The dogs were sacrificed after one week.

Histological examination of pancreas revealed degranulation of the β-cells. The extractable insulin content of the pancreas was found to be only 15 per cent of the normal.

The histological appearance of the pancreatic β-cells in the glucagon-treated rats has been variable. In some instances these cells show degranulation and hydropic degeneration, in other cases the β-cells appear to be more intensely granulated than normal. In both dogs and rats, glucagon consistently produces marked degranulation and atrophy of the acinar cells. The significance of this observation is not evident.

Although the glucagon used in these investigations was considerably purified, it contained significant amounts of other proteins. The possibility that the diabetogenic effect was due to an unknown contaminant had to be considered. However, we have since found that pure crystalline zinc glucagon has the same diabetogenic action; thus we attribute our initial results to the action of glucagon alone. The results of these investigations clearly show that under our experimental conditions glucagon possesses marked diabetogenic properties when administered to force-fed rats and to dogs fed *ad libitum*. It is not known, at this time, that a permanent diabetes can be produced with the pancreatic hyperglycaemic factor.

The mechanism(s) through which glucagon acts to produce diabetes is unknown. The effect of this substance on extrahepatic carbohydrate utilization remains a controversial subject. Studies carried out *in vitro* by Candela [648] and Snedecor, De Meio, and Pincus [716] indicate that glucagon inhibits the stimulating effect of insulin on glucose uptake and glycogen synthesis by the isolated rat diaphragm. However, Smith working with Dr. F. G. Young [822] has been unable to confirm this observation and Clarke of our department finds that the stimulating effect of insulin on glucose uptake by the rat diaphragm *in vitro* is enhanced if the animals are pretreated with glucagon.

Drury, Wick, and Sherrill [265] have reported that the hyperglycaemic factor slightly inhibits the disposal of blood glucose in eviscerated rabbits while Ingle, Nezamis, and Humphrey [416] claim that it has no effect on glucose utilization in eviscerated rats. Studies of a-v differences led Elrick *et al.* [282; 283; 284; 285] to conclude that glucagon enhances peripheral utilization in normal human beings and in normal or depancreatized dogs. The observations made by Elrick in normal humans have been confirmed and extended by Van Itallie, Morgan, and Dotti [764]. Bondy and Cardillo [138] could find no evidence of inhibition of glucose utilization in glucagon-treated humans. In our own department Dr. Margaret Henderson, working with Dr. G. Wrenshall, has found in one experiment using C^{14}-labelled glucose an increase in the utilization of glucose following the administration of glucagon to depancreatized dogs.

Although a definite conclusion cannot be reached, the experimental data at present available do not favour the view that the genesis of glucagon diabetes in the intact animal is due to a reduction in peripheral glucose utilization.

Our own data indicate that increased gluconeogenesis contributes to the glucagon-induced diabetes. Figure 49 shows the average urinary nitrogen excretion of intact fasting control rats and of comparable animals treated with glucagon. It is apparent that the fasting glucagon-treated animal excretes about 40 per cent more nitrogen than the controls. Under these conditions no glucosuria or hyperglycaemia occurs. The glucagon-induced

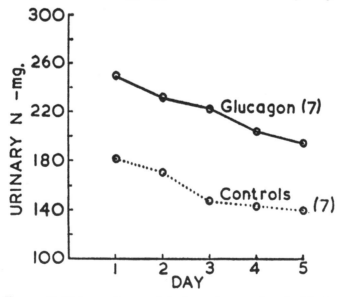

FIGURE 49. Urinary nitrogen of fasting male controls and of fasting
rats injected every eight hours with 400 gamma of glucagon.

increase in nitrogen excretion can be almost completely attributed to the increase in urea excretion.

Figure 50 shows the changes in the amino acid and sugar levels in the blood of controls and in rats injected with 1 mg of glucagon suspended in saline. The blood amino acids fell much more rapidly in the glucagon-treated animals and remained lower throughout the five-hour observation period. The blood sugar rose immediately after glucagon administration but

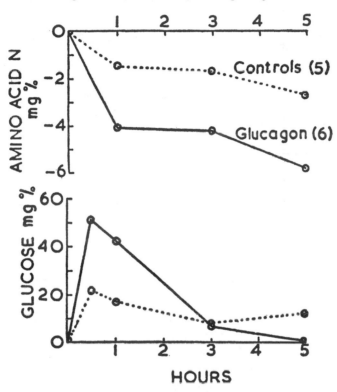

FIGURE 50. Changes in the blood amino acid and sugar levels of male control rats and of comparable animals given one subcutaneous injection of 1 mg glucagon suspended in neutral saline.

fell within three hours to normal levels. It does not appear that the glucagon-induced fall in blood amino acids can be attributed to an increase in the rate of peripheral utilizations since urinary nitrogen excretion also increased during this period.

In some respects the changes induced by glucagon administration are similar to those induced by adrenal glucocorticoids. The possibility that the marked increase in gluconeogenesis following glucagon administration was due to stimulation of the adrenal cortex was investigated.

Figure 51 shows the total nitrogen and urea nitrogen excreted by adrena-

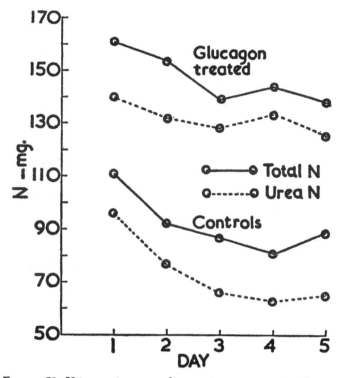

FIGURE 51. Urinary nitrogen and urea nitrogen excretion of seven male adrenalectomized rats (maintained on saline) injected with 400 gamma of glucagon every eight hours and of seven adrenalectomized pair-fed controls.

lectomized glucagon-treated rats and adrenalectomized controls. The food intake of the controls was limited to the amount consumed by the treated animals. It is apparent that the glucagon-treated adrenalectomized rats excreted about 50 per cent more nitrogen and urea than the controls.

Figure 52 shows the average urinary nitrogen excretion of fasting adrenalectomized rats treated with glucagon and of the fasting controls. The glucagon induced a marked increase in nitrogen excretion the first day but the effect became progressively less until on the fourth day there was no significant difference between the amounts of nitrogen excreted by each group. It will be recalled that in the fasting intact rat the glucagon-induced increase in nitrogen excretion was undiminished at the end of five days (see Figure 49).

The results of these last two experiments indicate that the catabolic action of glucagon is not mediated by way of the adrenal gland. However, the effect of glucagon on the catabolism of amino acids during the fasting state is partly dependent upon the presence of adrenal cortical secretions. Recent experiments have shown that the diabetogenic actions of glucagon

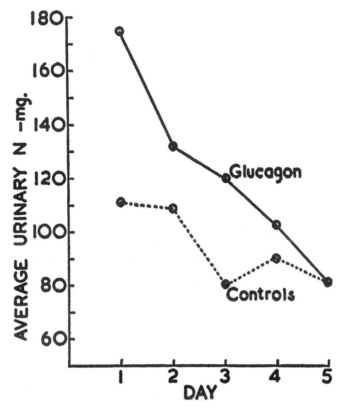

FIGURE 52. Urinary nitrogen excretion of five fasting adrenalectomized rats injected with 400 gamma glucagon every eight hours
and of five fasting adrenalectomized controls.

and cortisone are markedly synergistic. Rats treated with both substances
develop severe diabetic symptoms despite a 75 per cent reduction in their
food intake. Weight loss is precipitous and death occurs in from five to
seven days.

SUMMARY

The data presented show that glucagon when administered in large
amounts has a marked diabetogenic action in force-fed rats. It produces
intense glucosuria, hyperglycaemia, and weight loss. Preliminary experiments indicate that glucagon has a diabetogenic action in dogs fed *ad libitum*. The specific mechanisms responsible for glucagon diabetes are not
known, but the data strongly indicate that glucagon induces a marked
increase in gluconeogenesis and suggest that overproduction of glucose
contributes to this phenomenon. The protein catabolic effect of glucagon
is not mediated by the adrenal glands although a synergy between the
actions of adrenal cortical secretions and glucagon appears to exist.

ONE OF THE PHYSIOLOGICAL EFFECTS
of continued injections of glucagon is the production of a diabetic condition which persists after the injections have been discontinued. This condition, known as metaglucagon diabetes, is discussed in Paper 21.

In the study of the production of metaglucagon diabetes in rabbits, my colleague John Logothetopoulos has been the moving spirit. It should be possible to produce permanent diabetes in other species with greater susceptibility, but great care and a goodly supply of glucagon will be needed. The study of permanent diabetes produced by anterior pituitary extracts (F. G. Young) or somatotropin, has yielded valuable results. Equally important effects will doubtless accrue from the study of animals with permanent metaglucagon diabetes.

21. Glucagon and Metaglucagon Diabetes in Rabbits

J. LOGOTHETOPOULOS, M.D.

B. B. SHARMA, M.D.

J. M. SALTER, PH.D.

C. H. BEST, M.D.

Early attempts in this and other laboratories to demonstrate a diabetogenic action of glucagon have met with limited success. It was found that in order to produce a temporary diabetes with glucagon it was necessary either to force-feed [662; 178] the animals or to administer cortisone simultaneously [490].

Investigations described here differ from previous ones in that glucagon administration began on the second postnatal day and was continued for many months. Our purpose was to obtain additional information concerning the atrophy of alpha cells which follows prolonged treatment with glucagon [508]. We were, however, surprised to find that the anorexia produced by glucagon in adult rabbits did not occur in immature animals. The treated rabbits ate as much and grew nearly as well as their littermate controls. By the end of ten weeks seven of the nine glucagon-treated rabbits had blood sugar levels of about 300 mg per 100 ml throughout the day and were excreting 5 to 15 g of glucose daily. Continuation of the treatment caused a slow but progressive aggravation of the diabetic condition in five; in these cases, after the last injection of glucagon, the diabetes persisted for 63, 50, 30, 20, and 18 days, respectively. A preliminary account of these findings has been published elsewhere [509].

The results of additional studies, which confirm and extend our original observations, are presented here.

METHODS AND PROCEDURES

Litters of albino rabbits of mixed origin were used. The injections of glucagon started on the second postnatal day. A total daily dose of 2 mg of

Originally appeared in *Diabetes*, IX (1960), 278–85. Presented at the Symposium on Changing Basic and Clinical Concepts of Diabetes Mellitus sponsored by the Clinical Society of the New York Diabetes Association, Inc., on October 16, 1959.

glucagon per kilogram of body weight was given at seven to ten-hour intervals. The glucagon was suspended in sterile saline containing about 1,000 units of penicillin per millilitre. Saline containing penicillin was injected in the control animals. The young rabbits were weaned between the fortieth and fifty-fifth days and placed in individual metabolism cages. The food consumption and urine volume were measured daily, and every ten to fifteen days blood sugar levels were estimated at intervals throughout the day. The concentrations of glucose in urine and blood were determined by the Benedict [62] and Somogyi [726] techniques respectively. The classical staining techniques of Gomori [326; 327] as well as the Masson-trichrome method for pancreas fixed in Bouin's and Zenker-formol solutions were used for the investigation of the alpha and beta cells of the islets. Sections from pancreas fixed in Gendre's solutions at −10° C were stained with the periodic acid Schiff method.

Sections of unfixed pancreatic tissue cut at 7.5 μ with a cold knife technique were mounted in glycerin and examined by dark field illumination. In a background of slightly refracting nuclei of β cells and acinar cells, the α cells of control rabbits appear very prominent with their cytoplasm filled with white-silvery granules. [Fifteen figures have been omitted dealing with the histology of pancreatic islets of rabbits before and after treatment with glucagon.]

To secure an estimate of islet tissue concentration a ratio of islet to acinar tissue area was determined planimetrically on random sections of a piece of pancreas taken from the centre of the splenic portion.

A histological study was also made of specimens taken from practically all organs, including endocrine glands. (See Plates VII and X.)

RESULTS

Transient hyperglycaemia, of varying degree and duration, followed each injection of glucagon during the initial phase. The blood sugar level always returned to normal between injections. Figure 53 illustrates the patterns of hyperglycaemia and glucosuria observed in individual rabbits when the transition from intermittent to sustained hyperglycaemia was occurring. It can be seen that two of the four litter mates which had been treated for ten weeks had already developed a sustained hyperglycaemia and severe glucosuria, a third was showing intermittent hyperglycaemia and moderate glucosuria, and the fourth had become definitely resistant to the injections of glucagon.

The pancreases of the treated rabbits killed during the initial phase (fourth to eighth week) and during the transition period (eighth to twelfth

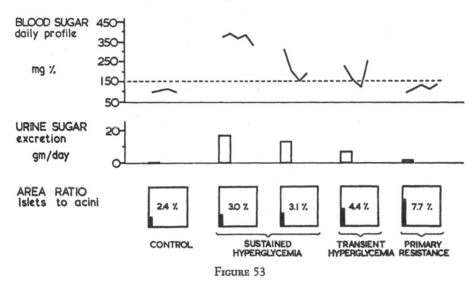

FOUR LITTER MATES TREATED WITH GLUCAGON FROM BIRTH
(10 weeks)

FIGURE 53

week) showed an increased concentration of islet tissue, partial degranulation and hypertrophy of the β cells, and a marked atrophy of the α cells.

The increased concentration of islet tissue was due to an increased number of islets and to an enlargement of individual islets. The rabbits which had become resistant to the hyperglycaemic effects of glucagon showed an equally marked hyperplasia of islet tissue. In some cases (Figure 53) this was more pronounced than in the animals exhibiting severe hyperglycaemia.

The degranulation of the β cells was of varying degree and did not appear to be correlated with the severity of the hyperglycaemic effect. The extreme atrophy of α cells made it impossible to distinguish them from marginal endothelial or connective tissue cells. Even from the fifth week of treatment many sections from the pancreas had to be searched to find a few α cells retaining specific staining characteristics.

Glycogen in the form of fine granules was found in the cells of the islets of rabbits which had just developed a sustained hyperglycaemia. The density varied in individual cells, and one could not be absolutely sure about a definite polarity towards the vascular pole. Glycogen infiltration was also found in cells of the ductules of the pancreas, in a few centro-acinar cells and in the ascending portions of the Henle loops and the distal tubules of the kidney.

Thus far, nine rabbits have been observed for periods of more than three months. Two remained resistant to glucagon treatment. Of the seven which entered the phase of sustained hyperglycaemia, two showed a period of decreased food intake, after which they could not be brought back to the previous diabetic level by continued administration of glucagon. In the other five rabbits there was a progressive aggravation of the diabetes. All these rabbits were kept for five to seven months before glucagon treatment was stopped.

The growth rate varied in the glucagon-treated rabbits and was on the average slightly less than in the controls. The loss of glucose in the urine was fully compensated by the increased food intake (Figure 54).

AVERAGE FOOD INTAKE OF RABBITS DURING GLUCAGON TREATMENT (5th and 6th MONTH)

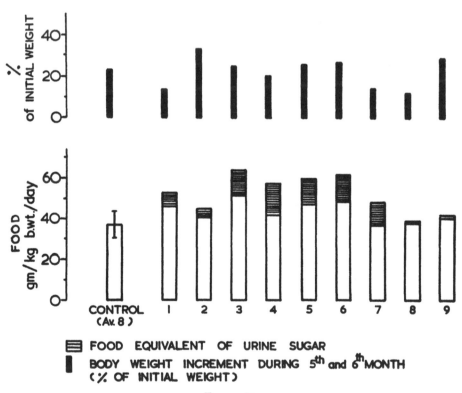

FIGURE 54

The diabetic animals had severe polyuria and polydipsia. The Rothera test for ketone bodies was occasionally positive during the last weeks of treatment. The progress of metaglucagon diabetes is shown in Figure 55. Zero day represents the day on which the last injection of glucagon was

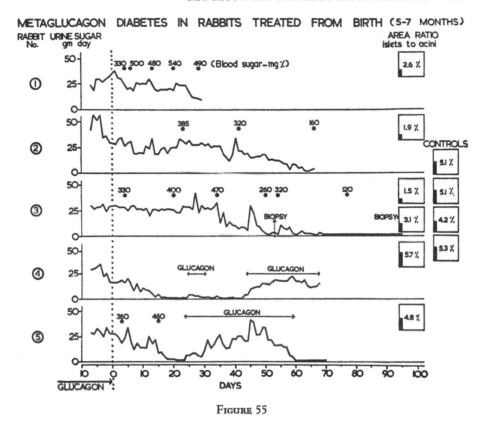

METAGLUCAGON DIABETES IN RABBITS TREATED FROM BIRTH (5-7 MONTHS)

FIGURE 55

given. There was no dramatic change in the diabetic state when the glucagon injections were stopped.

The first and second rabbits were sacrificed on the thirtieth and sixty-third day when the diabetic state was subsiding. A biopsy from the pancreas was taken from the third rabbit on the fifty-third day and the animal was then allowed to survive for one month and a half before it was sacrificed. The fourth and fifth rabbits had short periods of "metaglucagon" diabetes. In both, diabetes was re-established when glucagon treatment was resumed. Ratios of islet to acinar area in the first three rabbits were smaller than in controls.

The histological changes in the pancreases removed from the first and second rabbits when sacrificed were the same as those found in the biopsy specimen taken from the third animal on the fifty-third day after the cessation of glucagon injections.

Most islet cells appeared vacuolated and very few had a homogeneous cytoplasm. Aldehyde fuchsin stained granules were occasionally seen in the cytoplasmic rims of the vacuolated cells. The islet cells, however, which appeared vacuolated were found to be filled with masses of glycogen when sections from pancreas were fixed in alcoholic picric acid and stained by the periodic acid Schiff technique. Digestion with diastase brought back the vacuolated appearance. Glycogen was found also in cells of the ducts and ductules of the pancreas, in centro-acinar cells and in the kidney.

The histological appearance of the islets of two other rabbits sacrificed during glucagon treatment was similar to the one described.

The β cells of Rabbit 3, sacrificed six weeks after the biopsy had been taken, were free of glycogen and fully granulated. Normal β cells free of glycogen and fully granulated were also found in Rabbit 5, killed ten days after glucagon had to be stopped because of a sudden loss of appetite. The food consumption of this animal remained low until it was sacrificed.

Identifiable α cells were not seen for the first three or four weeks after the cessation of treatment. They started to appear by the fourth and fifth week but never seemed to be as numerous as they were in the controls.

DISCUSSION

The duration and magnitude of the hyperglycaemia following each injection of glucagon depends on many factors of which the nutritional state of the animals and compensatory insulin release appear to be very important.

The eventual fusion of hyperglycaemic waves into a sustained hyperglycaemia, observed in some of the rabbits, may be explained by the ultimate failure of the animals to produce adequate amounts of insulin. It would appear that a relative lack of insulin may be established, but, because of the high level of glucose in the extracellular fluids, the over-all glucose utilization seemed to be maintained at a normal level. A similar metabolic state has been reported in guinea pigs treated with cortisone [379].

Evidence for a peripheral anti-insulin effect of glucagon is controversial [60] and an inhibitory effect on the activity of the β cells has not been demonstrated. The experiments of Dohan and Lukens [258], of Brown et al. [152], leave no doubt that hyperglycaemia per se may eventually have a deleterious effect on the islets of Langerhans in many species. A reduced insulin secretion, that would follow as a consequence, would in turn aggravate the hyperglycaemia. This cycle may be operating in the "metaglucagon" diabetic rabbits when glucagon injections have been discontinued and endogenous glucagon production has been suppressed. An interesting possibility is that glycogen infiltration of the β cells may be a factor in the vicious cycle. It appeared quite early and paralleled the severity of the diabetes. The glycogen infiltration in the β cells may not be an innocuous deposition comparable to glycogen deposition in the liver, muscle, or in cells of the pancreatic ducts. In the advanced stages of the infiltration with glycogen there may be a mechanical interference with the function of the β cells.

In the "glucagon" and "metaglucagon" diabetic rabbits the β cells were the only endocrine tissue showing this glycogen deposition. The physico-chemical factors involved in this phenomenon are poorly understood and merit further investigation [272; 489].

The three rabbits with the prolonged periods of metaglucagon diabetes had a low islet concentration compared with the untreated controls. It is difficult to determine by histological examination whether this was the outcome of a slow progressive loss of β cells or was due to a failure of the formation of new β cells. Whatever the cause the process is extremely slow, compared with the rapid destruction of β cells in dogs treated with growth hormone [351; 639].

The failure of many glucagon-treated animals to develop a sustained hyperglycaemia or even to maintain intermittent hyperglycaemia may be attributed either to an effective compensatory hyperplasia of islet tissue or to a progressive loss of sensitivity to glucagon. The fact that all resistant rabbits had a high degree of islet hyperplasia favours the first view. Atrophy of α cells occurred during the first weeks of glucagon treatment and persisted throughout the period of treatment. We are unable to state whether they disappear, fail to grow, or become inconspicuous because of shrinking and degranulation. The observation that the α cells were apparently the only ones in the body which atrophied suggests that it was a true compensatory change and supports the view that they manufacture glucagon. Since the argentaffin cells of the gastrointestinal tract were fully granulated and well preserved, it seems unlikely that they possess metabolic characteristics similar to those of the α cells.

The atrophy of the α cells was unrelated to hyperglycaemia. It was equally prominent in the resistant and the diabetic rabbits. The reappearance of α cells on cessation of treatment was a very slow process.

As has previously been reported the islets of alloxan diabetic rabbits contain a large number of α cells [271]. This was strikingly demonstrated in fresh-frozen sections examined under dark field illumination. Agglomerates of fully granulated α cells made up most of the islets. In contrast the islets of the metaglucagon diabetic rabbits were free from identifiable α cells during the first weeks after cessation of treatment, yet the severity of the diabetes in these animals was comparable to that of the alloxan diabetic. The significance of α to β cell ratios in diabetic states becomes very doubtful as a result of these observations.

In conclusion we wish to stress that the experiments described do not provide evidence for or against the role of glucagon in human diabetes. The glucagon-induced diabetes in young rabbits, however, may become a useful experimental tool for the investigation of some basic problems in experimental diabetes. It is quite possible that the prolonged metaglucagon diabetes may be made permanent by intensified treatment of susceptible animals.

Summary

Rabbits were injected subcutaneously at eight-hour intervals with a total daily dose of 2 mg crystalline glucagon per kilogram body weight. Treatment commenced on the second postnatal day and continued for periods up to seven months. Initially the rabbits had intermittent hyperglycaemia and mild glucosuria but after eight to twelve weeks about 40 per cent of the animals developed sustained hyperglycaemia and severe glucosuria. The remaining animals became refractory to glucagon treatment. The diabetes grew progressively worse in five of the seven rabbits that were treated continuously for five- to seven-month periods. When glucagon treatment was stopped the diabetes persisted in these five rabbits for periods varying from eighteen to sixty-three days. The following observations were made:

1. The growth rate of the glucagon-treated rabbits was slightly less than that of the controls. The diabetic rabbits during and after the injections of glucagon compensated for the loss of glucose in the urine by consuming more food.

2. Hyperplasia of the islets, partial degranulation, and hypertrophy of the β cells and a marked atrophy of α cells was seen in all treated rabbits, refractory and diabetic alike.

3. Glycogen-deposition in the β cells was first evident at the time the sustained hyperglycaemia was developing. In the diabetic rabbits glycogen eventually filled most of the cytoplasm of the β cells. In the two rabbits killed when the severity of the metaglucagon diabetes seemed to subside sixty-three and thirty days after the last injection of glucagon, and in the pancreatic biopsy taken from one of the rabbits on the fifty-third day of the metaglucagon period, the infiltration of the majority of β cells with glycogen was still extensive. These three rabbits showed also a decreased concentration of islet tissue in comparison with the controls.

4. The α cells remained inconspicuous throughout the period of glucagon treatment and seemed to recover their normal appearance extremely slowly when the injections were stopped.

WHEN THE EXPERIMENTAL AND *clinical studies on insulin were no longer uppermost in Banting's mind, he developed a keen interest in tumours of experimental animals. Chickens, mice, and rats were used in his cancer research. Although he later became concerned with silicosis and other problems an interest in experimental tumours persisted throughout his life. Dr. W. R. Franks, Professor in the Banting and Best Department of Medical Research, is Banting's heir in this field. He is at least equally well known for his development of the Franks anti-gravity suit, certain details of which Banting was taking to England when his plane crashed in Newfoundland on February 21, 1941.*

Most medical research workers have dreams about cancer and many of them have tested the possibility that the metabolic process or chemical substance in which they have particular interest may play a role in tumour growth. Three substances of special favour in our laboratories are insulin, glucagon, and choline. Each of these has been shown to have some, probably quite indirect, influence on the growth of certain experimental tumours. R. De Meyer, a pupil and colleague of my close friend Professor J. P. Hoet of Louvain, Belgium, joined Dr. Salter to study the interesting inhibitory effects of insulin and glucagon discussed in Paper 22.

22. Effect of Insulin and Glucagon on Tumour Growth

J. M. SALTER, PH.D.

R. DE MEYER,* M.D.

C. H. BEST, M.D., F.R.S.

During the past few years we have been working on certain problems related to both insulin and glucagon (Salter and Best [660]; Salter et al. [661; 662]; Davidson et al. [247]). There is considerable evidence in the earlier literature that insulin may cause some inhibition in the growth of malignant tissue (Piccaluga and Cioffari [621]; von Witzleben [812]; Silberstein et al. [704]; Gomes da Costa [325]).† The results of experiments carried out in this laboratory are in general agreement with these earlier reports. We find that, although the effects of giving insulin to rats bearing the Walker carcino-sarcoma vary considerably, a small but significant inhibition of the growth of this tumour is produced in most instances. The findings presented in this preliminary communication show, for the first time, that glucagon alone also produces a significant inhibition in the growth of this tumour, while the simultaneous treatment with both glucagon and insulin consistently causes an inhibition that is considerably greater than the sum of their individual effects.

METHODS

Female Wistar rats weighing approximately 150 g were used in all experiments. The animals were fed powdered Purina chow containing 5 per cent corn oil.

Walker carcino-sarcoma tissue was collected from several donor rats, pooled and macerated with three parts (by weight) of 0.9 per cent saline until the resultant brei would pass through a 23-gauge hypodermic needle. Each

Originally appeared in the British Medical Journal, II (1958), 5–7.

*On leave of absence from Professor J. P. Hoet's Department, University of Louvain, Belgium.

†Our former colleague, Dr. Spencer Munroe, now of the Sloan-Kettering Institute for Cancer Research, has recently discussed with us his observations on the dramatic inhibition by insulin of the growth of Rous sarcoma in chickens.

animal was then injected in both gastrocnemii with 0.2 ml of the suspension. Treatments were started three days after the inoculations. At this stage the tumours were just palpable. In every experiment all rats had palpable tumours at the start. Protamine-zinc insulin (PZI) was injected once daily at 3 P.M. Crystalline glucagon suspended in 0.9 per cent saline was administered subcutaneously at 9 A.M., 3 P.M., and 9 P.M. The rats were sacrificed after 10 to 15 days of treatment. The back legs were skinned, carefully disarticulated at the hip-joint, and removed. Tumour weights were determined by subtracting from the weight of the tumour-bearing leg the average weight of the normal hind limb in rats of the same size. The doses of insulin and glucagon and other relevant data are given in Table 22.I.

RESULTS

The results of the experiments are also presented in Table 22.I. In Experiment 1 the administration of insulin inhibited the growth of the tumour by 10 per cent, while in Experiment 5 no inhibition was discernible. In a large series of other trials, not reported here, insulin consistently produced a small but significant slowing of the tumour growth. This inhibition occurred only when the food intake of the treated animals was restricted to the level of the controls.

The retardation of growth of the tumour induced by glucagon alone has varied from 20 to 40 per cent. This inhibition can be attributed, in part, to the reduction in food intake and the adverse effect of glucagon on the growth of the rat as a whole [662]. Although the rats treated with both insulin and glucagon lose less weight than animals given glucagon alone, inhibitions of tumour growth of 60–70 per cent have been obtained invariably. The inhibition is not therefore proportional to the weight loss. In each experiment the carcinostatic action of the combined therapy has been much greater than the sum of the individual effects of the two substances.

DISCUSSION

The data show that both insulin and glucagon produce some inhibition, which is, on the average, about 10 per cent for insulin and approximately 30 per cent for glucagon. Together they exert from 60 to 70 per cent inhibition of growth of this particular tumour. [Two figures have been omitted showing the inhibitory effect of treatment with glucagon and insulin on the development of tumours in the hind legs of rats.]

We have thus far only established that the inhibition persists while insulin and glucagon are being administered. Cessation of treatment is

TABLE 22.I

RESULTS OF EXPERIMENTS

Exp. No.	Treatment	No. of Animals Initial	No. of Animals Final	Days Duration	Av. Daily Food Intake (g)	Final Wt. (g)	Wt. Change (g)	Tumour Wt. (g S.E.)	Inhibition (%)
1	None	25	25		12.8	156‡	+14	13.4±0.42	
	P.Z.I. (1.6 u/day)	50	35	10	12.8*	154	−16	12.0±0.33	10
2	None	25	25		10.3*	151	+3	16.4±1.00	
	Glucagon (150 µg/day)	25	25	12	10.3*	142	−10	13.1±0.78	20
3	None	25	20		9.5*	138	−6	18.2±2.10	
	Glucagon (300 µg/day)	20	20	15	6.8	111	−29	13.2±1.00	27
	,, (300 µg+P.Z.I. 3 u/day)	50	28†		9.5	129	−13	6.1±1.18	67
4	None	20	20		10.5*	148	−5	13.5±1.67	
	Glucagon (900 µg/day)	20	20	10	5.6	116	−39	9.2±0.88	32
	,, (900 µg+P.Z.I. 3 u/day)	40	25†		10.5	132	−18	5.4±1.35	60
5	None	27	27		10.1	159	−10	7.0±1.12	
	P.Z.I. (1.6 u/day)	30	16	10	11.6*	150	−3	7.0±0.81	
	Glucagon (210 µg/day)	25	22		9.4	121	−33	4.1±0.93	40
	,, (210 µg+P.Z.I. 1.4 u/day)	34	24†		10.3	130	−18	2.1±0.48	70

*Food intake restricted to this amount.
†All deaths due to hypoglycaemia.
‡Figure represents weight of carcass exclusive of tumour.

followed by resumption of growth of the tumour. There has been a suggestion in a few cases that a prolonged remission may have taken place, but there is no proof as yet that this can actually be made to happen.

Hypoglycaemia still presents a serious problem, but the experience we have gained enables us to control the level of blood sugar better than was possible initially. A long-acting glucagon would be of great value in these studies.

If we consider for the moment only the control animals and those which have received insulin and glucagon together there have been in all 67 controls and 77 treated with the two substances. The inhibition of tumour growth produced by glucagon and insulin together has been remarkably consistent, but a great deal of further work will have to be done on this tumour and on others to determine the maximum extent and duration of the inhibition and the frequency with which it takes place in various species of animals. Dr. E. S. Goranson, of the Ontario Cancer Institute, working with one of us (J. M. S.), has already repeated our experiment, and has found that an extensive inhibition (80 per cent) is exerted by insulin and glucagon together on the growth of the Novikoff tumour in rats. There was a negligible difference in the weight of the control and test animals at the end of the experiments. Studies of various other tumours are under way.

It is abundantly clear that these findings demand, and that they will probably stimulate, an even more vigorous exploration of the metabolic effects of insulin and glucagon given together. No attempt will be made here to review the controversial literature on this subject. If glucagon supplements the peripheral action of insulin on normal tissue, the effects of the two together in "starving" the tumour may be supplementary. Equally plausible suggestions may be based on the possible katabolic effects of glucagon on the tumour itself. Both mechanisms could be involved.

The field of tumour growth is notorious for the frequency of pitfalls. We have seen no indication that the effect we are investigating is due to a contaminating infectious agent or to other artifacts. These may, of course, emerge later and necessitate a change in the interpretation of our findings. We have obtained glucagon from two sources—Indianapolis and Toronto. The various lots of insulin have been made in Toronto.

It is obvious that, if this phenomenon of the extensive inhibition of tumour growth by insulin and glucagon together is observed in a large number of other tumours in various species of animals, a clinical trial of the substances may become very tempting. Some aspects of the investigation would be easier to control in the hospital than in the experimental laboratory. Clinically the two substances *could* be given by continuous intravenous drip and the hypoglycaemia which has plagued us could be detected at an early stage. Frequent blood sugar estimations have not been considered advisable in the small animals. A sufficient number to establish low blood sugar as the cause of death in the insulin-treated animals which succumbed have been made. A great deal more should be learned in experiments on animals before any clinical study is seriously considered. An inhibition which persists only during the administration of the substances would be of limited clinical interest. The obvious possibility of using other substances to supplement the inhibition produced by insulin and glucagon is being explored.

ACKNOWLEDGMENTS

We are indebted to Mrs. H. Viilup, Mrs. C. Hooper, and Mr. Gunther Brunet for their efficient technical assistance. This work has been supported in part by funds from the Foster Bequest of the University of Toronto and the National Research Council of Canada. We wish to thank the Connaught Medical Research Laboratories for the insulin and some of the glucagon which we have used. Our major source of glucagon has been Eli Lilly and Company.

OVER THE YEARS SYNTHALIN, MYRTI-lin, and numerous other disappointing hypoglycaemic agents raised false hopes in the minds of many diabetics. There is no doubt that a new era of oral hypoglycaemic therapy is here. There is every indication that, if certain of the modern drugs are carefully used, a great deal of comfort and help can be given to properly selected patients.

One of the beneficial effects of the pioneer work of Dr. A. Loubatières in France and of Dr. F. Bertram in Germany has been the acceleration of interest in the diabetic state and in the mechanism of liberation of insulin from islet cells. My colleagues Dr. Anna Sirek and Dr. Otakar Sirek, with the co-operation of several others, have made detailed studies of the toxicity and anti-diabetic action of several of the oral hypoglycaemic agents. Paper 23 reports a study on the use of Tolbutamide.

It is extremely fortunate that after five years of use of Tolbutamide in human diabetes little or no evidence of toxicity has been seen. The picture in another species, the dog, is quite different.

23. Effect of Prolonged Administration of Tolbutamide in Depancreatized Dogs

ANNA SIREK, M.D.

OTAKAR V. SIREK, M.D., PH.D.

Y. HANUS

F. C. MONKHOUSE, PH.D.

C. H. BEST, M.D.

In a preliminary communication [712] we have reported that depancreatized dogs treated with tolbutamide for prolonged periods showed derangements of liver function. The present paper gives a detailed account of our studies on twelve depancreatized dogs treated orally with various doses of the drug. When given relatively large doses, the animals required appreciably smaller amounts of exogenous insulin to maintain a standard degree of control.

MATERIALS AND METHODS

The series represents a total of sixteen dogs and consists of the following groups of animals:

1. Depancreatized adult dogs:

(*a*) Two dogs maintained on 150 mg per kilogram body weight of tolbutamide; (*b*) three dogs on 100 mg per kilogram body weight; (*c*) three dogs on 30 mg per kilogram body weight; (*d*) two controls.

2. Depancreatized pups:

(*a*) Three pups maintained on 70 mg per kilogram body weight; (*b*) one control.

3. Partially depancreatized adult dogs (approximately 50 per cent of pancreatic tissue removed from the splenic end):

(*a*) One dog maintained on 30 mg per kilogram body weight; (*b*) one control.

Originally appeared in *Diabetes*, VIII (1959), 284–8.

The adult animals weighed about 10 kg and the pups, which at the time of pancreatectomy were approximately six months old, about 5 kg. The diabetic dogs were fed measured amounts of a commercial ration supplemented with raw pancreas. They were kept in metabolism cages and the urine was collected daily. The total amount of sugar was determined by Clinitest [Ames Company, Inc.] tablets. Regular and protamine-zinc insulin were administered daily, prior to feeding, in two separate subcutaneous injections in amounts required to keep blood sugar levels on the average below 200 mg per 100 cc and the glycosuria very slight. Because of considerable fluctuation from day to day and week to week, it was found more convenient to express the effect of tolbutamide upon blood sugar in terms of the amount of insulin spared. The diabetic dogs were kept under these standard conditions for at least two weeks and in some cases much longer before treatment was commenced.

Blood samples were obtained frequently before and during the test period. Blood sugar was determined by the micro-method described by King [454]. Bromsulphalein clearance tests were performed according to Gornall and Bardawill [328]. Serum bilirubin was determined according to Malloy and Evelyn [547]. Prothrombin clotting time was determined in whole plasma and in 25 and 50 per cent saline dilutions by the one-stage method of Quick [625]. Total cholesterol was determined by a modification of the method of Bloor, Pelkan, and Allen [131]. Total serum protein was determined by the method of Weichselbaum [783]. Serum albumin was determined by salt precipitation with 26 per cent sodium sulphate [546; 566] and the precipitated globulins were separated by centrifugation under ether according to Kingsley [456]. Serum alkaline phosphatase was estimated by the amount of phenol liberated from a phenol-phosphate substrate and expressed in King-Armstrong units per 100 ml of serum [455]. Serum glutamic-pyruvic and glutamic-oxalacetic transaminases (TGP and TGO) were determined by a procedure in which the oxalacetate and pyruvate formed an intensely brown-coloured hydrazone; the serum levels were expressed in Sigma-Frankel units per 1 ml of serum [703]. Total serum protein-bound hexose was determined with the orcinol reagent according to Lustig and Langer [521] using Winzler's modification [810].

RESULTS

The first change in liver function noted at any dose level was usually an elevation of the serum alkaline phosphatase. Figure 56-a,b,c shows the behaviour of the alkaline phosphatase in the first two groups of animals. The same elevation was observed in the partially depancreatized dog. A

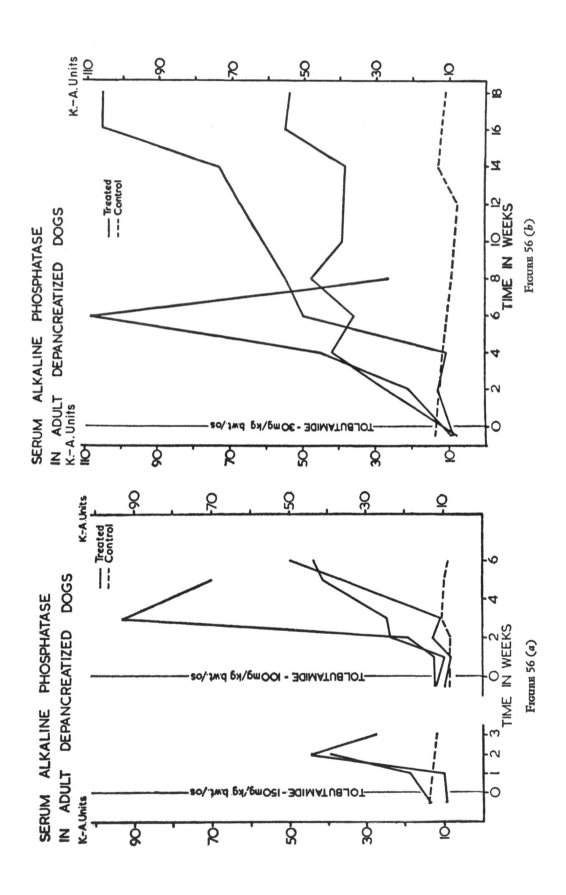

SERUM ALKALINE PHOSPHATASE
IN ADULT DEPANCREATIZED DOGS

Figure 56 (b)

SERUM ALKALINE PHOSPHATASE
IN ADULT DEPANCREATIZED DOGS

Figure 56 (a)

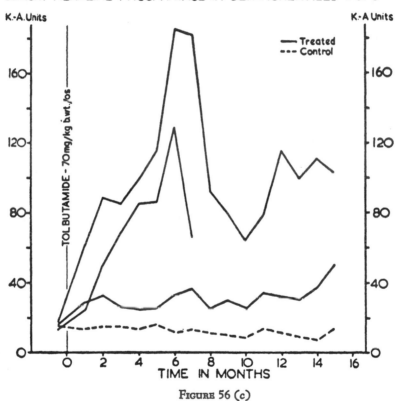

SERUM ALKALINE PHOSPHATASE IN DEPANCREATIZED PUPS

FIGURE 56 (c)

fall in total serum proteins was also encountered which was due to a decrease in serum albumin. Figure 57-a,b,c presents the results obtained in the same groups of animals. Again, the partially depancreatized animal showed the same change. The glutamic-oxalacetic and glutamic-pyruvic transaminase levels became elevated and the highest values as well as the normal ones are recorded in Table 23.I. The serum cholesterol levels were not followed closely, but in several dogs a profound fall was encountered in the terminal stages. The lowest figures as well as the control values for each animal are included in Table 23.I. Total protein-bound hexose was determined on a number of blood samples and an elevation from the average normal of 106 mg per 100 cc up to 153 mg per 100 cc was found in all our dogs treated with tolbutamide.

TABLE 23.I

SERUM TRANSAMINASE AND CHOLESTEROL VALUES
BEFORE AND DURING TOLBUTAMIDE TREATMENT

Dose mg/kg b.wt.	TGO—Units		TGP—Units		Cholesterol—mg %	
	Control	Highest	Control	Highest	Control	Lowest
150	31	1,010	20	230	306.2	65.9
	21	660	21	200	400.5	67.6
100	—	25	—	28	—	229.6
	—	14	—	18	—	156.6
	—	380	—	200	—	—
70	16	71	18	72	194.0	156.6
	14	78	24	240	288.4	131.0
	11	98	11	120	201.1	34.6
30	17	194	19	800	314.0	120.0
	23	155	21	670	251.0	90.8
	15	130	3	120	261.7	184.2
	*—	1,102	—	960	—	27.3

*Partially depancreatized.

Bromsulphalein clearance tests were performed on all animals frequently and the results were found to be within normal limits, i.e., less than 10 per cent retention fifteen minutes after injecting 10 mg per kilogram body weight.

The insulin requirements are recorded in Figure 58. It can be seen that those dogs which were maintained on 100 mg or 150 mg per kilogram body weight of tolbutamide required, after a certain time, considerably less insulin. The insulin requirements of the puppies which have been maintained on 70 mg of tolbutamide per kilogram body weight for almost sixteen months (and thus are now adult dogs), and the insulin require-ments of the dogs maintained on 30 mg per kilogram body weight have

SERUM ALBUMIN
IN ADULT DEPANCREATIZED DOGS

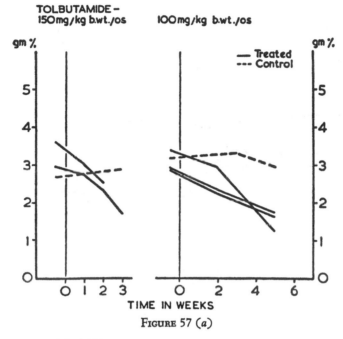

FIGURE 57 (a)

SERUM ALBUMIN
IN ADULT DEPANCREATIZED DOGS

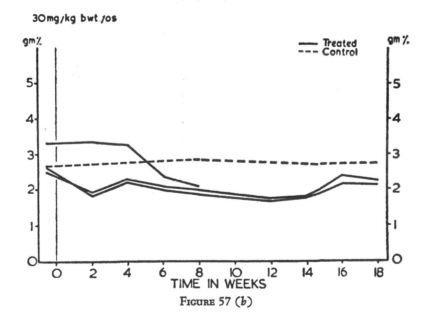

FIGURE 57 (b)

SERUM ALBUMIN IN DEPANCREATIZED PUPS

TOLBUTAMIDE - 70 mg/kg b.wt./os

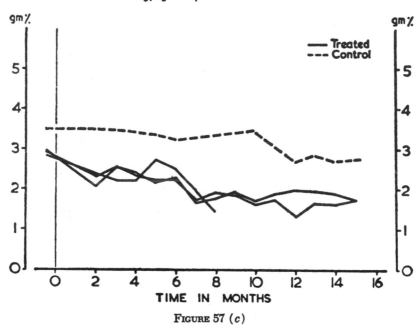

FIGURE 57 (c)

INSULIN REQUIREMENTS
OF ADULT DEPANCREATIZED DOGS

TOLBUTAMIDE —
150 mg/kg b.wt /os   100 mg/kg b.wt./os

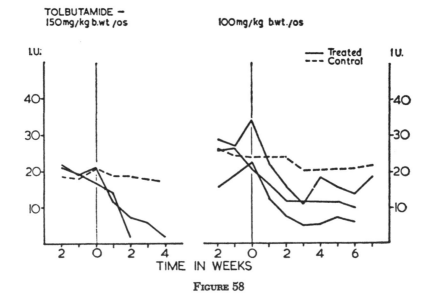

FIGURE 58

not appreciably changed. These figures are omitted from the graph. The partially depancreatized dog did not require exogenous insulin at any time and showed a moderate but substantial fall in blood sugar directly after the first dose of tolbutamide. In the totally depancreatized dogs which responded to the drug with a fall in blood sugar, there was no immediate drop after the first dose, but the blood sugars gradually fluctuated at lower levels and thus enabled us to decrease the daily amount of injected insulin.

The prothrombin clotting time in plasma diluted with saline to 25 per cent was in some cases prolonged to 300 seconds, in comparison with about twenty seconds for normal dogs. This prolongation usually could be eliminated by parenteral administration of vitamin K_1. In two animals the prothrombin clotting times were elevated in the terminal stages and here vitamin K_1 was without effect. In two other animals bleeding into various organs and into the peritoneal cavity was encountered but the prothrombin clotting time was normal. The dying animals were always jaundiced. The elevation in serum bilirubin levels was due to a rise in direct reacting bilirubin. It appears then that bleeding tendencies, prolonged prothrombin clotting times, and jaundice were abnormalities which occurred independently of each other but a final conclusion on this point is not possible in this small series of animals.

All five dogs treated with 100 or 150 mg tolbutamide per kilogram body weight deteriorated within three to six weeks and either died or had to be sacrificed. One animal in each of the other groups, i.e., those receiving less than 100 mg tolbutamide per kilogram body weight, followed the same course as those receiving the higher doses. The gross and microscopic findings in all of our autopsied animals will be reported in a separate communication. The completeness of the pancreatectomy was verified in each case.

Discussion

The data presented above indicate that the livers of our experimental animals have been seriously affected by tolbutamide. The data also show that prolonged administration of the drug in doses of 100 mg and 150 mg per kilogram body weight may produce a fall in blood sugar in depancreatized dogs and diminish but not abolish their requirements for exogenous insulin. A fall in blood sugar after prolonged administration of tolbutamide to depancreatized dogs was observed by Ricketts and associates [641] and Schambye [670]. Bleeding into organs of depancreatized dogs treated with large doses of tolbutamide was reported previously by Schambye [671], but he did not conduct any extensive study of liver function.

In another study Tarding and Schambye [746], using C^{14}-labelled glucose, were able to demonstrate a reduction in hepatic glucose output after a single injection of tolbutamide to normal dogs. Ashmore, Cahill, Earle, and Zottu [26], by cannulating the portal and hepatic veins, provided direct evidence of a diminished glucose output from the liver when normal dogs were given a single intravenous injection of tolbutamide. These results would suggest that an analogous situation may have existed in our depancreatized animals receiving 100 mg or more per kilogram body weight of the drug for prolonged periods. The diminished insulin requirements of our animals may prove to be due to a diminished glucose output from the liver. It would also be indicated that doses such as 30 mg or 70 mg per kilogram body weight, while effective in producing the described changes in liver function, were perhaps insufficient to interfere with glucose output as judged by the relatively steady blood sugar levels and insulin requirements. This suggestion is strengthened by the numerous reports on experiments with liver slices. Tolbutamide had to be present in the incubation medium in rather large concentration in order to depress the activity of enzymes involved in the release of free glucose from this organ [27; 66; 763; 766; 782].

It might be argued that the derangements in liver function observed in our dogs are the result of nutritional deficiencies due to malabsorption. All our depancreatized animals were kept under standard conditions for from several weeks to one year before they were given tolbutamide. None of the dogs showed any evidence of digestive or hepatic disturbance during the control period and these observations and the results of our previous experiences with depancreatized dogs on similar diets and insulin therapy tend to rule out nutritional deficiencies as a cause of the hepatic changes. In the partially depancreatized dog the pancreatic tissue was unable to protect the animal from the toxic effects of the drug. In recent experiments we have observed that even normal dogs, when treated with small amounts of tolbutamide, may show derangements in liver function similar to those described in the depancreatized animals.

The severe change in liver function found in dogs is in a striking contrast to the results of similar studies in human subjects. We have carried out the same liver function tests in a series of human diabetics treated with tolbutamide by our clinical colleague, Dr. B. Leibel, and in accord with other authors [825] have thus far seen no abnormalities. The results of the study of Mohnike and Wittenhagen [573] indicate that in the dog this drug is metabolized in a different way from that occurring in man. The possibility that the tolbutamide-treated dog produces a toxic metabolite either in the form of para-toluol-sulphonamide or some other by-product is now being investigated.

Summary

Tolbutamide (Orinase-Hoechst) was given in various doses orally to twelve depancreatized dogs for prolonged periods of time. All the animals suffered derangement in liver function, two died and six had to be sacrificed because they became jaundiced and were deteriorating rapidly. It was observed, in confirmation of other authors (Ricketts, Schambye), that depancreatized animals when treated with relatively large doses of tolbutamide may require appreciably smaller amounts of exogenous insulin to maintain a standard degree of control. The present findings are discussed in the light of those of other workers.

PAPER 24 IS OF GREAT INTEREST TO ME and takes me back to the early days of 1922 when Banting and I debated the pros and cons of using our most potent and pure preparation of insulin for the first clinical trial. I am indebted to my colleagues for permission to include this report of the re-investigation of extracts of foetal calf pancreas on experimental animals and of the first use of this material in human patients.

24. A Clinical Assessment of Foetal Calf Insulin

J. M. SALTER, PH.D.

O. V. SIREK, M.D., PH.D.

M. M. ABBOTT, M.D.

B. S. LEIBEL, M.D.

Early in their original work with insulin, Dr. Banting and Dr. Best were confronted with the problem of discovering a source of the hormone to meet the inevitable demands of the diabetic population throughout the world. At that time, the extraction of insulin seemed to depend upon the prior elimination of the external secretory portion of the pancreas. With this in mind Banting and Best, while working alone, explored the possibilities that foetal pancreas, before the development of its exocrine function, might provide a useful source of the hormone. Although foetal calf insulin was prepared in 1921 and used with dramatic success in diabetic dogs, it was never tested clinically, presumably because of an abundance of insulin soon made available from the adult cattle by alternative techniques [75]. Now, almost forty years later, a series of clinical trials of this substance have been initiated in order to fill this gap in the history of insulin.

METHODS

Banting's and Best's original notes were consulted and the insulin was prepared according to the procedure they used in 1921. Banting and Best used the pancreas immediately after they had removed it from the foetuses. Since we wished to prepare relatively large amounts of foetal insulin at regular intervals, it was necessary to collect and freeze the glands whenever they became available.

Two hundred grams of frozen foetal pancreas were cut into thin shavings and extracted for four hours in 200 ml of acid alcohol (95 per cent ethanol, 0.6 concentrated HCl). The extraction was performed with continuous agitation at a temperature of 5 degrees C. The mixture was then

Originally appeared in *Diabetes*, X (1961), 119–21.

filtered (later lots were centrifuged) and the filtrate was saved. The tissue debris was re-extracted for four hours with another 200 ml of acid alcohol. The filtrates from the extractions were combined and evaporated nearly to dryness in a small vacuum still. The residue was dissolved in 50 ml of saline. The insulin content was assayed by the mouse convulsion technique and was found to be 24 units per ml. Berkefeld filtration provided sterility.[1] The insulin solution administered to the children (patients R.K. and I.D.) was diluted to 12 units per ml while that administered to the adults was diluted to 20 units per ml.

Prior to its clinical use, two volunteers received small subcutaneous or intracutaneous injections of the foetal insulin extract on four separate occasions. It produced no detectable irritation or side effects.

RESULTS

At the Hospital for Sick Children, Toronto,[2] three children with diabetes of recent onset, while in the hospital for stabilization, volunteered for this experiment. They were treated with diet and were receiving 12 to 25 units of Lente and crystalline zinc insulin. The material to be tested was injected in the morning, twenty to twenty-four hours after the last dose of insulin. The patients were fasted overnight and their breakfast consisted only of eight ounces of unsweetened orange juice, given approximately two hours before the experiment.

Foetal calf insulin, Lot CHB-2, was injected subcutaneously in a boy, R.K., and in a girl, I.D. Both were seven years old. Figure 59 shows the effect of this material upon blood sugar concentration and the precipitous fall is quite evident when compared to the blood sugar curve obtained on a thirteen-year-old diabetic boy who received 0.5 cc of saline under the same experimental conditions. The material was well tolerated and there were no side reactions of any kind.

It was possible to compare foetal calf insulin with the action of crystalline zinc insulin at the Baycrest Hospital[3] for the chronically ill in Toronto.

---

[1]Recent experiments carried out in this laboratory indicated that the original procedure also extracts a substance (possibly an enzyme) that destroys insulin over a three- to four-month period. This slow inactivation was not evident during the early work because preparations were used promptly. Heating the insulin preparation rapidly to 70° C for three minutes and then cooling, prevents subsequent deterioration and allowed more prolonged storage of the foetal insulin. This heating procedure was used in the preparation of the later lots of material.

[2]The facilities of the Hospital for Sick Children were provided by Professor A. L. Chute.

[3]The clinical investigations of diabetes at Baycrest Hospital are supported by the S. Lunenfeld Charitable Foundation.

At this institution, the patients are in permanent residence and physical activity, emotional environment, and dietary intake are constant within practical limits. The subjects selected for study were changed from their usual depot insulin to divided doses of crystalline zinc insulin. A baseline was established by determining their blood sugar profiles which were

EFFECT OF FETAL CALF INSULIN IN CHILDREN
WITH DIABETES OF RECENT ONSET

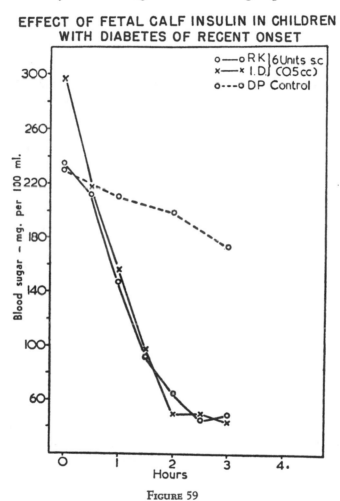

FIGURE 59

repeated at three widely spaced intervals. These were followed in each case by a similar survey after the patient had been receiving the same doses of foetal insulin for a period of two weeks. The results of these investigations are displayed in Figures 60 and 61. During the course of the latter therapy no local irritation at the sites of injection was seen, nor were there any remote toxic effects from the foetal calf insulin.

Mrs. E.W., aged seventy-seven years, was discovered to be suffering from diabetes seven years ago. Twenty years ago she had a myocardial infarction and developed congestive cardiac failure which has been controlled satisfactorily. Three years ago she fractured her left hip which was pinned successfully. The control of her diabetes mellitus has been uneventful.

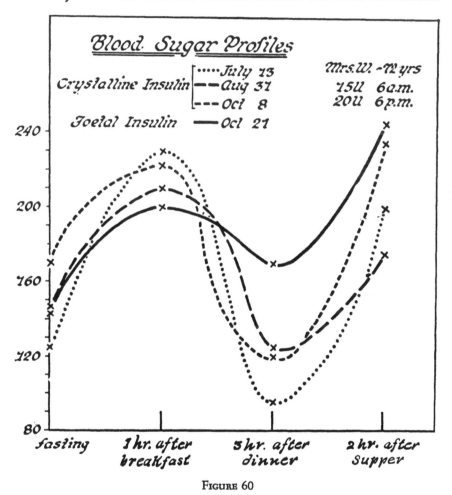

FIGURE 60

Mrs. J.M., aged seventy-five years, developed diabetes six years ago. At first she was controlled by diet alone, but subsequently also required insulin. In 1957 she was changed to tolbutamide therapy. Following a good response initially, she relapsed in six months and was then placed on insulin therapy. Nine years ago she had a posterior myocardial infarction and in recent months has been under therapy for essential hypertension and cerebrovascular disease.

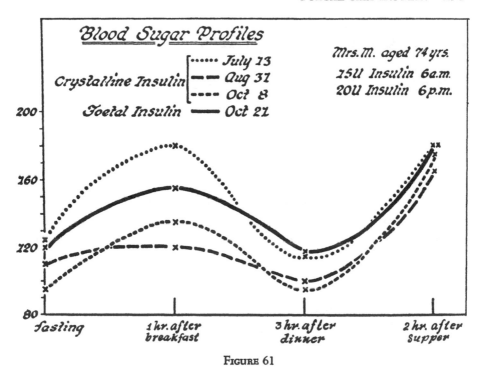

FIGURE 61

CONCLUSIONS

Foetal calf insulin, prepared by the original technique of extraction and purification used by Banting and Best in 1921, exerts the same effect in diabetic patients as does modern crystalline zinc insulin. The foetal calf insulin produced no local reactions and presumably would have provided a useful source of hypoglycaemic material for the initial treatment of cases of diabetes mellitus in Toronto in 1922 if a more readily available source (adult beef pancreas) had not proved satisfactory.

ACKNOWLEDGMENT

This work was supported in part by the Samuel Lunenfeld Charitable Foundation.

25. The Late John James Rickard Macleod, M.B., CH.B., LL.D., F.R.C.P., F.R.S.

C. H. BEST

John James Rickard Macleod spent ten of the most active years of his life in the University of Toronto. His research work was extensive and productive and his lecturing programme heavy. He was a particularly able teacher and his classes will long be remembered by those students who were fortunate enough to pass through his hands.

Professor Macleod was born in Cluny, near Dunkeld, Scotland, September 6, 1876. He received his early education in Aberdeen Grammar School and later graduated in Medicine from Aberdeen University. He was awarded the Anderson Travelling Fellowship and spent a year in the Physiology Institute, Leipzig. On returning to England he continued his postgraduate studies in Cambridge where he took his Diploma of Public Health. Professor Macleod went to the United States in 1903 as Professor of Physiology, Western Reserve University. He held this chair for fifteen years prior to coming to the University of Toronto in 1918 as Head of the Department of Physiology. One of the outstanding physiologists of the day, Professor Macleod received many honours from various scientific societies. He was elected in 1923 Fellow of the Royal Society, London, of which he had been MacKinnon Scholar from 1900 to 1903. He was President of the American Physiological Society in 1922, and in 1923 was awarded, jointly with Dr. F. G. Banting (now Sir Frederick), the Nobel Prize in recognition of the discovery and development of insulin. In 1925 Professor Macleod was elected President of the Royal Canadian Institute in which he was always keenly interested. Perhaps the honour which meant most to Professor Macleod came when he was invited to return to his own university, Aberdeen, as Regius Professor of Physiology. This post he held until his untimely death on March 16, 1935. Professor Macleod's main researches lay in the field of carbohydrate metabolism, but he did valuable work in many other fields. His publications are an indication of his wide range of interests, including as they do work on the chemistry of carbamates and purine metabolism, physiology of the intra-

Originally appeared in the *Canadian Medical Association Journal*, XXXII (1935), 556.

cranial circulation, ventilation, and surgical shock, etc. His textbook on physiology is one of the most popular in English-speaking countries today. Professor Macleod will long be remembered in the University of Toronto as a man who devoted his mental and physical strength without reserve to the advancement of scientific knowledge and to the instruction of students. His own achievements in medical research, and the work done by young men trained under him, will perhaps constitute the memorial which he himself would have most highly prized.

26. Frederick Grant Banting, 1891–1941

C. H. BEST

Frederick Grant Banting was born on November 14, 1891, on a farm near the town of Alliston, Ontario. His father, William Thomas Banting, was of Irish extraction, and his mother, Margaret Grant, of Scottish ancestry. Banting attended the rural school and the high school in Alliston. He had a remarkably robust physique and a most inquiring mind, both of which were to stand him in good stead in later life. He was fond of athletic exercise in his early days, but in later life spent little time in recreations with the exception of drawing and painting. He entered the University of Toronto, Victoria College, in 1912. Banting was not a brilliant medical student but his inquiring mind impressed his instructors and his classmates. There are many stories about the small impromptu investigations which he conducted as a part of his undergraduate course. His studies were interrupted in 1915 when he joined the R.C.A.M.C. as a private. He was later sent back to complete his course in medicine, and he was given his commission in the Medical Corps immediately after his graduation in 1916. He saw service in England and in France, and received the Military Cross for exceptional bravery while attending the wounded under fire. He was wounded at Cambrai and for a time it was thought that he would lose his right arm.

He returned to Canada after the First Great War and was appointed Resident in Surgery in the Hospital for Sick Children, Toronto. He became a well-qualified surgeon with particular interest in orthopaedics, which he had developed as a result of his contacts with Professor C. L. Starr, Professor W. E. Gallie, and Dr. D. E. Robertson. In 1920 he began the practice of medicine in London, Ontario, but his practice grew very slowly and he obtained a position as part-time demonstrator in the University of Western Ontario. He conducted some research work there in the Department of Physiology, 1920–21, but the results were not published until after the work on insulin was well under way. While preparing a lecture on diabetes Banting was greatly stimulated by the idea that failure by previous workers to obtain the hormone of the pancreas was due to the fact that the enzymes of the external secretion might have destroyed the hypothetical internal

Originally appeared in *Obituary Notices of Fellows of the Royal Society*, IV (1942), 21–6.

secretion during the course of preparation of the extract. The formulation of this idea was really the turning-point of his life. It forced him to give up his practice and his position in London to seek the opportunities available in Toronto for the testing of his hypothesis. These facilities were provided by Professor J. J. R. Macleod, Head of the Department of Physiology. The year 1921 was certainly one of the most strenuous and the most productive of Banting's life. He demonstrated at that time four great traits of his character—courage, persistence, scientific ingenuity, and industry. He sold his personal effects to secure money, and he threw himself wholeheartedly into medical research which was to become his life's work.

In his Cameron Lecture in 1927 Banting described in detail the start of the investigations which led to the discovery of the internal secretion of the pancreas. This work was begun on May 16, 1921, in collaboration with the writer, who had been asked by Professor Macleod to participate. The memory of the intimate association with Banting during that spring, summer, and autumn, when it became clear that an active diabetic principle could be prepared from degenerated or from normal pancreas, will always be cherished. The intense excitement and pleasure with which we watched the depth of colour in the sugar reagent fade as the blood sugars of the diabetic animals became reduced under the action of insulin, is difficult to describe. At the beginning of the investigation the surgical aspects of the problem were entirely in Banting's hands, while more chemical procedures fell to my lot. Later he taught me the essentials of surgical technique, and he acquired considerable skill in the estimations of sugar and of the other constituents in which we were interested. We were soon completely convinced that success had been achieved and looked forward with eager anticipation to the application of our findings to the human diabetic. In those days most of our time was spent in the laboratory where we frequently slept and prepared our meals.

Banting was light hearted and easily amused when the research was progressing favourably. He was inclined to be silent and preoccupied when advances were not being made. The mental stimulus furnished by a new idea was remarkably well demonstrated in his attitude toward life in the summer and autumn of 1921. He worked unceasingly under all conditions. Failures made him dourly determined that something must be done to push the problems ahead.

Banting was genuinely fond of the experimental animals with which he worked. The dogs were trained to put out their paws and to hold them steady while blood was removed from their veins. He was loath to sacrifice an animal, even though it was necessary to prove the validity of the conclusions which had been drawn from the experiments. He felt that no animal should be subjected to pain which the human experimenter would not willingly bear himself.

When Professor Macleod returned to his laboratory in the autumn of 1921 the work was continued under his general direction. Banting was given an appointment as lecturer in the Department of Pharmacology under Professor V. E. Henderson. During the following year, when he became interested in the clinical application of insulin, he was appointed senior demonstrator in the Department of Medicine under Professor Duncan Graham, a position which he held until 1923 when the Banting and Best Department of Medical Research was created and he was installed as Director. The chair was supported in part by an annual grant voted by the legislature of the Province of Ontario. In the same year the parliament of Canada provided Banting with a life annuity.

In the years following the discovery of insulin the whole scientific world joined to honour Banting with a galaxy of awards and medals. It will always be a source of gratification to his colleagues in the University of Toronto that they were among the first to recognize the greatness of the man. In 1922 he received the Starr Gold Medal for his M.D. thesis and the George Armstrong Peters Prize for his important contributions to surgical science. In 1923 he received the Reeve Prize, which is awarded for a published report of the best scientific research accomplished in any department of the Faculty of Medicine by a junior member of the staff, and in the same year the Charles Mickle Fellowship, which is awarded to that member of the medical profession (anywhere) who is considered by the Council of the Faculty of Medicine of the University of Toronto to have done most during the preceding ten years to advance sound knowledge of a practical kind in medical art or science. The Nobel Prize in medicine was awarded to Dr. Banting and Dr. Macleod in 1923. Banting, with characteristic generosity, immediately divided his share equally with the author, and Professor Macleod with Dr. J. B. Collip who joined our group in the autumn of 1921 and who had made several very important contributions within a short period of time.

Banting became an honorary member of most of the outstanding scientific and medical societies of the world. Awards followed each other in rapid succession: the Johns Scott Medal (Philadelphia) in 1923, the Rosenberger Gold Medal (Chicago) in 1924, the Cameron Prize (Edinburgh) in 1927, the Flavelle Medal of the Royal Society of Canada in 1931, the Apothecaries Medal (London) in 1934, and the F. N. G. Starr Gold Medal of the Canadian Medical Association in 1936.

In recognition of his great service to science and humanity Dr. Banting was created Knight Commander of the civil division of the Order of the

British Empire in June 1934. In the following year he was elected a Fellow of the Royal Society of London.

The first problem which he attacked after the experimental work on insulin reached a stage at which he felt that he could leave it, was the physiology of the adrenal cortex. He made strenuous efforts to prolong the lives of adrenalectomized dogs by giving extracts of various types. None of these attempts were successful, but he did advance our knowledge of the adrenal cortex and showed that with appropriate treatment the lives of these animals could be greatly prolonged.

The creation of a research department provided Banting with excellent facilities and enabled him to secure an adequate number of collaborators. In the course of the eighteen years in which he held the post as Director of this department, a great many researches were undertaken. Banting did not believe in the publication of results which did not materially advance the field. He had an aversion to a thorough search of the literature before a problem was undertaken. He felt that this procedure blunted the imagination. He was determined that young investigators with new ideas should be given the opportunity to investigate their problems. As was inevitable some of the studies yielded no valuable results but there were many which repayed his confidence. He became tremendously interested in work on silicosis. Interesting and valuable results were obtained in this field and a goodly portion of the credit belongs to Banting, who gave the investigators his support and enthusiastic help.

He divided his department up into several sections—one devoted to physiology, one to biochemistry, and one in which the work was largely pathological. He spent much of his own time on cancer research and devoted himself to this field with great enthusiasm and energy. He did much of this work with his own hands and derived great satisfaction from the slow but steady progress which he made in this difficult field. He would occasionally break away from his own researches and throw himself wholeheartedly into problems which his younger colleagues had initiated. He earned and deserved the affection and admiration of a great many young men who were at one time or another attached to his department.

Although Banting's great energies were devoted for the most part to scientific research on medical problems, he had many other interests in which he always hoped to indulge more fully after he had retired from active work. A member of the Arts and Letters Club of Toronto, he was one of Canada's most accomplished amateur painters. His oils of Quebec scenes, of Arctic life, and of the Canadian Rockies, form a valuable addition to the artistic records of those regions. Mr. A. Y. Jackson has written: "Banting's interest in art was something much more serious than is generally realized. Through pressure of work and the war he had done little sketching during the last three years of his life. He intended to devote much more time to painting when the war ended. He was not merely the amateur who paints as a hobby. He showed the same enthusiasm for painting as he did for research and much of the same enquiring spirit. When he took his sketch out of the box his invariable question was, 'Now what's wrong with it?' And in the next sketch he would show that all you had told him had been remembered. He loved the country and found sketching very exciting. With his energy, his active mind, his dislike of anything but honest work, he might have achieved fame in yet another field."

Banting interested himself in various aspects of Canadiana. He collected books and old manuscripts and various articles associated with the development of the practice of medicine in Canada. He made trips to the far north and thoroughly familiarized himself with the lore of the earlier explorers of that region.

Banting preserved his association with his old colleagues and particularly his classmates of 1917. He looked forward to his class reunions, to informal gatherings with his close friends, many of whom were classmates. He was fond of singing and had a good baritone voice.

The exceptional mental equipment with which Banting was endowed enabled him to overcome many obstacles which would have deterred a less forceful personality. His scientific curiosity was never satisfied and his energy was boundless. His training as a practical surgeon served him well on numerous occasions and he was always interested in the fundamental aspects of the problems which he attacked. His experiences during the great war as a battalion medical officer made a lasting impression on his mind. He was never too busy to leave the laboratory in order to set a fracture or to perform a surgical operation on one of his army comrades or on some patient who was in need.

The Second World War found Banting occupying the leading place in Canadian medical science and in the esteem of the Canadian people. He was almost immediately made the head of the Central Medical Research Committee of the National Research Council of Canada. Banting was ready for this new responsibility because, from the time of Munich, he had made up his own mind that war was inevitable and he had taken steps to initiate aviation medical research in his own department. This is not the place to describe in detail his tireless efforts from one coast of Canada to the other, to stimulate research workers to undertake problems of national importance. He was able, through his popularity with men in other fields and his unceasing efforts, to secure funds and to organize the work of a large group of scientists who devoted themselves to war problems.

When it became necessary in 1940 to effect a liaison with medical workers in Great Britain, Banting insisted on going himself. He carried valuable information in both directions, and on his return to Canada he threw himself again into research and organization. No risks were too great for him and he undertook many hazardous investigations in which he himself was the subject. When a second trip to England became necessary he welcomed the opportunity, but he had a premonition that the end was near. He died in a remote spot in Newfoundland on February 21, 1941, when the bomber in which he was travelling crashed in a forced landing. Banting died as he had lived—in the service of his country and of humanity. He is survived by his wife, the former Henrietta Ball, whom he married in 1939, and by one son of a previous marriage, William Robertson Banting, born in 1929.

The Banting Institute, the Banting Foundation, and the Banting Memorial Lectureship have been created in the University of Toronto as tangible tributes to him, but his name will live for ever in the hearts of successive generations of diabetics and in the minds of young investigators who will be stimulated by his brilliant and fearless career.

PUBLICATIONS OF F. G. BANTING

1922. (With C. H. BEST.) Internal secretion of pancreas. *Trans. Acad. Med. Toronto* 3: [pages not numbered]. (Publication of material presented orally, Feb. 7.)

—— (With C. H. BEST.) Internal secretion of pancreas. *J. Lab. Clin. Med.* 7: 251–66. (A summary of this paper was presented to the American Physiological Society at the meeting in New Haven, Dec. 1921: F. G. Banting, C. H. Best, and J. J. R. Macleod. *Am. J. Physiol.* 59: 479P.)

—— (With C. H. BEST, J. B. COLLIP, W. R. CAMPBELL, and A. A. FLETCHER.) Pancreatic extracts in the treatment of diabetes. *Can. Med. Assoc. J.* 12: 141–6.

—— (With C. H. BEST.) Pancreatic extracts. *J. Lab. Clin. Med.* 7: 464–72.

—— (With C. H. BEST, J. B. COLLIP, W. R. CAMPBELL, A. A. FLETCHER, J. J. R. MACLEOD, and E. C. NOBLE.) The effect produced on diabetes by extracts of pancreas. *Trans. Assoc. Am. Physicians* 37: 337–47.

—— (With C. H. BEST, J. B. COLLIP, and J. J. R. MACLEOD.) The preparation of pancreatic extracts containing insulin. *Trans. Roy. Soc. Can.,* 16, Sect. V: 27–9.

—— (With C. H. BEST, J. B. COLLIP, J. J. R. MACLEOD, and E. C. NOBLE.) Effect of insulin on normal rabbits and on rabbits rendered hyperglycemic in various ways. *Trans. Roy. Soc. Can.,* 16, Sect. V: 31–3.

—— (With C. H. BEST, J. B. COLLIP, J. HEPBURN, and J. J. R. MACLEOD.) The effect produced on the respiratory quotient by injections of insulin. *Trans. Roy. Soc. Can.,* 16, Sect. V: 35–7.

—— (With C. H. BEST, J. B. COLLIP, J. J. R. MACLEOD, and E. C. NOBLE.) The effect of insulin on the percentage amounts of fat and glycogen in the liver and other organs of diabetic animals. *Trans. Roy. Soc. Can.,* 16, Sect. V: 39–41.

—— (With C. H. BEST, J. B. COLLIP, and J. J. R. MACLEOD.) The effect of insulin on the excretion of ketone bodies by the diabetic dog. *Trans. Roy. Soc. Can.,* 16, Sect. V: 42–4.

—— (With F. R. MILLER.) Observations on cerebellar stimulations. *Brain* 45: 104–12.

—— (With C. H. BEST, J. B. COLLIP, J. J. R. MACLEOD, and E. C. Noble.) The effect of pancreatic extract (insulin) on normal rabbits. *Am. J. Physiol.* 62: 162–76.

—— (With C. H. Best, J. B. Collip, J. J. R. Macleod, and E. C. Noble.) The effect of insulin on experimental hyperglycemia in rabbits. *Am. J. Physiol.* 62: 559–80.

—— (With W. R. Campbell and A. A. Fletcher.) Insulin in the treatment of diabetes mellitus. *J. Metabolic Research* 2: 547–604.

1923. (With W. R. Campbell and A. A. Fletcher.) Further clinical experiences with insulin in the treatment of diabetes mellitus. *Brit. Med. J.* 1: 8–12.

—— Insulin. *J. Mich. Med. Soc.* 22: 113–24.

—— (With A. McPhedran.) Insulin in the treatment of severe diabetes. *Intern. Clinics* 2: 1–5.

—— (With C. H. Best and D. A. Scott.) Insulin in blood. *Trans. Roy. Soc. Can.*, 17, Sect. V: 81–5.

—— (With J. A. Gilchrist and C. H. Best.) Observations with insulin on Department of Soldiers' Civil Re-establishment diabetics. *Can. Med. Assoc. J.* 13: 565–72.

—— (With J. J. R. Macleod.) The antidiabetic functions of the pancreas and the successful isolation of the antidiabetic hormone—insulin. *Beaumont Foundation Annual Lecture Course*, Ser. II. St. Louis: C. V. Mosby.

—— The use of insulin in the treatment of diabetes mellitus. The Nathan Lewis Hatfield Lecture. *Trans. College Physicians, Philadelphia* Ser. 3, 45: 153–64.

—— (With C. H. Best and E. C. Noble.) Pancreatic extracts in the treatment of diabetes mellitus. *Bull. Battle Creek San. and Hosp. Clinics* 18: 155–70.

—— The value of insulin in the treatment of diabetes. *Proc. Inst. Med. Chicago* 4: 144–57.

—— (With Sir Thomas J. Horder, et al.) Discussion on diabetes and insulin. *Brit. Med. J.* 2: 445–51.

1924. (With C. H. Best.) The discovery and preparation of insulin. *Univ. Toronto Med. J.* 1: 94–8.

—— Medical research and the discovery of insulin. *Hygeia* 2: 288–92.

—— Insulin. *Intern. Clinics* Ser. 34. 4: 109–16.

—— Glandular therapy: pharmacologic action of insulin. *J. Am. Med. Assoc.* 83: 1078.

—— (With S. Gairns.) Factors influencing the production of insulin. *Am. J. Physiol.* 68: 24–30.

—— Canada's record in research. *Maclean's Magazine* 37: no. 22 (Nov. 15): 22, 44.

1925. Medical research. *Ann. Clin. Med.* 3: 565–72.

—— Diabetes and insulin. *Les Prix Nobel* 1924–25. Stockholm: Norstedt.

—— Diabetes and insulin (Nobel Prize Lecture). *Svenska Läk. Sällsk. Handl.* (in English) 51: 189– 201.

1926. Diabetes and insulin (Nobel Prize Lecture). *Can. Med. Assoc. J.* 16: 221–32.

—— (With S. Gairns.) Suprarenal insufficiency. *Am. J. Physiol.* 77: 100–13.

—— Medical research. *Can. Med. Assoc. J.* 16: 877–81.

1929. History of insulin. *Edinburgh Med. J.* 36: 1–18.

1930. With the Arctic patrol. *Can. Geograph. J.* 1: 19–30.

—— (With S. Gairns.) The antitryptic properties of blood serum. *Am. J. Physiol.* 94: 241–6.

1931. (With S. Gairns, J. M. Lang, and J. R. Ross.) A study of the enzymes of stools in intestinal intoxication. *Can. Med. Assoc. J.* 25: 393–9.

1932. Medical Research. *N.Y. State J. Med.* 32: 311–5.

1934. (With S. Gairns.) Resistance to Rous sarcoma. *Can. Med. Assoc. J.* 30: 615–19.

—— (With S. Gairns.) A study of serum of chickens resistant to Rous sarcoma. *Am. J. Cancer.* 22: 611–14.

—— (With D. Irwin and S. Gairns.) A study of Rous sarcoma tissue grafts in susceptible and resistant chickens. *Am. J. Cancer* 22: 615–19.

1935. Silicosis. *J. Indiana Med. Assoc.* 28: 9–12.

—— (With A. R. Armstrong.) The site of formation of the phosphatase of serum. *Can. Med. Assoc. J.* 33: 243–6.

—— (With J. T. Fallon.) The cellular reaction to silica. *Can. Med. Assoc. J.* 33: 404–7.

—— (With J. T. Fallon.) Tissue reaction to sericite. *Can. Med. Assoc. J.* 33: 407–11.

1936. (With G. E. HALL and G. H. ETTINGER.) An experimental production of coronary thrombosis and myocardial failure. *Can. Med. Assoc. J.* 34: 9–15.

—— In Memoriam: Ivan Petrovitch Pavlov, 1849–1936. *Am. J. Psychiatry* 92: 1481–4.

—— (With G. H. ETTINGER and G. E. HALL.) Effect of repeated and prolonged stimulation of the vagus nerve in the dog. *Can. Med. Assoc. J.* 35: 27–31.

—— Science and the Soviet Union. *Can. Business* 9: no. 2, 14–15, 67–9.

—— Silicosis research. *Can. Med. Assoc. J.* 35: 289–93.

1937. (With G. E. HALL.) Experimental production of myocardial and coronary artery lesions. *Trans. Assoc. Am. Phys.* 52: 204–9.

—— Early work on insulin. *Science* 85: 594–6.

—— (With G. W. MANNING and G. E. HALL.) Vagus stimulation and the production of myocardial damage. *Can. Med. Assoc. J.* 37: 314–18.

1938. (With G. E. HALL, J. M. JANES, B. LEIBEL, and D. W. LOUGHEED.) Physiological studies in experimental drowning. *Can. Med. Assoc. J.* 39: 226–8.

1939. Walter Ernest Dixon Memorial Lecture: Resistance to experimental cancer. *Proc. Roy. Soc. Med.* 32: 245–54.

O N LOOKING BACK OVER THE INSULIN reprints which I have chosen to include in this volume it occurs to me that there are several recollections, partly personal and partly scientific, which have not been mentioned either in the papers or in the connecting bridges. For example, some of Banting's close friends knew that a part of his motivation stemmed from an interest in a schoolmate in Alliston, Ontario, who died of diabetes. Recently my wife and I went to Alliston and helped to dedicate a portrait of Fred Banting which is to hang in the entrance hall of the Banting Memorial High School. We saw again the farm where he was born; where I first met his fine parents; and where our friend, Fred's older brother Thompson Banting, now lives. We drove along the road where Fred Banting walked to school and passed the house which, we were told, was the home of the diabetic little girl.

Banting and I frequently went together to the abattoir to collect foetal pancreas or glands from adult animals. Finally the time arrived when we were to make an extract to be tried on a diabetic patient. On this particular occasion I went alone. The abattoir authorities kindly immobilized a recently killed steer in a fairly convenient position so that I could remove the pancreas with aseptic precautions. This was taken back to the laboratory in a sterile container and worked up.

The records in our notebooks show that we had been making insulin by macerating whole beef pancreas, immediately after removal, in an equal volume of 95 per cent alcohol made acid by the addition of 0.2 per cent of concentrated hydrochloric acid. After thorough grinding of the mixture with mortar and pestle, the acid alcoholic extract was filtered and the clear filtrate evaporated to dryness at first in a warm-air current, and later in an efficient laboratory vacuum-still which I had used during the previous year.

In our second paper (Paper 5 above), which I have looked at again recently, it is noted that on December 15, 1921, 200 mg of the dried residue of ox pancreas extract were washed twice with toluol and then in 95 per cent alcohol and then dried again, and the resulting powder dissolved (or emulsified) in saline.

We had previously shown that it was possible to put the aqueous solution made from our acid alcoholic extract of normal beef pancreas through a Berkefeld filter. The final material in the first sample to be used clinically was a reasonably good-looking product although of course it contained a great deal of inert protein. Banting gave the first injection to himself and the second one to me. The next morning we had rather red arms but there was no other effect. We did not follow our own blood sugars. However, we did test the material on one of our diabetic dogs. Intravenous injection of this preparation caused the blood sugar to drop from 0.37 per cent to 0.06 per cent in four hours. Our notes indicate that the improvement in the dog's condition was as dramatic as the fall in sugar. Thus we established the potency of this extract which was sent over to the Toronto General Hospital and which was administered to several of the patients under the supervision of Dr. W. R. Campbell and Dr. A. A. Fletcher in Professor Duncan Graham's department. The first injection of insulin was given to Leonard Thompson by the Senior Houseman on that particular ward, Dr. Edward S. Jeffrey, a close friend of Fred Banting's and of mine, who told us all the details surrounding this first clinical trial.

After a relatively short period, however, as I have mentioned elsewhere, serious difficulties in the preparation of active material developed. The supply of insulin for the Clinic completely stopped. Several of the patients, including a young girl in whom my wife and I were particularly interested, died from lack of insulin after having been dramatically improved by the first injections which they received. Fred Banting insisted, in such a major crisis, that I should temporarily abandon the basic research I was doing towards my M.A. and that I should concentrate on the large-scale preparation of insulin. In the absence of advice from experienced chemical engineers we waged a night-and-day struggle in the hope that we might again hit upon an effective procedure. The secret of the success that we achieved after a few weeks may have been due to a return to the use of 0.2 per cent of concentrated hydrochloric acid in the extractive, or to the substitution of a lower boiling solvent (acetone) for alcohol in the original extraction. Possibly the introduction of an efficient wind tunnel for the rapid evaporation of the extracts was equally important. With the consistent production of reasonable amounts of insulin, the clinical work was started over again. The recovery, during the spring of 1922, of the process for making insulin bridged the gap between the laboratory preparation and the subsequent large-scale commercial production by the Insulin Division of the Connaught Laboratories and by Eli Lilly and Company at Indianapolis. A little later, valuable contributions came from Great Britain and many other countries.

27. Reminiscences of the Researches Which Led to the Discovery of Insulin

C. H. BEST

The Editor's invitation to contribute some "personal notes" for the Banting Memorial Number of the *Canadian Medical Association Journal* stimulated me to look over the notebooks which Banting and I kept in the Department of Physiology from May 17, 1921, to January 1, 1922.

Banting's modesty was apparent from the very start of the investigations. Our first problem was to look over the literature in the attempt to get a better idea of the various operative procedures which had been used in work on the pancreas. Professor Macleod informed me that Banting felt he would have to depend entirely upon me for the translation of articles in the French literature. I found, however, that when I secured the publications of Hédon and other French workers in this field, that Banting's knowledge of French was of the same order as my own. We translated these articles together and the information secured provided a basis for our first attempts to produce the diabetic state upon which we wished to study the effect of the pancreatic extract. The operating facilities, however, were not satisfactory during the hot summer months of 1921 and we eventually abandoned the Hédon procedure of removing the pancreas in two stages and adopted a technique, which Banting developed, for complete pancreatectomy at one operation.

The blood sugar estimations, in which the Myers and Bailey modification of the Lewis-Benedict method were used, ran smoothly throughout the investigations but we had some preliminary difficulties with the D/N ratio. Banting had understood from Professor Macleod that the D/N ratio of the completely depancreatized dog must be 3.65 to 1 before a maximum degree of diabetes could be assumed. Actually, this ratio is the one which may be obtained in phloridzinized animals, but it is never exhibited for prolonged periods by the completely depancreatized dog. After a great deal of discussion of the results of the glucose and nitrogen estimations a search of the literature revealed the above-mentioned facts and Banting was then happy

Originally appeared as a special contribution to the Banting Memorial Number (November) of the *Canadian Medical Association Journal*, XLVII (1942), 398–400.

to proceed with the injections of extract into animals which had a much lower D/N ratio. [The D/N (or G/N) ratio refers to the proportion of sugar (dextrose, sometimes called glucose) to nitrogen excreted in the urine.] The results in the notebooks show that very definite lowering of blood sugar, decrease of sugar excretion, and improvement in the general condition of the diabetic animals were secured in July 1921. Even more definite results were obtained in August and one of the curves drawn by Banting is reproduced here (Figure 62).

On August 14, 1921, an experiment was made to investigate the effect of what we then considered to be an overdose of the extract. The blood sugar was lowered from 0.22 per cent—a definitely diabetic level—to the hypoglycaemic figure of 0.06 per cent. A reproduction of this page from the

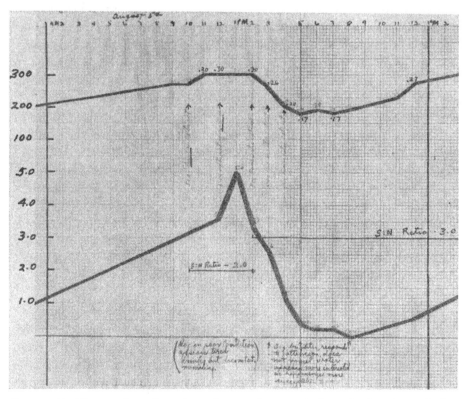

FIGURE 62. Photographic of portion of page from original notebook: chart of data obtained from dog 408 on August 5, 1921, by Banting and Best. Some parts have been inked over by C. H. Best to increase the legibility of the lines in the original notebook. The upper curve shows the effects of injecting 5 cc doses of various tissue extracts (liver, spleen, and 3 of pancreas). The pancreatic extract caused prompt lowering of the blood sugar from 300 to 170 mg per 100 cc. The lower curve shows the dramatic drop in the amount of sugar excreted in the urine. The figures in the upper scale on the left axis represent the blood sugar in mg per 100 cc; the lower figures are the percentage of sugar in the urine.

notebook is shown in Figure 63. A little later this experiment was repeated and a note was made that the animal with a low blood sugar appeared much brighter after the administration of glucose.

We were also interested, at an early phase of the study—August 17, 1921 —in the effect of whole fresh gland extracts and a page from the first notebook (Figure 64) shows that on this date a very definite fall in blood sugar was obtained with an extract made up in Ringer's solution, and with one which had been acidified. The alkaline extract apparently did not produce any definite effect. It may be noted, however, that the figure for the blood sugar before this extract was given has been omitted.

It will be observed in Figure 64, at the bottom of the page, that Banting recorded the fact that the steam shovel had arrived for the excavation of a basement for the new Anatomy Building. There are a number of notations of this type throughout the notebooks.

Dean Mackenzie, the Acting President of the National Research Council, in the course of the first Banting Memorial Lecture at the University of Toronto, referred to Banting's affection for the animals with which we worked. He did develop a tremendous attachment for a number of dogs. Most of them were trained to put out their paw and to hold it steady while samples of blood were taken from their veins. Plate II(a) shows a picture taken on the roof of the Medical Building in July, 1921. The dog was the first whose life, we felt, had been saved by the administration of insulin. This picture has not hitherto been published. The animal did not live for a long period as the supply of potent extract was inadequate. The first one which was kept alive for what was considered an indefinite period—some seven weeks—was maintained in excellent condition and probably could have been kept alive for many months or years.

There are some notes in this first book which remind me of the fact that the supply of animals was not always satisfactory. Suggestions have been made by poorly informed authors that dogs were appropriated from the street with very little ceremony. This is not true, but there were occasions when we made a tour through various parts of the city and bargained with owners of animals. They were paid for by funds which we took from our own pockets. This money may have come from the sale of Banting's automobile. Neither of us received a stipend during the summer of 1921 and for a time I used funds which he loaned me. A part of this money certainly came from the sale of his Ford car.

These notebooks have brought back many other memories—of meals prepared in the night over the Bunsen burner, of a minor operation performed on a friend balanced precariously on the animal operating table, and of the many long chats with Banting about what the future might hold

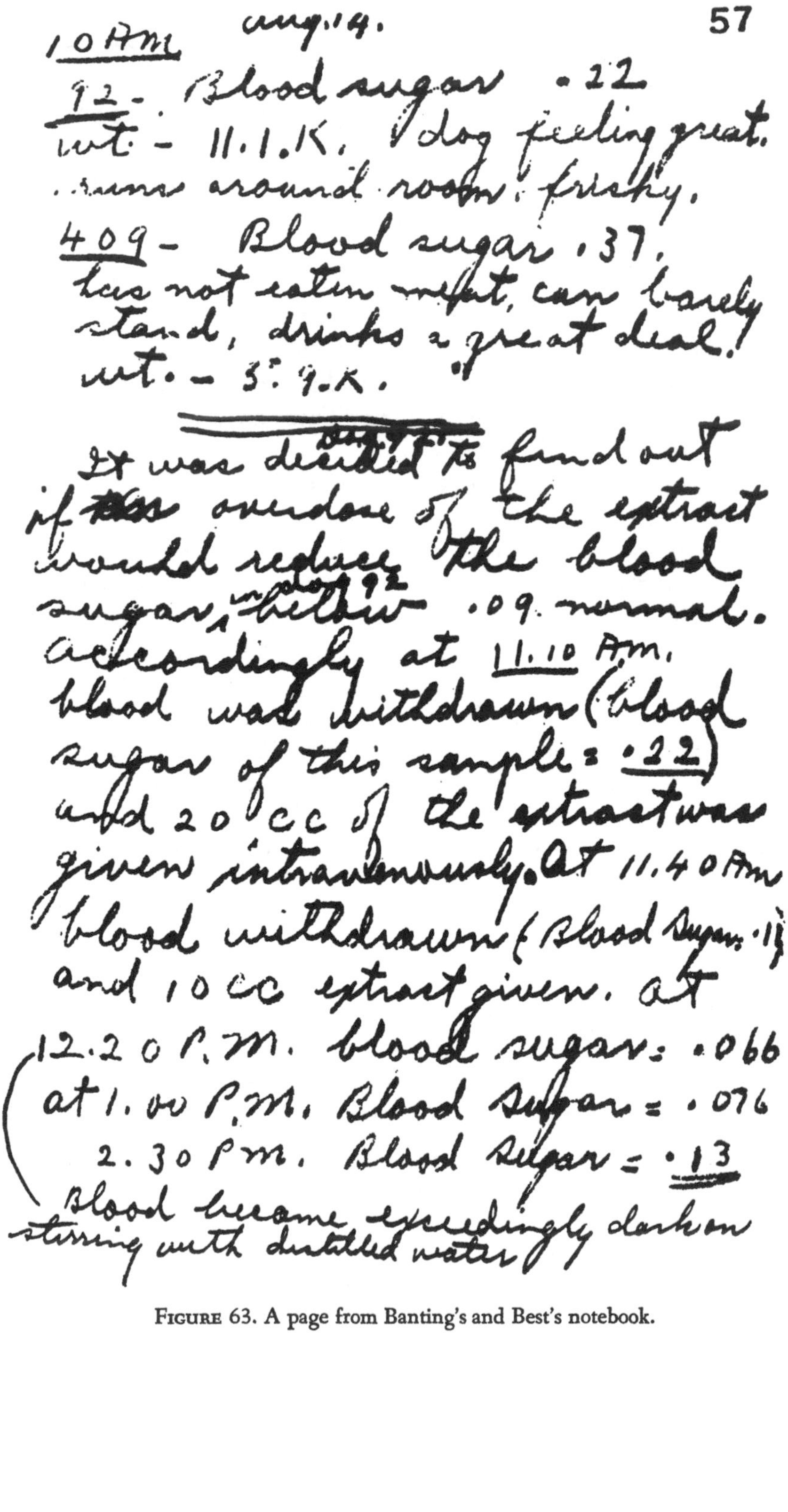

10 AM.   aug. 14.   57

92 - Blood sugar .22
wt. - 11.1.K. dog feeling great.
..runs around room. frisky.

409 - Blood sugar .37.
has not eaten meat, can barely
stand, drinks a great deal.
wt. - 3: 9.K.

It was decided to find out
if this overdose of the extract
would reduce the blood
sugar, below .09. normal.
accordingly at 11.10 A.m.
blood was withdrawn (Blood
sugar of this sample: .22)
and 20 cc of the extract was
given intravenously. at 11.40 Am
blood withdrawn (Blood Sugar. .1)
and 10 cc extract given. at
12.20 P.m. blood sugar: .066
at 1.00 P.m. Blood Sugar = .076
2.30 Pm. Blood Sugar = .13
Blood became exceedingly dark on
stirring with distilled water

FIGURE 63. A page from Banting's and Best's notebook.

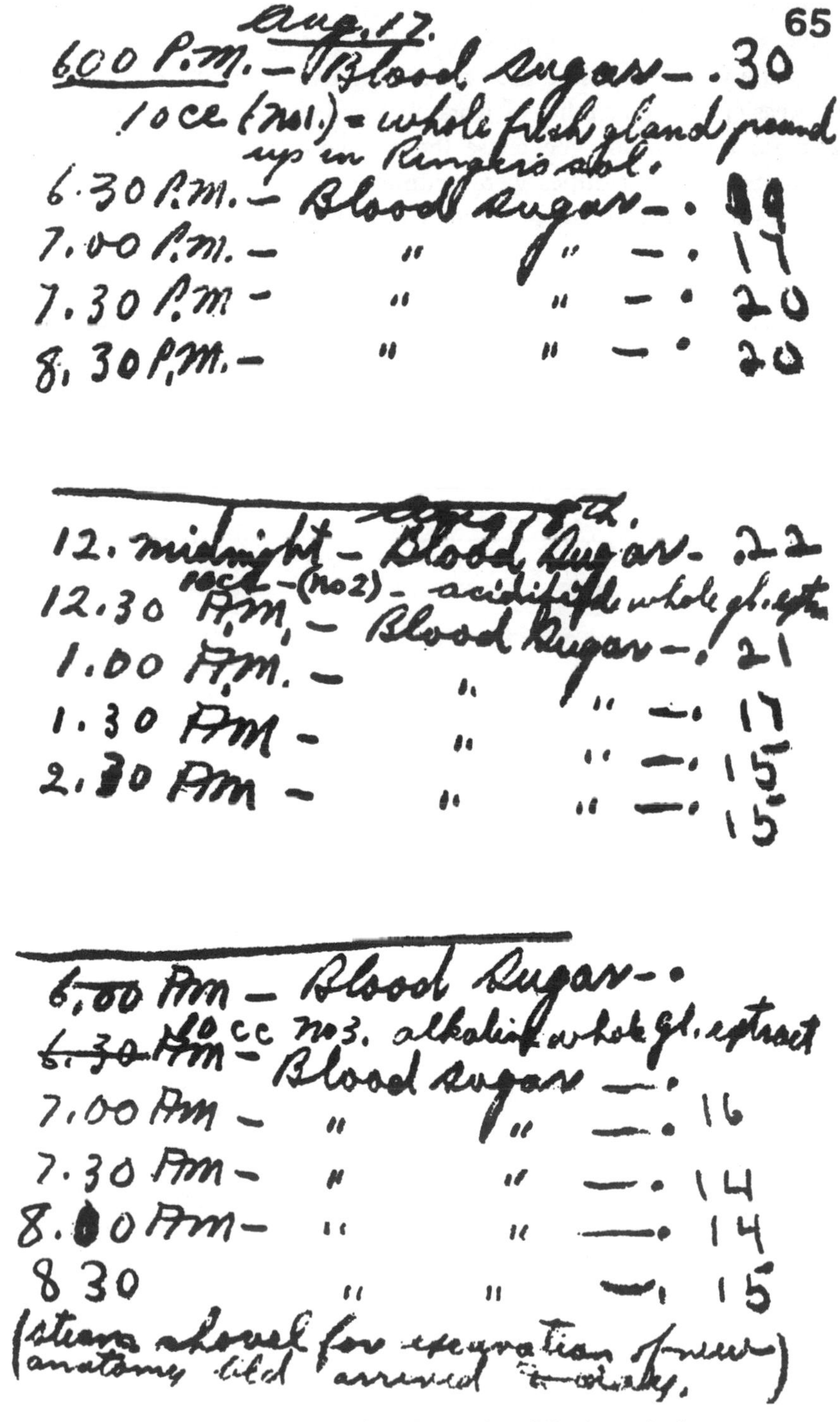

65

aug. 17.

6.00 P.M. — Blood sugar — .30

10 cc (no 1.) = whole fresh gland pound
up in Ringer's sol.

6.30 P.M. — Blood sugar — . 19

7.00 P.M. —   "   "   — : 17

7.30 P.M. —   "   "   — : 20

8.30 P.M. —   "   "   — : 20

12. midnight — Blood sugar — 22

12.30 P.M. — (no 2) — acidified whole gl. extr.
         Blood sugar — : 21

1.00 P.M. —   "   "   — : 17

1.30 P.M. —   "   "   — : 15

2.30 P.M. —   "   "   — : 15

6.00 Am — Blood sugar — .

6.30 Am — 10 cc no 3. alkaline whole gl. extract
         Blood sugar — :

7.00 Am —   "   "   — : 16

7.30 Am —   "   "   — : 14

8.00 Am —   "   "   — : 14

8.30   "   "   — : 15

(steam shovel for excavation (new)
 anatomy bld arrived today.

FIGURE 64. A page from Banting's and Best's notebook.

when unlimited amounts of insulin would be available. These and many other points may some day be the subject of a more detailed reminiscence.

During the years just before the present war Banting and I discussed on several occasions the possibility of working together again in a research on carbohydrate metabolism. We chose the problem and made preliminary arrangements, but other duties were permitted to interfere until, with the outbreak of war, it was too late to carry out our plans.

28. Insulin and Diabetes—in Retrospect and in Prospect

SURGEON CAPTAIN C. H. BEST, C.B.E., F.R.S.*

In this fourth Banting Memorial Lecture we again pay tribute to the accomplishments of our late colleague. As I wrote at the time of his death, his chief monument will be in the minds of young men stimulated by his brilliant and fearless career and in the hearts of successive generations of diabetics who owe so much to him. The number of more tangible tributes steadily increases. In addition to those in our own University[1] which are well known to you, there are: the Banting Memorial Lecture of the American Diabetes Association, the Banting Memorial Home for Convalescent Diabetics—projected by the British Diabetic Association—and the Sir Frederick Banting Memorial Hospital in Newfoundland erected by the Royal Canadian Air Force not far from the scene of the fatal accident.

There are few memorials which could give as much satisfaction to a scientist as the furtherance of researches which he has initiated. I am going to discuss certain aspects of the insulin studies this afternoon and I will take the opportunity, as we did in the introduction to the first paper on the anti-diabetic hormone, to pay tribute to a few of the many deserving scientists who made possible the culmination here in Toronto of the prolonged search for the internal secretion of the pancreas.

I would commend to students of medicine Paul Langerhans' thesis, presented in 1869, and reprinted in English in 1937 with an introductory essay by Dr. H. Morrison. This young man, as a medical student, discovered the structures which were later named in his honour by Laguesse, the islands of Langerhans. Langerhans had no knowledge of the actual function

Originally appeared in the *Canadian Medical Association Journal*, LIII (1945), 204–12. A part of the material in this lecture was later presented before the Société Canadienne d'Endocrinologie, in Montreal, and also to the Alpha Omega Alpha Honorary Medical Fraternity of the University of Western Ontario.

*Director, Banting and Best Department of Medical Research and Department of Physiology, University of Toronto. At present on Active Service with the Royal Canadian Navy as Director of the R.C.N. Medical Research Division.

[1]The Banting Institute, the Banting and Best Department of Medical Research, the Banting Research Foundation, and the Banting Memorial Lecture.

of the islets and indeed it was not until a year after his death that von Mering and Minkowski proved that complete removal of the pancreas invariably produces diabetes in some species of animals. Von Mering died in 1908, but Minkowski lived for ten years of the insulin era and was appointed chairman of the German Insulin Committee, which received as a gift all the rights which the University of Toronto had acquired in Germany as a result of the discovery. After his work with von Mering in 1889, Minkowski tried very hard, as hundreds of others did, to detect the internal secretion in extracts of pancreas. One has a very keen sympathy for these scientific workers who so narrowly missed the goal towards which their own findings had partially paved the way. I have been told many times by German scientists of the meeting at which one of their members made, perhaps with some justification, an impassioned plea for recognition of the priority of his work on pancreatic extracts. Minkowski listened attentively and at the end rose and said very simply, "I too regret that I did not find insulin."

Minkowski, one of the great students of diabetes, died in 1931, but his wife lived to be a victim of Nazi oppression. It is a source of gratification to all of us that funds made available by the Insulin Committee of this University played a part in her rescue. After her arrival in South America she wrote as follows:

Executive Secretary, Insulin Committee,
University of Toronto.

After a very unhappy time I had to pass before I could leave, I finally just now arrived here, where I am happy to see my children after long years of separation.

It is only now that I got to know, that your great kindness enabled me to come here at all and to have the best possible opportunity for travelling in these times. So I have arrived in pretty good health, though with all my belongings, even luggage, lost.

My first action here is to thank you and the Insulin Committee from all my heart for helping me so generously in remembrance of all my husband once did for medical science and mankind.

I remember the great pleasure my husband had, when you came to see him. For him it was good luck, that he had not to live through these terrible years.

Very faithfully yours,

MARIE MINKOWSKI

In the last decade of the nineteenth century and in the first two of the present one, many workers in Germany, in France, Italy, Great Britain, and the United States, whom I will not even attempt to name at this time, contributed in a great variety of ways to the knowledge of the diabetic state. Operative procedures for complete or partial pancreatectomy were elaborated. The effects of tying the pancreatic ducts, which produced a rapid degeneration of the cells which make the external secretion and a slower disappearance of the islands of Langerhans, were studied. The technique of metabolic investigation was improved and advances of the greatest importance were made in the procedures for estimating sugar, ketone bodies, nitrogen, etc., in small amounts of blood. Thus in 1921 we had great advantages over previous investigators.

The details of Banting's initiation of the work and a description of the procedures which resulted in the isolation of insulin, are to be found in our early papers. They have been fully discussed in a number of lectures, some of which were given by Banting. His address in Stockholm when he received the Nobel Prize in 1925, or his Cameron Prize Lecture, delivered in Edinburgh in 1928, provide excellent descriptions. A detailed and accurate account of the early work is also to be found in Professor J. J. R. Macleod's book, *Carbohydrate Metabolism and Insulin*, published in 1926. There are, of course, many interesting sidelights which have as yet been preserved only as rough notes or as a part of personal correspondence. These will some day be of historical importance, and could provide material for several lectures.

Preparations of Insulin for the Treatment of Diabetic Patients

I would like this afternoon to outline very briefly the improvement in the insulin preparations from the first crude ones which we had available in 1921 to the pure products of today. In the following figure (Figure 65) the lowering of blood sugar produced by one of the earliest extracts from the degenerated pancreas of the dog is illustrated and there are some relevant comments in Banting's handwriting. The impurities present in these extracts may have delayed the liberation of the insulin even when administered intravenously but this was much more apparent when similar material was given subcutaneously. The first extracts from normal beef pancreas, prepared with the modifications and improvements made by Professor Collip in the procedure which we originally used, had an appreciably longer duration of action than an equivalent amount of the purer insulin now available. I do not wish to imply that the early extracts were not effective in the treatment of depancreatized dogs or of diabetic people. They were amazingly good and a part of their effectiveness, when administered subcutaneously, was undoubtedly due to the gradual and therefore prolonged period of absorption of the potent material.

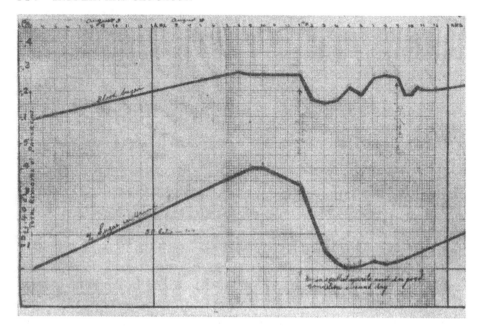

FIGURE 65. Effect of early insulin preparation (Banting's and Best's notebook, 1921). Photograph of another portion of the chart showing the data obtained from dog 408 (cf. Figure 62). These values are from 2.00 P.M. on August 3 until midnight on August 4, 1921. Portions have been inked over to increase the legibility of the lines in the original notebooks. One can see faintly, in Banting's writing, "5 cc of pancreatic extract 4 days old" under each of the arrows below the upper curve, and below the lower curve, "Dog in excellent spirits and in good condition, wound dry." As shown by these curves injections of the extract at 1.00 P.M. and 9.00 P.M. on August 4 caused small but definite decreases in the blood sugar. A dramatic fall in urine sugar also occurred after the first injection.

The natural goal of the chemist is to prepare substances in their purest form and insulin soon attracted the attention of a very competent group under the leadership of the late Professor J. J. Abel who obtained insulin in crystalline form in 1926 (Plate V(a)). A little later my colleague of long standing, Dr. D. A. Scott, showed that these crystals are the zinc salt of the insulin protein. These zinc insulin crystals are made up of twin plaques which can be clearly seen as the crystals rotate. Crystalline insulin has been prepared not only with zinc but Scott and Fisher have successfully used other materials. [Three figures have been omitted showing insulin crystals prepared with piperidine, normal amylamine, and isoamylamine, respectively.]

The first international standard of insulin adopted by the Health Organization of the League of Nations (which has brought order out of chaos in the whole field of biological standardization) was non-crystalline and had a potency of 8 units per mg. The present standard—the material for which was made in the Connaught Laboratories of our University—is composed of the zinc insulin crystals and has a potency of 22 units per mg. The creation of these international yardsticks has been largely responsible for the uniform potency of insulin the world over and the accurately predictable effect it has exerted on the uncomplicated case of diabetes.

Crystalline insulin is made up entirely, as far as can be ascertained, of protein, and contains the following amino acids in the percentages shown: serine 3.6, threonine 2.7, glutamic acid 21, cystine 12.9, leucine 30, lysine 1.3, arginine 3.3, histidine 4, phenylalanine 8.4, tyrosine 12.8, proline 10. (The total accounted for, 110.0 per cent, includes the water added as each peptide linkage was split.)

The number and complexity of these building stones make the possibility of synthesis of insulin remote. These amino acids are presumably joined together in one special manner by nature to form the insulin molecule. There are many thousands of ways in which the building stones might be united.

From the practical viewpoint, i.e., of the treatment of diabetes, the successful purification of insulin was not an unmixed blessing. Solutions made with the crystals had a shorter duration of action than many of the less pure preparations. Having completed the task of purifying insulin it was necessary to replace the impurities by a harmless and inert substance which would delay the absorption of the active material, i.e., to add a pure "impurity" which would form a compound with insulin from which the latter would slowly be liberated. Many attempts were made to accomplish this objective but the first practical solution came from Hagedorn and his group in Copenhagen who developed protamine insulin. Protamine insulin was a most valuable, but relatively unstable material and it was greatly improved when Dr. D. A. Scott and Dr. Albert Fisher of the Connaught Laboratories added a small amount of zinc. A comparison of the compositions and properties of protamine, and protamine zinc insulin, is given in Table 28.I. More than half the insulin now used in Canada or in the

TABLE 28.I

COMPARISON OF COMPOSITIONS AND PROPERTIES OF PROTAMINE
INSULIN AND PROTAMINE ZINC INSULIN

	Protamine Insulin	Protamine Zinc Insulin
Vials per dose	two	one
Stability	unstable	moderately stable
Appearance	cloudy suspension	cloudy suspension
Reaction	pH 6.9 to 7.4	pH 7.1 to 7.4
Protamine (per 100 units of insulin)	0.8 mg	1.25 mg
Zinc	little or none	0.2 mg
Potency left in supernatant	small amount	insignificant amount

United States is protamine zinc insulin (Table 28.II). Many attempts to improve this product have been made. Clear solutions of relatively slow-acting insulin, such as globin insulin, have been prepared. Clinical opinion, however, is still largely in favour of protamine zinc insulin but slight changes such as an increase in the insulin to protamine ratio may be introduced.

TABLE 28.II
USE OF INSULIN PREPARATIONS
RELATIVE YEARLY VALUES
(*Considering 1937 as 100*)

1924	9	
1934	69	
1937	100	(Protamine zinc insulin = 25%)
1940	172	(Protamine zinc insulin = 49%)
1944	278	(Protamine zinc insulin = 54%)

There are many clinical results which demonstrate the more gradual and prolonged effect of the protamine insulins. The contrast with regular insulin is well illustrated in Figure 66 made from data obtained on a diabetic dog in the Department of Physiology.

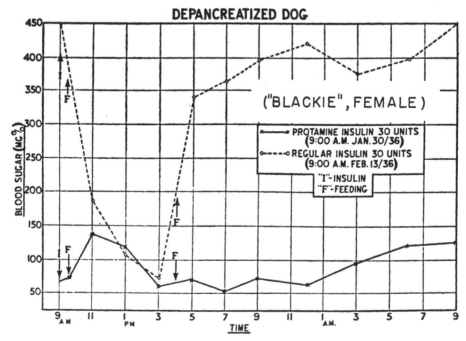

FIGURE 66. More gradual and prolonged effect of protamine insulin (From Kerr and Best [449].)

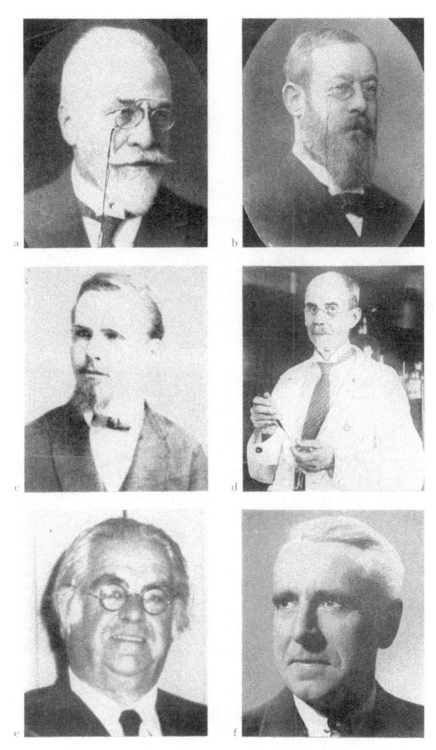

PLATE III. Some of the important contributors to the development of insulin: (a) Professor Oskar Minkowski (1858–1931). (b) Professor Joseph von Mering (1849–1908). (c) Dr. Paul Langerhans (1849–88). (d) Professor J. J. Abel (1857–1936) (e) Dr. H. C. Hagedorn (1888–   ). (f) Dr. D. A. Scott (1892–   ).

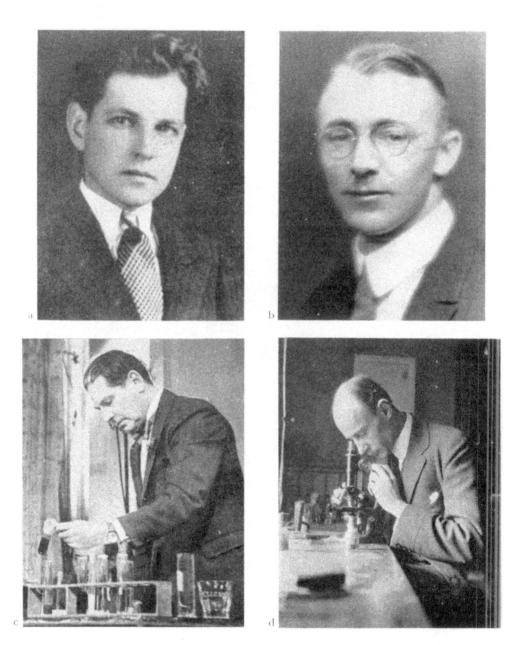

PLATE IV. (*a*) Leonard Thompson (1908–35). First patient to receive insulin. (*b*) Dr. Joseph Gilchrist (1893–1951). First diabetic physician to receive treatment with insulin. (*c*) Dr. Robin Lawrence (1892–   ), who received his first insulin in May 1923, is one of the most famous diabetic specialists in the world; he was the founder of the British Diabetic Association and the first president of the International Diabetes Federation. (*d*) Dr. George Minot (1885–1950). A patient of Dr. E. P. Joslin and one of the early diabetics to receive insulin in the United States. He became the co-discoverer of the liver treatment of pernicious anaemia.

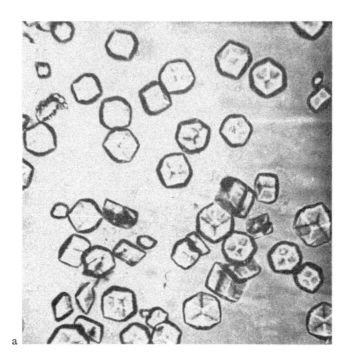

a

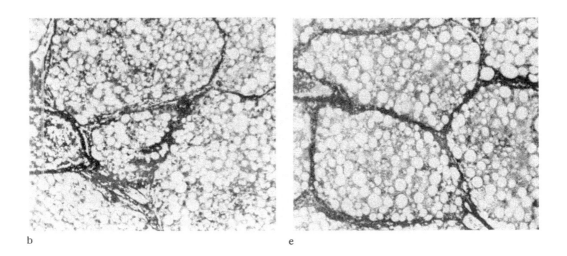

b   e

PLATE V. (a) Insulin crystals prepared with zinc (from Scott). (b) Well-defined fibrosis in liver of a rat fed basal diet and given 15 per cent alcohol in place of drinking water (Paper 44). Paraffin section: azocarmine, aniline blue, and orange G. ($\times$ 80.) (c) Well-defined fibrosis in liver of rat fed basal diet and sugar. Paraffin section: stained as in (b) ($\times$ 80) (Paper 44).

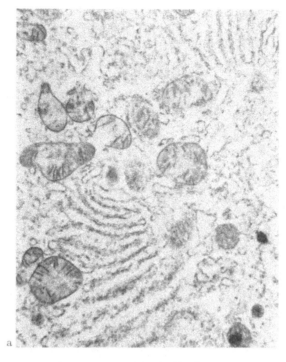

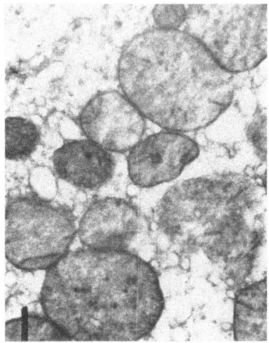

PLATE VI. (*a*) Appearance of mitochondria and ergastoplasmic sacs in a parenchymal cell of the liver of a control rat fed the basal choline-deficient food mixture supplemented with adequate choline (0.5 per cent). (*b*) Liver of a choline-deficient rat (fed the basal diet without choline for three weeks) showing the tremendous enlargement of the mitochondria ("megamitochondria") and the vacuolation of the ergastoplasmic sacs with loss of DNA-particles. Both electron-micrographs ($\times$ 20,000) have been provided by Dr. J. W. Grisham, formerly of the Department of Pathology, Washington University Medical School, St. Louis, Missouri.

The Supply of Insulin

When our only source of insulin was from dog's pancreas the ducts of which had been tied some 8 or 10 weeks previously, Banting and I visualized herds of cattle upon which this operation had been performed at the appropriate interval before their demise. Indeed, we went as far as obtaining some steers at the country seat of the Connaught Laboratories and after anaesthetizing them we rearranged their internal structure to suit our convenience. Happily, from all viewpoints, this procedure on a large scale was not required and after passing through a phase when foetal calves were at a premium, we found that commercial beef pancreas extracted with alcohol provided us with a readily available source of the internal secretion. Now, the pancreas from one steer may weigh approximately one-half a pound and will provide enough insulin to treat the average diabetic patient for about two weeks. Obviously, therefore, the number of cattle available in the world acquires an additional interest in the minds of many millions of people.

The discovery of a readily available source of insulin in 1921 did not immediately remove all the obstacles to a more satisfactory rate of production. The advances in methods of purification which Professor Collip made were of great importance but knowledge of the properties of insulin was so meagre that, even after treatment of patients had commenced, the secret of securing active material was lost for weeks—which seemed years! The struggle in the sub-basement of the Medical Building during the winter and spring of 1922, deserves a chapter for itself. The wind tunnel in which acetone extracts of pancreas were evaporated with the help of hot (and unprotected) electric wires, the gigantic glass flask which exploded, the first metal still whose hungry condenser demanded and received two tons of ice per day (delivered by hand), the floods, and the wild rats, all these made lasting impressions on me and on my first scientific colleague, D. A. Scott, in what was then called the insulin division of the Connaught Laboratories. Production gradually improved, as you will see from Tables 28.III and 28.IV. The insulin supplied at this time contained only from five to ten of the present units per cubic centimetre in contrast with the 40, 80, or 100 unit material now available.

The primitive insulin plant in the Medical Building was followed by a much more efficient one constructed in the house which had previously accommodated the university Young Men's Christian Association. Many of you do not remember this little structure which stood in the shade of some fine elms somewhere between the present School of Hygiene and the Engineering Building. This unit continued to serve a most useful purpose until the insulin plant was transferred to the School of Hygiene in 1927.

TABLE 28.III

INSULIN SUPPLIED TO DR. BANTING

	cc
June 1922	122½
July 1922	512
August 1922	390
September 1922	1,682

TABLE 28.IV

INSULIN SENT OUT, OCTOBER 1922

Name and address	Total
	cc
Dr. Banting, Toronto	696
Diabetic Clinic, Toronto General Hospital	932
Soldiers' Civil Re-establishment, Christie Street Hospital	1,120
Laboratory, Toronto	331
Hospital for Sick Children, Toronto	76
Mr. Havens, Rochester	48
Dr. Black, Hespeler	4
Total	3,207

If one had been asked to predict the curve of insulin distribution from 1922 to 1945, many of us would have suggested a very steep rise during the first five or six years and a much more gradual increase from there on. This has not been the case, and the total distribution of insulin in Canada and the United States has doubled every five years for the past fifteen years. While a small proportion of the insulin used has been for non-diabetic, particularly mental, cases, the main demand has been for the treatment of the rapidly increasing number of diabetics. The dramatic lowering of the mortality rate of young diabetics and increase of the life span of diabetics in all age groups has been recently summarized by the Metropolitan Life Insurance Company.

Today, the average diabetic child of ten may be expected to celebrate his fiftieth birthday, whereas just prior to 1922 most diabetic children lived little more than one year after the onset of their disease. At age thirty expectation of life is now twenty-seven and one-half years, compared to little more than six years in the days before insulin. Even at age fifty the improvement is sizable, with an expectation of life of fourteen and one-half years today which is 50% more than in the pre-insulin era. And these added years of life are useful and active, not years of invalidism. Moreover, this great improvement in the active life of the typical diabetic is of particular importance, because the number of these persons in the population is actually increasing through the aging of the population and through the increased survivals of younger diabetic patients to older ages.

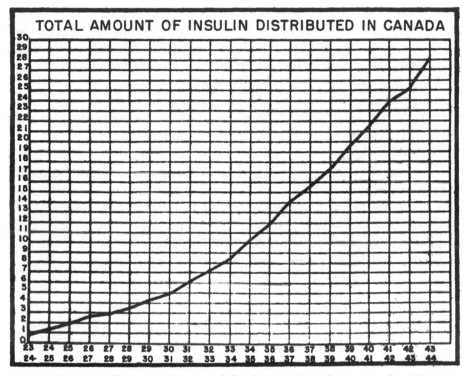

FIGURE 67. Curve illustrating the rate of distribution of insulin in Canada. (Abscissae refer to years 1923–1944, ordinates are arbitrary units.)

This paragraph based on accurate statistics describes the complete realization of all that Banting and I hoped and planned for in the summer of 1921. The curve illustrating the rate of increase of insulin distribution in Canada (the one for the United States is essentially the same) is shown in Figure 67.

The demand for insulin has placed a heavy strain on the source of the material, and the shortage of pancreas threatened to become acute just before the present war. Although certain steps can be taken to make more of the smaller sources of supply available, the situation will become critical again in the not distant future if the demand for insulin continues at the present rate.

The war has had a favourable effect on the supply of pancreas for the production of insulin in the United States and Canada, since the amount of raw material shipped to Europe from the Western Hemisphere has decreased. But the diabetics of the occupied countries of Europe have suffered from a lack of insulin and for many cases there has been none available. Through the kindness of Sir Henry Tidy, President of the Royal Society of Medicine, London, I was given the opportunity, slightly more

than a year ago, to discuss the insulin situation with the medical representatives of the "governments in exile" of practically all of the countries
which were at that time occupied. The lack of insulin was only one of their
many woes, but as some of them expressed it: "To have our children thrust
back to before the 'insulin era' is hard to bear."

Matters have now improved. The Canadian Red Cross sent insulin to
Greece, the first lot arriving not long after the German occupation. Several
shipments have been made more recently. Supplies have now reached
France and Belgium from various sources. Full details of the present
situation are, of course, not yet available. Germany may have had adequate
reserves of insulin for Aryan diabetics and certain satellite countries may
have attempted to purchase unusually large amounts during this war.

There has been no lack of insulin in England but on one occasion two
of their main supply depots were destroyed by bombs. An adequate amount
of insulin powder was dispatched immediately by air from the United
States and the situation was saved.

The Action of Insulin

As a bridge between what we know and what we hope to know about
insulin, let us consider the mechanism of its action in the body. The broad
over-all picture seems bright and clear. The administration of insulin to
the recently depancreatized dog or to the uncomplicated case of human
diabetes, completely restores the organism and if the treatment is carefully
continued and no accidents or complications occur, the patient may proceed
with an essentially normal existence. If further proof were needed for this
statement, the war has provided it, since, although diabetics are not
accepted in the Services, a few have evaded their medical colleagues and
have served as pilots over Germany with the Royal Air Force, as captains
of ocean liners during the worst of the submarine menace, and in other
positions of great responsibility.

We, as medical men, have been greatly impressed by the scientific
accomplishments of our diabetic medical colleagues—the greatest of these
is the liver treatment of pernicious anaemia, in the discovery of which Dr.
George Minot was the senior partner. Many diabetic physicians[2] treat the
condition which they have learned to control in themselves. My friend
Dr. Robin Lawrence has set a fine example during the war, as he did before
it, to his fellow members of the British Diabetic Association, the President
of which is Mr. H. G. Wells (who writes that he has found diabetes "an
invigorating diathesis").

[2]Including the first physician treated with insulin—Dr. Joseph Gilchrist of Toronto.

The detailed mechanism of the action of insulin is by no means as clear as its specific effect on diabetes might suggest. We soon learned that the formation of the key polysaccharide glycogen was stimulated by insulin and that the burning of sugar was accelerated. The wasteful and dangerous breakdown of protein to sugar and fats to ketone bodies in the liver was checked. More recently direct evidence of an action previously postulated, i.e., the acceleration of the formation of fat from sugar, has been obtained. It is now possible to label the sugar molecule and, in part, to follow it while it is changed to fat under the influence of insulin. Some of the phosphate compounds of paramount importance in provision of energy for muscular contraction hasten their rate of interchange when insulin is present. Thus we know many interesting effects of insulin but we have much more to learn before the picture is complete.

The provision of exogenous insulin rests the pancreatic islets and their stores of insulin decrease.

The Prospects

The prospects of obtaining a more complete knowledge of the action of insulin, and of improving in many ways the treatment of diabetic patients, are very bright.

The intelligent use of such labelling agents as radioactive phosphorus and the stable isotopes of carbon, nitrogen, sulphur, and other elements, is certain to illuminate many of the dark passages through which insulin passes in producing its effect on diabetes. We can confidently expect further advances in this field which has been widened and cleared even during this war.

The fact that in the diabetic patient or in an experimental animal, eight-tenths of the insulin-producing capacity may have disappeared before it is possible to detect this by any procedure except direct examination, which of course is not feasible in a patient, presents a challenge to clinician and experimentalist alike. It is inconceivable to me that a clear-cut problem of this kind can long resist the onslaught of fresh and vigorous minds which we hope will attack it and other "Islands of Resistance" when peace comes. There are many physiological and chemical avenues of approach which have not been explored.

We have no reliable methods for the estimation of insulin in small quantities of blood. Mastery of this technique would help in diagnosing the type of diabetes and perhaps in the treatment. We need either a sensitive and specific chemical test or a micro-biological procedure which is capable of detecting the small amounts of the anti-diabetic hormone which are certainly present in varying quantities in blood. Relatively few vigorous attacks have been made on this problem.

Experimental evidence suggests that diabetes may be produced by an excess of the secretions of the anterior pituitary or adrenal glands. We must develop accurate procedures for the assay of these diabetogenic materials in blood. It has already been shown that diabetes may be most favourably affected by removal of the exciting cause which has been found in a few clinical cases in one of the adrenal glands.

We can look forward with confidence to the development of better diets for diabetics. A lead has been supplied recently by English workers who, confirming the well-known favourable effect of diets rich in fat on the diabetes of experimental animals, have suggested that certain fats may be used as a source of energy without the production of excessive amounts of the dangerous ketone bodies. The role of some of the new accessory food factors on the intensity of diabetes is just beginning to be studied and the use of small animals made diabetic by the injection of alloxan, a chemical which selectively destroys the insulin-producing cells, will be of great value.

We know that there will be better control of infections, which produce the main problems in the treatment of many diabetics. Penicillin by its gentle and effective action should introduce a new era of progress in relation to the control of infection in diabetic patients.

The problem of giving insulin in a more physiological way presents many difficulties. It will not be easy to make a compound of insulin which is susceptible to the sugar content of the tissues. This compound should free insulin more rapidly as the sugar content of its environment increases and thus simulate conditions in the normal pancreas. Improvements over protamine-zinc insulin are quite possible and should certainly engage the attention of those who have already made such strides in this field. Insulin by mouth for mild cases of diabetes is by no means an impossibility although it will probably always be a wasteful procedure and perhaps a hazardous one, when the dose of insulin must be very accurately regulated.

If insulin could be given by mouth, the difficulties of supply, which I have already emphasized, would be increased. Perhaps there is some short cut to the synthesis of insulin, or perhaps only certain of the chemical groupings in the complicated formulae which I showed you, are necessary for the anti-diabetic effect. We may well have to utilize the large amounts of insulin which could be collected from the bony fishes who manufacture and store their insulin in an organ devoted exclusively to this task. Perhaps some of the more primitive but readily available forms of life make something which is either insulin or which can be readily transformed into it.

In many of the chronic cases of diabetes, the insulin-producing capacity of the islet cells is irretrievably lost and we can work only to improve the replacement therapy, i.e., the procedures by which insulin is given. In the mild or new cases and perhaps in some of the older patients, there is hope that a cure will be discovered. This problem, and the prevention of the disease, are two of the most urgent ones which face workers in this field.

In experimental animals the diabetes resulting from partial removal of the pancreas or from administration of the diabetogenic hormone of the anterior pituitary gland may now, under certain conditions, be prevented or in its early stages cured by the appropriate use of insulin and diets which do not tax the capacity of the remaining islets of Langerhans.

The prevention and cure of diabetes in experimental animals arouses hope that application of similar procedures may some day be made in the human subject. This will not be easy until the potential human diabetic can be recognized much earlier than is possible at present and until much more light is thrown on the etiology of the diabetic state in man. In spite of the obvious difficulties I have no doubt that some enterprising clinician will determine, by actual trial, the extent to which the results of the animal experiments are applicable to the human subject. In the meantime further experimental research may help to clarify the situation.

In conclusion, the experiments begun in the building across the campus in May 1921 resulted in the isolation of the anti-diabetic hormone, the administration of which to completely depancreatized dogs restores these animals to perfect health, which can be maintained indefinitely. A great deal has been learned about the action of insulin. The purification of the active principle has made available the pure crystalline insulin protein. The clinical application of the experimental findings, dating from January 11, 1922, has created an ever-increasing demand for insulin which threatens to outrun the immediate source of supply.

Many of the gains made in the field of insulin and diabetes are well consolidated but a host of new problems, on a much broader front, have appeared. This is a healthy situation which should attract many young minds in what we hope will soon be a great post-war period of medical research.

29. Insulin

CHARLES H. BEST, c.b.e., m.d., f.r.s.

The personality of Frederick Grant Banting made such a lasting impression upon those of us who knew him well that it is difficult to realize that it is more than eleven years since he left us. These memories, obtained from many points of vantage, will all be clear and in the forefront of our minds. Some of you knew him when he was fulfilling the promise of his earlier years. A few of us knew him before he became Canada's most famous scientific son. I have my own vivid memories, particularly of our work together in the spring, summer, and autumn of 1921.

There are two very high peaks which feature the brilliant record of Banting's achievements. The first was in that intensive period preceding the discovery of insulin, when all considerations were laid aside except those which advanced the research. The second came just before and in the early phases of the Second Great War when he gave inspired leadership in the effort to develop the full potential of Canadian medical research for the emergency. His courage, vigour and perseverance were abundantly demonstrated on both these occasions. In the latter, maturity and administrative ability had been added to his younger qualities of greatness. Last year I had the honour of unveiling a bust to Fred Banting which now stands in our Simcoe Hall. The sculptress, Miss Frances Loring, captured and preserved for posterity those characteristics of youthful vigour and mature strength combined with complete courage and firmness of purpose which made Banting the great man he was.

When the Programme Committee of our Council invited me to give this lecture I did not look far for a title. A perfectly objective approach to the historical aspects of this subject is obviously impossible for me. It has been attempted in our columns by others with, as would be expected, different degrees of success. There have been a few interesting statements about the early development of insulin which I completely fail to recognize. Objective descriptions are, of course, invaluable and there are some who are particularly well qualified to make them in this field. The names of Dr.

Originally appeared in *Diabetes*, I (1952), 257–68.

Elliott P. Joslin in this country, Sir Henry Dale in England, and Dr. Bernardo Houssay in the Argentine come to my mind. I will not attempt to select any names from an even younger group, but there are many in this Association who are interested and well informed on these matters.

The facts are simple and straightforward. The young surgeon formulated a hypothesis which was vital to his initiation of the work and it thus completely fulfilled its function. He obtained permission to explore this hypothesis in the physiological laboratory of his Alma Mater and he received some excellent general advice from the Head of the Department. The fundamental working hypothesis was that an internal secretion of the pancreas existed and that it could be captured. Banting and I shared in its exploration. We formed a partnership which was based on the new knowledge and experience which we gained together. We had no stipends, but the facilities of Professor Macleod's deserted department were at our disposal. We worked completely alone during the four summer months of 1921 without any verbal or written advice from any senior investigator and until well after the salient facts, consistent dramatic lowering of blood and urinary sugars and complete recovery of our moribund depancreatized dogs, had been repeatedly demonstrated.

In the spring of 1923 the first recognition of our work came with the award of the Reeve Prize of our Faculty of Medicine to Banting and myself for the discovery of insulin. The prize was $50 and was "awarded annually on the basis of a published report of the best scientific research accomplished in any department of the Faculty of Medicine by a research fellow or junior member of the staff." Later in the same year The Banting and Best Act of the Ontario Legislature, creating a Chair of Medical Research with the same names, was passed.

Banting and I had hoped that our article on "The Internal Secretion of the Pancreas," which appeared in the February 1922 issue of the *Journal of Laboratory and Clinical Medicine* [40] would be universally accepted as the original record of our work. However, a summary of this paper, sent for publication some weeks later, and bearing in addition the name of the Head of the Department, actually appeared in print first [49].

Banting generously stressed our fraternal partnership and the interdependence of the surgical and biochemical techniques in several public announcements and in unpublished letters. When Professor Macleod asked me if I would like to volunteer for the work with Banting, I was not actually a medical student. Rather, after five years of university study, and a year in the Canadian Army, I was a very recent graduate in the Arts course of Physiology and Biochemistry. I was deeply interested in physiology, and for family reasons particularly interested in diabetes. I had been a part-time research worker on diabetes and a demonstrator in physiology to the medical students during 1920–21. I was registered for an M.A. in Physiology during the year Banting and I worked together and was awarded this degree in June 1922. In September 1922, sixteen months after Banting and I began our work, I decided to proceed towards an M.D. rather than a Ph.D. degree and registered for the first time in the Medical Faculty of the University of Toronto.

As the representative of the staff of the Department of Physiology when insulin was discovered, and of the staff of the Department created in 1923 by the Banting and Best Act of the Ontario Provincial Legislature, I have a sensation of giving an account of my stewardship—not only to the present membership of the American Diabetes Association, but to some who are no longer with us.

THE SOURCE OF INSULIN

A good starting point for a discussion of insulin is the Islands of Langerhans. After a brief historical review I will select, for emphasis, certain aspects of this interesting subject. In 1869, in the introduction to his article entitled "The Microscopic Anatomy of the Pancreas," [484], Paul Langerhans wrote: "There is indeed hardly another organ in which there is such glaring contrast between the brilliant results of physiological research and the complete darkness in the realm of anatomical knowledge." The pancreas was known merely as a racemose gland in spite of the very early work of the Dutch investigator Regner de Graaf [330] and Claude Bernard's demonstration [63] that its secretion played a vital role in the digestion of carbohydrates, proteins, and fats. Langerhans was a very young man, 22 years old, when he published this, the third of his scientific papers, and he was appropriately modest. He wrote: "I can describe at most a few isolated observations which suggest a much more complicated structure of the pancreas than hitherto accepted." In introducing the newly recognized bodies he stated: "The cell is a small irregularly polygonal structure. . . . The cells lie together, generally in considerable numbers, diffusely scattered in the parenchyma of the gland." There is no suggestion anywhere in this article that Langerhans had any idea of the physiological significance of his cells, but the more experienced histologist Laguesse did suggest an endocrine role. "Dans le pancreas d'un homme adulte (supplicié) je retrouve ces îlots très nombreux et volumineux (je les désignerai provisoirement sous le nom d'îlots de Langerhans)." Thus we read the thoughtful words which immortalized Langerhans. They appear in one of a series of short articles by Laguesse in *Mémoires de la Société de Biologie*, 1893 [478].

In 1907 M. A. Lane [481] a pupil of R. R. Bensley's, made an important advance in knowledge of the islands. He developed more definite procedures for the differentiation of the alpha and beta cells. The granules of the alpha cells are relatively large and have large spherical nuclei with little chromatin. The granules are precipitated by 70 per cent alcohol. The granules of the beta cells are soluble in this concentration of alcohol but are precipitated by aqueous chrome sublimate. They are much more numerous and considerably smaller than those of the alpha cells and contain higher concentrations of chromatin.

Professor R. R. Bensley, a graduate from Toronto in 1892 who has spent most of his active life in the U.S.A., has perhaps more than any other person of his generation informed us regarding the minute structure and interrelationship of the cells in the islands of Langerhans. His work widened and strengthened the foundation upon which our present conceptions are based. One of Bensley's contributions was the clear demonstration of a system of fine anastomosing tubules about the pancreatic duct which are in continuity with the islands Langerhans. . . . I wrote to Professor Bensley to secure his reaction to the present situation. He answered promptly in his own firm hand:

I am afraid that my knowledge of recent developments is too meagre to give you much help. . . . The record of the medical profession in the management of diabetes, both pre-insulin and post-insulin, has been a magnificent one and has my enthusiastic admiration. In the fundamental sciences, however, the tendency to a narrow point of view has been ever manifest. The preoccupation at the present time with the alloxan phenomenon is, to my mind, an evidence of this since most modern workers in this field seem to be unaware that in the pre-insulin era cases of diabetes of the greatest severity, proceeding rapidly to a fatal issue, occurred in which no indication of histological changes in the islands of Langerhans or in the pancreas as a whole could be discovered. I investigated several such cases myself with the most advanced techniques. I examined these pancreases with the full co-operation of the physician as to promptness of autopsy and methods of preparation. In that period the pathologist felt a sort of compulsion to adapt his findings to a popular theory and this compulsion spoilt his objectivity. In those cases where reduction in number or size of the Islands was not reported, obviously the pathologist was at his wit's end to explain the disease. I think that it is important that workers in the fundamental sciences who are engaged in this field should be made to realize that, while plus or minus insulin is an important factor, the situation is far more complex. The recent experiences with ACTH and cortisone help us to appreciate these facts, although I am sorry to say that the medical profession has not exercised the restraint and caution in the use of these hormones which was imposed in the case of insulin by the dramatic results of over or under dosage.

I will bring to your attention today some evidence supporting, in a general way, Professor Bensley's view. There are many facts, as he states, which emphasize the complexity of clinical diabetes. As a physiologist one could not, of course, accept the normal appearance of a gland as a complete proof of normal function. The histologist and the physiologist are not now, as in the past, commonly integrated in a single individual, but they can work together most profitably. Using appropriate stains, my colleagues Dr. Hartroft and Dr. Wrenshall find that the granule count in the cells may frequently run parallel to the amount of insulin extractable. Indeed, this had been observed in the earlier work on diet and insulin content of pancreas which Haist and I discussed some years ago. Similarly, in meta-diabetes produced in dogs by purified growth hormone or by alloxan, the histologist can predict with reasonable accuracy what the insulin content will prove to be. This is also true in "growth onset" type of human diabetes, where the lesions in the cells are always advanced and the insulin content is consistently low. But difficulties were encountered when the pancreas of "maturity onset" diabetics were studied, and the correlation of granule counts and insulin content was not nearly as satisfactory as in cases exemplifying other types of diabetes. The basic cause of this situation is, quite probably, that an extensive depletion of granules becomes obvious and unmistakable, but when the decrease is slight various other factors affect the picture and it is impossible for the histologist always to make an accurate interpretation.

It is important and interesting to ask: "In how many diabetic patients is there no evidence of any abnormality in the manufacture or liberation of insulin?" Professor Bensley had referred to the fact that he was unable to detect any islet cell abnormalities in some diabetic patients at autopsy. Shields Warren [779] states that 26 per cent of the autopsies in his series of diabetics revealed essentially normal islets. Wrenshall, Bogoch, and Ritchie [815] found the average insulin content of the pancreas of "maturity onset" diabetics approximately half that of non-diabetics. Based on units of insulin per gram of pancreas, 6.8 per cent of the diabetics had values falling *above* the average of non-diabetics. Based on units of insulin per square metre of surface, 3.4 per cent had values above the non-diabetic average. The number of cases of "maturity onset" diabetics falling within the standard deviation range of non-diabetic controls was 32 per cent based on units per gram of pancreas, or 21 per cent based on units per square metre of body surface. Three diabetics out of 59 had more total insulin in their pancreas than the average non-diabetic. Twelve had values falling within the range of standard error of the non-diabetics.

We are interested in the histological appearance of the islets and in their insulin content, but the question which we hope will be answered by these studies is: "How much insulin in relation to the normal amount was this subject's pancreas providing for the tissues of the body?" The level of blood insulin will give us an important part of the answer we seek, but this has yet to be placed on a quantitative basis. Mr. J. M. Salter, in our department, is just beginning to achieve satisfactory assays using the Gellhorn-Bornstein technique with some slight modifications and improvements. He has successfully alloxanized his hypophysectomized rats. I have been talking about blood insulin for a long time and I congratulate Dr. Gellhorn, Dr. Anderson, Dr. Bornstein, Dr. Groen, and the others who have made the present methods available. Bornstein and Lawrence [141] have already provided us with some information on the level of blood insulin which can be maintained by the "maturity onset" diabetics who have, as I have mentioned [815] about half the normal pancreatic insulin. This average figure may well prove to have little clinical significance since each case will have to be considered as an individual. Some cases with high blood insulin may prove to require more exogenous insulin than others with a lower blood level. As I have discussed elsewhere [72] we must also learn to assay the insulin antagonists in blood. Dr. Donald Clarke, in our department, has been attempting to concentrate plasma insulin using a Kirkwood electrophoretic cell. He has secured as high as a sixfold increase in potency per unit volume with added insulin and his recent figures indicate that a similar procedure may produce a several-fold concentration of natural insulin. Perhaps he will be able to use normal or diabetic mice, more readily available test objects than can now be used to estimate the insulin content of blood. . . . In the normal guinea pig's pancreas stained by Gomori's haematoxylin ephloxine procedure there is no difficulty in distinguishing alpha and beta cells. [Nine coloured figures have been omitted, including one to illustrate this point.] Similarly in the normal rat pancreas the peripheral alpha cells stand out clearly from the centrally located beta type (Plate VIII(d)). As originally shown by Arnozan and Vaillard [18] and by Schulze [680], ligation of the pancreatic ducts isolates the islets with waves of fibrous tissue. It was from degenerated pancreas like this that Banting and I extracted our first insulin in 1921. The historical importance of this fact is not decreased by the knowledge that the exact procedures which we used for the degenerated gland would have given us more insulin from the intact dog or ox pancreas.

Professor Lyman Duff, whom we are proud to claim as a Toronto graduate in Medicine (he is now Dean of Medicine at McGill), has kindly sent me examples of what we used to call hydropic degeneration, but now know from the work of Duff and Toreson [272] to be glycogen infiltration. Similar conditions can be demonstrated in metapituitary diabetes in dogs where the glycogen is found in the degenerated islet and duct cells. Preparations illustrating this were made available to me by Professor James Campbell, whose studies on the production of permanent diabetes in dogs by injection of highly purified growth hormone are now appearing in press from our Department of Physiology. In a case of spontaneous diabetes in a dog studied by Dr. Wrenshall, glycogen infiltration of the duct cells was observed. Dr. Hartroft studied many sections of this pancreas before he found any islets. We have many other interesting pictures confirming the effect of alloxan on beta cells and the recent findings of our Belgian colleagues of cobalt on alpha cells, but I must not pause to show them here.

Turning now to human cases, I would like to record the fact that Leonard Thompson, the first diabetic patient treated with insulin, who died of bronchopneumonia some eleven years after January 11, 1922, the day he received his first injection, had an atrophied pancreas in which it was difficult to find any islet tissue. The beta granules stand out beautifully in the *normal* pancreas stained by the Wilson-Gomori procedure (Plate IX(*a*)). The shrunken islet lacking beta granulation, illustrated in Plate IX(*b*), is from Leonard Thompson's pancreas. (I am indebted to both Dr. Walter Campbell and to the Department of Pathology, University of Toronto, for permission to use this illustration.) I have recorded elsewhere that it fell to my lot to remove the normal pancreas from a steer, make the partially purified insulin and establish its potency in diabetic dogs before Banting and I took our first injections. We gave the rest of this material to Dr. Campbell and Dr. Fletcher for the first clinical trial. The insulin was crude but active, and certain features of its preparation, such as the concentration of ethyl alcohol for the initial extraction of that normal adult beef pancreas, which I adopted after preliminary trials and testings on diabetic dogs, have been almost universally used for the past 30 years in the large-scale production of insulin.

Plate IX(*c*) shows the granules in the islet cells of the first doctor to receive insulin. Banting's friend and mine—Joseph Gilchrist—lived for nearly 30 years after we gave him his first injection of insulin in our laboratory in the winter of 1922. I followed his blood sugar downward and his expired air was collected for gas analysis. He had an attack of hypoglycaemia about midnight on his way home from the Physiological Laboratory that night. If a pathologist studied only a limited number of islets such as the one illustrated, he might conclude that this pancreas should contain appreciable amounts of insulin. But there proved to be relatively few normal islets and the insulin content of the pancreas was 0.3 units per gram instead of the normal 2.4 units. The total insulin content of the pancreas was 9.8 units instead of about 200 units. The gland weighed 35 g in contrast to a normal weight of 80 g. We can only guess at the output of insulin, but it was presumably a very small fraction of the normal. The figures were obtained by my colleagues Wrenshall and Hartroft from the specimen made available by Dr. A. J. Blanchard of the Sunnybrook Military Hospital in Toronto.

The first case in which an excessive secretion of insulin was established by clinical and necropsy findings was that of Wilder, Allan, Power, and Robertson [796]. This patient, also a physician, had profound hypoglycaemia and an exploratory operation revealed a tumour mass in the pancreas with metastases in the liver. Insulin was found in one of the liver metastases as well as in the primary tumour (cf. Plate IX(d)).[1]

The first case of islet cell tumour to recover after surgical removal of the growth was that reported from Toronto by Howland, Campbell, Maltby, and Robinson [410]. A tumour about 1.5 cm in diameter was removed by my close friend the late Roscoe Graham, and although it was originally considered probably to be carcinomatous in nature, the pathologist Dr. W. L. Robinson, who also made many contributions during the early insulin investigations, now considers that it may be classified as benign (Plate VIII(a)).

In the most recent collection of cases with islet cell tumours, 398 in number [404], there were 313 benign adenomas. The carcinomas numbered 37 and the others were questionably malignant. In 12.6 per cent of cases there was more than one adenoma present.

Various tissue culture experts have attempted to grow islet cell tumour tissue *in vitro* and to transplant the cells, which have been "acclimatized" in serum from the potential recipient, to diabetic patients. Professor Gaillard in Leiden had a few encouraging results. Dr. Marjorie Murray at the Presbyterian Hospital in New York also secured good growth but on transference to patients there was no evidence of persistent growth of insulin-producing cells [792].

One of the most interesting sections of islets which I have seen is from a case of hyperinsulinism in a child studied by Dr. W. L. Donohue of the Toronto Sick Children's Hospital (Plate VIII(b)). Our Mr. Wilson cut many sections before he demonstrated an afferent and an efferent capillary in the same picture. One can almost see all the 16 amino acids hurrying in to keep their precise appointments with the many coupling enzymes in the busy beta cells and the purposeful outward march of the complete molecules of insulin within the efferent vessel. . . .

Another interesting pancreas, also obtained through the kindness of Dr. Donohue [260], shows a large part of the field taken up with islets—

[1]Dr. Allen O. Whipple's recent review "Islet Cell Tumours of the Pancreas" [792] gives an excellent account of the historical and present aspects of this field. See also Dr. Russell Wilder's paper "Hypoglycemia" [795].

there is obviously a tremendous increase in islet tissue (Plate VIII(c)). No histological evidence of either pituitary or adrenal overactivity was found.

Dr. Haist and I made a series of studies on the effects of diet on the insulin content of pancreas [345]. Fasting or feeding diets rich in fat greatly reduces the amount of insulin extractable. Insulin administration lowered the insulin content but removal of the pituitary or adrenals had no effect. In metadiabetes of all types, i.e., permanent pancreatic diabetes produced by chemical or hormonal agents, the insulin in the pancreas is greatly reduced or completely absent.

Since insulin is a product of the islets of Langerhans, and we believe that most cases of diabetes are characterized by either an absolute or a relative insulin deficiency, it is important to learn more about the factors which control the total amount of islet tissue. This problem has been approached by measuring the volume or weight of the islets of Langerhans under a variety of experimental conditions. The weights have been estimated, in work directed by Haist, by a special technique employing intravenous injection of neutral red, fresh tissue preparations, and the planimetric method of measurement. Both dietary and hormonal factors influence islet growth. If the intake of a balanced diet is so reduced that the individual fails to gain weight the islets fail to grow [348]. Tejning (1947) [747] found that in rats fed *ad libitum* there was a greater islet weight when the diet was high in carbohydrate than when the diet was rich in fat. Other evidence for a stimulating effect of carbohydrate is to be found in the increase in islet tissue which results from the continuous infusion of glucose (Woerner [813], Haist and colleagues [348]).

The hormonal factors influencing the islets are also numerous. Insulin, itself, when given in very large amounts, depresses the growth of the islets [293]. The hormones which are apparently antagonistic to insulin tend to stimulate islet growth.

In most instances where a trophic effect of the pituitary on a gland has been established, removal of the pituitary leads to its atrophy. Hypophysectomy prevents the islets from growing normally and thus may lead to some reduction in islet weight as compared with paired-fed control animals, but this difference is small when considered in relation to the decrease in size of adrenals or gonads after pituitary removal. Hypophysectomy results in an atrophy of the acinar tissue of pancreas [332; 470] and thus increases the ratio of islet to acinar tissue in the hypophysectomized rats, even though the islet tissue itself has not increased in amount. As Haist [348] points out, this illustrates one reason for not accepting a change in islet to acinar ratio as an adequate *sole* criterion for a change in islet volume.

In intact rats, the islets can be made to grow by the injection of crude saline extracts of the pituitary gland (Richardson and Young [638], Haist and colleagues [348]) and in hypophysectomized rats also the injection of crude saline extracts or of purified growth hormone preparations, leads to an increase in islet tissue.

The thyroid gland also influences the islets and probably the pituitary thyrotropic material would do likewise. The administration of desiccated thyroid for 40 days or longer caused an increase in the weight of islet tissues as well as an increase in pancreas weight [348]. In one small series of hypophysectomized animals, thyroid administration was found by Haist and his colleagues to cause both islets and pancreas to increase in weight (personal communication).

A considerable amount of work on the influence of the gonads on carbohydrate metabolism and the islets of Langerhans has been carried out by Ingle [414] and by Houssay and his group. Cardeza [174] reported an increase in islet to acinar ratios in the pancreatic remnants in rats with 95 per cent of pancreas removed following the administration of estrogens. Dr. Haist's group found that injection of large doses of diethyl stilbestrol into female rats led to an increase in islet weight and in the ratio of islet weight to unit of body weight which was statistically significant, as was the increase in islet to pancreas ratio. Under the conditions of the Toronto studies, progesterone in large doses also caused an increase in islet weight. Removal of the gonads had no significant effect on islet growth. A valuable review of the effects of sex hormones on experimental diabetes has recently been published by Houssay [400].

It was well established, of course, by the brilliant work of Herbert Evans and his colleagues, that the anterior pituitary provides a factor vital to the growth of the animal as a whole. Since the islet volume is so well correlated with body weight, it may be that islet growth is related to the growth of the animal as a whole and to the effect which body growth has on insulin requirements. Procedures which prevent body growth, such as restriction of caloric intake, also interfere with islet growth. The manner in which the demand for insulin is transmitted from the cells of the body to those of the islets is not known. It is possible that, directly or indirectly, an increase in blood sugar level or a change in blood insulin may set in motion physiological events which affect islet activity. This is yet another set of obviously related physiological facts for which the mechanism of interrelation remains obscure. Insulin may be the most essential anabolic hormone, and processes relating to fat, glycogen, or protein formation may call for an increased supply.

ON THE CHEMISTRY OF INSULIN

For many of us, insulin is the most interesting of all proteins. It obviously has a charm also for the protein chemists, for they know more about its structure than about that of any other protein.

The protein chemist says that he is devoted to insulin not because of its physiological significance and therapeutic value, but because its peptide chains are relatively short! It is stable in acid and reversibly inactivated in mild alkali. It can be readily crystallized. It is practically the only protein which can be purchased in large amounts in a pure form. In spite of this array of facts, I still feel that the chemist's interest is subconsciously catalysed by the realization that in the completely diabetic organism one molecule of insulin accounts for the utilization of some 15,000,000 molecules of glucose per hour [262] and that the lives of many people are prolonged by its daily use.

It was first isolated in crystalline form by Abel in 1926 [2]. In 1934, David A. Scott showed that it could be readily crystallized as the zinc salt and that Abel's crystals contained zinc. Nickel, calcium, and cobalt also aid in effecting crystallization of insulin preparations [682; 683]. There is about 0.5 per cent of metal in the crystals. The "salts" of the insulin protein may appear in various forms—the zinc compound usually as twin plate-like rhombohedra. Chemical analysis by Brand [147] and by the Cambridge workers under the leadership of A. C. Chibnall [758; 544; 634] indicate that the insulin molecule is built up entirely or almost entirely of amino acids. Insulin is richer in the amino acids leucine, glutamic acid, and cystine than most other proteins; methionine, tryptophane and hydroxyproline, which are common in many proteins, are absent from the insulin molecule.

When insulin is in solution at a protein concentration between 0.4 and 0.9 per cent, and pH between 7.0 and 7.5 the maximum molecular weight of insulin is 48,000. However, when more dilute solutions of the hormone are used below pH 4 or above 7.5 the insulin molecule dissociates into subunits having a molecular weight of about 12,000 (Gutfreund [339]). This is probably the physiological form of insulin although the physical chemists are actively debating the possibility of a smaller unit.

When insulin is oxidized with performic acid the molecule is split into its separate polypeptide chains. Two fractions can be isolated: A, an acidic fraction containing no basic amino acids and B, a basic fraction. These two physiologically *inactive* components are normally linked together by the -S-S- bridges of cystine and perhaps by other as yet unknown bonds. This work of Sanger's [666] led to the conclusion that the 12,000 molecular weight insulin is composed of two identical A chains and two identical B chains. Sanger made a great contribution by introducing the use of partial hydrolysis of dinitrophenyl derivatives of the fractions to determine the sequence of the amino acid components. He had available the invaluable tool of paper chromatography of Martin and Synge [556] and the newer knowledge of the chemical linkages attached by specific enzyme systems, such as pepsin, trypsin, and chymotrypsin. The exact sequence of all the amino acids in the two chains of insulin is now known but we are still far removed from the knowledge of how the chains are formed and joined together in the beta cells of the islets.

When a dilute acidic solution of insulin containing a small amount of salt is heated, a flocculant precipitate forms [772]. In experiments in which slightly different conditions were used, Waugh [781] has shown that the insulin can be modified to yield fibrils. The rate of fibril formation increases with increasing hydrogen ion, salt, and protein concentration, and with temperature. In fibril formation two reactions are involved. First the formation of active centres, and second the elongation of these into fibrils. These fibrils have little or no anti-diabetic activity but can be converted into active insulin, as can the so-called heat precipitate of insulin, by changing the reaction to the alkaline side. Seeding an insulin solution with fibrils may bring about a complete conversion of the active insulin into inactive fibrils.

This brief and inadequate glimpse of a few of the chemical properties of insulin may stimulate those of us whose activities lead us far away from this highly specialized and fascinating field.

On the Action of Insulin

The dramatic fall in blood sugar, the cessation of glucose excretion, and the even more exciting recovery of our moribund diabetic dogs when insulin was given, stimulated Banting and me to ask ourselves in July 1921: "How does it act?" Banting asked me: "How can we tell what it actually does to the sugar which disappears from the blood?" I suggested that we should determine the oxygen consumption and carbon dioxide output before and after insulin in our depancreatized dogs. This was the first exploration of the action of insulin ever proposed. Banting was interested but as he remarked: "I know just as much about respiratory quotients as you do about intussusception." I had never heard of the latter until one of our depancreatized dogs exhibited the signs which Banting suggested and later demonstrated were caused by this condition. With the help of Dr. John Hepburn, these respiratory studies were made on diabetic dogs and on the first diabetic doctor to receive insulin. Dr. Gilchrist's respiratory quotient mounted as his blood sugar fell. I used some of these initial findings on respiratory exchange after insulin in man and dogs as part of my M.A. thesis in Physiology. It was a sketchy effort written at the last moment in a single evening, for we had at that time again completely lost the long-buried secret of how to make insulin in sufficient amounts for the treatment of diabetic patients. Some of the patients who had been "brought back" by insulin died, and our struggles to regain the necessary knowledge made even the fascinating pursuit of physiological action impossible at that time.

However, before many months had passed, the Toronto group had established a number of points about the action of insulin. Banting and I, in addition to discovering its effect on blood and urinary sugar, had secured preliminary indications of decreased nitrogen and ketone body excretion. We had, of course, repeatedly demonstrated the complete and prolonged "clinical" recovery of our depancreatized dogs when treated with an alcoholic extract of commercial beef pancreas. We noted the more normal, less yellow appearance of the livers of our treated dogs. With Professor Macleod, Collip, Noble, and Hepburn we reported the formation of liver glycogen, the abrupt cessation of ketosis, the rise in R/Q, the fall in blood and liver fat, and the gain in weight and strength after insulin administration. At one time I had hoped to present a brief sketch in this lecture of the efforts of the many individuals and laboratories that have given us our present knowledge of the effects of insulin on carbohydrate, fat, protein, phosphorus, and potassium metabolism. This is out of the question; but it seems to me that a picture of insulin as perhaps the central anabolic hormone is being drawn. Many of the great names in present-day research on metabolic processes have contributed to and discussed this general subject which, in its broader aspects, is of course the integration of many, perhaps all, endocrine-stimulated anabolic processes. I did make a list of twenty prominent names among those interested in the mechanism of action of the pituitary growth hormone, the adrenal corticoids, the sex hormones, and the thyroid hormone, and in the part which the presence of insulin may play in many of these activities. But this making of "lists" is a dangerous practice! I hope to know a lot more about these subjects before the end of July when many of those whom I listed, and others equally interested, will have devoted two weeks in London and in Leiden to discussions of carbohydrate metabolism. Professor Frank G. Young and I have been named as chairmen of these two conferences.

We have become actively interested recently in the extent to which other anabolic hormones may depend on insulin for the production of their effects. I will have to refer you to the articles written by workers who have contributed much more to this subject than we have. Mirsky, Evans and Li, Young, Evans, Long, Lukens, Milman and Russell, de Bodo, Cori, Stadie,

Lotspeich, De Jongh, Wilhelmi, and many others have discussed aspects of this matter in recent years.

It may be that many of the previous conclusions about purified growth hormone preparations will have to be revised when the Raben-Astwood material, which has been stated not to be diabetogenic, has become available. The changes may, however, merely affect the names of the fractions responsible for the effects produced by cruder extracts. It is obvious that someone must determine (a) what constituent of pituitary exerts the insulin-reversible inhibition in Cori's cell-free hexokinase system; (b) what properties are responsible for the differences between the *in vitro* effects of crude pituitary extract and purified growth hormone on glycogen formation in the diaphragm in Stadie's experiments; (c) whether the same constituent lowers the blood sugar in normal rats (Milman and Russell) but fails to do this in normal dogs (de Bodo, Sirek); (d) whether the increased volume of the islet cells and perhaps their insulin output, produced by the pituitary principle or principles, are the result or the cause of the augmented appetite and food intake. In one of Dr. Sirek's studies in my laboratory, the same purified growth hormone preparation which produced no change in blood sugar in the normal dog caused a prompt and extensive rise in the same animal after complete pancreatectomy. What prevented the rise in blood sugar of the intact animal? Could it have been the liberation of insulin or do these pituitary preparations contain both a hyperglycaemic and a hypo-glycaemic factor with the "balance of power" dependent on the state of the field of action? De Bodo only obtained a fall in blood sugar after growth hormone in depancreatized dogs when the material was given soon after pancreatectomy. Sirek has now demonstrated this with one growth hormone preparation much longer after pancreatectomy. There may, of course, have been a trace of natural or exogenous insulin present under both these conditions. Krahl's work demonstrates an insulin-like effect of purified growth hormone on blood sugar and diaphragm in alloxan-diabetic rats. It is abundantly apparent that more good chemistry is needed before the physiologist and biochemist can push forward with confidence.

Under the standardized conditions of Sirek's experiments, purified growth hormone preparations do not lower the blood N.P.N. of normal dogs. Testosterone does lower the N.P.N. of normal dogs but not of depancreatized dogs without insulin. Insulin lowers the N.P.N. of depancreatized dogs and testosterone does not supplement the insulin effect.

Mr. Salter and I thought it would be interesting to study the growth effect of insulin in the absence of the pituitary gland. This has not been investigated because everyone knows how very sensitive hypophysectomized animals are to insulin. Some species die in hypoglycaemia without administered insulin if fasted for even a relatively short period. Now the tests for the pituitary growth hormone utilize principally the weight increase in "plateaued" hypophysectomized rats, increase in body and tail length, increase in organ size, widening of the epiphyseal line of the tibia, and nitrogen retention. When in our initial experiment a small dose of insulin was given to a hypophysectomized rat, his appetite and food intake were increased and he began to grow. The dose was rapidly stepped up from 1 unit to 6 units of protamine-zinc insulin per day. The animal put on weight, his body and tail increased in length, his organs (liver, heart, and thymus) gained in weight, his epiphyseal line widened and from later determinations on other comparable animals, he undoubtedly retained a lot of nitrogen, presumably in large part as protein. These preliminary findings will, of course, be extended and published in due course (Figure 68). This

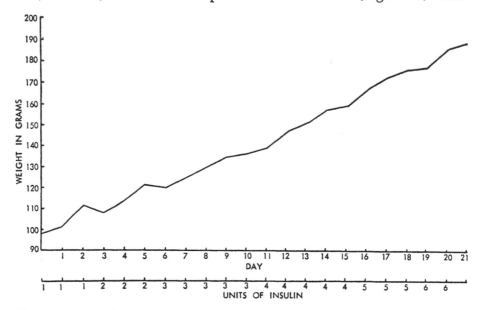

FIGURE 68. Weight changes induced in a hypophysectomized rat by daily administration of protamine zinc insulin. This animal showed no weight change during a five-month period prior to insulin treatment. Throughout its life it was fed *ad libitum* on a complete diet.

work proves that insulin is a growth hormone which apparently can operate in the absence of the pituitary gland. Before insulin was given the rats did not grow. Their sex glands and adrenals continued to decrease in weight in spite of the growth effect of insulin. At autopsy their *sella turcicae* confirmed the absence of appreciable amounts of pituitary gland and serial sections are in process. It would appear, judged by the criterion of independent action, that in the rat, insulin is a more indispensable growth hormone than somatotropin. Perhaps one of the causes of cessation of growth after removal of the pituitary is decreased secretion of insulin. The islets do not atrophy but some essential stimulus for the liberation of insulin may be lacking. A small amount of somatotropin may have remained in our experiments, although this appears unlikely; but no one would suggest that insulin exerts its anabolic effects through increased liberation of somatotropin. The two hormones are certainly essential synergists for normal growth, but we wish to know just how much insulin is liberated in the hypophysectomized animal. To what extent could decreased insulin secretion account for the lack of growth in hypophysectomized animals? To what extent can large unphysiological doses of insulin compensate for the lack of physiological amounts of the growth hormone? My young colleague, Mr. Salter, has found that all the hypophysectomized rats die if given even very small amounts of regular insulin. A slow acting insulin and a high carbohydrate diet constantly available in an attractive form are essential. The first insulin we used may have contained a very little hyperglycaemic factor. The last series of rats were given insulin free of this material and the results are similar. This work opens up a new vista to us. We must study the effect of insulin on growth, nitrogen retention, etc. in the hypophysectomized depancreatized preparations. We must know the extent of the participation of each of the other hormones in the growth effect of insulin and we must compare the results of forced feeding and of pituitary growth hormone administration with those of insulin under exactly comparable conditions in normal, depancreatized, hypophysectomized and Houssay animals. Several of these studies are in progress.

Thus the thirty years since Banting and I discussed how insulin acts have not witnessed the solution of all the problems. The current literature is full of valuable articles on this subject. Not long before his death Banting and I discussed working again together in the laboratory. We had selected a problem in carbohydrate metabolism and had planned a combined surgical and chemical approach.

Acknowledgments

I am deeply indebted to all my colleagues whose names appear in the text of this article and to Mrs. Margaret Cornell and Miss Linda Mahon for their help with the manuscript. I have drawn particularly heavily on Professor W. Stanley Hartroft's time and skill.

30. Diabetes since 1920

CHARLES H. BEST, c.b.e., m.d., d.sc., ll.d., f.r.s.

I would like to begin by making one deferential bow to the past, to the work of Professor Oskar Minkowski who, with von Mering, laid the foundation for the study of experimental diabetes [561]. The University of Toronto donated all of its rights for insulin in Germany to an Insulin Committee formed in that country in 1922, and Professor Minkowski was the first chairman. Recently my friend, Dr. Martin Goldner, told the story of his own observations on the day when Professor Minkowski received his first small parcel of insulin from Toronto. The professor held up a vial of insulin for his large class to see and said: "Gentlemen, I had hoped to be the father of insulin but I am now delighted to be its grandfather." At that time I was Director of the Insulin Division of the Connaught Laboratories and I remember vividly when this insulin was sent to Professor Minkowski.

It is unnecessary for me to describe the clinical treatment of diabetes in 1920. The drastic dietary procedures, which were used in the effort to prolong life, are well known. I shall not attempt any analysis of the results, but many of us remember diabetics who were on the starvation regimen.

Two great physiologists, Professor Ernest H. Starling and Professor J. J. R. Macleod, published editions of their textbooks in 1920, and these provide us with outlines of the knowledge of experimental diabetes at that time. Professor Starling [733] wrote and taught as follows: "We do not yet know how the pancreas affects sugar production or utilization in the normal animal. It is generally assumed that it secretes into the blood stream a hormone which may, according to the view of the nature of diabetes which we adopt, pass to the tissues and enable them to utilize sugar, or pass to the liver and inhibit the sugar production in this organ. A very small portion of the pancreas is sufficient for this purpose, but we have been unable to imitate the action of the pancreas still in vascular connection with the body by injection or administration of extracts of this organ."

Professor Macleod [537] wrote and taught in 1920 that, "The most recent work has shown that injection of pancreatic extracts into a de-

Originally appeared in the *Canadian Medical Association Journal*, LXXXII (1960), 1061–6. Read at the plenary session, Joint Meeting of the British and Canadian Medical Associations, Edinburgh, July 1959.

pancreatized animal produces no change in the respiratory quotient, although injections of extracts of pancreas and duodenum may cause a temporary fall in the excretion of glucose in the urine on account of the alkalinity of the extract. Neither have experiments with blood transfusions yielded results that are any more satisfactory. . . . The removal of some hormone necessary for proper sugar metabolism is, however, by no means the only way by which the results can be explained, for we can assume that the pancreas owes its influence over sugar metabolism to some change occurring in the composition of the blood as this circulates through the gland—a change which is dependent on the integrity of the gland and not on any one enzyme or hormone which it produces."

There is more behind these statements than appears in the textbooks. Knowlton and Starling [460], in 1912, had reported that a boiled extract of pancreas restores to the heart of a diabetic dog the power of utilizing the glucose of the circulating blood. Professor Macleod, lecturing in 1920, stated that he found the evidence for this statement quite unconvincing. Macleod and Pearce [541], in 1913, had reported that in the "liverless" diabetic animal the rate of disappearance of sugar from the blood was the same as in the normal preparation. Later in 1913, Patterson and Starling [613] re-investigated in greater detail the effects of pancreatic extracts and abandoned the conclusion that they exerted a beneficial effect on the diabetic heart. Thus it was with this background that Starling and Macleod wrote as they did, and these circumstances also may have contributed to make Professor Macleod very cautious and conservative when an unknown young surgeon approached him with a working hypothesis. The idea that ligation of the pancreatic ducts might be helpful, a thought which was formulated independently by Fred Banting and which was responsible for the initiation of the work in Toronto and for many of the procedures which we employed, had been previously tested by several groups of workers without success. This latter fact must have been in the back of Professor Macleod's mind, but you will find no specific mention of it in any of the records which he made at the time. We had very little correspondence with Professor Macleod during the summer of 1921, when he was in Scotland for three months.

The main findings which Banting and I established in July, August, and September of 1921 were that neutral or acid saline or alcoholic extracts of degenerated dog pancreas, foetal calf pancreas, or normal beef pancreas consistently gave us a dramatic lowering of the blood sugar in completely depancreatized dogs. There was frequently a corresponding improvement in their clinical condition. We demonstrated the effects of insulin on 75 consecutive occasions [41], without any failure, and we had available constantly, from July 30, 1921, a method on which we could completely rely to make small lots of potent insulin.

Our results of the effect of insulin on blood sugar and urine sugar of depancreatized dogs were not preliminary in nature as one poorly informed or misguided individual has suggested, but were actually final and conclusive. We spent ten times as much effort on this point as we felt was necessary, but we were determined not to permit ourselves to explore the innumerable fascinating new pathways until we had established beyond any doubt our primary objective—a consistent demonstration of the presence of an anti-diabetic substance in extracts of pancreas. We worked alone for six months, and then a group under Professor Macleod was formed which, with the collaboration of Professor Collip, quickly made a number of other advances in the purification of insulin and established many of its effects which Banting and I could not explore in the time or with the facilities available to us. It was shown that glycogen was formed in the liver, that the respiratory quotient was raised, that liver fat was decreased, that ketosis was abolished, that normal animals reacted to insulin and could be used as test objects, that the hypoglycaemia produced by excess insulin could be dramatically alleviated by sugar [43; 44; 45; 46; 47; 207]. Banting and I had first produced hypoglycaemia in a diabetic dog by a very large dose of insulin on August 14, 1921.

In mentioning very briefly the contributions to our knowledge of diabetes made by various schools, we should note not only the advances in fundamental physiology and biochemistry, but the discovery of various hormonal factors in addition to insulin that may play a role in the diabetic state.

The contributions of Carl and Gerti Cori [225] and their pupils are many and of very great importance. Their work on the absorption of sugars and on the metabolic and enzymatic pathways from glucose-1-phosphate to glycogen is epoch-making. Their findings include the discovery of the enzyme phosphorylase and the effects of adrenaline and glucagon on its activity, the elucidation of the mechanism of formation and breakdown of glycogen and of its structure, the investigations of the mechanism of action of insulin and emphasis on the possibility that the activity of glucokinase may play a key role in explaining hormonal effects in the normal and diabetic organism. These and many other advances justify calling this group of investigators one of the most productive of our era. Pupils and colleagues of Dr. and Mrs. Cori have originated new areas that have been relevant to the field of diabetes. Colowick, Krahl, Sutherland, Park, Bornstein, and others have lighted new beacons in their laboratories.

Experimental surgery has contributed in many important ways to our knowledge of diabetes. Dr. B. A. Houssay [399], who is one of the greatest contemporary physiologists, established the hypersensitivity of hypophysectomized toads and dogs to insulin, and proved for the first time that experimental diabetes produced by total extirpation of the pancreas can be ameliorated by hypophysectomy. Houssay and his colleagues also provided evidence that it is the anterior lobe of the hypophysis which is potentially "diabetogenic" in the sense that extracts of this lobe injected into depancreatized-hypophysectomized animals aggravate the diabetes. Houssay and his group, Magenta, Biasotti, Rietti, Lewis, Leloir, Foglia, Martinez, Rodriguez, and others, have sharply focused the attention of experimentalists and clinicians on the potential importance of hormones other than insulin on the production and course of diabetes. In recent years, this group has contributed a great deal to our knowledge of the role of the thyroid and sex hormones in this field.

F. G. Young [821], in 1937, in extension of the work of Houssay and Herbert Evans, was able for the first time, by injecting large doses of pituitary extract into normal dogs, to produce consistently metahypophyseal diabetes. Similar results were later obtained with the highly purified preparations of growth hormone of Li and Evans [501]. Young's work has increased our knowledge of the role of the pituitary in experimental diabetes and has stimulated a great deal of productive research on the interrelation of the anterior pituitary and pancreatic hormones.

The diabetogenic effect of extracts rich in ACTH administered to normal human subjects was shown by Conn. With Fajans and others, he has pioneered in the elaboration of tests for the prediabetic state [296].

In 1936, Long and Lukens [510] demonstrated convincingly that in adrenalectomized-depancreatized cats receiving daily injections of cortical extracts, the intensity of the diabetes is dramatically less than in the depancreatized animal. The excretion of glucose, nitrogen, and ketone bodies was decreased and the survival rate was increased. Long and his colleagues of different times, White, Russell, Wilhelmi, Sayers, Engel and others, have brilliantly illuminated many other aspects of adrenal, pancreatic, and liver physiology. Dohan and Lukens [257] have demonstrated that continuous hyperglycaemia produced by intraperitoneal administration of glucose may produce damage to the beta cells and permanent diabetes.

The importance of the insulin content of blood as an index of the balance between insulin formation and destruction was obvious long before suitable methods were available to study the problem. Although there is no chemical method for the determination of insulin, techniques of bio-assay by which insulin-like activity can be estimated with considerable accuracy are available. The principal investigators have been Gellhorn, Anderson, Bornstein, Groen, Randle, Vallance-Owen, Renold, and their colleagues. Much further work, however, is necessary to determine exactly the role of insulin alone in the total insulin-like activity detectable in blood. Extraction procedures such as that developed by Bornstein, which separate insulin from other factors, will probably be helpful. Recently, several investigators have utilized the formation of insulin antibodies as an assay procedure for insulin. An excellent re-evaluation of the various *in vitro* methods for the bioassay of insulin has recently been published by Piazza, Goodner, and Freinkel [620].

The physiological significance of insulinase and insulinase inhibitors, discovered and developed by Arthur Mirsky [567], who is a pioneer also in the study of the action of insulin on blood amino acids, remains to be fully understood and appreciated. Robert Williams and his colleagues have recently added a great deal to our understanding of this field.

The discovery of glucagon marked the beginning of an epoch in the history of diabetes. Kimball and Murlin [451] were the first to appreciate that the initial rise in blood sugar, seen after insulin injections, might be due to a new substance. In 1930 Bürger and his colleagues established this hypothesis as a reality by their chemical and physiological studies. They separated glucagon from insulin. Sutherland, Cori, and De Duve have extended this work and have elucidated the action of glucagon on phosphorylase. Sutherland and his colleagues have recently provided evidence for the presence of glucagon in blood. Staub, Sinn, and Behrens obtained glucagon in crystalline form, and Bromer has determined the position of the constituent amino acids. Very recently metaglucagon diabetes, i.e., prolonged diabetes after cessation of glucagon injections, has been demonstrated for the first time by a group in our laboratory [509].

The discovery of the diabetogenic action of alloxan has provided us with a most valuable tool for the investigation of carbohydrate metabolism [273]. There is now a long list of chemical compounds which damage the beta cells of the pancreas.

Crystalline insulin was first prepared by Abel [2] of Johns Hopkins, in 1926. My Toronto colleague, D. A. Scott [682], proved that the crystals were the zinc salt of the protein.

A special section should be devoted to the recent outstanding contributions of the chemists who have revealed the structure of insulin. The earlier work has been reviewed by Sanger, who has himself advanced this field dramatically. The elucidation of the structure of insulin by the Cambridge workers [667] is a prominent milestone in protein chemistry and in the history of diabetes.

Scott and Fisher, in Toronto, showed that the addition of zinc to insulin solutions slowed the rate of absorption. Hagedorn's group, in Copenhagen, produced the first long-acting insulin of therapeutic value by adding prota-mine to insulin, and Scott and Fisher obtained an even more sustained hypoglycaemic action by using zinc as well as protamine. Bauman should be credited for the development of globin insulin and Hagedorn's group for NPH insulin. Recently, the lente insulins, developed by Hallas-Møller and his colleagues, in which zinc alone, i.e., without protamine, provides the desired slowing of absorption, have added further to the physician's armamentarium. There will be many further improvements in insulin as a therapeutic agent and some day we will approach physiological perfec-tion.

The availability of insulin promptly initiated a search for the mechanism by which it acts. After the effects on blood and urinary sugar and on the clinical condition of our diabetic dogs were established, the first experiment on the site of the action was performed when Banting and I noted the absence of any effect of a potent extract on the rate of disappearance of sugar from blood *in vitro*. The search for loci of action of insulin has con-tinued and this field obviously has attracted many of the finest workers in physiology and biochemistry. Stadie, Hastings, Levine, Park, Ross, Mirsky, Krahl, Wick, Chaikoff, Gemmill, Drury, Stetten, Ingle, Gurin, Randle, Weinhouse, De Bodo and Steele, Fisher, Miller, Chain, Kipnis, and many others have elucidated the effect of insulin on the fate of dextrose, acetate, pyruvate, amino acids and other metabolites in the intact and eviscerated organism; in cardiac, diaphragmatic and skeletal muscle, in perfused livers, in liver slices and in other preparations. The work of Wertheimer and his colleagues, on the effect of insulin on adipose tissue, has focused the attention of experimenters and clinicians on a previously neglected but very important field. A fascinating new chapter on the action of insulin on adipose tissue is now being written by Cahill, Renold, and their colleagues. The same may be said of Foley's studies on the mammary gland, Dole's and Gordon's work on unesterified fatty acids, and that of Dorfman on the tissue mucopolysaccharides.

Three of my senior colleagues have established international reputations in the field of experimental diabetes. Professor R. E. Haist [345; 346] has contributed a very large portion of our knowledge of the insulin content of pancreas and of factors which affect the growth of the islands of Langer-hans. Professor James Campbell [162; 164] is an authority on fat mobiliza-tion and ketosis and on the diabetogenic properties of somatotropin. Professor Gerald Wrenshall [815] has provided most of the data on insulin extractable from human pancreas, and his finding that the pancreas of "adult onset" diabetes contains approximately 40 per cent of the normal amount of insulin, has stimulated a great deal of further work.

The effects of insulin upon oxidation of glucose, glycogen formation, and upon fat synthesis are well established, and the metabolic pathways are in large part known. The situation is not clear with respect to the effect of insulin upon protein synthesis. The work of Krahl and associates on the action of insulin upon the amino acid uptake of muscle in the absence of glucose in the medium, strongly suggests a protein anabolic effect of insulin which operates independently of glucose utilization. Two valuable papers by Manchester, Young, and Randle have recently extended our knowledge of this subject. More has to be learned about these matters as well as about the mechanism by which carbohydrates exert their "protein sparing" effect. Levine and co-workers [496] have established that insulin accelerates the "transport" of glucose through the cell membrane of muscle and a number of other tissues. Park, Kipnis, and others have developed this concept and have shown that lack of insulin decreases the rate of entry of glucose into the cell to a greater extent than it does the activity of hexokinase. In insulin deficiency, the rate-limiting step in the glucose uptake of muscle appears to be the "transport" of glucose into the cell. In the presence of insulin, the rate-limiting step may prove to be the first stage in the utilization of sugar, i.e., phosphorylation by hexokinase. Recent work from Montreal suggests that insulin may accelerate the rate of entry of a wide variety of substances into cells.

The effects of insulin upon the liver are manifold: increase in phosphorylation of glucose, decreased gluconeogenesis, decrease in the activity of glucose-6-phosphatase, increase in glucose-6-phosphate dehydrogenase and enhanced utilization of glucose via the phosphogluconate oxidation pathway are but a few of the established effects of this hormone. An effect of insulin upon liver slices with respect to glucose uptake, glycogen synthesis and synthesis of protein and fatty acids has been demonstrated by De Duve and others. However, the balance of evidence indicates that these phenomena measured *in vitro*, but produced by the injection of insulin into the intact animal, are, in large part, indirect effects of insulin, i.e., the result perhaps of a general stimulation of carbohydrate metabolism. There are some indications of a more direct effect of insulin on the liver.

The evidence [519] indicates that cell "permeability" to glucose in the liver is not influenced by insulin as it is in muscle and adipose tissue, i.e., insulin presumably alters intracellular enzyme activity rather than "transport" through the membrane of the hepatic cell. In other words, the "permeability" of the liver cell to glucose is not lost in diabetes. The possibility that small amounts of insulin liberated by the pancreas decrease hepatic glucose output rather than stimulate peripheral utilization has become a major interest with respect to the mechanism of action of the oral hypoglycaemic agents. The question is whether the effect upon liver is a direct one or mediated by insulin. This is difficult to answer until the effect of insulin upon the liver is fully understood.

The first report of the hypoglycaemic effect of a sulphonyl compound was made in 1930 by Ruiz and his co-workers [657]. The accidental observation by Jambon and his colleagues, in 1942, of the hypoglycaemic effect of thiodiazol derivatives and the fine experimentation in 1944 to 1946 of Loubatières [511; 512], which revealed many of the essential facts concerning the action of these agents, marked the dawn of a new era. It is interesting to note that, in 1946, Chen and co-workers [201] in the United States also studied the hypoglycaemic action of a sulphonamide (sulphanilamidocyclopropylthiazole) in rabbits, and since the effect was not seen after administration of alloxan they concluded (as Loubatières did) that these substances may stimulate insulin secretion. These observations had no practical application until 1955, when German physicians [309] saw and established the potentialities of the urea derivative, carbutamide, in the oral treatment of diabetes mellitus. Subsequently many different sulphonylureas have been tested for their hypoglycaemic effect with the aim of finding a drug of superior potency, greater duration of action, and minimal side effects. Tolbutamide is undoubtedly the drug selected by most physicians at the present time. In spite of the fact that these drugs are approved by the medical profession, little is known with certainty about their mode of action. Functioning beta cells are necessary for the immediate hypoglycaemic effect of the sulphonylureas, and in pancreatectomized or alloxan-diabetic animals the drugs are inactive. In the presence of intact beta cells, hypoglycaemia develops even if the liver is removed. There is considerable evidence that the drugs, in the presence of functioning beta cells, release from the pancreas a hypoglycaemic substance, presumably insulin. After administration of these drugs the pancreatic venous blood has been found to have increased insulin-like activity. Injections of that blood have produced hypoglycaemia in mice and in cross-circulation experiments have produced hypoglycaemia in normal and in recipient alloxan-diabetic dogs. This endogenous insulin, which is supposedly released by the drug, has not as yet been shown to produce a complete insulin-like effect on the peripheral tissues [732]. On the other hand, conclusive evidence has been secured that the sulphonylureas reduce the rate of glucose release from the liver. Thus these drugs exert an action not only on the pancreas but also directly or indirectly on the liver. It is probable that a slight increase in peripheral utilization of glucose will also be shown to be an indirect effect of their administration but this may depend upon the amount of the hormone released and the duration of the effect.

348 INSULIN AND GLUCAGON

INSULIN RESISTANCE

Owing to its low molecular weight (just under 6000), insulin is only weakly antigenic but the formation of antibodies in the course of prolonged insulin therapy is well established. These antibodies are the commonest cause of insulin resistance. Space does not permit description of the fascinating and important work of my old friend and colleague Dr. Peter Moloney [574] or the great new contribution to this field of Doctors Berson and Yalow [65]. The short-lasting insulin resistance of the patient in diabetic coma is due to a "humoral antagonist" which is quite distinct from antibodies. Although it is a protein, it has a different electrophoretic mobility from the insulin-antibody complex. Also, this factor does not prevent insulin from binding to the muscle. An insulin "antagonist" has also been found to be present in the poorly controlled diabetic patient and it is not known whether this factor is identical with that found in the comatose subject. "Contra-insulin" factors have been found in plasma of experimental animals made diabetic by alloxan or pancreatectomy, and these tend to disappear after adrenalectomy and hypophysectomy. These "antagonists" must be identified and their relationship to each other established. Recently, Australian workers have found a "contra-insulin" factor in the blood of diabetic patients with retinopathy and nephropathy. While some authorities contend that the disturbing vascular degeneration in some diabetics is unrelated to the extent of the control of the disorder by diet and insulin, no physician will blame himself, whatever may prove to be true, if he has done his utmost to attain and maintain the physiological state.

Many of the specific clinical advances over the last 40 years have resulted from the experimental findings. The benefits to diabetics of the antibiotics and the general advances in medical and surgical knowledge are obvious and well appreciated. I can merely mention the improved classification of diabetics resulting from the work of Robin Lawrence, and the more accurate recognition of the pancreatic lesions in diabetics owing to the studies of Torenson and Duff, Ogilvie and Maclean, Bell, Gepts, and others. While it used to be stated that *no* pancreatic lesions could be found in a large proportion of diabetics, now the expert pathologist can detect abnormalities in most cases. My Edinburgh friend, Dr. Robertson Ogilvie, is my chief authority for this statement, but other leading investigators in this field agree. The improvements in the treatment of diabetics are well discussed in the latest and finest edition of Dr. Elliott P. Joslin's book.

I predict that we will have much better forms of insulin. My main objection to the oral agents is that they have diverted our attention from the problem of making insulin available in a more physiological way. The

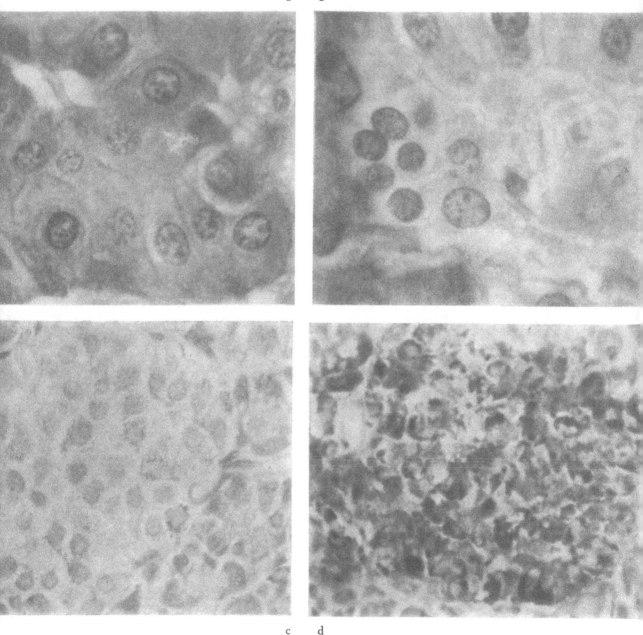

c   d

PLATE VII (Paper 21). (a) Peripheral portion of pancreatic islet of control rabbit. Active alpha cells (red) with broad granulated cytoplasm, paranuclear macula, and negative Golgi image. (Gomori's chrome alum haematoxylin. × 775.) (b) Pancreatic islet of rabbit treated with glucagon for 24 days. A group of five atrophied alpha cells at the margin of the islet. (Gomori's chrome alum haematoxylin. × 775.) (c) Pancreatic islet of rabbit (10 weeks old) treated with glucagon since birth. Fine granules of glycogen in the cytoplasm of most beta cells. (Periodic acid Schiff, haemalum. × 265.) (d) Metaglucagon diabetes. Pancreatic islet of a rabbit treated with glucagon for five months; thirty days after cessation of treatment. All cells of the islet are densely filled with glycogen. (Periodic acid Schiff. Fixed in Gendre's fluid. × 380.)

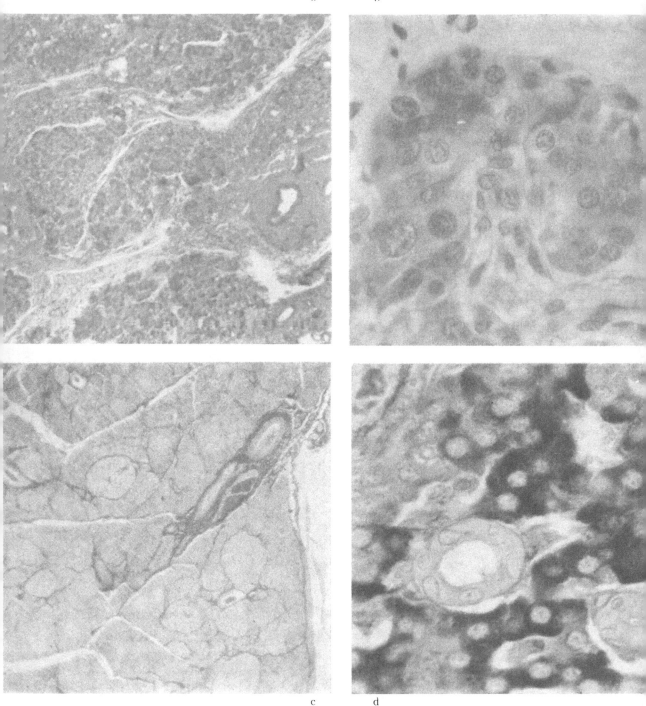

PLATE VIII (Paper 29). (*a*) Masses of islet tissue are present in this section prepared from the pancreas of the case reported by Howland, Campbell, Maltby, and Robinson (see text). Haematoxylin and eosin stain. (× 100.) (*b*) Afferent and efferent vessels to this small islet are included in the same section. Pancreas of a case of hypoglycaemia in an infant autopsied by Dr. W. L. Donohue. Gomori's chromium haematoxylin and phloxine stain. (× 1000.) (*c*) There is a striking increase in the number and size of the islets of Langerhans in this section of the pancreas from the case of "dysendocrinism" reported by Dr. W. L. Donohue. Wilson's modification of Gomori's aldehyde-fuchsin stain. (*d*) Normal islet from pancreas of rat. Two small ducts in cross-section appear surrounded by islet cells. The beta granules are stained deep purple, while the cytoplasm of the alpha cells is Green. Wilson's modification of Gomori's aldehyde-fuchsin stain. (× 1000.)

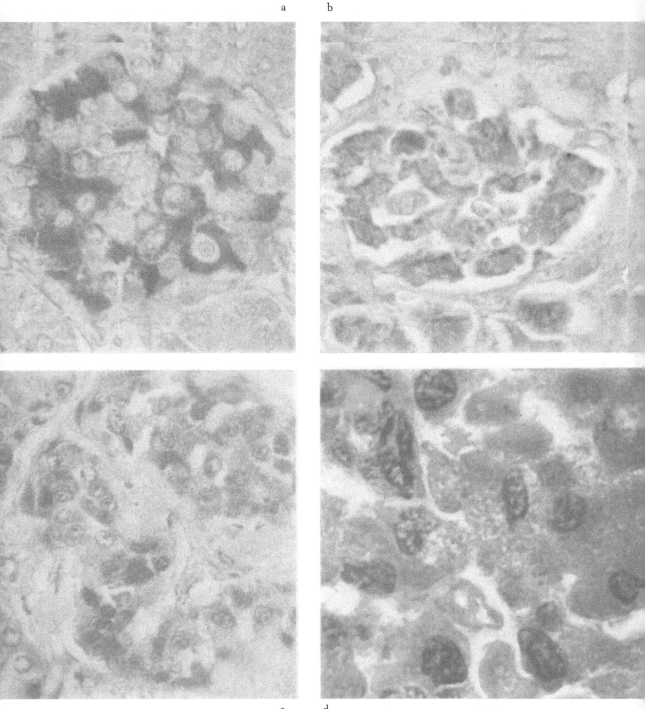

PLATE IX (Paper 29). (*a*) Granules in the beta cells of this islet from a normal man are stained deep purple. The granules may frequently lie massed along that boundary of the cell which abuts on a sinusoid. Wilson's modification of Gomori's aldehyde-fuchsin stain. (× 1000.) (*b*) An atrophic islet from the pancreas of Leonard Thompson, the first diabetic to receive insulin. Very few granules are present in the scanty rims of cytoplasm which surround the nuclei of the islet cells. Stain and magnification as for VII(*a*) above, with which this photomicrograph should be compared. (*c*) Pancreatic islet from the case of Dr. J. Gilchrist. Beta cells containing granules (greyish-brown) are present, but the ratio of alpha cells (red) to beta cells is higher than normal. There is hyalinization of the sinusoids throughout. Gomori's chromium haematoxylin and phloxine stain. (× 1000.) (*d*) Beta cell tumour similar to that reported by Wilder, Allan, Power, and Robertson (see text; [796]). Scattered granules (purple) are present in the beta cells. Wilson's modification of Gomori's aldehyde-fuchsin stain. (× 700.)

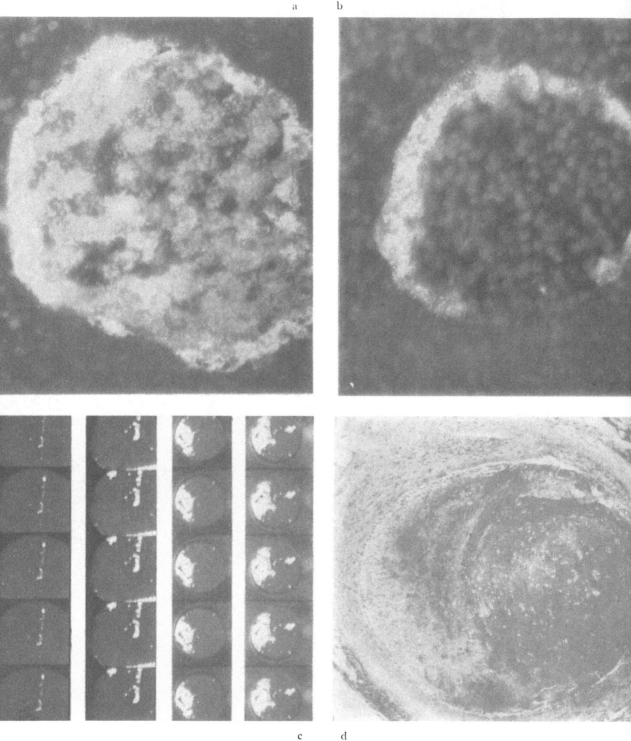

PLATE X. (*a*) Pancreatic islet of control rat infused with dithizone. Fresh-frozen section mounted in glycerol. Dark field illumination. Granular precipitate of zinc-dithizonate in peripheral alpha cells (+ + +) and beta cells (+). Photomicrography does not reproduce orange colour of zinc dithizonate granules. (× 230.) (*b*) Pancreatic islet of insulin-treated rat infused with dithizone. Fresh-frozen section mounted in glycerol. Dark field illumination. Granular precipitate of zinc-dithizonate in the peripheral alpha cells only. Beta cells contain no reactive zinc, indicating absence of secretion granules. (× 200.) (*c*) Growth of white thrombi forming upon a scratch made on the inner surface of a glass tube. Frames from a motion picture film showing that the thrombus grows "down-stream." (See Paper 55.) Heparin prevents the formation of these thrombi. (*d*) Thrombus completely occluding injured blood vessel of a dog; in the presence of heparin no trace of thrombus could be found. (Paper 55.)

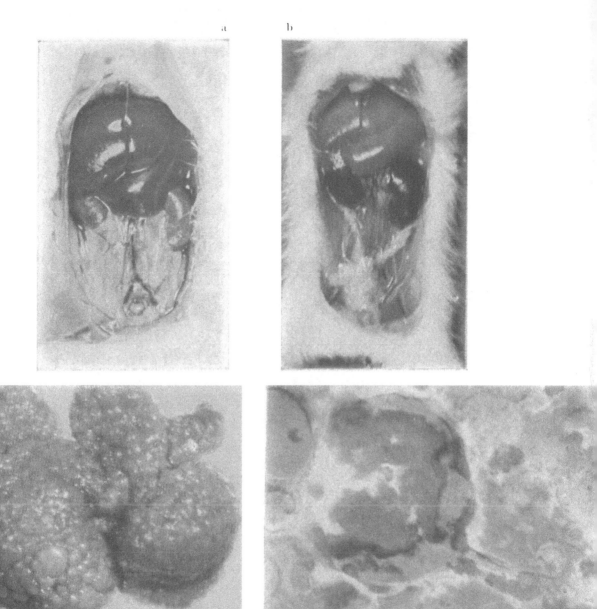

PLATE XI. (*a*) Normal liver and kidneys of young rat. (*b*) Tawny-coloured fatty liver and enlarged haemorrhagic kidneys produced by dietary means (choline deficiency). (Paper 48.) (*c*) Dietary cirrhosis in rat fed choline-deficient diet for six months. The majority of the nodules (regenerating parenchymal tissue) are of monolobular dimensions as in monolobular (Laennec) cirrhosis associated with alcoholism in man. There are, however, nodules of multilobular proportions as in the Marchand type of cirrhosis. Thus monolobular cirrhosis is, in some instances, a stage in the development of a coarse, Marchand type in the rat. Popper has reported similar data in man. (*d*) A possible mechanism of the formation of fat emboli in choline deficiency is suggested by this section which illustrates a free communication between the lumen of a liver sinusoid and that of a fatty cyst. Both the cyst and the sinusoid are filled with a mixture of fat (red) and erythrocytes (green).

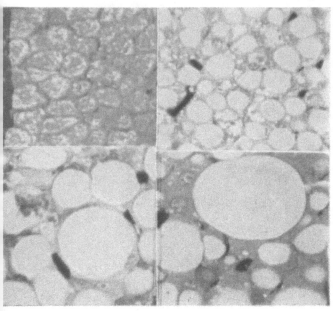
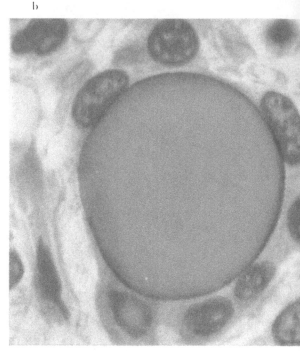

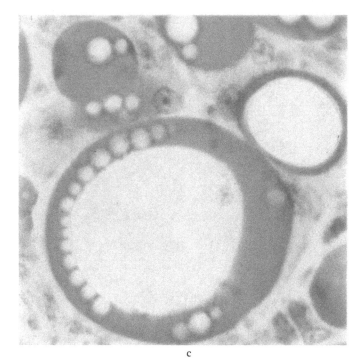

c

PLATE XII. (*a*) Composite photomicrographs of livers of four rats (same magnification) illustrating forms in which lipid appears in choline deficiency. Upper left: control rat fed complete diet. The others are from rats fed the same diet lacking choline. Upper right: intracellular accumulation of fat in spherules filling cytoplasm and displacing nucleus. Septa of adjacent fat-filled cells rupture to form cysts. These cysts are filled with lipid and their walls are formed by parenchymal cells. Fusion of adjacent cysts shown in both lower sections. (Paper 48.) (*b*) Fatty cyst in human alcoholic: the nuclei of some seven liver cells forming the wall of the cyst can be seen. These fatty cysts are regularly present in the livers of alcoholics; when found in and around the edges of fibrous trabeculae they have considerable etiological significance. (Frozen section stained with Oil Red O.) (*c*) Effect of choline therapy on fatty cysts: lipid can be mobilized rapidly from intracellular positions but more slowly from fatty cysts. Cysts appear partially empty; lipid remaining adjacent to wall is vacuolated and foamy in appearance. When observed in biopsy material of fatty and cirrhotic livers in man, this appearance is almost certainly pathognomonic of the effects of treatment.

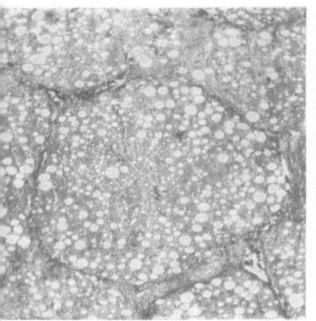 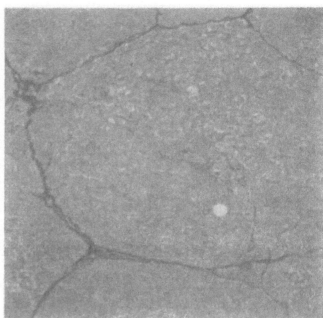

a   b

PLATE XIII. (*a*) Biopsy specimen showing fatty liver with moderate cirrhosis in rat fed choline-deficient diet, low in protein, for four months. (Paper 48.) In the transition from a fatty to a fibrotic and cirrhotic liver in choline deficiency, the early trabecular pattern assumes this characteristic annular form, as a result of cyst-atrophy and stromal condensation in the non-portal regions of the hepatic lobule (Rappaport). Eventually these trabeculae extend to portal triads (one in centre of field) giving an appearance of splitting the conventional hexagonal lobule. Thus a monolobular lesion resembling Laennec's cirrhosis develops. Comparable stages in the development of alcoholic cirrhosis in man have been observed in biopsy material. (Paper 48.) (*b*) Dietary treatment of early cirrhosis: specimen from same rat showing almost complete absence of fat and only slight residual excess fibrous tissue after feeding diet with improved protein and supplementary choline for nine months. (Paper 48.) *In the early stages* of cirrhosis induced in rats by choline deficiency, complete reabsorption of abnormal fat and excess fibrous tissue is possible. Intracellular fat is mobilized within days, extracellular fat within weeks, and abnormal fibrous tissue within a few months. The fine strands of fibrous tissue, stained blue, would have soon disappeared completely. If treatment is delayed until the cirrhosis reaches a multilobular (Marchand) stage with advanced architectural distortion, it will progress, as Grisham and Hartroft have shown.

oral hypoglycaemic agents available at present will probably disappear and be replaced by others which act on a variety of biochemical mechanisms. Modified forms of insulin may become available for oral administration. While this will not enhance the intrinsic therapeutic value and may well involve a considerable wastage of the hormone, as do the present methods of administration, there is no doubt that elimination of the needle will be popular with both patient and physician.

There have been 70,000 to 80,000 publications on the subject of insulin since 1921, and many times that on the various other factors involved in diabetes. These fields are still being cultivated vigorously and productively, and to miss a month of reading is to be out of date.

31. Insulin and Glucagon: A Review

ROBERT METZ, M.B., B.CH., M.S.

CHARLES H. BEST, C.B.E., M.D., F.R.S.

Ever since 1921 successive attempts to delineate the place of insulin in the physiology of the mammalian organism have been characterized by marked shifts in emphasis as new aspects of its action have come to light. The pace of discovery has been accelerating in recent years, but much remains to be elucidated. By what mode, or modes, of action insulin brings about its bewildering variety of effects will not, in all probability, be known for many years. Neither the mechanism of its secretion from the beta-cell, nor the factors concerned with "resistance" to the hormone are well understood.

The discovery of glucagon, or at least of a hyperglycaemic-glycogenolytic contaminant of insulin, was made as long ago as 1923, but only in the last twelve years has interest in this substance quickened. Nevertheless, in one respect information concerning glucagon has outstripped that on insulin, in that an action of glucagon on one specific enzymatic reaction has been clearly demonstrated. As with insulin, however, new metabolic effects of glucagon have recently been discovered, and their mode of action and relative importance await elucidation. This review is designed to present a survey of the current situation with respect to both of these secretions of the islets of Langerhans [12; 17; 77; 472; 744].

INSULIN

Sanger's analysis of the insulin molecule, in terms of the sequential arrangement of its constituent amino-acids, represents one of the major scientific achievements of recent years, but the application of this knowledge to an understanding of the unique biological properties of this protein awaits further advances in the fields of physiology and of protein chemistry. The insulin molecule consists of 51 amino-acid residues arranged in two chains, connected by disulphide linkages. Apart from a recent and as yet unconfirmed report to the contrary, the evidence has indicated that neither chain alone possesses insulin activity. The molecular weight is approxi-

Originally appeared in "Symposium on Endocrinology" in *The Practitioner*, CLXXXV (1960), 593–601.

mately 6,000, but whether insulin exerts its characteristic effects in the monomeric form is not known. Recent evidence indicates that in the blood it is complexed with other substances, probably basic proteins, and that this may also obtain in the beta-cells. It would be of the greatest interest to know if an insulin-protein complex in the beta-cell is split enzymatically before the release of free insulin. The insulin content (or, more properly, the extractable insulin) of the pancreas is about 2.5 units per g of pancreas (about 200 units per pancreas in the adult) in non-diabetic subjects, and, on the average, somewhat less than half of this in the adult diabetic. Virtually no insulin can be extracted from the pancreas in cases of established juvenile diabetes.

Secretion and Degradation of Insulin

A large body of work over a period of more than thirty years has established that the blood sugar exerts a controlling influence on the rate of secretion of insulin into the blood. It has recently been shown in the dog that insulin output from the pancreas is a continuous function of the blood-glucose concentration, this mechanism probably serving as a negative feed-back arrangement, contributing to the regulation of the blood-sugar level. The dog pancreas appears to have an enormous capacity to vary the ouput of insulin. Insulin secretion virtually ceases during hypoglycaemia, and in severe hyperglycaemia is estimated to be as high as 160 milli-units per minute, or almost 10 units per hour from the pancreas as a whole. Both clinical and experimental evidence indicates that galactose may also provoke the secretion of extra insulin, and even the pentose, d-ribose, may do so. This has led to the suggestion that the secretion of insulin is stimulated by sugars the utilization of which is influenced in turn by the hormone.

In recent years interest has centred on other substances which may stimulate insulin secretion [562]. Chief among these are the sulphonylurea compounds. There is general agreement that probably the most important action of these drugs is to stimulate insulin secretion, both from the normal pancreas and, in a proportion of cases, from the diabetic pancreas, which presumably does not respond to glucose in a normal manner. Another field of unusual interest has opened up with the discovery that in a large percentage of cases of idiopathic hypoglycaemia in infants, the hypoglycaemic episodes follow the ingestion of foods containing the amino-acid, l-leucine, and there is a recent report of an increase in blood insulin following leucine administration in these patients [205]. Equally fascinating are the reports of patients with islet-cell adenomas exhibiting leucine sensitivity. The pituitary growth hormone also appears to stimulate insulin secretion in some species.

Insulin degradation in the tissues is apparently brought about mainly by the action of insulinase, a relatively specific enzyme which is found in highest concentration in liver, kidney, muscle, and, interestingly enough, in placenta. There is, however, no evidence as yet of any diseased state arising from alterations in insulinase activity.

METABOLIC EFFECTS OF INSULIN

The research on insulin in recent years has largely been concerned with the attempt to track down its manifold physiological properties to its effects on isolated tissues, and to the cellular and subcellular elements thereof. The mechanism by which the classic physiological effect on the blood sugar is brought about has not yet been completely elucidated. Experiments utilizing a great diversity of techniques have led to conflicting conclusions about the relative importance of the uptake of glucose by the peripheral tissues and of the suppression of glucose output by the liver. Recent work in our laboratories by Wrenshall and Hetenyi [818], using a method of successive injections of labelled glucose for the study of transfer rates, has clarified the respective roles of the liver and extra-hepatic tissues in the production of insulin hypoglycaemia. They found that after insulin administration in the dog, hepatic glucose output was transiently reduced, increasing subsequently to higher than normal as the blood sugar fell to low levels, while the over-all glucose uptake by the extra-hepatic tissues increased greatly. The fact that endogenous insulin is secreted into the portal vein, in contradistinction to injected insulin which first enters the systemic circulation, may be significant in this regard. In 1958 Madison and his colleagues [545] presented evidence indicating that the intraportal administration of insulin results in a proportionately greater hepatic effect than does systemic administration. If these quantitative differences are physiologically important, the replacement therapy of diabetes with injected insulin may provide the appropriate substance by an inappropriate route. When referring to exogenous insulin as the appropriate replacement for the endogenous hormone, it should be borne in mind that there are immunological differences between the insulins of different species, and insulin antibodies may modify the action of the exogenous hormone. Furthermore, the rate of entry of administered insulin into the blood stream does not vary with fluctuations in the blood-sugar level.

Insulin has several "target organs" and more than one effect in some of them. Table 31.I lists most of the known effects on isolated mammalian

TABLE 31.I

Effects of Insulin on Mammalian Tissues

Tissue	Insulin Effect
Striated muscle	(a) Accelerates glucose uptake and the uptake of certain other sugars. (b) Increases glycogen and oligosaccharide formation, the oxidation of glucose and the incorporation of glucose into glucose-peptide complexes. (c) Accelerates amino-acid uptake, even in the absence of glucose. (d) Stimulates the incorporation of amino-acids into muscle protein. (e) Increases resting membrane potential. (f) Accelerates K^+ and PO_4 uptake.
Adipose tissue	(a) Accelerates the uptake and utilization of glucose, and, to a lesser extent, of mannose and fructose. (b) Stimulates lipogenesis and glycerol formation from glucose, and from acetate and pyruvate in the presence of glucose. (c) Stimulates the oxidation of glucose, particularly via the direct pentose-phosphate oxidative pathway. (d) Promotes the uptake of fatty acids. (e) Inhibits the release of fatty acids. (f) Stimulates pinocytosis (the engulfing by the cell of a liquid droplet enclosed in an envelope derived from the cell membrane). COMMENT. The effects of insulin on muscle and adipose tissue appear rapidly *in vitro*. The ability of adipose tissue to synthesize fat is completely dependent upon the presence of insulin.
Liver	(a) Reduces glucose output *in vivo*. (b) Addition of insulin to normal rat liver *in vitro* stimulates the formation of fatty acids from acetate in the presence of glucose. (c) Addition of insulin *in vitro* does not correct the abnormally low net glucose uptake, glycogen, or the fat and protein synthesis in liver slices from diabetic animals, but injection of insulin into the animal several hours before sacrifice does correct these abnormalities. (d) Previous injection of insulin into the rat enhances the incorporation of amino-acids into protein by hepatic-cell ribosomes (microsomal particles) *in vitro*.
Other tissues	(a) Stimulates fat synthesis in lactating mammary gland in some species. (b) Accelerates glucose transport into white, but not red, blood cells. (c) Accelerates glucose transport through the lens. (d) The synthesis of mucopolysaccharides in connective tissue of skin is depressed in diabetic animals, and this defect is corrected by insulin treatment. (e) Glucose (and galactose) uptake by brain and spinal cord is probably not affected by insulin. (f) Glucose transport in gut and kidney is apparently independent of insulin. (g) The growth of various tissues in culture is stimulated by insulin in the culture medium.

tissues. Whether these apparently diverse effects, on different effector organs, are dependent upon a single mechanism of action is not known. As yet we do not even have a really satisfactory unified theory of insulin action, although many stimulating speculations have been published. It is generally accepted that there has been no convincing demonstration of an action of insulin on a specific enzymatic reaction in a cell-free system.

There is abundant evidence that insulin enhances the passage of glucose and certain other substances into the cell, and it appears to do so by altering the permeability of the cell membrane to these substances. The recent demonstration, by means of the electron microscope, that insulin stimulates pinocytosis in the adipose tissue cell, provides direct evidence of an insulin-induced morphological change in the membrane. Another finding implicating this structure as a site of action is the increase in the transmembrane potential in the muscle cell in the presence of insulin. This hyperpolarization of muscle, which occurs even in the absence of glucose, seems to be the cause, and not the effect, of the increased potassium uptake under the influence of insulin.

The fact that insulin affects cellular transport, probably by a direct action on the cell membrane occupies a central place in present-day theories of its mode of action [38]. Nevertheless, it seems unlikely from the available evidence that all its effects on protein and fat metabolism are entirely due to an effect on cellular transport. Indeed, Chain [183] has presented evidence to suggest that the permeability theory is inadequate to explain all the effects on the metabolism of even glucose itself. It is possible, however, as has been suggested, that a sort of chain reaction of molecular rearrangement in the interior of the cell might be set off by changes in the membrane. Certainly the findings of Korner [469], in a series of very fine experiments, that the previous injection of insulin in the rat promotes the incorporation of amino-acids into protein in isolated hepatic-cell microsomes, would seem to demand an explanation other than an effect purely on the cell membrane. It has been shown by others that the intravenous administration of I^{131}-labelled insulin is followed by fixation of the labelled insulin to various subcellular fractions in the liver cell, particularly the microsomes and mitochondria. It is possible that these are sites of insulin degradation, but an action of insulin on subcellular particles seems probable.

The metabolic abnormalities of liver slices from a diabetic animal are largely corrected by the previous injection of insulin into the animal, but not by the addition of insulin to the slices *in vitro*. This discrepancy remains an unsolved problem. It may be seen from Table 31.I, however, that much progress has been made towards uncovering the intimate metabolic responses to insulin that are responsible for its major physiological effects; namely, the acute reduction of the blood levels of glucose, fatty-acids, amino-acids, potassium, and phosphorus, and the long-term preservation of the fat depots, of liver glycogen and of a positive nitrogen balance. The stimulation of amino-acid incorporation into microsomal protein (which, in all probability, reflects an increased net synthesis of protein) may go a long way towards explaining the role of insulin as a growth hormone.

INSULIN ASSAYS

A major field of interest during the past decade has been the development and application of *in vitro* techniques for estimating the insulin content of blood. The use of the isolated rat diaphragm for the bio-assay of insulin grew out of attempts to demonstrate an action of insulin *in vitro*. In 1941, Gemmill and Hamman [319] reported that insulin accelerates the disappearance of glucose from the medium in which the diaphragm is incubated. Gemmill had previously shown that glycogen formation in this tissue is stimulated in the presence of insulin. These phenomena were subsequently adapted by others for an assay method when it was shown that there is a proportionality between the concentration of insulin in the medium and the magnitude of the biological effect. The rat diaphragm method is sensitive and probably specific when applied to undiluted plasma, but it is not very precise, and the result of any assay is only likely to be correct within half and twice the actual value. In the last few years several workers have used the epididymal fat pad of the rat as the insulin-responsive tissue. This method would seem to provide a more sensitive and convenient, and possibly more accurate, assay procedure, but doubts about its specificity remain.

Obviously the bio-assay procedure can measure only the biologically active insulin in the plasma, unless steps can be taken to inactivate the insulin inhibitors which may be present. The new immunochemical assay technique of Yalow and Berson [820] promises an answer to this problem. Their method, which employs insulin antibody and I^{131}-labelled insulin, appears to provide an exquisitely sensitive, highly accurate, and practicable procedure for assaying the total insulin content of plasma. For proper evaluation of the plasma insulin in the diabetic patient, both bio-assay and immuno-assay should probably be employed, the former for estimating the effective, and the latter for estimating the actual, concentration. The simultaneous use of the two methods would thus permit an estimation of the insulin inhibitors present in the plasma. It may well be that the methods developed for assaying insulin will find their most important application in the estimation of the various circulating insulin antagonists present in different pathological and physiological conditions. It has been suggested that an understanding of the role of inhibitors of insulin action may provide the key to the problem of the retinal, renal and vascular complications of diabetes.

GLUCAGON

Several observations reported during the two decades following the discovery of insulin had indicated the presence in insulin preparations of a hyperglycaemic-glycogenolytic factor, to which Kimball and Murlin, in 1923, applied the name glucagon [451]. During the following twenty-five years interest in glucagon was kept alive mainly by Bürger. In 1948, Sutherland and his colleagues extracted this material in partially purified form, and a few years later a group at the Lilly Research Laboratories were able to crystallize it, and subsequently to determine its amino-acid sequence. Glucagon is a polypeptide of 29 amino-acid residues (including methionine and tryptophan which are not present in insulin) arranged in a single chain, and having a molecular weight of about 3,500. Present-day American and Canadian commercial preparations of insulin contain less than 0.5 per cent glucagon, while Danish and British preparations are virtually glucagon free.

ORIGIN, SECRETION, AND DEGRADATION OF GLUCAGON

The available evidence overwhelmingly favours the alpha-cell of the islet of Langerhans as the prime, if not the only, site of production. The evidence for other sites of origin is controversial. It is generally accepted that glucagon is a hormone, although strict criteria require that a deficiency state be demonstrable in the absence of a substance so defined. Unequivocal evidence of glucagon deficiency has not been obtained, although a few cases have been reported of familial hypoglycaemia in infants who lack alpha-cells. On the other hand, a depancreatized animal or human being can be managed quite adequately on glucagon-free insulin; indeed the insulin requirements are lower following total pancreatectomy than after removal of 90 to 95 per cent of the pancreas, and this may possibly be construed as indicating a glucagon "deficiency." In any event it would seem that there are three possibilities to account for the absence of clear-cut evidence of deficiency: glucagon is produced in sites other than the pancreas, or it is dispensable because its role is only a subsidiary one, or its absence results in subtle changes which, although important, are not easy to detect. The recently developed immunochemical method for assaying glucagon in blood should make possible an investigation of its role in diabetes and in various other metabolic disorders, such as the Zollinger-Ellison syndrome and other conditions associated with non-insulin-containing adenomas of the pancreatic islets. Evidence of abnormalities due to deficiency and, perhaps, to overproduction, may soon be forthcoming.

It has recently been shown that the output of glucagon from the pancreas is increased in the presence of hypoglycaemia, the increase being rapidly reversed by intravenous glucose. The secretion of glucagon and of insulin would thus appear to be reciprocally stimulated by the blood sugar. By virtue of their respective effects on the blood sugar in turn, each hormone would tend to stimulate the secretion of the other. Obviously such an intimately connected system of counter-regulatory effects could provide for a most efficient maintenance of blood-glucose homeostasis. The evidence concerning the effects of other substances on glucagon output is inconclusive. The sulphonylureas have not been shown to suppress glucagon secretion. Growth hormone administration results in the appearance of a hyperglycaemic-glycogenolytic substance in the pancreatic venous effluent, but studies in our laboratories suggest that this substance is not glucagon.

Plasma-glucagon levels, as determined by the immuno-assay technique, were found to average about 27 mcg per 100 ml in fasted human subjects. The transient effects of an injection of glucagon are probably due to its rapid destruction in the blood as well as in the tissues. In the blood, hydrolysis of the polypeptide is probably brought about by the plasmin system. The nature of the tissue glucagonolytic system, found in highest concentration in the kidneys and liver, has not been identified.

METABOLIC AND PHYSIOLOGICAL EFFECTS OF GLUCAGON

The most conspicuous result of the administration of an adequate dose of glucagon is a prompt rise in blood sugar, the magnitude of the effect being largely determined by the store of liver glycogen. In 1948, Sutherland and his colleagues elucidated the mechanism of this effect. They found that glucagon acts to bring about the conversion of liver phosphorylase from the inactive to the active form. This process involves the formation of a specific nucleoside, but not all the steps in the reaction are known. Muscle glycogen is uninfluenced by glucagon. The available evidence, although conflicting, would seem to indicate that glucagon does not influence carbohydrate metabolism in the extra-hepatic tissues, except indirectly by mobilizing liver-glycogen stores. This effect of glucagon in making substrate available to the tissues suggests that it may act as an adjuvant to insulin. The schema shown in Figure 69 depicts the possible interrelationship between the action of insulin and glucagon. With every turn of the cycle the magnitude of the responses would decrease, and thus, as suggested by Anderson and his colleagues, there would be a smooth approach to carbohydrate depletion without the intervention of the adrenal medulla.

In attempting to define a physiological role for glucagon, consideration must be given to its other known effects. Our laboratories, amongst others, have been interested in the effects of glucagon on protein metabolism. Under its influence protein catabolism is accelerated, with a consequent increase in urea formation and gluconeogenesis. The level of blood amino-

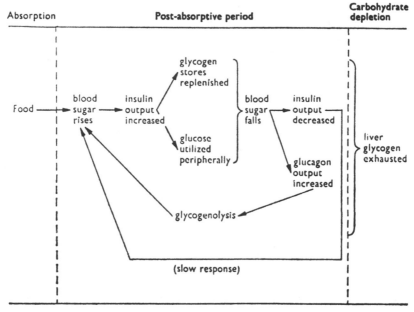

FIGURE 69. Postulated interrelationship of the actions of glucagon and insulin on the utilization of carbohydrate.

acids falls, and creatine excretion is depressed, possibly because of the decreased availability of the necessary amino-acids for the synthesis of creatine. These effects of glucagon are similar to those of the glucocorticoids (except for an opposite effect on creatine excretion) but are not mediated via the adrenal glands. The addition of glucagon *in vitro* brings about an increase in urea production, both in liver slices and in the isolated perfused liver. The increased gluconeogenesis is probably responsible for the "rebound" of liver glycogen to above the resting level following the initial glycogenolysis brought about by glucagon. The mechanism of action of these effects on amino-acid metabolism is quite obscure at present.

Little is known of the possible influence of glucagon on fat metabolism except that it is strongly ketogenic, in both man and dog, when administered in large doses. Glucagon causes a fall in the fatty acids in blood, but this appears to be an indirect effect of hyperglycaemia. An interesting and puzzling property of glucagon is that it produces a prompt and considerable increase in the metabolic rate when administered to intact rats in large doses. The presence of the thyroid and adrenal cortex, but not the adrenal medulla, is necessary for this effect, which is apparently not related to the glycogenolytic action of glucagon.

Several other interesting and possibly important effects of glucagon have been observed in the intact animal. A severe reduction in blood flow has been reported to occur in the hindquarter of the dog upon intravenous administration of glucagon. On the other hand, its effect on the liver, in both man and dog, is to increase blood flow, and recent studies in the dog indicate that this may be the case in the kidney as well. The hepatic and hindquarter flow changes do not occur in the fasted animal. Neither the mechanism nor the physiological importance of these haemodynamic effects, which would tend to bring about a redistribution of cardiac output, is known. One other property of glucagon is its markedly depressant effect on appetite and on gastric motility, possibly by a direct action on the stomach.

Clinical Uses of Glucagon

Glucagon has proved very useful in the treatment of insulin shock. The advantages claimed include ease of administration, relative promptness of response, and little disturbance of the patient's carbohydrate balance. The usual dose is about 0.2 mg of crystalline glucagon per kg body weight, administered intravenously. Care must be taken to feed the patient upon recovery, to prevent a possible relapse into coma. There is a report of one patient who suffered a severe hypotensive episode following a very large dose of glucagon given to relieve hypoglycaemic coma. The only other established clinical use of glucagon is in the diagnosis of glycogen storage disease. Glucagon therapy does exert a favourable effect on the arthritic manfestations of rheumatoid arthritis, but the hyperglycaemia, and the nausea and anorexia experienced by the patients so treated, render this form of therapy impracticable at present [664].

32. The Future in the Field of Diabetes

CHARLES H. BEST

Many people have asked me what advances are likely to be made in the field of diabetes. Predictions in this field cannot be made with any more certainty than other prognostications, but after forty years I may be justified in hazarding some guesses as to the course developments will take. In recent years I have recorded a series of unsolved problems which the presentations of my colleagues and surveys of the literature have brought to my mind. Hundreds of useful investigations became obvious but I shall attempt here to list only a few of the important advances which will, I trust, be made. Apropos the literature, few people realize that about seven new papers on insulin appear every day. If one included all aspects of diabetes this figure would be multiplied many times. With such a vigorous and sustained study of the disorder important advances are certain.

For a number of reasons, surveys of the prevalence of diabetes have been conducted in only a few parts of the world. People have not as yet been convinced of the great advantage to themselves of the early detection of a deviation from the normal healthy state. The large-scale organization of detection drives is a time-consuming, expensive, and complicated matter, and there is, of course, never complete co-operation between the private physician and the public health services of a country. However, physicians and organizations devoted to the study of diabetes have made a great deal of progress with detection campaigns. In countries where state medicine exists, comprehensive surveys of the prevalence of diabetes have not been conducted. Under the very best conditions, detection drives now test only approximately 1 per cent of the population; the good which they undoubtedly do could be multiplied by one hundred. As the tests for the detection of diabetes are improved, the time will come when most individuals who will later develop frank diabetes can be recognized at an early stage. Facilities for obtaining and recording this type of information must be provided by the health services of the country. Our goal should be more complete knowledge of the situation throughout the world. Some day all countries will know the incidence of diabetes and the identity of most of the diabetics in their population. Then we will be able, readily, to trace hereditary influences.

When the causes of all types of diabetes mellitus are discovered (defects in storage, liberation, and transport of insulin must be considered as well as failure in formation) I hope that the abnormalities will not all be found to reside entirely in the genes. Although modern studies point that way, great strides are being made in finding nutritional or other procedures that minimize the disability associated with such biochemical lesions. Specific drugs may some day be available which prevent or correct the undesirable manifestations resulting from the genetic defect.

At one time diabetes mellitus was considered to be due solely to a lesion of the pancreas, involving only malfunction of the beta cells of the islands of Langerhans. In support of this idea is the fact that competent histologists can find abnormalities in the beta cells of every case of diabetes. But in many adults the lesion in these cells is not advanced. The insulin content of the pancreas in most juvenile (growth-onset) diabetic individuals is extremely low, while in maturity-onset cases some 40 per cent of the normal insulin remains in the beta cells. Most of these adult cases were, however, carefully treated with insulin. What would have been the picture if they had had no insulin? It is now recognized that in many human diabetics there are ample stores of insulin and the insulin-like activity of blood may be high. In these diabetic persons the lesion does not appear to involve interference with the production of insulin by the beta cells. In juvenile diabetic patients failure of insulin production is more the rule. But in some untreated cases of juvenile diabetes there is evidence that there may be an increased level of insulin-like activity in the blood. This may be due to a hormonal imbalance, that is, to an excessive production of insulin under the stimulus of a physiological agent whose function is to maintain a normal blood sugar by opposing the action of insulin. Whether the excessive response is due to an excess of the agent acting upon normal beta cells or whether over-sensitive beta cells are reacting abnormally to a normal amount of the insulin-opposing agent is not yet clear.

In the future, the different tissues of diabetics must be tested for their response to insulin and to other hormones. A beginning has been made in this study, but we can no longer assume that skeletal muscle, adipose tissue, and liver are always equally affected by the diabetes-producing lesion.

Following total pancreatectomy the blood sugar of many patients is maintained in the normal range by about 40 units of insulin daily. These observations provide the best estimate of the daily production of insulin by the normal human pancreas. The daily dose of insulin required by most diabetics is also about 40 units although a small proportion (less than 1 per cent) require much more. These so-called insulin-resistant cases presumably have some other defect: either the insulin becomes bound and is less physiologically available or there may be faulty utilization of the hormone or an excessive destruction. These few abnormal cases must not blind us to the fact that many millions of patients respond well to about the same amount of insulin that is secreted daily by the normal pancreas. This does not mean that the primary seat of the disorder is necessarily in the beta cells. One of the most puzzling facts is that there is so little evidence of an increased demand for insulin in human diabetics. There should be more emphasis, therefore, as my colleague, Dr. R. E. Haist, has frequently stated, on diabetes as a disease of compensation.

We know only a little about the control of the liberation of insulin but current studies are providing valuable leads. Sugar and the pituitary growth hormone produce an increase in plasma insulin but we have as yet only a superficial understanding of how they act. Knowledge of the neurogenic control of insulin liberation has advanced very little during the last 35 years. These problems are now being forced on our attention by the evidence that the sulphonylureas liberate insulin. The direct experimental findings establish only a rapid and transient effect. The indirect clinical evidence suggests a mild but prolonged action. Attempts to demonstrate an effect of the oral hypoglycaemic agents through the vagus fibres going to the islets have failed. A direct chemical action is assumed by some investigators.

Great progress has been made in the chemistry of insulin. The brilliant work of Sanger is a landmark, but there is still much more to be done before the orientation of all the links in the chains is perfectly understood. Insulin may, of course, be made synthetically eventually, but it would appear that this is not just around the corner. Dickson and Wilson, working in the Connaught Laboratories of the University of Toronto, have confirmed the fact that the two chains of insulin, when separated, are inactive. They have been able to reunite these chains with a recovery of a definite amount, albeit small, of physiological activity. (DeWitt Stetten and his colleagues have made similar observations.) This is not what we mean when we speak of the synthesis of insulin, but it is a great advance.

I have discussed many times the possibility that insulin, or an active derivative, will eventually be given by mouth, and I am still persuaded that this is by no means an impossibility. There will be, I trust, a breakthrough in this area and the results will affect the treatment of diabetes in many ways. The necessity of giving insulin by injection has stood in the way of important clinical investigations.

We must keep in mind the possibility that some physiological substance, or mixture of substances, will be found which acts as a more potent stimulant of insulin liberation than any of the oral hypoglycaemic agents. It will be unfortunate, but not unexpected, if the hormonal physiological stimulant of insulin liberation turns out to be ineffective when administered by mouth.

The invention and development of new apparatus, automation if you wish, is affecting many aspects of medical research and treatment. A brief description of the contrast between a laboratory in which I worked in 1921 and one which I am now equipping and in which I would like to work for the next twenty years, may be interesting. The problems of the two periods are rather similar. I wish to follow blood sugars, liver fat, and glycogen, certain aspects of protein metabolism, to analyse expired air, to look at histological preparations of the islands of Langerhans, to assay the insulin in the pancreas and other tissues—in short to advance knowledge of the physiological significance of insulin.

In 1921 we had the first model of the Duboscq–Leitz colorimeter, our most expensive apparatus, costing possibly $250. The microscope cost $100. The standard glassware and reagents, the metabolism cages, the syringes, sterilizers, etc., may have pushed the total to nearly $1,000. We had no technical assistance and for the first several months received no stipends. Later we were given $60 a month. This was perfectly normal for the times. The same pattern would have been followed in most other countries. (It was not normal, nor did it prove possible, to continue these arrangements in the Department of Physiology after we had established the effects of insulin on depancreatized dogs. Banting and I were given appointments in other University departments soon after we presented our first paper on November 14, 1921, but that is another story.)

In 1961, in large part through the generosity of the Wellcome Trust, several new research laboratories were constructed for the Banting and Best Department of Medical Research. In the one which is for my own use I hope to have available the following standard equipment: an auto-analyser for the continuous recording of blood sugar ($5,000); an amino acid analyser ($15,000); gas chromatography apparatus for fatty acids ($4,500); recording apparatus for oxygen and carbon dioxide in expired air ($3,500); automatic scintillation counter ($10,000); a recording spectrophotometer ($10,000); an electron microscope ($36,000); centrifuges for the preparation of cell fractions ($7,500); and standard apparatus for paper chromatography ($1,000). All of these are or will be available (but admittedly are not, and will not all be, concentrated in my personal laboratory). The total cost with the usual accessories will be about $95,000. This is not an extravagant plan. Laboratories devoted to other types of research would require even more expensive apparatus. The contrast with 1921, however, needs no emphasis.

We must have a great deal more clerical and mechanical help in scanning, selecting, summarizing, and cataloguing the huge volume of relevant scientific literature which confronts us.

We must be able to formulate our problems clearly and to plan the attack on them with first-rate scientific strategy. Then the mechanical devices, kept in perfect order, can be the tireless servants of the investigator who must not inundate his mind with more data than it can evaluate and utilize. In the future the mechanical aids to research will be more complicated, more expensive, possibly more efficient, and we hope more productive. It is our duty to attract, select, and train investigators who can use these devices intelligently and who place the real advance of knowledge above a mere demonstration of the amazing capacity of new apparatus to perform wonders. The advance in knowledge of diabetes will continue, as it has in the past, to throw light on the whole field of medicine.

One may savour the memory of the "good old days" of research in diabetes, but the promises of the present situation are immense and wonderful.

Part II: CHOLINE
AND LIPOTROPIC PHENOMENA

33. A Brief History of the Discovery of the Lipotropic Factors

CHARLES H. BEST

Professor C. C. Lucas, Dr. Jessie H. Ridout, and I had planned for many years to write, and had even started, a book entitled "Choline and its Dietary Precursors: The Lipotropic Factors." The following account of certain historical aspects and of the personalities involved in the lipotropic story is taken, with the consent of my colleagues, from that unborn monograph.

The centres of interest in the ground to be covered are now so numerous that some aid to orientation is a necessity for newcomers to the field. It may be helpful to mention some of the explorers whose efforts have contributed to the charting of the main features. Sometimes we, and others too, temporarily mistook dusty detours for the main road. At times, sidetrials beckoned temptingly, appearing to offer possibilities fully as rewarding as those on the main highway. Not infrequently it has been almost impossible to determine which of several paths was the most important. But in spite of many unprofitable side excursions great progress has actually been made.

In 1932 a compound that had been known to chemists for nearly a century was discovered to be an important new dietary factor. We found that choline prevents and cures fatty changes in the liver. It prevents cirrhosis in animals and cures it if the lesion is not too far advanced. It has provided a new link between fat and protein metabolism. Choline has played a part in the recognition of the phenomenon of transmethylation. It is associated in an interesting way with other dietary factors, particularly folic acid and vitamin B_{12}. Choline deficiency causes kidney changes in young rats, and renal injury resulting in hypertension has been produced by its absence. Choline is a vital factor in poultry nutrition. The clinical implications have been stimulating but no entirely satisfactory clinical trials have been conducted. It has been impossible to justify anything but a complete diet for sick individuals and for this reason the effect of this single dietary factor has not been determined.

When insulin became available in 1921, scores of attractive avenues for research in the field of carbohydrate metabolism appeared and a link with fat metabolism was soon established because of its dramatic effects on ketone bodies and blood lipids. To some extent at least, certain of the new findings were the predictable outcome of a successful frontal attack on diabetes, a problem of long standing. However, the isolation of insulin had many other effects as well—it stimulated a great deal of research on other endocrine glands and led, quite unexpectedly, to the recognition of a group of new dietary factors, the lipotropic agents.

At first Banting and I were mainly interested in the observations that the excretion of sugar and the rapid deterioration in the condition of depancreatized dogs could be arrested by injections of extracts of pancreas prepared in certain ways and that upon cessation of the injections all the signs of diabetes promptly reappeared. During these early phases of the work the investigators were concerned with short-term experiments. Once the effectiveness of the extracts had been firmly established and methods of preparation and purification had been improved, attention turned on the clinical front to therapeutic applications of insulin, and on the experimental side to the observation of depancreatized dogs maintained with insulin for long periods. We had made plans for such long-term experiments but this work was actually conducted by new members of the group—particularly by a young medical graduate, F. N. Allan, now a senior physician at the Lahey Clinic and one time editor of the *Journal of the American Diabetes Association*.

The knowledge of the nutritional requirements of dogs was not what it is today. The existence of most of the accessory food factors that are now so well known had not even been suspected. Possibly by good fortune (in the light of subsequent events), the diets offered the dogs were not always adequate. Moreover, as had been well recognized ever since the first production of experimental diabetes by von Mering and Minkowski in 1890, the digestive function of the depancreatized dog is seriously affected by the absence of the digestive ferments of the pancreas. Administration of insulin does not, of course, improve this aspect of the situation. Thus, impaired digestion and absorption of food is a complication in these animals which is not usually encountered in the spontaneously diabetic dog or in the human diabetic. The significance of this was not at first fully appreciated. It was during this phase of the study of experimental diabetes that the lesions now known to be characteristic of choline deficiency were first encountered.

One of the more striking abnormalities in the untreated depancreatized dog is a large, yellow liver which is produced by distension of the hepatic cells with fat—a picture originally described by von Mering and Minkowski in 1890. Restoration of the diabetic fatty liver to normal by insulin was first reported by the Toronto group in 1922. The dramatic change produced in the very fatty liver by insulin made a lasting impression on me in 1921 and this action of the hormone has played an important part in my continued interest in the factors which control deposition of fat in the liver cells. Banting and I fully realized, as the notes made in 1921 reveal, that prolonged observations on completely depancreatized dogs treated with insulin might provide fascinating new facts, but the development of a large fatty liver, *which was independent of the supply of insulin*, was unexpected. This abnormal liver and signs of failure of hepatic function appeared eventually in animals receiving as much insulin as they could tolerate in two doses daily.

It was reported independently in 1924 from Toronto by Allan, Bowie, Macleod, and Robinson and from Chicago by Fisher, that when depancreatized dogs were maintained for long periods (seven months or more) with insulin, the animals sickened and died and enlarged, yellow livers were observed consistently at autopsy. Many possible explanations came to mind. Lack of pancreatic enzymes was at first believed to be the most likely cause of the abnormality. Support for this idea was forthcoming when it was found that if raw beef pancreas was included in the diet of lean meat and cane-sugar, fatty livers did not develop. Whether or not a lack of pancreatic enzymes was the fundamental defect, it was by this time clear that the abnormalities were related to the absence of the pancreas.

The next step seemed obvious: to identify the factors in the pancreas that are responsible for the protection of the liver. Crude preparations of pancreatic lipase and of trypsin were found to be beneficial in protecting the livers of depancreatized dogs, according to Dr. Jacob Markowitz who was working in the laboratory at that time, but three or four years later attention turned suddenly to an entirely different type of pancreatic component.

Employed in the insulin-testing laboratory was a young man, James Melford Hershey, who had been given permission to work towards an M.A. degree. Prescribed reading in *The Fats* by J. B. Leathes and H. S. Raper, led Hershey to contemplate the suggestions of Bloor and of MacLean and MacLean that phospholipids are concerned in the transport and mobilization of fat. Sometime late in 1927, Hershey formulated the hypothesis that a failure in fat transport or metabolism rather than a defect in digestion might be responsible for the condition of the animals. Therefore, he added crude egg-yolk "lecithin" to the daily rations of eight insulin-treated, depancreatized dogs that had developed typical signs of liver dysfunction (jaundice, bile pigments in the urine, etc.) on the basal diet of lean meat and sucrose. The animals were maintained in an apparently healthy condition and when two of them were sacrificed a year later the content of fat in the liver was normal. Hershey concluded that the pancreatic enzymes are not essential to life in the depancreatized dog.

Samuel Soskin, a recent medical graduate who was working towards his Ph.D. in Physiology, joined Hershey in this problem and they extended these observations. It was at this stage of the study (1929) that Professor Macleod returned to his native heath to occupy the Chair of Physiology in the University of Aberdeen. I was recalled from postgraduate studies with Sir Henry Dale at the National Institute for Medical Research, Hampstead, England, to fill the vacancy in Toronto. Professor Macleod was not convinced that the findings of Hershey and Soskin were new or significant. He advised me to assure myself by repetition of the work, and by personal observation, that the liver damage was not due to the lack of some well-recognized dietary constituent which might be contained in the crude lecithin. The observations were, therefore, continued for more than a year before the first report of this work was made by Hershey, from my department, in 1930.

It was noted by Hershey and Soskin that the addition of cod liver oil and brewer's yeast or marmite (a concentrated yeast extract) to the diet improved the condition of the dogs greatly without altering the essential finding, viz. that crude lecithin regularly alleviated signs of liver dysfunction which developed in the insulin-treated depancreatized dogs maintained on the diets then in vogue in this laboratory. Their conclusion that the pancreatic enzymes are not essential in the depancreatized dog receiving lecithin appeared to be supported by an earlier observation of Penau and Simonnet in France. They had kept a depancreatized dog alive and well for over two years by giving insulin without supplying any raw pancreas or the enzymes from it. A fact which later proved to be of greatest significance was that the ration fed their dog contained large amounts of milk and bread. In 1929 Soskin obtained his Ph.D. and left Toronto to become Director of Metabolic and Endocrine Research at the Michael Reese Hospital in Chicago.

In 1931 Miss Mary Elinor Huntsman came into the Department of Physiology as a graduate student and joined me in an attempt to determine the factors involved in the production and cure of fatty livers. Progress had, up to this time, been very slow because in depancreatized dogs the desired lesion required from three to eleven months to develop on the rations then in use. These experiments were not only very time-consuming, but the variability of the results made the use of large numbers of animals imperative, while limitations of space as well as the cost of rations and of salaries for attendants made this difficult to attain.

Following up the observation that the presence of fat in the diet of depancreatized dogs aggravated the liver damage, rats were placed on high fat (and incidentally low protein) diets. In the relatively short period of three weeks, fatty livers developed in rats fed a diet containing mixed grains and bone meal with 40 per cent of beef dripping. With this contribution by Best, Hershey, and Huntsman in 1932 the tempo of the study was suddenly accelerated: new facts became available in weeks where formerly months or years had been required.

Mr. Hershey now decided to complete his medical course. He obtained his M.D. in 1934, his Ph.D. in Physiology in 1936, and his Diploma of Public Health in 1936. He continued to contribute to the development of the problem throughout these years, but eventually went into public health work in western Canada. In October 1951, Dr. Hershey relinquished his post as Director of Regional Services of the Saskatchewan Health Department to become Medical Defence Hospital Consultant in the New York State Health Department.

The reduction of the fat content of the livers by ingestion of commercial lecithin was apparently not due to a contaminant in the crude egg-yolk lecithin since Hershey, Huntsman, and I found that a sample of crude beef-liver lecithin had the same effect, and the activity was retained by both materials after purification by the cadmium chloride method of Levene and Rolf. Those were exciting days in the laboratory. Within a month the same three workers were able to publish a note identifying choline as the active constituent of the lecithin molecule; betaine was found to have a similar effect on liver fat.

During the next seven years (up to the outbreak of war in 1939) several senior colleagues and numerous junior members of the Department of Physiology and in the School of Hygiene helped in the further elucidation of the increasingly fascinating "fatty liver" problem. Omand McKillop Solandt and Miss Huntsman investigated the effect of choline chloride on the deposition of fat in the livers of species other than the white rat while Dr. George C. Ferguson assisted in the study of the efficacy of choline in depancreatized dogs maintained with insulin. Mice developed fatty livers readily on the high fat, mixed grain diet and choline prevented this; puppies sometimes developed fatty livers, chickens did not, on the same diet. More dietetic research was considered desirable before conclusions could be drawn in these and other species. Soon after this Solandt went to England for further study. Later, as Director-General of the Defence Research Board of Canada, he had more weighty matters on his mind. He is now Vice-President of the Canadian National Railways in charge of research.

The July 1933 issue of the *Journal of Physiology* carried an article by Best, Ferguson, and Hershey in which choline was shown to cure as well as to prevent the development of fatty livers in depancreatized dogs. Thus the effect of choline, observable in rats within a test period of several weeks, was shown to resemble that obtained in dogs after 250 to 330 days.

Meanwhile Dr. Jessie Hamilton Ridout had joined the group and (except for a hectic period devoted to supervising the preparation of dried blood serum during the Second World War) she has been actively engaged in the study of lipotropic phenomena since about 1933. In 1933 Professor Harold John Channon of the University of Liverpool accepted my invitation to visit the University of Toronto. He spent three months working with us on problems of mutual interest in the lipotropic field. After his return to England, Channon and his colleagues carried on parallel studies for some six years, especially on the role of dietary proteins and amino acids in lipotropic phenomena. At about this period, or within a year or two, Dr. Earle Willard McHenry, Dr. Donald Logie MacLean, and Dr. Hugh Massey Barrett became interested in different aspects of the fatty liver problem and contributed their special knowledge and experience.

Dr. McHenry, after collaborating with me for several years on the study of histamine and histaminase, became curious as to the cause and cure of fatty livers and for more than ten years this subject occupied a prominent position in the research program which he followed. In 1941 with Dr. Gertrude Gavin, he discovered the lipotropic activity of inositol in a fat-free diet. In 1942 he was made Associate Professor of Physiological Hygiene in charge of Nutrition, and in 1946 Professor of Public Health Nutrition in the School of Hygiene.

Dr. D. L. MacLean, with his special training in pathology, assisted on many occasions by studying tissues from animals on hypolipotropic diets. The first illustration to be published showing the early signs of cirrhosis in choline-deficient animals was in a paper with him.

Dr. H. M. Barrett was largely responsible for the first use of isotopes (fatty acids labelled with deuterium), in the study of lipotropic phenomena. About 1940, however, Dr. Barrett began work on problems of chemical warfare which displaced his interests in lipotropic factors. In due course Dr. Barrett became the Director of the Canadian Establishment for Defence Research at Suffield, Alberta. Later he was "loaned" to the British government and was Superintendent of the Defence Laboratories at Porton in England. He is at present a very senior scientist in the Defence Research Board of Canada.

About 1934 Arnold deMerritt Welch was doing postgraduate work towards a Ph.D. degree in the Department of Pharmacology, University of

Toronto, and his wife Mary Scott Welch was registered for an M.A. in the Department of Physiology. Although the Toronto group can claim no credit for the clear, incisive thinking and excellent experimental work done by Welch in the field of the lipotropic factors, it is of interest to record the influence of personal contacts and the maintenance of cordial relationships between research departments.

Another name prominent among those investigating lipotropic phenomena is that of Thomas Hughes Jukes, who was registered in the School of Graduate Studies of the University of Toronto about the same time. He took the course in Advanced Physiology given by me in 1930–31. A doctorate from the Department of Biochemistry (1933) and subsequent research on the nutrition of poultry led back unexpectedly to a field which former colleagues had developed and which he had heard much about as a graduate student.

I. L. Chaikoff, now a Professor of Physiology in the University of California and the leader of one of the most active groups studying certain aspects of the lipotropic phenomena, graduated in Medicine from Toronto in 1927. He received his first training in physiological research with Professor Macleod with whom he took his Ph.D. in 1924. His interest in diabetes and in fat metabolism dates from that time.

The term "lipotropic" used to describe the newly found activity of dietary factors such as choline and betaine, first appeared in 1935 in a note published by Best and Ridout. Three months later the first definition is to be found in a footnote to a paper in *Nature* by Best, Huntsman, and Ridout in which they explained that "the term 'lipotropic' is used to describe substances which decrease the rate of deposition and accelerate the rate of removal of liver fat." Many words constructed from various Greek and Latin roots had been considered before it was decided to adopt "lipotropic," at the suggestion of Dr. Norman B. Taylor, then one of the professors of physiology in the University of Toronto. The derivation from *lipos* (fat) and *tropeo* (to affect or change) seemed obvious, and the word was simple and easy to pronounce compared with "pymyelodiathetic" and other monstrosities which were proposed only to be discarded. Further, the word "lipotropic" did not appear in several dictionaries that I consulted. However, years later it was brought to my attention that the word had appeared earlier in at least one medical dictionary with a different meaning, relating to the affinity of basic dyes for fat in tissue. In current medical literature the word is used almost exclusively to refer to the action of choline (and other *dietary* factors which act as its precursors) on liver lipids.

Certain unexpected results in one of the experiments conducted by Best and Huntsman in Toronto indicated that the nature or amount of dietary protein might be an important factor in lipotropic studies. This observation led to a detailed examination, particularly in the Biochemical Laboratory in Liverpool, of the lipotropic effect of various proteins and of individual amino acids. An anti-lipotropic effect of cystine was noted by Beeston and Channon in 1936 but the Liverpool group were unsuccessful in accounting for the lipotropic action of some proteins and the inactivity of others. Then in 1937 came the report from Ann Arbor that methionine exerts a strong lipotropic effect. This discovery of Tucker and Eckstein was confirmed in 1938 in Liverpool by Channon, Manifold, and Platt, and in Toronto by Best and Ridout in 1940.

The brilliant studies of Dr. Vincent du Vigneaud and his colleagues have been largely responsible for the elucidation of the mechanism by which dietary methionine and betaine exert their lipotropic effect. This is not the place to discuss in any detail the discovery of transmethylation and the many outgrowths from this interesting biochemical process. The role of folic acid and vitamin B_{12} in the biosynthesis of methyl groups is also another story.

Because we are concerned here with the role of choline in lipotropic phenomena we shall only mention the fatty liver caused by protein deficiency or by an imbalance of the essential amino acids in the diet. Under these dietary conditions, the fatty droplets appear in a different part of the liver lobule and their appearance is not prevented by the presence of choline in the diet.

Looking back from our present vantage point it is apparent that the problem of the lipotropic activity in minced beef pancreas might have been productively attacked in any one of several ways. If the protein fraction of the pancreas had been fed to rats on diets rich in fat the lipotropic activity of methionine-containing protein might have been found earlier. If a more thorough study of the administration of enzymes obtained from the pancreas had been carried out in the insulin-treated depancreatized dogs, the indirect lipotropic action of these substances, later so effectively elucidated by Chaikoff and his colleagues, would presumably have been found. We have described the route which actually was followed in the recognition of the lipotropic activity of choline, betaine, and methionine, the physiological lipotropic agents. It has become more and more apparent that choline provides an essential part of the pathway by which the other lipotropic agents exert their effects.

34. The Effect of Lecithine on Fat Deposition in the Liver of the Normal Rat

C. H. BEST

J. M. HERSHEY

M. ELINOR HUNTSMAN

The very interesting effects of some component of crude lecithine upon the condition of diabetic animals have been discussed in previous communications from this laboratory (Hershey [387]; Hershey and Soskin [388]; Best and Hershey [89]). The symptoms exhibited by these animals and the autopsy findings indicate that the characteristic condition is largely attributable to failure of liver function. The results of these studies suggested that an investigation of the effect of lecithine on deposition of fat in the livers of normal animals might be profitable. The literature relevant to this subject has been reviewed in the monographs by Leathes and Raper [491] and by MacLean and MacLean [534]. As far as we know, the particular problem in which we are interested has not been investigated by previous workers. The experiments were planned with a view to obtaining deposition of large amounts of fat in the livers of a group of control animals. This was accomplished by feeding a diet high in fairly saturated fats. A second group of animals comparable in every way, as far as we could determine, with the controls, received the same amount of fat as those in the control group and *in addition* varying amounts of crude or purified lecithine. The results demonstrate, among other points, that crude and purified lecithine influence the accumulation of fat in the livers of the test group of animals.

METHODS

White rats of the Wistar strain, weighing between 150 and 230 g, were used as test animals. Previous to the experiment they had been receiving a stock diet which was adequate in all respects. All the animals used in the

Originally appeared in the *Journal of Physiology*, LXXV (1932), 56–66.

experiment were apparently healthy, and great care was taken to ensure that the various groups into which they were divided for any one experiment were as similar as possible. Much time was wasted in preliminary experiments in which attempts were made to use groups of animals in one cage, but this procedure was not found to be feasible. In all the experiments reported in this paper individual cages were used, and notes on the condition of each animal were made throughout the experiment. Every animal in any experiment ate approximately the same amount of the stock diet, which has the following composition: 32.5 per cent of each of the following—whole cracked wheat, rolled oats, and corn meal, and 2.5 per cent of bone meal. The amounts of fat and of the lecithine under test are given in each of the tables or summaries. In all cases the fat was provided in the form of beef dripping, which has an iodine number of approximately 40. The food was prepared daily. The dripping was melted and added to the stock diet. The mixture was then heated in a boiling water bath for two hours, with intermittent stirring. The stirring was continued during the subsequent cooling to ensure the equal distribution of the added fat. The lecithine was thoroughly mixed with the other food by prolonged grinding. The diet for each rat was carefully weighed each day, and in cases where food was left in the cage at the end of 24 hours the amount was determined by weighing. The food trays were designed so that there was little or no food spilled, and the construction of the cages made it possible to recover any spilled food without difficulty. Fat estimations on the food residue showed that the fat had been thoroughly mixed with the other constituents. At the end of the experiment the animals were stunned and decapitated. The animals were not fed on the day on which they were killed. Blood samples were collected from the severed carotid arteries. The livers were removed as soon as the animals were dead, and the content of fatty acid determined by the Leathes and Raper modification of Liebermann's saponification method. The iodine number of the fatty acid of the liver was determined by Wijs' procedure, as outlined by Leathes and Raper. The phospholipines of the liver and blood were calculated from the phosphate content as determined on the alcohol-ether soluble portion by the Briggs modification [148] of the Bell-Doisy method. Glycogen was estimated by the Pflüger technique.

EXPERIMENTAL RESULTS

Egg-yolk lecithine. In the first experiment ten rats were used in each of the two groups. The details of the experiments and the results are shown in Tables 34.I and 34.II. The egg-yolk lecithine used in these experiments was secured from a commercial firm and was prepared from dried egg-yolk,

TABLE 34.I

STOCK DIET WITH FAT
(40 per cent of total food)

Rat no.	Length of Experiment (days)	Av. Fat Eaten Daily (g)	Wt. of Rat before (g)	Wt. of Rat after (g)	Wt. of Liver (g)	Fatty Acids in Liver (%)
1	36	2.8	170	188	7.77	20.50
2	36	2.6	154	167	5.02	5.88
3	35	2.6	152	160	4.71	4.20
4	36	2.6	178	175	5.58	4.05
5	35	2.8	155	167	4.42	5.52
6	36	2.6	135	144	4.78	5.12
7	38	2.6	121	135	4.51	3.67
8	38	2.6	150	144	5.22	6.87
9	38	2.6	149	152	6.44	11.30

Average = 7.36

TABLE 34.II

STOCK DIET WITH FAT (40 PER CENT), SUPPLEMENTED WITH CRUDE EGG-YOLK LECITHINE

Rat no.	Length of Experiment (days)	Av. Fat Eaten Daily (g)	Wt. of Rat before (g)	Wt. of Rat after (g)	Lecithine Daily (g)	Wt. of Liver (g)	Fatty Acids in Liver (%)
11	35	2.9	181	185	1.4	7.32	3.20
12	36	2.5	149	150	1.2	4.57	3.78
13	36	2.5	162	157	1.2	6.33	3.38
14	38	2.7	193	189	1.3	7.34	3.09
15	38	2.4	154	148	1.2	6.86	3.29
16	35	2.7	190	182	1.3	7.61	3.30
17	35	2.6	144	135	1.3	6.37	3.75
18	38	2.5	140	147	1.2	5.48	3.12
19	38	2.6	176	170	1.3	6.59	3.97
20	38	3.1	185	192	1.5	6.85	3.50

Average = 3.38

after removal of the fats with benzene, by alcoholic extraction of the phospholipines and subsequent removal of the alcohol *in vacuo*. The results of the experiments in which this material was used appear to demonstrate in a convincing manner that some component of lecithine modifies the deposition of fat in the livers of the test animals. The figures also illustrate the very important fact that there is a tremendous variation in the deposition of fat in the livers of different members of a group of animals, each of which is receiving approximately the same amount of fat in the diet.

In most of the experiments all the rats consumed a satisfactory amount of fat. In certain cases, however, the quantity eaten by some of the test animals was not of the same order as that ingested by the controls. The figures for these animals have not been included in the results.

The effects of smaller amounts of lecithine. To study the effects on fatty acids of the liver when small amounts of lecithine were provided, a group of thirty white rats was used. The animals were divided into three groups of ten each, care being taken that the groups were as similar as possible.

Ten rats received 6.15 g of stock diet *plus* fat 3.5 g (beef dripping, iodine number 40). Fat formed 40 per cent of the total food. The experiments lasted 26 days. The average amount of fat taken daily was 3.4 g. The average weight of the rats initially was 190 g, and at the end 182 g. The percentage of fatty acids in the livers varied from 7.0 to 25.3 per cent (average 15.7 per cent). The iodine numbers varied from 78 to 108 (average 95).

In the second group all rats received the same amount of stock diet and fat, and in addition egg-yolk lecithine. The lecithine formed 9.4 per cent of the total food. The average fat eaten daily was 2.97 g, lecithine intake was 0.85 g. The average weight of the rats initially was 191 g, and at the end was 177 g. The percentage of fatty acids in the liver varied from 3.3 to 5.1 (average 3.7 per cent). The iodine number varied from 101 to 136 (average 129).

The diet for the third group was exactly the same as that of the second, except that lecithine formed 4.9 per cent of the diet instead of 9.4 per cent. The average amount of fat eaten daily was 3.12 g, the average lecithine was 0.44 g. The average weight initially was 191 g, and at the end 187 g. The percentage of fatty acid in the liver varied from 3.1 to 8.2 per cent (average 4.6). The iodine numbers varied from 83 to 107 (average 98).

These results appear to furnish evidence that as little as 0.44 g of crude egg-yolk lecithine daily is sufficient to prevent the deposition of large amounts of fat in the liver of a rat under the conditions of these experiments. It will be observed that the rats in the test groups in this series did not eat quite as much added fat as the controls. We have no hesitation in reporting these results, however, for the following reasons: (1) In many other experiments rats from the same colony have invariably shown as high an average fat content of the liver as the test animals in this particular experiment. In these other experiments the controls have eaten even less fat than that taken by the test animals of this experiment. (2) The figures for the individual rats show that many of the animals did eat as much fat as the controls. (3) The test animals ate a certain amount of fatty material in the crude lecithine, which can perhaps be placed to their credit. (4) Furthermore, a study of the tables which contain the results of the determinations made on the control rats demonstrates that the extent of the deposition of liver fat is not proportional to the amount of fat eaten when this amount varies between 2 and 3.5 g per day. For example, rats which ate 2.3 g of fat daily showed a much higher fat content than several which ate 2.5 g.

The effects of purified lecithine. Crude egg-yolk lecithine was purified by the cadmium chloride procedure of Levene and Rolf [495]. This fractionation was carried out by one of us (M.E.H.) in the Department of Biochemistry under the direction of Professor H. D. Kay. The purified lecithine (iodine number 65) obtained was tested on a group of animals. The results in Tables 34.III and 34.IV establish the fact that purified egg-yolk lecithine exerts the same effect as that produced by the crude material.

TABLE 34.III

STOCK DIET WITH FAT (40 PER CENT OF TOTAL FOOD) FED FOR 22 DAYS

Rat no.	Av. Fat Eaten Daily (g)	Wt. of Rat before (g)	Wt. of Rat after (g)	Fatty Acids in Liver (%)	Iodine no.
1	2.48	300	253	6.35	105
2	2.48	202	174	19.2	100
3	2.47	190	194	27.6	—
4	2.46	179	171	19.3	97
5	2.43	189	172	16.2	102
6	2.40	180	177	20.5	95
7	2.48	177	180	15.9	96
8	2.40	169	166	28.2	102
9	2.45	162	160	12.5	104
10	2.44	150	150	17.2	77
				Average = 18.3	

TABLE 34.IV

STOCK DIET WITH FAT (40 PER CENT) SUPPLEMENTED WITH PURIFIED LECITHINE FED FOR 22 DAYS

Rat no.	Av. Fat Eaten Daily (g)	Wt. of Rat before (g)	Wt. of Rat after (g)	Av. Lecithine Daily (g)	Fatty Acids in Liver (%)	Iodine no.
11	2.40	278	257	0.48	3.49	137
12	2.43	203	177	0.49	3.65	107
13	2.35	190	150	0.47	7.4	113
14	2.38	180	171	0.48	3.15	117
15	2.41	199	186	0.48	3.98	118
16	2.13	184	164	0.43	3.58	124
17	2.22	180	166	0.44	3.74	139
18	2.40	170	167	0.48	8.4	76
19	2.34	160	155	0.47	4.05	129
20	2.44	160	151	0.49	4.11	128
					Average = 4.5	

Lecithine from beef liver. In the next series of experiments, lecithine prepared from fresh beef liver, was tested. The lecithine fraction was prepared in the following manner: fresh beef liver was minced and dried in a vacuum oven at low temperature. The dried material was ground and then thoroughly extracted with absolute ethyl alcohol. The material was filtered through paper and the filtrate evaporated to small volume in an efficient vacuum still. The residue was evaporated to a syrup in a large glass flask, and ether was then added until no more material would go into solution. The mixture was allowed to stand overnight in a cold room, and then filtered through paper. The clear ethereal solution was added with stirring to three volumes of acetone. After 48 hours the supernatant fluid was decanted, and the precipitate removed. This material was then stored over paraffin in an atmosphere of nitrogen. This was the material which was subsequently purified by the cadmium chloride procedure. We are indebted to the Connaught Laboratories for the fresh beef liver, for the various reagents, and for the use of the large apparatus required in the preparation of the lecithine.

The effect of crude beef liver lecithine. The results demonstrated that 1 g and 0.5 g of lecithine from this source daily are capable of preventing the deposition of fat in the liver of normal white rats. [Two tables were given here in the original paper, showing that the average liver fatty acids were reduced from 17.3 per cent (7.8–29.6 per cent) in the controls to 4.8 per cent (3.1–9.5 per cent) in those given the crude beef liver lecithine; the iodine values of the isolated fatty acids averaged 110 and 185, respectively.]

Purified beef liver lecithine. Some 340 g of purified lecithine (iodine number 75) were obtained by fractionation of the lecithine according to the Levene and Rolf cadmium chloride procedure. Varying amounts of this lecithine were added to the stock diet in the manner described above. The smallest effective daily dose studied was 0.1 g. The results of the experiment in which 0.25 g was given daily were slightly more consistent, however. [Two tables have been eliminated; these showed that the purified beef liver lecithine reduced the hepatic fatty acids from 14.4 per cent (8.2–28.2 per cent) to 5.8 per cent (4.3–6.6 per cent); the iodine numbers of the isolated fatty acids averaged 98 and 112, respectively. The fat eaten daily by controls averaged 2.50 g and the fat excreted was 0.16 g; in the animals given purified liver lecithine the corresponding values were 2.48 g and 0.17 g per day.]

Proof that the excretion of fatty acids plays no part in the effects of lecithine. Although these results may be shown subsequently to have little physiological significance, they are of considerable interest provided that the effect of lecithine is not due to some relatively unimportant mechanism. The only obvious pitfall seems to be that the lecithine might increase the excretion of fat. In preliminary experiments in which the food residue and faeces were examined for fat, no evidence could be obtained that more fat was lost in the animals on lecithine than in others. In an attempt to make this point perfectly clear, however, the fat in the faeces has been estimated by the saponification method, for each of the members of control and test groups of animals, in three experiments. The faeces were collected daily and were immediately placed in the alkali. There is no difference in the fat excretion of the control and test groups—very strong evidence that fat excretion is not a significant factor in the interpretation of these results. In the other experiments in which phospholipines prepared from beef liver and egg-yolk lecithine prevented deposition of liver fat, the fat excretion of the animals which received the lecithine was of the same order as that of those on the control diet. The figures for the experiment in which egg-yolk lecithine was used are given in Tables 34.V and 34.VI. These results, in addition to the data on fat excretion which they provide, furnish further evidence of the effect of phospholipines derived from egg-yolk on deposition of liver fat.

Lecithine in liver and blood. Determinations of alcohol-ether soluble phosphorus on samples of liver and blood from control and test animals

TABLE 34.V

STOCK DIET WITH FAT (40 PER CENT OF TOTAL FOOD) FED FOR 21 DAYS

Rat no.	Av. Fat Eaten Daily (g)	Av. Fat Excreted Daily (g)	Wt. of Rat before (g)	Wt. of Rat after (g)	Fatty Acids in Liver (%)	Iodine no.
1	2.50	0.12	171	150	8.9	110
2	2.43	0.11	155	145	21.5	86
3	2.48	0.14	158	148	14.8	106
4	2.48	0.13	200	195	17.3	100
5	2.50	0.12	174	170	12.3	89
6	2.43	0.13	165	150	27.7	84
7	2.50	0.12	163	160	25.0	97
	Average = 0.13			Average = 18.2		

TABLE 34.VI

STOCK DIET WITH FAT ADDED (40 PER CENT) SUPPLEMENTED WITH CRUDE EGG LECITHINE FED FOR 21 DAYS

Rat no.	Av. Fat Eaten Daily (g)	Av. Fat Excreted Daily (g)	Wt. of Rat before (g)	Wt. of Rat after (g)	Lecithine Daily (g)	Fatty Acids in Liver (%)	Iodine no.
11	2.43	0.10	153	150	0.49	3.75	—
12	2.32	0.08	177	162	0.46	3.50	133
14	2.47	0.16	181	175	0.49	3.32	140
16	2.38	0.12	161	137	0.48	3.15	137
20	2.45	0.11	150	148	0.49	3.50	114
	Average = 0.11					Average = 3.44	

were very kindly made for us by Dr. Kay of the Department of Biochemistry. The average liver value, calculated as lecithine, in four control animals was 2.94 per cent. In four test animals each of which ate approximately 0.85 g of egg-yolk lecithine daily the value was 3.38 per cent, and in four test animals which ate 0.44 g of the same material 3.20 per cent. We are not prepared to conclude without further experiments that the difference between control and test animals is significant, but it is interesting to note that a very large proportion of the total fatty acid in the livers of the test animals must have been derived from the phospholipines. The livers of test animals which contained 3.38 per cent lecithine showed an average value of 3.85 per cent fatty acid, those with 3.20 per cent lecithine 3.80 per cent fatty acid. The livers of the controls contained 2.94 per cent lecithine and 11.2 per cent fatty acids.

The results for the phospholipines, calculated as lecithine, in blood samples from control animals, demonstrate that these values are definitely lower than those obtained from the animals given lecithine. While the animals were not fed on the day on which they were killed, and while we are certain that some of the animals did not eat anything for at least five hours previous to their death, we cannot conclude that absorption of lecithine from the intestine did not influence these values obtained for the blood.

Glycogen. Glycogen determinations on samples of the livers of control and test animals have been made for us by our colleague Dr. E. T. Waters. The results thus far obtained do not suggest that there is any significant difference in the amounts of liver glycogen in the two groups.

Fatty acid content of whole animal. In several experiments the total fatty acid content of control and test animals has been determined by the saponification procedure. These figures suggest that the animals which had lecithine do not contain as much fatty acid as the controls. The difference is not great, however, and further experiments are required to settle the point. The iodine numbers of the fatty acids obtained from the bodies (livers excluded) of the control and test animals were of the same order.

DISCUSSION

A review of the literature shows that there is very little information available concerning the effects of diets rich in fat on the deposition of fat in the livers of various species of animals. In the experiments which we carried out during the hot summer weather, difficulties were encountered in securing a high average fat content in the livers of white rats. During the autumn and winter, however, a daily ration containing approximately

2.5 g of fairly saturated fat has consistently produced a high average fat content in the livers of the control animals (Tables 34.I, 34.III, and 34.V). These results are so consistent that it might be considered unnecessary to provide a group of control animals for every new test if one could be absolutely certain that the rats were from the same colony and had received the same diet and attention. It is certain, however, that rats from one colony cannot be used as controls on those from another. In one experiment in which a series of rats from a new colony was used the results had to be discarded because we made the mistake of assuming that the control group would exhibit fatty livers on the same diet as that received by the control rats referred to in the above tables. None of the rats from the new colony which were used as controls had a high liver fat. The cause for this great difference between rats from various colonies would be an interesting subject for further study.

The results of the experiments reported in this paper provide evidence that the addition of crude and purified lecithine from egg-yolk and from fresh beef liver to the diet of normal white rats prevents the accumulation of liver fat. These results are very clear-cut. The evidence appears satisfactory that the effect is not due to excretion of fat by the animals on the "lecithine" diet. The faeces were carefully examined by one of us each day, and it appeared probable, even before the actual estimation of the faecal fat in the control and test groups had been made, that fat excretion by the test animals was not a significant factor in the interpretation of the results. It is in the highest degree unlikely that the saponification method would fail to detect fatty material in one case and not in the other. It is also most improbable that the fat in the intestine of the lecithine-fed animals would be decomposed beyond the fatty acid and glycerol stage.

In the determination of the iodine numbers of the fatty acids from various sources the reagents and the technique have been repeatedly checked by determination of the iodine absorption of a sample of Merck's oleic acid. The iodine number of the beef dripping has ranged between 39 and 41. The tables demonstrate that the iodine number of the fatty acids from the livers of the lecithine-fed animals are on the average considerably higher than those of the control groups. While the average figures may have no great significance in this connection, calculation of these values from the experiments which are reported in this paper shows the following result—control rats 100, lecithine-fed rats 132. The iodine number of the faecal fat varied between 20 and 50, and was usually between 30 and 40. An interesting point arising out of the determination of the iodine numbers is the very high figures obtained for the fatty acids of the liver of certain of the rats which received lecithine prepared from beef liver. These estimations were made with the same reagents and at the same time as those on the control animals. These high figures suggest that the livers of certain of the animals receiving crude lecithine may contain a large proportion of highly unsaturated fatty acid, but further study is required on this point. If this result can be confirmed, however, in experiments on larger animals, a good opportunity might be provided for the isolation and identification of the fatty acid or acids responsible.

In an investigation of the effects of the components of lecithine on deposition of liver fat, the results of which will be published shortly by two of us (C.H.B. and M.E.H.), evidence has been obtained that the active component of lecithine is choline. In view of this finding a discussion of the physiological significance of the results given in this paper will not be included here.

SUMMARY

When white rats weighing between 150 and 230 g receive a daily ration containing 2.5 g of fairly saturated fat (iodine number approximately 40) for 3 weeks, their livers may be found to contain very large amounts of fatty acids. The average value of the iodine number of these fatty acids in our experiments was approximately 100. Comparable groups of animals receiving the same diet as above, and in addition varying amounts of crude or purified lecithine prepared from egg-yolk or beef liver, do not exhibit this increase in liver fat. The values obtained may be as low or lower than those of animals fed on a normal mixed diet. The average value of the iodine numbers of the fatty acids of this group was approximately 132. No evidence could be obtained that increased excretion of fat plays any part in the interpretation of the effect of lecithine.

The results of a preliminary investigation of the effects of lecithine upon liver glycogen and phospholipines, and upon the distribution of fat in other parts of the bodies of the test animals, are briefly discussed.

ACKNOWLEDGMENTS

We would like to express here our appreciation of the expert technical assistance given us by Miss G. I. Harpell.

A part of the expense of this research has been defrayed by a grant from the Banting Research Foundation.

35. The Effects of the Components of Lecithine upon Deposition of Fat in the Liver

C. H. BEST

M. ELINOR HUNTSMAN

The results of the experiments in which purified lecithine from two sources, egg-yolk, and fresh beef liver, has been shown to prevent deposition of fat in the livers of normal rats (Best, Hershey, and Huntsman [91]) have led us to study the effects of feeding various components of lecithine. It appeared possible that the oleic or other unsaturated fatty acid, the glycerophosphate, the choline, some combination of two or more of these factors, or the whole lecithine molecule, might be the active agent. The general procedure in this series of experiments has been to substitute for the lecithine in the daily diet of each rat the amounts of glycerophosphate, oleate, or choline, which it is calculated might be derived from 0.5 g of purified lecithine. This amount of lecithine was previously found to be effective in preventing the deposition of fat in the livers of normal white rats, each of which ingested daily for three weeks approximately 2.5 g of fairly well-saturated fat.

METHODS

The methods used in this study were in general similar to those discussed in the preceding paper. Any slight change will be noted in the description of each experiment. The required amount of the material under test was dissolved in water, except in the case of sodium oleate, and thoroughly mixed each day with the diet, which contained approximately 40 per cent fat (beef dripping).

EXPERIMENTAL RESULTS

Glycerophosphate. In the first experiment the effect of sodium β glycerophosphate was tested; 0.12 g was added to the daily diet of each rat. [Four

Originally appeared in the *Journal of Physiology*, LXXV (1932), 405–12.

tables have been eliminated. The first showed data for 10 rats fed the high fat basal diet, the second the results of adding sodium β glycerophosphate: average fatty acids in livers of control rats 15.6 per cent (7.6–23.5 per cent), with glycerophosphate 18.1 per cent (7.4–36.3 per cent).]

In another series of experiments in which calcium α glycerophosphate was used the average liver fatty acid of the control group was 17.3 per cent and that of the test group 19.5 per cent. These results indicate that deposition of fat in the liver is not prevented by the glycerophosphoric acid derived from the lecithine. In some preliminary experiments performed several years ago, in which sodium phosphate was added to a diet high in fat, Hershey and Soskin obtained similar negative results.

Sodium oleate. Approximately the amount of sodium oleate which might be formed as a result of the decomposition of 0.5 g of purified lecithine was added to the daily ration of each test rat in this series. [The second pair of tables showed that the average fatty acids from the livers of 10 rats fed the basal diet was 14.4 per cent (8.2–28.2 per cent), with added oleate 12.2 per cent (7.5–18.2 per cent).]

These results demonstrate that sodium oleate does not inhibit fat deposition in the liver under the conditions of these experiments. In other experiments in which much larger amounts of sodium oleate were provided, negative results were also obtained.

Choline. The effects of various amounts of choline have been studied. The largest amount given, 117 mg daily, appeared to be fairly well tolerated. The smallest dose used (10 mg daily) produced a definite effect on deposition of liver fat, but the average value in this series was considerably higher than in other animals from the same colony which received larger amounts of choline. The average figures for the fatty acid content of the livers of all the control and test animals are given in Table 35.I, while the results for the individual rats in one series are given in Table 35.II. The controls for this group are the same as those receiving sodium glycerophosphate and sodium oleate. Figures for daily fat excretion are given in Table 35.I. *In each of the seven experiments in which choline was administered, deposition of liver fat was unmistakably less than in the control animals.*

The Effect of Choline Administered Subcutaneously

In two short series of experiments the effect of choline injected subcutaneously has been studied. In the first series 5 mg administered in one dose daily produced no detectable effect upon the deposition of liver fat. In the second series 10 mg were administered at each injection, and each test rat received for a period of three weeks two injections on Saturdays and Sundays, and four on other days. This treatment resulted in average liver

TABLE 35.I

STOCK DIET WITH FAT ADDED (40 PER CENT FINAL MIX) SUPPLEMENTED
WITH CHOLINE. SUMMARY OF RESULTS

Choline per Day per Rat(mg)	No. of Rats	Av. Fat Eaten per Diem (g)	Per cent Fatty Acids in Liver	Iodine no.
0	37	2.5	16.2	97
10	10	2.5	9.7	95
20	9	2.5	4.9	102
40	9	2.5	5.5	110
66	6	2.5	3.5	135
70	10	2.5	5.2	103
100	5	2.4	3.4	—
117	10	2.4	5.1	111

TABLE 35.II

STOCK DIET WITH FAT (40 PER CENT OF TOTAL FOOD) SUPPLEMENTED WITH CHOLINE

Rat no.	Fat Eaten per Diem (g)	Fat Excreted per Diem (g)	Wt. of Rat before (g)	Wt. of Rat after (g)	Choline per Diem (g)	Per cent Fatty Acids in Liver	Iodine no.
51	2.5	0.19	210	206	0.07	3.8	112
52	2.5	0.15	170	168	0.07	5.6	98
53	2.1	0.17	170	164	0.06	6.1	98
54	2.5	0.15	178	158	0.07	5.4	91
55	2.5	0.16	182	180	0.07	6.2	100
56	2.5	0.12	190	190	0.07	3.2	126
57	2.5	0.15	210	210	0.07	5.6	106
58	2.5	0.16	212	198	0.07	3.9	109
59	2.5	0.16	242	218	0.07	8.0	88
60	2.5	0.23	240	222	0.07	4.2	104
					Average = 5.2		

fatty acids of 3.8 per cent in the 10 test rats. The control animals of this series received the same volume of saline and the same number of injections as those to which the choline was administered. This treatment did not agree well with either the control or test animals, and they were not in good condition at the end of the experiment. The average liver fatty acid of the control animals was 7.4 per cent. Since a comparable group of animals receiving the same diet, but no injections of saline, had an average liver fatty acid content of 15.6 per cent, it is apparent that the frequent handling and subcutaneous injections interfered with deposition of liver fat. The choline chloride may have been slightly more irritating on subcutaneous injection than the saline, but the animals which received choline were in quite as good condition as those that had saline at the termination of the experiment. It appears, however, that choline administered subcutaneously does inhibit fat deposition in the liver under the conditions of this experiment. Another group of ten animals in this series received subcutaneously 0.5 cc each day of a suspension containing 50 mg of purified beef liver lecithine in distilled water. The lecithine was not well absorbed, and lumps developed at the sites of the injections. The average liver fatty acid content at the end of three weeks was 5.2 per cent (controls 7.4 per cent). The results of these preliminary experiments suggest that the subcutaneous administration of the factor or factors which affect deposition of liver fat in the white rat is unlikely to be satisfactory.

Effect of Some Other Substances

Amino-ethyl alcohol. Since the purified lecithine which has been used contained a small amount of amino-nitrogen, the effect of amino-ethyl alcohol was studied. The results obtained in the test animals are given in Table 35.III; the liver fatty acids of the controls averaged 14.4 per cent.

TABLE 35.III

STOCK DIET WITH FAT ADDED (40 PER CENT OF TOTAL FOOD) SUPPLEMENTED WITH AMINO-ETHYL ALCOHOL

Rat no.	Length of Exp. (days)	Total Fat Eaten (g)	Fat Eaten per Diem (g)	Wt. of Rat before (g)	Wt. of Rat after (g)	Amino-Ethyl Alcohol per Diem (g)	Per cent Fatty Acid in Liver	Iodine no.
51	20	47.5	2.4	170	167	0.036	11.0	107
52	20	50.0	2.5	196	208	0.038	10.7	104
53	21	52.5	2.5	198	190	0.038	12.7	95
54	21	52.5	2.5	185	175	0.038	10.6	92
55	21	52.5	2.5	170	172	0.038	14.4	87
56	21	51.0	2.4	164	160	0.037	16.7	90
57	21	52.5	2.5	164	170	0.038	14.8	97
58	21	52.5	2.5	194	—	0.038	6.2	86

Average = 12.1

TABLE 35.IV

STOCK DIET WITH FAT ADDED (40 PER CENT OF TOTAL FOOD) SUPPLEMENTED WITH BETAINE

Rat no.	Fat Eaten per Diem (g)	Wt. of Rat before (g)	Wt. of Rat after (g)	Betaine per Diem (g)	Per cent Fatty Acids in Liver	Iodine no.
101	2.5	160	164	0.12	5.6	70
102	2.5	158	168	0.12	10.7	79
103	2.3	170	170	0.11	6.1	116
104	2.5	180	178	0.12	3.6	114
105	2.4	190	182	0.12	4.6	120
106	2.5	200	200	0.12	5.5	98
107	2.5	212	202	0.12	3.8	146
108	2.5	216	206	0.12	7.8	96
109	2.5	212	202	0.12	5.0	109
110	2.5	234	226	0.12	5.8	137

Average = 5.9

Betaine. The activity of choline in preventing deposition of liver fat immediately focused our attention on substances of similar chemical constitution. A comprehensive study of related compounds is contemplated. It is very interesting that an apparently positive result has been obtained with betaine. The results for the betaine test animals are given in Table 35.IV (controls 15.6 per cent, ranging from 7.6 to 23.5 per cent).

DISCUSSION

The results of the experiments reported in this paper establish the fact that neither sodium nor calcium glycerophosphate nor sodium oleate, when fed daily in amounts which might be derived from 0.5 g of lecithine, inhibits the deposition of fat which takes place in the livers of control white rats under the conditions of our experiments. Choline chloride, however, added to the stock diet inhibits in some way this accumulation of fat in the liver. The possibility that oleate or glycerophosphate may influence this action of choline has not yet been investigated.

The fact that amino-ethyl alcohol, when fed daily in amounts which might be derived from 0.5 g of kephaline, does not inhibit deposition of fat in the livers of rats, suggests that kephaline plays no part in the "lecithine" effect. The apparently positive result obtained when betaine was added to the diet indicates that other compounds containing pentavalent nitrogen should be investigated.

$$(CH_3)_3 \equiv N < ^{OH}_{CH_2-CH_2OH} \qquad (CH_3)_3 \equiv N < ^{OH}_{CH_2-COOH}$$
$$\text{Choline} \qquad\qquad\qquad \text{Betaine}$$

It may be necessary to determine the relative potencies of betaine and choline and perhaps of other compounds before proceeding with the study of the physiological significance of the factor or factors which modify deposition of liver fat.

In the previous paper [91] a number of very high iodine numbers were reported for the liver fatty acids of one group of animals which received crude liver lecithine. We have encountered similar very high values in only one of the choline-fed series. While we have no ground, other than that of improbability in the light of present knowledge, for suspecting the reliability of these high iodine numbers, we wish to reserve judgment on their probable significance until a more adequate study of this aspect of the problem has been carried out. These very high values are not included in Table 35.I. In addition to the great variation between animals from different colonies and individuals from the same colony, the possibility of irregular physiological activity in commercial choline preparations must be considered in attempting to locate the causes of aberrant results. The possibility that certain specimens of liver may contain substances which interfere with determinations of iodine numbers by Wijs' procedure merits further investigation.

Since we intend to follow several of the leads suggested by the results of the experiments reported above, it will be advisable to wait for further information on certain points before expressing an opinion on the physiological significance of this action of choline chloride. We are at present attempting to determine the action of choline in various species of small animals. The deposition of liver fat in mice is apparently influenced by choline in the same way as in rats. Experiments are also already well under way in which the effect of choline (1) on the lipaemia which may be produced in diabetic dogs and (2) on the condition in these animals characterized by fatty degeneration of the liver, which has been referred to in previous communications, may be studied. Until the action of choline on depancreatized dogs has been thoroughly investigated there is no direct evidence for the attractive assumption that the mechanisms of the "lecithine" effects in diabetic dogs and normal rats are essentially similar. The results of one experiment on a depancreatized dog suggest, however, that this may prove to be the case.

While it is obvious that the effects of choline or other active substances on fatty changes in the livers of experimental animals produced by various means (phosphorus or chloroform poisoning) may prove interesting fields of investigation, it is equally evident that much more information on normal animals can profitably be obtained before studies of that kind are initiated.

In interpreting the results of these experiments, the values obtained from the analyses of the livers for total fatty acid are the only ones upon which we have relied. It is interesting, however, that in an experiment in which adequate amounts of a substance under test have been provided, the results can always be predicted from the appearances of the livers of the control and test animals. Livers containing large amounts of fatty acid are yellowish in colour, and those in which the fat content is extremely high are very friable. The livers from the test animals are approximately normal in colour, and are smaller and firmer than those from the controls.

SUMMARY

The effects of the various constituents of lecithine upon the deposition of fat in the livers of normal white rats have been determined.

The results indicate that neither the unsaturated fatty acid (sodium oleate) nor the glycerophosphate (sodium or calcium glycerophosphate) is the active factor in the "lecithine" effect. Since our purified lecithine contained a small amount of amino-nitrogen, the action of amino-ethyl alcohol was also determined. Here again the results were negative. Choline (choline chloride), on the other hand, administered by mouth has consistently inhibited the deposition of fat in the livers of the rats under the conditions of our experiments. No evidence has been obtained that choline increases the excretion of fat. In one experiment positive results have been obtained with betaine. This finding indicates that further investigation of compounds containing pentavalent nitrogen may be profitable.

36. Choline and the Dietary Production of Fatty Livers

C. H. BEST

H. J. CHANNON

JESSIE H. RIDOUT

The production of fatty livers in rats by the administration of a diet consisting of mixed grain and 40 per cent of beef fat has been demonstrated by Best, Hershey, and Huntsman [91]. The work of other authors has shown that fatty livers may be produced by feeding animals on diets containing cholesterol. Thus the results of Chalatow [184], Anitschow and Chalatow [14], Bailey [36], McMeans [543], Yuasa [823], and Kimura [452] all show directly or indirectly that diets containing cholesterol cause a change in the nature or an increase in the amounts of the liver lipoids. More recently Okey [603] showed that the dietary administration of 1 per cent of cholesterol to rats caused a large increase in the lipoid content of the liver, and in particular a remarkable rise in the amount of total cholesterol, far the greater part of which was present as cholesteryl esters. Similar results have been reported by Chanutin and Ludewig [196]. Thus fatty livers may be produced either by feeding to animals certain diets of high fat content or by inclusion in the diets of a relatively small amount of cholesterol, methods which are far less unphysiological than the action of the drugs commonly used for this purpose. Their importance is emphasized by the finding that the inclusion of choline in the diets in the relatively small amount of about 1 per cent prevents the appearance of the fatty liver which they would otherwise cause (Best and Huntsman [94]; Best and Ridout [111]). Dietary methods are now therefore available, both for producing fatty livers and for preventing them by the use of substances, sterols, fats and phosphatides, which are normal constituents of both plant and animal cells. Further, although the amounts in which these substances have been experimentally employed may be greater than are usually present in a diet, they are such as to lead one to believe that the mechanism involved

Originally appeared in the *Journal of Physiology*, LXXXI (1934), 409–21. From the School of Hygiene, University of Toronto, and the Department of Biochemistry, University of Liverpool.

may perhaps finally prove to be one of those which occur in the normal animal, and which have come to light because of the unbalancing by experiment of two factors which are antagonistic.

Best and Huntsman [94] and Best and Ridout [111] in investigating this action of choline used the Liebermann saponification method as modified by Leathes and Raper, but without removal of unsaponifiable matter, for the determination of the amount of "fat." Since the figures obtained by this method give merely the sum of the total fatty acids and the unsaponifiable substances, their results, although effectively demonstrating the preventive action of choline, provided no evidence of the changes undergone by the individual components of the "fat." The subsequent publications of Okey [603; 604] showed that the fatty liver induced by cholesterol is characterized by the appearance of large amounts of cholesteryl ester. It became of importance, therefore, to determine whether the fatty liver caused by the feeding of diets high in fat bore any relation to that caused by cholesterol feeding. This was necessary in order further to investigate the action of choline in preventing fatty livers from both these causes, since choline might be preventing the occurrence of the fatty liver because it was involved in the metabolism either of glycerides or of cholesterol, or possibly of both. Because choline occurs in the tissues generally as lecithine and sphingomyeline, it was also important to determine whether the amounts or nature of these substances in the tissues was modified by adding choline to the diet. We have therefore carried out a comprehensive study of the effects of various diets on the nature and the amounts of the individual constituents of the lipoids of different tissues of groups of rats, and at the same time have attempted to investigate the modifications of these constituents caused by giving to other groups of animals the same diets supplemented by choline. Three diets have been employed. Of these, two have been such as to cause fatty livers, one containing a high percentage of fat, the other added cholesterol, whilst the third has been an ordinary stock diet which results in no accumulation of fat in the liver. In these investigations the total ether-soluble material of the livers, hearts, lungs, spleens, kidneys and carcases of groups each of twenty to thirty animals, on the three diets, with and without added choline, has been investigated. The tissues from each group have been pooled in order to permit of the investigations being as complete as possible, and because the very large number of determinations on individual livers already carried out has shown that both the high fat diet and that containing cholesterol will cause intensely fatty livers and that choline added to these diets prevents this. In the present paper we record only the results which have been obtained on the livers, because they seem to us to advance the subject sufficiently to warrant their publication at the present stage in view of the delay which the tedious nature of the investigation of the other tissues entails.

METHODS

The diets used were based on the grain diets previously employed (32.7 per cent each of oatmeal, cornmeal, and cracked wheat with 1.9 per cent of bone meal), modified for the different experiments as set out in Table 36.I, where the other relevant figures are recorded.

TABLE 36.I
DIETARY CONDITIONS AND CHANGES IN BODY WEIGHT

Diet	No. of Rats	Average Weight before Exp. (g)	Average Weight after Exp. (g)	Duration in Days	Average Food Consumption per Day (g)
F: grain 60%, beef dripping 40%	20	188.2	193.9	23	7.8
G: as F, with 0.1 g choline chloride per rat per day	20	188.3	195.2	23	8.9
H: grain 78%, "Crisco" 20%, cholesterol 2%	29	169	165	26	9.1
J: as H, with 0.23 g choline chloride per rat per day	29	175	169	26	9.4
L: grain	20	195.5	205.1	21	11.0
M: grain, with 0.1 g choline chloride per rat per day	20	191.7	205.2	21	12.5

The animals were killed by a blow on the head 18 hours after their last meal, and the livers removed.

The weighed livers were minced with sand immediately under five volumes of absolute alcohol. The mixture was heated to boiling and filtered. Two further treatments with hot alcohol were then given, followed by one with ether. At this stage the material was reground and further extracted three times with hot ether. The combined alcohol–ether extracts were evaporated to dryness *in vacuo*, and the residue extracted with warm ether several times and the mixture filtered. Such an extract will, of course, contain large amounts of materials not of lipoid nature, nor soluble in pure ether, but soluble in ethereal solutions of phosphatides such as these. The combined ethereal extracts were concentrated and transferred to a standard flask, from which suitable aliquots were withdrawn for analysis. The unsaponifiable fraction and fatty acids were prepared as described by Channon and El Saby [187]. Free cholesterol and total cholesterol were estimated by the digitonin method on the original material and on the unsaponifiable fraction respectively. Ether-soluble phosphorus was determined by the colorimetric method after perhydrol oxidation. The total choline in the extract was assayed on the rabbit's intestine after conversion to acetylcholine.

After determination of the required fat constants, the remainder of the solution was evaporated to dryness. The residue was dissolved in four volumes of ether and precipitated by excess of acetone at room temperature. After standing for some hours, the mixture was filtered, and the residue, after washing with acetone, was redissolved in 25 per cent solution in ether and reprecipitated by acetone. After filtration, the phosphatide was dissolved in ether and its weight obtained after evaporation to dryness. The fat fraction contained in the acetone ether mother liquors was also weighed. These two fractions were then hydrolysed by boiling with a solution of sodium ethylate in absolute alcohol. From the fat fraction the unsaponifiable fraction was removed after hydrolysis and the fatty acids prepared. The fatty acids were also prepared from the phosphatide fractions. Iodine values (Rosenmund and Kuhnhenn [654]) were determined, and a separation into solid and liquid acids by the Twitchell process carried out in some cases, with subsequent determination of the iodine values of the solid and liquid acids.

RESULTS

In Table 36.II are recorded the weights of the livers of each group of experimental animals and the percentage yield of extract, together with its percentage composition; in Table 36.III the quantity of certain components in 100 g of liver is given.

TABLE 36.II

WEIGHTS OF LIVERS, YIELD AND PERCENTAGE COMPOSITION OF EXTRACTS

	F	G	H	J	L	M
Wt. of livers, g	135	133.8	246.2	220.5	132.5	132.5
Wt. of extract, %	16.86	6.46	17.93	9.40	5.42	5.27
The extract contained, %						
fatty acids	82.77	46.67	70.44	46.60	50.99	48.98
unsaponifiable matter	5.55	9.42	18.48	18.44	7.99	6.25
free sterol	1.31	3.04	1.61	2.91	3.57	3.80
total sterol	1.87	3.17	16.02	14.10	4.24	3.95
ester sterol	0.56	0.13	14.41	11.19	0.67	0.15

The method of calculating the amount of the various fatty constituents of the liver, which are shown in Table 36.III, needs a word of explanation.

TABLE 36.III

YIELDS PER 100 G OF FRESH LIVER

	F	G	H	J	L	M
Total fatty acids	13.96	2.98	12.63	4.38	2.76	2.58
Neutral fat	12.76	1.09	9.50	1.51	0.40	0.27
"Lecithine"	2.39	2.76	2.36	3.08	3.36	3.29
Total sterol	0.315	0.206	2.872	1.323	0.230	0.205
Free sterol	0.221	0.196	0.289	0.273	0.194	0.197
Cholesteryl oleate	0.158	0.020	4.350	1.768	0.036	0.008

Groups G, J, and M received choline.

The figures for "lecithine" given in that table have been calculated from the estimation of phosphorus in the original ether extract upon the arbitrary assumption that all the phosphorus was present as dioleyl lecithine (P 3.86 per cent). Calculations have also been made from the yield of fatty acids on hydrolysis of the crude acetone precipitate upon the same assumption. From comparison of the results obtained by these two methods it appears that in the case of F and H all the phosphatide has been precipitated by acetone, but that in the case of G, J, L, and M some phosphatide has remained in the mother liquor, for the figures are 11, 17, 9, and 6 per cent lower respectively than when calculated by the former method. This inference is confirmed when the calculation is made from the phosphorus content of the fractions into which the original ethereal extracts were separated. It is immaterial which figure is taken inasmuch as the effect on the figure for neutral fat is less than 0.2 per cent of the liver weight and accordingly the figure based on the ether-soluble phosphorus has been used in the calculations in Table 36.III.

The figures for neutral fat have been obtained by subtracting from the total fatty acids those present as "lecithine" (70.4 per cent oleic acid) and as cholesteryl ester (ester $\times$ 282/650), and multiplying the difference by 1.045 to convert oleic acid into triolein.

DISCUSSION

The Effects of High Fat and Cholesterol Feeding

In discussing these results, the figures for group L, which was the only group receiving a normal diet, may be taken as the standard. If we confine our attention to the two groups F and H which received diets high in fat and containing added cholesterol respectively, it is seen that although the combined figures for the fatty acids and unsaponifiable matter which would have been obtained by the Liebermann saponification method yield very similar total figures, i.e., 14.9 and 15.97 per cent respectively, these two means of producing fatty livers have given a markedly different distribution of the constituents. High fat feeding in the conditions of these experiments has caused something like a 25 per cent greater rise in neutral fat than has cholesterol administration. This large increase in neutral fat has resulted in an insignificant rise in free sterol (cf. F 0.221 with L 0.194) and a small but definite rise in cholesteryl ester (cf. F 0.158 with L 0.036). In the cholesterol-fed series H, however, the most striking effect in spite of the large increase in neutral fat is the increase in cholesteryl oleate from 0.036 in the control series L to 4.35 per cent. There is also an increase in free cholesterol to 0.289 per cent which although of smaller degree seems to be significant. It is not easy to interpret these different types of fatty liver. It rather looks as though the accumulation of free cholesterol in the liver was harmful and that its presence in abnormal amounts there caused a mobilization of neutral fat; such a mobilization might be of service for the conversion of cholesterol into its fatty acid esters and so lowering its melting point. In any case it appears to be significant that when cholesterol is fed to animals it does not appear in the liver in the free form in any greatly increased amount.

The Effect of Choline

Neutral fat. The effect of choline administered with high fat diet has been to reduce the glyceride fraction from F 12.76 per cent to G 1.09 per cent, and with the cholesterol diet from H 9.50 per cent to J 1.51 per cent. The livers of the animals receiving the stock diet (L) contained 0.40 per cent of neutral fat, and if this be taken as the control value, it is seen that although the daily amounts of choline chloride administered to the animals of these groups, G 0.1 g, J 0.23 g, respectively, have in very large measure prevented the accumulation of neutral fat, they have not quite caused a normal value. The clear deduction can be made, however, that choline administration prevents the appearance of neutral fat in the liver in diets which would otherwise cause fatty livers. Even in series M the neutral fat fraction (0.27 per cent) is less than that of L (0.40 per cent) by an amount which we are inclined to believe may be significant. If this be so, it seems forcibly to suggest that one very definite effect of choline at least is to decrease the neutral fat fraction of the liver, irrespective of the amount in which it would otherwise occur.

Cholesterol and cholesteryl esters. Choline has no effect on the free sterol of the livers of any of the groups. The slight fall in G (0.196 per cent) from F (0.221 per cent) is probably merely incidental to the fall in the neutral fat fraction. The effect on the ester fraction is, however, marked as is seen by comparing G 0.020 per cent with F 0.158 per cent, J 1.768 per cent with H 4.35 per cent, and M 0.008 per cent with L 0.036 per cent. The most striking feature of these results is that whereas choline has prevented the increase in the neutral fat fraction of the livers of the animals receiving cholesterol as effectively as it has done for those receiving the high fat diet, it has failed to prevent more than 60 per cent of the very large rise in the cholesteryl ester fraction which the former diet has caused, 1.768 per cent in group J compared with 4.350 per cent of series H, and 0.036 per cent of the control series L.

Blatherwick, Medlar, Bradshaw, Post, and Sawyer [128; 129] have produced evidence that feeding animals on whole dried liver, raw liver, or certain liver extracts causes fatty livers in rats. They found that the addition of 2 per cent of lecithine to the diet did not prevent the appearance of these fatty livers, and they contrast their results with those of Best and his colleagues. We believe that the explanation of their contradictory results may lie, in part at least, in the relatively small amount of lecithine administered. Thus the dried liver diet, as well as a number of other diets used by Blatherwick and his co-workers contain not only enough fat to cause a very fatty liver but also enough cholesterol. Hence the addition of 2 per cent of lecithine to the diets used by them, i.e. the ingestion of 30 mg of extra choline daily by each rat, is an amount which would not be expected to be effective, because it has to oppose the combined effects of the two different factors in their diets, each of which can independently cause fatty livers, since each rat receiving the dried liver diet ingested 4.16 g of fat and 87 mg of cholesterol daily. We shall defer further comment on the results of Blatherwick until certain additional experimental work has been completed.

The phosphatide fraction. The effect of choline administration is best seen from Table 36.IV, in which the figures for ether-soluble phosphorus are compared with the figures for the sum of the total fatty acid and total cholesterol contents arranged in descending order of magnitude.

These figures confirm existing knowledge that the percentage of phosphatide in general falls with fatty infiltration although the results with groups G and J are somewhat anomalous. They show that the percentage

TABLE 36.IV

LIPID COMPONENTS IN 100 G LIVER

	H	F	J	G	L	M
Sum of total fatty acids and cholesterol, g	15.50	14.27	5.70	3.19	2.98	2.78
Total fatty acids, g	12.63	13.96	4.38	2.98	2.76	2.58
Ether-soluble phosphorus, mg	91.1	92.3	119.0	106.5	129.7	127.0

Groups G, J, and M received choline.

of phosphatide is greater in the livers of the groups which received choline G and J, compared with the corresponding control groups F and H. On the other hand, choline administration has not affected the phosphatide percentage of group M. Bearing in mind that the water content of livers is reduced by fat infiltration, the phosphatide increases in groups G and J are actually much greater when referred to dry weight than appears when the phosphatide is expressed as percentage of the fresh tissue as in Table 36.IV. The lack of increase in group M compared with group L makes interpretation of these phosphatide changes difficult. It may suggest that the effect of choline in increasing the phosphatide percentages in groups G and J over groups L and M is possibly only an indirect one resulting from the action of choline in preventing the fatty liver.

The fatty acids. The iodine value of the fatty acids of the beef fat used for groups F and G was 40.4, and of the "Crisco" used for H and J 65.8. The stock diet of grain contained very little fat and its nature was not investigated. In Table 36.V are recorded the iodine values of the fatty acids of the fat and phosphatide fractions, together with those of the solid and liquid acids of the latter, determined by the Twitchell method.

TABLE 36.V

EFFECT OF DIETARY CHOLINE ON THE FATTY ACIDS OF THE PHOSPHATIDE
FRACTION OF THE LIVER LIPIDS

	Iodine Values of Fatty Acids		Phosphatide Acids		Iodine Values	
	Fat fraction	Phosphatide fraction	% solid	% liquid	Solid	Liquid
F	73.8	135	36.6	63.4	14	219.1
G	72.6	130.7	41.0	59.0	9	205.3
H	90.0	130.2	35.8	64.2	19	196.3
J	87.5	124.4	lost	61.7	21	176.2
L	92.0	—	42.6	57.4	16	186.2
M	88.4	—	43.1	56.9	12	179.5

The general deduction to be made from these figures is that choline administration has materially affected neither the distribution of the phosphatide fatty acids nor their iodine values. The iodine values of the fat fractions of F and G, and of H and J, reflect the influence of the dietary fats. The other variations which appear in the iodine values, such as that of the phosphatide fatty acids of J, 124.4, and in the relatively high values of those of the solid fraction of the phosphatide acids and the low value of the liquid acids of the phosphatide in J and M, we believe to be occasioned by unavoidable delays in working up of the small amounts of material available, and to be regarded as of no significance.

The choline content of the livers. Determinations were made of the choline in the total extracts and in the protein residues of the livers by biological assay on the rabbit's intestine after conversion to acetylcholine. These investigations, in which Mr. J. P. Fletcher has taken a considerable part, will be described in detail in a subsequent communication, in which the question of the amounts of free and combined choline present in tissues will be fully discussed. Acid hydrolysis of the protein residues and subsequent assay following conversion to acetylcholine showed that the amount of choline in the residues of F, G, H and J was on the average only 2.4 per cent of the total choline in the ethereal extracts prepared as described (extreme values 4.1 and 1.4 per cent). Further, the total choline content of the phosphatide precipitates averaged 92.4 per cent of that of the ethereal extracts from which they had been obtained (extreme values 87.3, 98.1 per cent). Attempts to determine the free choline in the ethereal extracts gave an average value of 4.92 per cent of the total (extremes 4.61, 5.82 per cent), and a similar small average figure for free choline, namely 5.5 per cent of the total, was found in the phosphatide precipitates. We thus incline to the view that it is probable that free choline is not present in liver in significant amounts, and that the amounts found have been produced by slight hydrolysis of the phosphatides present in the extracts. For the purposes of discussion, therefore, it appears legitimate to regard our extracts as having contained all the choline of the original tissues, and further that this choline is entirely present as phosphatide, for the small amount not present in the phosphatide fraction (7.6 per cent of the total) is explained by the fact that not all the phosphatide was precipitated by acetone as explained on p. 396. It is therefore possible to compare the effect of choline on the nature as opposed to the amount of phosphatide fraction, and to determine whether its administration has affected the amounts of lecithine or sphingomyeline at the expense of the kephaline and the other unknown constituents of liver phosphatides. In Table 36.VI are recorded the total amounts of choline found, the choline calculated on

TABLE 36.VI

EFFECT OF DIETARY CHOLINE ON THE CHOLINE CONTENT OF THE PHOSPHATIDES OF THE LIVER

	F	G	H	J	L	M
(1) mg P/100 g liver	92.4	106.6	91.2	119.0	129.5	127.0
(2) Choline (calc. P × 121/31)	361	416	356	465	506	496
(3) Choline found	177	219	201	252	266	281
Choline found as a percentage of (2)	49.1	52.7	56.5	54.3	52.6	56.6

Groups G, J, and M received choline.

the basis that the ether-soluble phosphorus is entirely present as lecithine, and the ratio of the choline found to the latter figure.

Comparison of G with F, and J with H shows that choline administration has not affected the proportions in which the choline-containing phosphatides occur in the general phosphatide mixture. The figures for M show a greater divergence from the control series L, but it appears tolerably certain that this difference is not outside the experimental error. We incline to the view, therefore, that the composition of the phosphatide mixture is unaltered by the administration of choline.

Conclusions

These findings therefore show essentially that the inclusion of suitable amounts of choline in the diet used will prevent that occurrence in the liver of the abnormal amounts of neutral fat and in part of the cholesteryl esters, which would otherwise result. It is early yet to form a view as to the mechanism of this action. Previous work in the Toronto Laboratories has shown that the fat excretion of animals on a high fat diet is not increased by choline administration and therefore neither the total absorption nor the excretion is involved. The results on the other tissues, so far as they are complete, suggest that the effect of choline is on the liver only, and for the purposes of discussion this will be considered as if it were proven. The role of the liver in the metabolism of fat is little understood beyond the essential fact that the liver appears of prime importance in this connection, as is shown by the mobilization of fat to it caused by the action of various drugs and pathological conditions and its ability selectively to absorb unsaturated acids from the blood after fat absorption. In the case of diets of high fat content the effect of choline might be concerned either with the transport of fatty acids from the liver or directly or indirectly with their oxidation. With the fatty livers induced by the cholesterol feeding the former hypothesis might be applicable, while the catabolism or excretion of cholesterol might also be involved.

The possible function of lecithine in the transport of fatty acids from the liver to the tissues for oxidative purposes has often been discussed, especially in the light of the hypothesis of Leathes that one of the functions of the liver may be the preliminary preparation of the fatty acids for more ready use by the tissues by rendering them less saturated. If lecithine does play an active role in fat transport, it is conceivable that the provision of extra choline in a diet containing much fat might explain the preventive action of choline. On the other hand, there is no obvious reason why fat should accumulate in the liver on a high fat diet. Further, the action of choline in preventing the "cholesterol" fatty liver is perhaps unlikely to be concerned in a mechanism involving lecithine as a carrier of fatty acids. These two types of fatty liver involve essentially two different substances, the fatty acid and cholesterol, and it seems reasonable to seek an explanation of the action of choline in a common process in which both may be concerned. The most probable suggestion appears to be that choline in some way or other accelerates either directly or indirectly the oxidation of fatty acids and cholesterol by the liver itself, and to this problem we are giving our attention.

But apart from speculations, the fact is established that even though the fatty liver contains its normal amount of choline as phosphatide it is yet fatty, and therefore if choline should prove to be normally involved in fat removal either directly or indirectly this implies that little of the liver phosphatide may be called upon to supply choline. Such a result is to be expected, because the studies of the French school of Mayer, Schaeffer, and Terroine have repeatedly shown that even in death from inanition, the phosphatides of such tissues as liver cannot be called upon for energy requirements. A further point emerges also. If choline provides in any way a means whereby fat infiltration in the liver is normally controlled, the occurrence of fatty livers produced by diet implies a limited ability of the animal to synthesize the base for this purpose. Apart from fat oxidation, choline might be counteracting some effect of fat infiltration in interfering with the formation or oxidation of carbohydrate by the liver, and in this connection the results of Best and Hershey [89] need consideration. These authors showed that when lecithine was given to depancreatized dogs which were showing the signs of failure of liver function, the urinary sugar excretion markedly increased. If carbohydrate formation or oxidation were involved, the removal of the two types of fatty liver by choline might result in this indirect manner.

These results also show that choline is far more active in preventing the accumulation of neutral fat in the fatty livers than of cholesterol. This is seen in the F and G and H and J series. In G 0.1 g of choline chloride per day has reduced the neutral fat fraction from 12.76 to 1.09 per cent, a reduction of 11.67 g/100 g liver; in J 0.23 g of choline chloride has reduced it by 7.99 per cent, approximately to the same level as that of G. From the results with G this fall in neutral fat by 7.99 per cent would require less than 0.1 g of choline chloride. The J series received, however, 0.23 g, and this increased amount has merely resulted in the removal from the liver of 2.58 g of cholesteryl ester, leaving still in the liver 1.768 g. It must not be overlooked, however, that the effect of choline may be on the fatty acids of the neutral fat only. Cholesterol may accumulate as ester only in the liver for reasons which have been mentioned on p. 397. If this were so, and if choline affected the oxidation or translocation of the neutral fat fraction only, possibly the removal of that fraction would entail the disappearance by excretion of the cholesteryl esters.

Summary

1. Three diets have been given for periods of 21–26 days to groups each of 20 or 30 rats. These diets have been (*a*) a diet containing 40 per cent of fat; (*b*) one containing 2 per cent of cholesterol; (*c*) the normal stock diet. In three other groups the animals have received similar diets over a similar period, but each rat has had also 0.1–0.23 g of choline chloride daily.

2. The total lipoid material from the pooled livers of each group has been prepared and analysed for its content of free and combined sterol, neutral fat, phosphatide, and choline.

3. The fatty liver caused by high fat feeding is occasioned entirely by increase in the neutral fat fraction. That caused by cholesterol feeding is characterized by the appearance of excessive amounts of cholesteryl esters, together with a large increase in neutral fat. The phosphatide content of both these types of fatty livers varies inversely with their total lipoid content.

4. Choline administration prevents the appearance of both types of fatty liver, from which it is deduced that choline is concerned in the metabolism both of neutral fat and cholesterol.

5. The percentage of phosphatide in the livers is increased by choline administration probably indirectly and because choline prevents the occurrence of the fatty liver.

6. Estimations of choline by biological assay after conversion to acetylcholine show that choline administration does not increase the proportions in which the phosphatides containing choline (lecithine and sphingomyeline) occur in the phosphatide mixture.

7. Choline administration has had no significant effect on the degree of unsaturation of the fatty acids of the fat or phosphatide fractions.

8. The possible mechanism by which choline exerts its effect on the amount of the liver lipoids is discussed.

Acknowledgments

We wish to express our gratitude to Dr. J. G. FitzGerald, Dean of the Faculty of Medicine in the University of Toronto, for his kind interest in this work.

We also wish to record our thanks to Mr. J. Truax for his valuable technical assistance.

37. The Distribution of Choline

JOHN PALMER FLETCHER

CHARLES HERBERT BEST

OMOND McKILLOP SOLANDT

Interest in the total choline content of animal and plant tissues has been aroused by recent investigations which have demonstrated the importance of choline as a dietary constituent. Previous estimates of the choline content of various tissues have been largely concerned with the determination of free choline (Alles [11]; Guggenheim [337]). More recently there have been some attempts to measure free and bound choline separately. The methods used for the separation of free and bound choline are complex and tedious and the separation is apparently unnecessary for the purpose of dietetic experiments on normal animals. Consequently an attempt has been made to evolve a reasonably accurate and rapid method for the estimation of the total choline content of foods. The present paper is concerned with the details of the method devised and some of the results obtained with it. In addition to measuring the total choline content of many materials which have been incorporated in experimental diets for rats and dogs, the total choline content of the different tissues of the normal white rat was investigated.

METHOD

After careful consideration of all the chemical and biological methods for the estimation of choline it was decided that extraction, acetylation and assay of the resultant acetylcholine, using the isolated intestine of the rabbit, was the most advantageous method for the present purpose. A description of the method finally evolved may be divided into two parts. First, the digestion of the tissue, hydrolysis of choline-containing compounds and extraction and acetylation of the choline; second, the biological assay of the resulting acetylcholine.

DIGESTION AND ACETYLATION

The hydrochloric acid digestion used by Best and McHenry [106] for the estimation of histamine in tissues has proved to be equally satisfactory

Originally appeared in the *Biochemical Journal*, XXIX (1935), 2278–84. From the Department of Physiological Hygiene, School of Hygiene, University of Toronto.

for the determination of choline. This procedure breaks up the tissue, hydro-lyses the choline-containing compounds and extracts the choline without destroying measurable amounts.

The technique finally adopted is as follows: 2–4 g or more fresh tissue or other material are rapidly weighed, minced, and transferred to a 1-litre, round-bottomed flask; 20–40 ml of 18 per cent HCl are then added and the mixture is boiled under a reflux condenser for 1 hour. After the boiling, 30–60 ml of 95 per cent ethyl alcohol are added and the mixture of water, alcohol, acid, and ester is removed *in vacuo* at about 90°. The residue is then extracted with a small amount of 95 per cent alcohol and finally with absolute alcohol. The alcohol is removed *in vacuo* as before.

The residue, which has been carefully dried after the final extraction with absolute alcohol, is then acetylated by the method of Abderhalden and Paffrath [1]. 25 ml glacial acetic acid and 5 ml acetic anhydride are added to the residue and the mixture is boiled under a reflux condenser for 2 hours. The acetic acid and anhydride are then removed *in vacuo* at about 90° and the residue extracted once with absolute alcohol. The acety-lated residue is finally transferred to a volumetric flask by alternate small washings of alcohol and water until the total volume is 100 ml. This alco-holic solution is then diluted as required for assay.

Each step in this procedure has been tested by control experiments. The results of these experiments may be summarized as follows.

1. Many experiments on the destruction of choline during tissue auto-lysis suggest that no special precautions are necessary to prevent loss of choline between the time of death of the animal and the beginning of diges-tion of the tissue.

2. Varying the time of acid digestion from 30 to 90 min. caused no change in the value for the choline content of pancreas, suggesting that hydrolysis and extraction are complete in the shorter time.

3. Pure choline chloride is not measurably affected by 90 min. boiling with 18 per cent HCl.

4. The method of acetylation repeatedly gave perfect acetylation of pure choline chloride solutions within the limits of accuracy of the biological assay.

5. Recovery of choline chloride added to tissues has always been complete within the limits of accuracy of the method.

THE BIOLOGICAL ASSAY

The isolated intestine of the rabbit was used as the test object for all assays. The intestine was mounted in a double intestine bath of conventional design and was bathed in Ringer-Tyrode's solution containing no glucose. It was found that better results were obtained with the duodenum than with any other part of the intestine. The intestine was definitely more reliable when removed under ether anaesthesia than when it was obtained from the dead animal. Purity of the Tyrode's solution and accuracy of temperature control are of course essential to satisfactory assaying.

All assays were done against a standard acetylcholine solution. The potency of this standard was frequently checked against fresh solutions and against freshly acetylated choline.

The accuracy of the biological assay was tested by assaying other dilutions of the standard against that ordinarily used. The results of these tests never showed an error greater than 10 per cent and there did not seem to be any significant constant error. To attain this accuracy it is essential that doses of acetylcholine be chosen which will cause a contraction which is about 75 per cent of the maximum. The concentration of acetylcholine necessary to elicit such a contraction varies considerably with different preparations but is usually one part of acetylcholine in 1 to 3×10^{-8} parts of solution.

In discussing the accuracy of the biological assay of the acetylated tissue residues, a great many interfering substances must be considered (Chang and Gaddum [186]). The prolonged heating and exposure to hydrochloric acid involved in the digestion process almost certainly destroy the adenosine derivatives (Drury and Szent-Györgyi [264]), the substance P (Euler and Gaddum [292]) and callicrein (Frey and Kraut [312]; Kraut et al. [473]). Two samples of creatinine were tested on the rabbit intestine. In doses up to 5000 times the usual dose of acetylcholine they caused no contraction at all.

The method of extraction used does not destroy histamine so that all the histamine from the tissues appears in the final solution. The rabbit intestine is very insensitive to histamine, but in order to be certain that the histamine would not have any significant effect on the results the histamine/acetylcholine ratio was determined by direct assay. Ratios were also obtained for choline and betaine. The results of these assays are given in Table 37.I.

Among other substances which might interfere are acetate ions and ethyl alcohol. In most of the assays performed the amount of acetylcholine present was so great that, in the solution actually used for assay, the concentration of these substances was entirely negligible. In all cases where the concentration of acetylcholine was low enough to suggest some danger of interference, the solutions were assayed both before and after the addition

TABLE 37.I

POTENCY RATIOS DETERMINED WITH THE
ISOLATED INTESTINE OF THE RABBIT

Material	Dose
Acetylcholine	1
Acetyl-β-methylcholine	1.7
Histamine	1,300
	2,700
	3,250
Choline	3,500
	4,200
	5,500
	6,100
Betaine	70,000

(The figures given are the dose of the
material required to cause a contraction of
the intestine of the same magnitude as that
caused by a unit dose of acetylcholine.)

of atropine to the perfusing fluid. In addition to the assay after atropine, some of the solutions were assayed before acetylation.

This combination of acid digestion, acetylation, and assay on the isolated intestine of the rabbit seems to result in a method for the estimation of the total choline content of tissues which is quite specific for choline. The accuracy of the results obtained is probably limited chiefly by the accuracy of the biological assay in all cases where the amount of choline in the substance being examined is moderately large. Where the amount of choline present is very small the presence of interfering substances may produce an appreciable error. The maximum error in the assay of the acetylated tissue residues is apparently about ±15 per cent since duplicate assays have occasionally differed by almost 30 per cent. With careful technique differences of this magnitude are very rarely encountered. In most of the present work duplicate assays were done on at least two samples of the material being analysed so that the average result should be correct within less than ±10 per cent.

RESULTS

The results which are reported here include the total choline content of the tissues of the normal white rat, of a variety of other animal tissues and of some materials used in experimental diets for rats and dogs. In addition, many other total choline determinations, done by the method which has been outlined, have been or will be reported in other communications. (Best et al. [80]; Best, MacLean and Ridout [108]; Best, Huntsman, McHenry, and Ridout [96]; McHenry [528], etc.)

The Total Choline Content of Rat Tissues

The results of the choline estimations on rat tissues are given in Table 37.II. The rats used were all young adult white rats of the Wistar Institute strain. They had been reared at the Connaught Laboratories Farm on a commercial "balanced ration." The average weight of the rats used was about 200 g. The rats were starved for 24 hours before use. In most cases corresponding tissues from several rats were pooled for the choline estimations.

TABLE 37.II

TOTAL CHOLINE CONTENT OF RAT TISSUES (Adult, white.)

No.	Tissue	No. of Exps.	Total no. of Rats	Average Choline Content mg/100 g
1	spermatic fluid	2	5	514
2	spinal cord	2	2	370
3	brain	4	10	325
4	adrenals	6	15	304
5	cerebellum	2	5	296
6	cerebral hemispheres	2	4	274
7	liver	28	28	260
8	pancreas	5	14	232
9	pituitary	4	8	224
10	kidneys	8	9	202
11	thyroid	4	11	167
12	lungs	3	5	164
13	heart	4	8	158
14	lymph glands	1	3	152
15	stomach	3	4	152
16	spleen	4	7	151
17	small intestine	5	6	142
18	large intestine	2	3	139
19	salivary glands	1	2	131
20	tongue	2	6	123
21	thymus	2	3	113
22	skeletal muscle	4	9	100
23	uterus	3	5	74
24	skin	2	2	64
25	bone	2	4	44
26	connective tissue	1	1	40
27	fat	5	6	23
28	blood—starved	3	4	22
	fed	1	1	31

No difference was detected between the choline contents of tissues from male and female animals.

The tissues are listed in the table in order of choline content. The results show that sperm-containing fluid from the seminal vesicles has the highest choline content of any tissue examined. This high choline content makes the values obtained for epididymis, ductus deferens and seminal vesicles of little significance since the result probably depends largely upon the content of seminal fluid.

The results obtained for the various parts of the central nervous system are quite in keeping with the high phospholipin content of these structures. It is interesting to note that the adrenal gland has approximately the same choline content as the other structures of nervous origin.

The average value given for the choline content of the liver is based on many more estimations than are the other results. In one experiment the livers of 24 rats were tested individually. These rats had been on an adequate mixed diet and were fully grown, averaging 250 g in weight. The average choline content of the livers of these 24 rats was 260 mg per 100 g of fresh tissue.

The figure for the choline content of rat's pancreas may be too low since considerable difficulty was experienced in separating the pancreas from the connective tissue in which it is embedded.

The acetylated product from the lymph glands gave a very large, delayed contraction of the intestine after the contraction due to acetylcholine had subsided. This delayed contraction was not eliminated by atropine. Although the delayed contraction was not considered in calculating the result it is possible that the substance causing the contraction may have affected the result obtained.

The fat used in the choline estimations was all intra-abdominal fat and was obtained from around the kidneys, testicles, or uterus and from the mesentery.

The Total Choline Content of other Animal Tissues

In Table 37.III are given the total choline contents of a variety of tissues from animals other than the rat. Most of these results require no comment. The results for the choline content of dog stomach were obtained

TABLE 37.III

TOTAL CHOLINE CONTENT OF VARIOUS ANIMAL TISSUES

Animal	Tissue	No. of Samples	No. of Determinations	Choline Content mg/100 g
Ox	liver	1	2	270
	pituitary—anterior lobe	3	3	259
	posterior lobe	3	3	217
	pancreas	7	26	230
	muscle	1	1	76
	blood (defibrinated)	1	2	13
	fat	2	3	0.5–2.6
Dog	liver	4	19	230
	stomach	2	4	90
	blood (whole)	5	10	34
Pig	pancreas	1	4	280
	bacon (cured side bacon)	1	1	44
	fat (from cooking bacon)	1	2	6
	lard	1	2	1
Codfish	muscle	2	2	78

on material prepared for histamine assay (Gavin *et al.* [318]). This process involves neutralization and filtration, which is not included in the ordinary technique for choline estimations, so the result may be slightly lower than would otherwise be the case.

The total choline content given for dog's blood is the average of 10 determinations on 5 samples of blood from 4 different dogs. The dogs were not starved before the blood was drawn. The results obtained ranged from 27 to 39 mg of choline per 100 ml of whole blood, with an average value of 34 mg per 100 ml.

The Total Choline Content of Various Foods

The total choline content of a considerable number of foods has been investigated in a search for suitable ingredients for low-choline diets for rats and dogs. The results of the total choline estimations on some of these materials are given in Table 37.IV. Those substances which are stated to contain no choline contain less than 0.1 mg per 100 g of material. The acetylated products from sugar and potato starch caused a smooth, rapid contraction of the intestine, not unlike that caused by acetylcholine, but

TABLE 37.IV

TOTAL CHOLINE CONTENT OF VARIOUS CEREALS AND OTHER MATERIALS
USED IN EXPERIMENTAL DIETS

Material	Remarks	Choline Content mg/100 g
Flour	White wheat flour	140
Dog biscuit	Spratt's commercial grade	130
Oxo	Commercial meat extract	105
Rice	Polished	94
Milk powder	Dried, skimmed milk	90
Bovril	Commercial meat extract	78
Rice flour	Various commercial brands	73–65
Caseinogen	"Lister's prepared casein"	70
Bone meal	Commercial grade	30
Washed bran	—	28
Corn starch	—	25
Cheese	Canadian cheddar	19
Egg albumin	—	18
Rice starch	Various commercial brands	15–4.3
Butter	Fresh creamery butter	13
Caseinogen	British Drug Houses, "fat- and vitamin-free"	3.5
Egg white	White separated from hard-boiled eggs	2.0
Cellu flour	Ground cellulose	1
Edestin	Pfanstiehl, "pure"	1
Agar-agar	Various commercial brands	1.6–0.8
Crisco	Hydrogenated vegetable oils	0.4
Potato starch	Various commercial brands	0
Cane sugar	Various commercial brands	0
Mazola	Refined corn oil	0
Olive oil	—	0

this contraction was not diminished by atropine. Hence sugar and potato starch were considered to contain no significant amount of choline.

In Table 37.V are given the total choline contents of a variety of vitamin-

TABLE 37.V

TOTAL CHOLINE CONTENT OF VITAMIN CONCENTRATES AND VITAMIN-RICH FOODS

Material	Remarks	Choline Content mg/100 g
Baker's yeast	Dried and powdered	270
Brewer's yeast	Dried and powdered	240
Radiomalt	—	64
Turnip	Fresh—used as source of vitamin C	42
Vitamin B₁ concentrate	Prepared according to method of Kinnersley and Peters (4 samples)	22–8
Cod-liver oil concentrate	Vitamin A—500,000, vitamin D—3,000 International Units per g	14
Tomato juice	Various commercial brands	9.8–6.6
Vitamin E oil	Unsaponifiable matter of wheat germ	4.0
Vitamin B₁ concentrate	Fuller's earth adsorbate from an extract of rice polishings	1.2

rich foods and vitamin concentrates which were investigated in connection with the preparation of the diets low in choline.

SUMMARY

A method for the estimation of the total choline content of tissues is described. The method consists of digestion of the tissue with hydrochloric acid, acetylation of the extracted choline, and assay of the resulting acetylcholine on the isolated intestine of the rabbit. The use of the hydrochloric acid digestion is the only novel part of the method. Acetylation and assay are carried out by well-established procedures.

The total choline contents of the various tissues of the normal white rat, of several tissues from other animals and of many dietary constituents of both animal and vegetable origin have been determined by this method.

38. The Effects of Cholesterol and Choline on Liver Fat

C. H. BEST

JESSIE H. RIDOUT

The results of the first investigation of this problem (Best and Ridout [111]) indicated that large doses of choline or betaine inhibited the deposition of "fat" in the liver produced by feeding cholesterol. These results were confirmed and extended by Best, Channon, and Ridout [80], who noted that under certain experimental conditions the esters of glycerol were more readily affected than those of cholesterol. Channon and Wilkinson [194] found, however, that in certain short-term experiments the rate of removal of cholesteryl esters was not accelerated by choline, while a very slight effect was exerted on the glyceride fraction. These results which have been discussed by Best and Channon [79] were due in part to the low glyceride content of the livers at the beginning of the experiment and in part to the short period of observation. Furthermore, added choline may exert relatively little effect when naturally occurring lipotropic factors are present in appreciable amounts in the diets used. Under more favourable conditions (Best and Ridout [112]) choline accelerates the removal of the esters of both glycerol and cholesterol. Beeston, Channon, and Wilkinson [59] have recently confirmed the finding that choline inhibits the accumulation of both kinds of ester which is produced by feeding large doses of cholesterol.

This paper contains a further study of the action of choline on cholesteryl esters and glyceride in the liver made fatty by cholesterol. Particular attention has been paid to the effect of choline on the rate of disappearance of cholesteryl esters. The use of smaller doses of cholesterol has enabled us to demonstrate a more rapid and more extensive action of choline on these esters than previously.

EXPERIMENTAL RESULTS AND COMMENTS

I. *Experiments with Continued Administration of Cholesterol*

(a) *Effect of choline when a relatively small dose of cholesterol is*

Originally appeared in the *Journal of Physiology,* LXXXVI (1936), 343–52. From the School of Hygiene, University of Toronto.

continued throughout experiment. In this experiment 109 rats were placed on a diet consisting of mixed grains, bone meal (2.5 per cent) and beef fat (20 per cent). Fifty mg of cholesterol were added to the daily ration of each rat. After 53 days the average liver fat in twenty of the animals was determined (Table 38.I). All of the remaining animals were transferred

TABLE 38.I

EFFECT OF CHOLESTEROL AND CHOLINE ADMINISTRATION ON LIVER LIPIDS

No. of Rats	Duration of Exp. days	Av. Change in Wt. (g)	Av. Daily Intake			Cholesterol		Glyceride as Triolein (%)	
			Food (g)	Cholesterol (mg)	Choline (mg)	Free (%)	Ester as Oleate (%)		
20	53	+2	10	50	—	0.25	1.81	5.44	Preparatory period
14	18	−17	8	41	—	0.28	3.27	9.67	Test period
14	18	−26	7	35	87	0.30	0.65	1.27	"
15	32	−35	7	37	—	0.28	3.16	7.15	"
15	32	−33	6	32	81	0.28	0.31	0.94	"
16	42	−44	7	37	—	0.29	3.44	3.63	"
15	42	−34	6	32	81	0.28	0.34	0.54	"

Average initial weight was 199 g

In this and the following tables under "Glyceride" is included that portion of the total fatty acids present as simple glyceride and not as phosphorylated fat (lecithine etc.) nor as cholesteryl ester. The figures for total fatty acid and for lecithine etc. are not dealt with in this paper and so are not included in the tables.

to a diet low in choline (casein 11.5 per cent, egg white 3.5 per cent, beef fat 20 per cent, sucrose 58.3 per cent, salt mixture 4.8 per cent, agar 1.9 per cent, and vitamins A, D, and B_1). Cholesterol feeding was continued and the various groups ingested from 31.5 to 40.5 mg daily: slight variation in cholesterol intake does not produce a significant difference in liver fat. Choline was added to the diets of half of the animals and groups were examined after 18, 32, and 42 days. The behaviour of the glyceride fraction of the livers is very interesting in this experiment. The preliminary rise after transfer of the animals to the diet low in choline is the usual reaction of liver fat when the supply of choline and other liptropic factors is reduced. This effect is consistently observed when animals are transferred from a diet rich in fat and naturally occurring lipotropic factors to one free from both, e.g., sucrose only (Best and Huntsman [95]). The subsequent fall in the glyceride content of the livers of the animals which did not receive choline may be due, in part, to the appropriation of fatty acid from the glyceride by the cholesterol. While it appears unlikely, from unpublished data, that this fall in glyceride is due to depletion of body fat the possibility must also be considered in this experiment. The effect of choline on the glyceride fraction is typical. The change in cholesteryl esters is very definite. Without choline there is a prolonged rise while with choline a decrease is observed.

(b) *Effect of choline when a larger dose of cholesterol is continued throughout experiment*. In this experiment 105 rats were placed on the low choline diet and 95 mg of cholesterol were added to the daily ration of each rat.

[A table and a figure have been omitted for brevity. After 24 days, liver fat was determined on 15 animals (glycerides 8.24 per cent, cholesteryl esters 3.10 per cent). The remaining rats were fed the same diet and choline (85 mg daily) was given to half the animals. An attempt was made to keep the caloric intake of the two groups the same. Groups of 15 rats were killed after 18, 27, and 58 days on the test diets. The cholesteryl esters at first increased rapidly even when choline was present. Later, the effect of choline, which in the case of glycerides was obvious from the first, was well demonstrated on the cholesteryl esters too. For instance, at the end of 58 days the glycerides and cholesteryl esters in the group without the supplement of choline were 6.10 and 7.59 per cent respectively; the corresponding values for those receiving choline were 2.67 and 3.96 per cent.]

(c) *Low choline diet with 10 per cent protein*. In this experiment seventy-five rats were placed on the diet low in choline, but the protein content was reduced from 15 to 10 per cent and the carbohydrate correspondingly increased. Each animal had 100 mg of cholesterol. After 25 days the liver fat was determined on the pooled livers of eighteen rats. Half the remaining animals were given choline. Some of the animals were killed after 18 days and some after 40 days (Figure 70).

There was no significant difference in the cholesterol (70 mg) intake of the four groups during the test period.

II. *Experiments with Cholesterol Administration Discontinued*

Three experiments of this type will be described briefly.

(a) In the first the animals were placed on the low choline diet, with 167 mg of cholesterol added, for 14 days. The test period, with cholesterol discontinued, was 12 days. Two groups received sucrose only, while two were given sucrose (80 per cent) and fat (20 per cent). One of each of the two groups was supplied with choline. The results are shown in Table 38.II.

(b) In the second of these experiments 112 rats were placed on the low choline diet with 200 mg of cholesterol added for a period of 23 days. At this time the cholesteryl ester in the pooled livers of fifteen rats had reached a value of 7.51 per cent and the glyceride 18.89 per cent. Cholesterol feeding was discontinued and choline (100 mg daily) was given to half the animals. A preliminary account of this experiment was reported previously (Best and Ridout [112]); the results are illustrated in Figure 71.

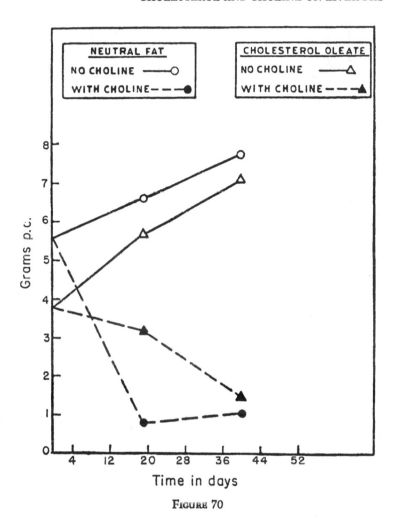

FIGURE 70

TABLE 38.II

EFFECT OF DIETARY CHOLINE ON LIVER LIPIDS

No. of Rats	Duration of Exp. days	Av. Change in Wt. (g)	Av. Daily Intake			Cholesterol		Glyceride as Triolein (%)	
			Food (g)	Cholesterol (mg)	Choline (mg)	Free (%)	Ester as Oleate (%)		
20	14	+4	10	167	—	0.24	2.58	6.09	Preparatory period
15	12	−32	10	—	—	0.24	3.83	6.81	Test period
14	12	−31	9	—	90	0.27	3.00	1.44	,,
13	12	−33	9	—	—	0.28	3.42	6.94	,,
14	12	−25	9	—	103	0.26	3.13	2.10	,,

Average initial weight was 190 g

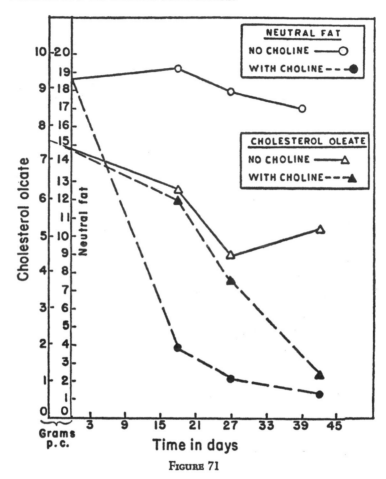

FIGURE 71

(c) In the third experiment an attempt was made to keep the glyceride at a low level during the preparatory period by supplying a small amount of choline (Table 38.III). During this time the animals received the stock

TABLE 38.III

CHOLINE IN PREVENTIVE AND CURATIVE STUDIES

No. of Rats	Duration of Exp. days	Av. Change in Wt. (g)	Av. Daily Intake			Cholesterol		Glyceride as triolein (%)	
			Food (g)	Cholesterol (mg)	Choline (mg)	Free (%)	Ester as oleate (%)		
20	45	—	9	46	23	0.26	1.02	4.43	Preparatory period
16	18	−10	9	—	—	0.23	0.38	6.74	Test period
16	18	−24	8	—	83	0.23	0.02	0.58	,,
17	27	−17	9	—	—	0.24	0.20	4.77	,,
17	27	−24	8	—	83	0.24	0.06	0.61	,,
			Average initial weight was 182 g						

grain diet, beef fat (20 per cent) and 23 mg of choline daily, together with 46 mg of cholesterol. In the test period the diet low in choline was provided and cholesterol feeding was discontinued; the choline for half the animals was increased and eliminated from the diet of the remainder. In both groups the cholesteryl esters of the liver decreased. The rate of fall was slightly but definitely greater in the animals receiving choline. The glyceride content in the rats without choline after a slight increase was at approximately the same level on the twenty-seventh day as at the beginning of the test period. These results provide further evidence that even in the absence of dietary choline the cholesteryl esters decrease rapidly when cholesterol feeding is discontinued. There is, of course, a certain amount of non-choline lipotropic factor present in this diet, but since it has not caused a decrease in glyceride there is no reason to believe that it is exerting any effect on the cholesteryl esters. All available data indicate that more choline is required to affect cholesteryl esters than glyceride.

DISCUSSION

The rapid decrease in the glyceride content of the "cholesteryl" fatty liver and the much slower fall in cholesteryl esters when choline is supplied appears to support the suggestion (Best, Channon, and Ridout [80]; Best and Ridout [112]) that the primary effect of this substance is on the glyceride fraction. In the short experiments referred to above (Exp. II *a* and Table 38.II), choline produced no effect on cholesteryl esters while the glyceride fraction was very definitely affected. Furthermore, it has been consistently observed that the dose of choline required to influence deposition of cholesteryl esters is appreciably greater than in the case of glyceride. All the results reported here may be interpreted on the basis that an effect on the neutral fat precedes that on the cholesteryl ester fraction, but the inference from this suggestion that the glyceride must be reduced to very low levels before an effect on the cholesteryl esters is observed is not justified. These latter have shown a definite fall in several cases while an abundance of glyceride is present—and presumably available. The possibility that choline affects both cholesteryl esters and glyceride directly has, therefore, not been eliminated. . . .

When cholesterol feeding is discontinued the cholesteryl ester content of the liver tends to fall, whether choline is given or not (Exp. II *b* and *c*), while the glyceride content, if choline is not given, is maintained at a high level until the supply of body fat is reduced to extremely low levels, when it falls rapidly [Best and Mawson, unpublished]. These results obviously indicate that for the maintenance of the high levels of cholesteryl esters and neutral fat a continued supply of the constituents is necessary. If the food contains no fat, fat may come from the depots, but this is not so with cholesterol; when very little of this is supplied by the food the amount found in ester form in the liver falls. We may assume that the accumulation of cholesteryl esters is limited by the supply of cholesterol; fatty acids in these experiments would not be lacking; they are even necessary for the absorption of the cholesterol from the gut, and could also have been supplied from the depots.

Histological evidence indicates that when livers become extremely fatty the blood supply to some areas may be seriously disturbed. This disturbance might well interfere with the movement of cholesteryl or glyceryl esters into or out of the liver. . . .

The duration of the test periods is a very important factor in experiments of this type. The amount of fat available from the depots and the ability of the liver cells to take up fat from the blood and to metabolize it may change as the experiment progresses.

SUMMARY AND CONCLUSIONS

1. When a fatty liver has been produced in rats by relatively small daily doses of cholesterol, the addition of choline to the diet causes a very definite fall in both glyceride and cholesteryl ester content of liver tissue.

2. When larger amounts of cholesterol are provided there may be an increase in cholesteryl esters even, during the early part of the experiment, in animals receiving choline. Later, the effect of choline may be clearly shown. Under these conditions the glyceride level of the livers may fall while the cholesteryl esters are increasing. In the control series of animals this effect is not attributable to choline and is perhaps due to an appropriation by the cholesterol of fatty acids from neutral fat.

3. When cholesterol feeding is discontinued during the test period, choline accelerates the fall in cholesteryl esters. The decrease, in the absence of choline, is probably due to cessation of cholesterol supply.

4. While the effect of choline on the glyceride fraction apparently always precedes that on the cholesteryl esters, large quantities of neutral fat may still be present in the liver when the action on the cholesteryl esters is well demonstrated. The possibility that choline affects these esters directly cannot be eliminated.

ACKNOWLEDGMENT

It is a pleasure to acknowledge the efficient technical assistance of Miss M. Luxton and Miss M. E. Hocking.

39. The Effect of Anterior Pituitary Extracts on the Liver Fat of Various Animals

C. H. BEST

JAMES CAMPBELL

In a previous investigation Best and Campbell [78] studied the action of a ketogenic extract of the anterior pituitary gland which produced an intense infiltration of fat and a rapid increase in the size of the livers of fasting rats. Daily administration of this extract for a period of 3 days to forty-seven fasting white rats resulted in a fourfold increase in total liver fat over the corresponding value in the same number of control animals. The subsequent observations of MacKay and Barnes [529] and of Fry [313] have confirmed these results.

The present study is chiefly concerned with the quantitative differences in response of various species to treatment with this extract. The increase in liver fat and in the ketonuria produced by the administration of the anterior pituitary extract has been investigated in rats, guinea-pigs, mice and chickens. The studies on chickens, which were obtained in collaboration with Dr. Leslie Kilborn, will be published in another communication.

METHODS

Both male and female animals have been studied, but in a single experiment only one sex was used. In nearly all instances the effect of fasting alone and of fasting together with the administration of anterior pituitary extract was observed. The fasting animals were given water *ad. lib.*

The methods for the determination of urinary ketone bodies, liver fat (fatty acids plus unsaponifiable matter) and body fat were similar to those described previously (Best and Campbell [78]). In the experiment described in Table 39.IV and 39.V where it was necessary to determine

Originally appeared in the *Journal of Physiology*, XCII (1938), 91–110. From the School of Hygiene, University of Toronto. A preliminary report of this work was made at the Annual Meeting of the American Physiological Society, March 1936.

the fats before hydrolysis and to determine the water, protein, and non-protein nitrogen fractions of the livers, the following procedure was employed. The livers were combined, weighed, minced three times in a fine grinder, and pulped in a mortar. Samples were dried at 110° C to constant weight. A sample (30 g) of liver pulp was extracted repeatedly with alcohol and ether. Five extractions with hot absolute alcohol and four with warm ether were made. The combined alcohol and ether filtrates were evaporated *in vacuo* to dryness, transferred with petroleum ether to a 100 cc volumetric flask and made up to volume. After standing until a fine precipitate of non-fatty solids had settled out, aliquots of the fat fraction were evaporated *in vacuo* in round-bottomed flasks to constant weight. The alcohol- and ether-insoluble residue consists mainly of protein, and its weight was determined after drying to constant weight in a vacuum desiccator.

The nitrogen content of each fraction was determined by the macro-Kjeldahl method: The non-protein nitrogen was determined in trichloracetic acid filtrates. To about 25 g of pulped liver 4.5 vol. of water were added and the mixture was well shaken for 10 min. One vol. of 25 per cent trichloracetic acid was added, the mixture was shaken and filtered after 15 minutes.

The preparation of the anterior pituitary extract was the same as that used in our previous work. The dry powder, which is termed the "anterior pituitary preparation" and is subsequently referred to as A.P.P., is stable and solutions of desired concentration can be made, clarified by centrifuging, and used for injection. One g of the preparation contains the active material derived from 100 g of fresh beef anterior pituitary glands. There appears to be little variation in activity between lots but one large sample was kept as a standard to control the potency of others.

The experimental animals were of uniform stock supplied by the Connaught Laboratories Farm. The rats were Wistar strain. Some of the mice were of the Webster strain while others were of a strain obtained from the Rockefeller Institute. The guinea-pigs were of an inbred albino strain.

EXPERIMENTAL RESULTS

In agreement with the conclusions of Mottram [581] we felt that the most satisfactory index of a change in liver fat was its relationship to the initial body weight and we therefore utilized this ratio in analysing our data on liver and kidney fat, liver and kidney weight, etc. This index was also used in determining the effect of the A.P.P. on ketonuria.

Effect on Liver Fat of Rats

(a) *Single injection.* The data in Table 39.I illustrate the effect of a single injection of saline (series I, 30 rats) and of the solution obtained

TABLE 39.I

FEMALE RATS

Series	No. of Rats	Initial Weight (g)	Time Elapsed after Injection (hr)	Loss of Weight (g)	Liver Weight per 100 g Initial Weight (g)	Total Liver Fat (mg)	Liver Fat per 100 g Initial Weight (mg)	Liver Fat (%)
I	6	253	0	—	3.21	339	134	4.17
	4	248	24	14	2.55	397	161	6.31
	5	235	48	25	2.41	333	141	5.85
	5	237	72	28	2.19	328	138	6.30
	5	247	96	39	2.35	412	167	7.11
	5	243	144	52	2.07	285	117	5.65
Ia	8	239	24	7	3.51	1137	475	13.6
	8	217	48	18	2.91	584	270	9.27
	8	244	72	26	2.65	511	210	7.91
	8	242	96	31	2.77	507	210	7.59
	8	239	144	53	2.40	311	129	5.41

Series I. Injected once with 3 cc saline.
Series Ia. Injected once with 3 cc extract equivalent to 62.5 mg of A.P.P. per 100 g. Fasted during the period of the experiment.

from 62.5 mg of A.P.P. (series Ia, 40 rats). The animals were fasted from the time of injection and groups were sacrificed at intervals for the determination of liver fat. There were only slight changes in the amount of liver fat in the control (fasting) rats injected with saline. This has been observed frequently in our studies on rats. If the data are calculated on the basis of the percentage of fat in the liver, however, an apparent increase during fasting is noted. This is due to the fact that the liver loses weight rapidly in the first 24 hrs of starvation.

The A.P.P. *caused a 3½-fold increase in liver fat in the first 24 hrs.* During the following 24 hrs a rapid decrease occurred. This decrease continued at a diminishing rate until at the end of six days the liver fat was again at the control level.

(b) *Repeated injections.* In Table 39.II the changes in the liver fat over a period of four days, when the injections of the A.P.P. were given daily to fasting rats, are described. Under these conditions a rise in liver fat occurred up to the third day, the bulk of the increase occurring on the first day. On the fourth day the amount decreased despite the continued injection of extract. A similar fall has also been noted in guinea-pigs receiving daily injections of extract.

TABLE 39.II

FEMALE RATS

Series	No. of Rats	Initial Weight (g)	Days of Fast and Injection	Loss in Weight (g)	Liver Weight per 100 g Initial Weight (g)	Total Liver Fat (mg)	Liver Fat per 100 g Initial Weight (mg)	Liver Fat (%)
II	5	203	0	—	4.40	331	163	3.71
	5	207	1	16	2.81	303	146	5.21
	2	187	2	19	2.78	321	172	6.20
	2	219	3	31	2.47	277	127	5.14
	2	187	4	30	2.51	197	105	4.20
IIa	7	198	1	—	4.08	1047	529	12.9
	8	199	2	22	4.24	1162	584	13.7
	8	197	3	28	4.23	1224	620	14.6
	8	199	4	34	3.93	1105	555	14.1

Series II. Injected once daily with 3 cc saline.
Series IIa. Injected once daily with 3 cc extract equivalent to 75 mg of A.P.P. per 100 g rat. Fasted during the period of the experiment.

(c) *Three daily injections of various amounts.* We desired to develop a method for assaying the material from the anterior pituitary gland which produces an increase in liver fat. As fasting female rats gave a maximum response after three subcutaneous injections at daily intervals, this procedure was used for the test. Fairly large groups were employed (usually twenty animals) to allow for individual variation. A group of twenty control animals was injected with a volume of saline corresponding to that of the extract given. There is undoubtedly more variation in the results than would have occurred if all the dosages had been tested at one time on one lot of animals.

The data in Table 39.III show that under the conditions of this experiment the liver fat increases with the amount of A.P.P. administered. Analysis

TABLE 39.III

FASTING FEMALE RATS

Daily Dose of Anterior Pituitary Preparation mg per 100 g Rat	No. of Animals		Difference in Liver Weight of a over b per 100 g Initial Weight (g)	Liver Fat mg per 100 g Initial Weight		
	a	b		a	b	Increase
6.8	19	19	−0.19	145	114	31
14.9	20	20	+0.39	181	107	74
30.5	18	16	+0.64	249	120	129
60.6	20	20	+1.26	444	113	331
96.8	19	20	+1.58	629	160	469

Series a. Injected daily for 3 days with varying doses of A.P.P.
Series b. Injected daily for 3 days with the corresponding volumes of saline.

of the data indicates that the dose-response curve (Figure 72) is best treated as a straight line of slope,

$$\frac{d(\text{increase in liver fat, mg 100 g rat})}{d(\text{dose, mg A.P.P. per 100 g rat})} = 4.5.$$

The statistical treatment of the results will not be discussed here as it soon became apparent that the test could only be used when doses of at least

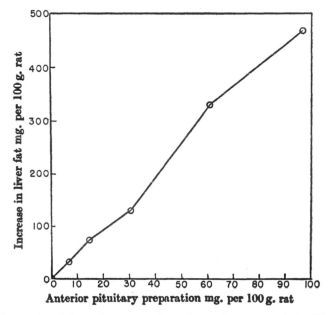

FIGURE 72. Effect of A.P.P. on liver fat in fasting rats (♀). The ordinates refer to the increments in liver fat due to A.P.P. (last column) in Table 39.III.

30 mg of A.P.P. per 100 g rat were given daily for three days. This dosage can only be attained when large amounts of concentrated extract are available.

Effect on the Liver Fat of Guinea-Pigs

The effect of the A.P.P. on the liver fat of fasting female guinea-pigs was determined in experiments somewhat similar to those carried out on rats. Groups of female guinea-pigs were injected daily with A.P.P. over a period of three days while the control animals received at the same time equal volumes of saline (Figure 73). The liver fat in a group of fed, untreated animals was determined to secure the initial value. We observed a great increase in the 24 hrs following the first injection and a lesser rise on the second day. On the third day, despite the continued injection of extract,

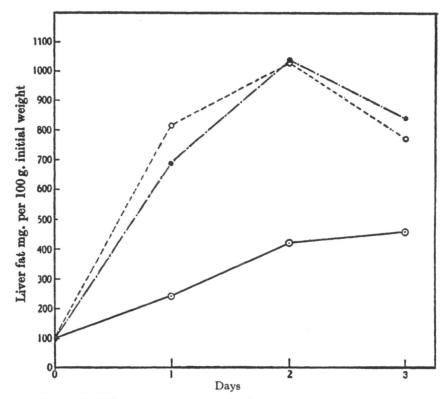

FIGURE 73. Effect of A.P.P. on fasting female guinea-pigs.
O - - - O Injected once daily with 10.0 mg A.P.P. per 100 g initial weight.
●— · —● Injected once daily with 3.8 mg A.P.P. per 100 g initial weight.
⊙ ——— ⊙ Injected once daily with saline.

the liver fat decreased. Thus an increase in liver fat occurs in fasting guinea-pigs receiving daily injections of the A.P.P. similar in general form to those obtained in female rats under similar conditions.

There are, however, notable differences between the responses of these two species to the extract. (1) The dose of extract required to produce a given increase in liver fat is much less in guinea-pigs than in rats. (2) There is a steady increase in the liver fat of guinea-pigs during three days of fasting. The liver fat, initially 3.0 per cent, rose on successive days of fasting to 8.1, 12.3, and 14.8. As was pointed out above, no definite increase in the amount of liver fat occurs in fasting rats under our experimental conditions.

It is, therefore, apparent that guinea-pigs exhibit a greater increase in liver fat due to (a) fasting, and (b) administration of anterior pituitary extracts than rats under similar conditions. The former species might therefore be used for assay of the potency of the A.P.P. If such a step were contemplated, it would appear that the liver fat should be determined 24 hrs after the injection of a sample. While the level of liver fat is greatest on the second day of injection the control (fasting) liver fat also increases markedly in this time and thus reduces the effect attributable to the extracts alone.

Effect on the Liver Fat of Mice

At the beginning of the work on mice, when the anterior pituitary extract was given daily, large variations in liver fat were encountered and

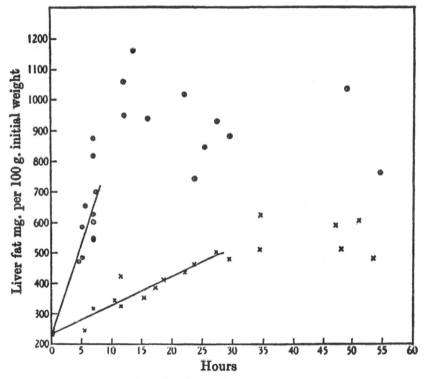

FIGURE 74. Effect of A.P.P. on fasting female mice.
× —— × Injected at 0 hr with 0.4 cc saline.
⊙ —— ⊙ Injected at 0 hr with 40.0 mg A.P.P. per 100 g initial weight.

some of the mice died. This was surprising at the time as the extract had never produced any apparent toxic effects in rats or guinea-pigs. It developed that the variable results and frequent deaths in mice were due to the fact that the extract had been given in too large a dose or was allowed to act for too long a period. This is illustrated by the curves shown in Figure 74. The data were obtained from three experiments carried out at different times and refer to the increase in liver fat due to fasting alone and to fasting after a single injection of 10 mg of A.P.P. From other data [161] it was known that this dose was approximately maximal for the mouse. The liver fat was determined in groups of four mice.

The lower curve shows that fasting causes a considerable increase in liver fat in 24 hrs. Within this period the values show a fairly uniform rise. After this time, however, large fluctuations are encountered and the liver fat may rise to very high or sink to very low levels. This behaviour seemed to be related to the amount of depot fat, for it was evident that in animals which had good stores, fatty livers were present and in those in which the fat reserves were depleted, the liver fat was low. Values illustrating this particularly well are those obtained from two groups of mice fasted for seven days. An active, healthy group of mice showed, at this time, ample stores of body fat and high liver fat, the values of which were 14.5 g and 1500 mg per 100 g of body weight, respectively. At the same time a group of weak mice with low body temperatures had 3.9 g of body fat and 175 mg of liver fat per 100 g of body weight. The high value of 1500 mg was equivalent to 28 per cent of fat in the liver. Good stores of body fat apparently in many cases are associated with a high level of liver fat under these experimental conditions.

In mice which were fasted after a single injection of 10 mg of A.P.P. a very sharp increase in liver fat occurred which was much greater than that due to fasting alone. The values showed more variation in this series than during fasting alone and in a shorter time, i.e., in 10 hrs, became even more variable than the fasting values. The fluctuations in this curve seem to be dependent not only on the stores of body fat but also on the "sensitivity" of the particular group or groups to the active substance. It was noted that after long periods of fasting certain groups of mice with good stores of depot fat showed as large amounts of liver fat as were obtained (within much shorter periods) in mice injected with the A.P.P. The response of mice to the materials in anterior pituitary extracts causing an increase in liver fat will be discussed more fully in a later paper [161].

Change in Liver Weight Due to Fasting

In mice, 7 hrs after the beginning of fasting the liver weight dropped to about 67 per cent of the initial value. After this abrupt fall the liver weight *increased* until after about 15 hrs of fasting it reached the initial or a slightly higher level. This new level seemed to be maintained up to three days of fasting. As is shown in Figure 74, the liver fat increased progressively from the beginning of the fast. Owing to the dispersion of the values it was not possible to find, in mice, any quantitative relationship between the secondary rise in liver weight and the rise in liver fat.

In guinea-pigs during the first 24 hrs of fasting the liver weight fell rapidly. Thereafter, the liver weight increased slightly up to the completion of the three days of fasting which ended the period of observation. During the fast the liver fat increased steadily (Figure 73) and the ratio

$$\frac{\text{increase in liver weight}}{\text{increase in liver fat}}$$

in the period 24–48 hrs was 3.5 and in the period 48–72 hrs was 4.1.

In fasting rats the liver weight fell rapidly in the first 24 hrs but, in contrast to the findings in mice and guinea-pigs, after the initial large drop the liver weight continued to decrease. The liver fat remained constant or decreased slightly (Tables 39.I and 39.II).

Changes in Liver Weight Due to Injection of A.P.P.

The administration of the A.P.P. to fasting rats, to fasting guinea-pigs, and to fasting mice produced increases in liver weights above the control fasting levels. The changes in liver weight of the animals which received daily injections of A.P.P. during fasting are given in Table 39.II. In Table 39.III the effect of varying doses of A.P.P. on liver weight are shown.

Comparison of the results of the three experiments shows that in fasting rats the injections of A.P.P. cause very similar changes in both the liver fat and liver weight.

The data of Table 39.III refer to the experiments in which various daily doses of A.P.P. were given for three days to fasting rats. When curves are drawn for the increase in liver fat and the increase in liver weight against dosage, the points seem to fit a straight line in both cases. From this experiment the ratio has the average value of 3.1. We find, therefore, that shortly after the administration of anterior pituitary extract to fasting rats, for every gram increase in fat (fatty acids plus unsaponifiable matter), the liver retains approximately 2.1 g of other materials.

In order to determine the quantitative relationship of the increase in liver fat to the increase in liver water and non-fatty solid constituents, the liver fats were determined as such by weighing after extraction with alcohol and ether. In this experiment female rats were fasted for 24 hrs previous to and after injection. A group of fifteen was injected with 150 mg each of A.P.P. and the fifteen control animals were given an equal volume of saline. Twenty-four hrs after the injection the livers were removed and fractionated. The data show (Table 39.IV) that when the A.P.P. was administered the fat fraction of the liver increased to the greatest extent, amounting to 51.3 per cent of the total increase in liver weight. The water content also increased to an amount corresponding to 43.8 per cent of the total increase. The alcohol-insoluble fraction represents the material not soluble in 89 per cent alcohol and in ether and consists chiefly of protein. This fraction increased only slightly, 4.85 per cent of the total increase, and the non-fatty solids soluble in 89 per cent alcohol and in ether increased by only 0.071 per cent. In this latter fraction would be found many non-protein nitrogenous constituents, and the carbohydrates would be accounted for in the alcohol-insoluble or the non-fatty, alcohol-soluble fractions.

TABLE 39.IV

FASTING FEMALE RATS

| | Weights of Fractions | | | | |
| | Series a | | Series b | | Percent of the Increase in Liver Weight (liver weight increase = 0.845 g per 100 g) |
Fraction of the Liver	g per 100 g initial weight	% of liver	g per 100 g initial weight	% of liver	
Non-fatty solids					
Alcohol insoluble	0.7200	19.70	0.6790	24.40	4.85
Alcohol soluble	0.0076	0.21	0.0070	0.25	0.071
Water	2.260	61.80	1.890	67.95	43.80
Fat	0.654	17.90	0.221	7.95	51.3
Totals	3.642	99.6	2.797	100.5	100.0

Series a. Injected once with 3 cc extract equivalent to 83 mg of A.P.P. per 100 g.
Series b. Injected once with 3 cc saline.
Composition of the livers 24 hrs after injection.

TABLE 39.V

FASTING FEMALE RATS

| | Weight of Nitrogen | | | |
| | Series a | | Series b | |
Fraction of the Liver	mg per 100 g initial weight	mg per 100 g liver	mg per 100 g initial weight	mg per 100 g liver
Non-fatty solids				
Alcohol insoluble	102.00	2790	97.90	3520
Non-protein nitrogen	6.56	179	6.03	216
Fat nitrogen	5.08	138	4.62	128
Totals	113.6		108.5	
Total nitrogen	113.5		105.4	

The distribution of nitrogen (Table 39.V) showed that the extracts produced an increase in the total nitrogen of the liver which amounted to an increase of 5.5 per cent over the control liver nitrogen. Due to the increase in fat and water there was a decrease in the percentage of total nitrogen in the liver. Similarly the non-protein nitrogen increased slightly in absolute amount but fell in terms of percentage of liver weight. It is evident that the increase in liver weight was due mainly to fat and water, only a small part being due to protein-like constituents. The increase in nitrogen of the alcohol-insoluble fraction × the factor 6.24 (Addis *et al.* [5]), represents an increase in protein of 25 mg per 100 g initial body weight.

Effect on Ketogenesis of Rats and Guinea-pigs

The data show (Table 39.VI) that in fasting rats receiving saline injections there is no perceptible increase in the excretion of ketones and no

TABLE 39.VI

FEMALE RATS

| Series | No. of Rats | Initial Weight (g) | Total Ketone Body Excretion mg per 100 g Initial Weight per Day Days | | | Liver Fat at End of 3 Days per 100 g Initial Weight (mg) |
			1	2	3	
V	17	159	0.70	0.63	1.13	219
Va	22	159	1.39	22.80	32.40	673

Series V. Injected once daily with 3 cc saline.
Series Va. Injected once daily with 3 cc extract equivalent to 94 mg of A.P.P. per 100 g initial weight.
Fasted during the period of the experiment.

increase in liver fat. The daily injection of anterior pituitary extract produces a striking excretion of ketones on the second and third days, but little increase on the first day. The liver fat, however (Table 39.II), rises sharply on the first day and continues to increase slightly on the second and third days. There is, therefore, a decided lag in the production of ketone bodies as compared with the rise in liver fat in this experiment.

Since guinea-pigs respond more readily than rats with an increase in liver fat during fasting or after the administration of anterior pituitary extracts, it might be expected that they would also excrete more ketone bodies. This does not appear to be the case (Table 39.VII). In these experiments the animals were fasted from the time of the first injection. The test animals received injections of A.P.P. daily for three days while the controls received saline. The ketone body excretion was followed from day to day, and at the end of three days the liver fat was determined. It can be seen (*a*) that in female guinea-pigs the liver fat is increased more readily than in males both by fasting and by fasting with the administration of anterior pituitary extracts; (*b*) the production of ketone bodies (due both to fasting and fasting with the administration of anterior pituitary

TABLE 39.VII

EFFECT OF A.P.P. ON KETONE EXCRETION AND HEPATIC LIPIDS

Animals (fasting)	No. of Animals	Daily Injection of Anterior Pituitary Preparation per 100 g Initial Weight (mg)	Total Ketone Body Excretion in 3 Days per 100 g Initial Weight (mg)	Liver Fat per 100 g Initial Weight (mg)	Liver Fat (%)
Female rats	11	94.0	82.0	430	10.70
	22	saline	2.46	138	5.50
Female guinea-pigs	5	4.6	7.44	647	17.10
	5	2.0	3.95	732	20.50
	5	saline	2.68	382	12.80
Male guinea-pigs	5	4.6	2.33	316	9.20
	5	2.0	2.08	244	7.80
	5	saline	1.86	157	5.62

extracts) is greater in female guinea-pigs than in males; (c) female guinea-pigs do not excrete more ketones than female rats during fasting, although the increase in liver fat is much greater in the former. It can be seen also that when a sufficient dose of A.P.P. is given to rats to increase the liver fat by an amount similar to that produced by a smaller dose in guinea-pigs, the ketone body excretion is much greater in the rats.

There are, therefore, some large quantitative discrepancies between the accumulation of liver fat and the ketonuria under the influence of fasting and of anterior pituitary extracts. There are obviously several points which suggest a relationship between the two.

Histological Observations on Kidney Fat and Liver Fat

Histological sections show that the livers of fasting rats, following injection of anterior pituitary extract, have a characteristic appearance due to the infiltration of fat. Using the haematoxylin-eosin stain, the fat is represented by vacuoles which are seen to be more numerous in the region of the portal veins than in the region of the central veins. The fat is distributed as fine globules scattered throughout the protoplasm of the cells and many examples can be picked out where the droplets form a ring around the nucleus. The appearance of this liver is different from a liver made fatty by diets poor in choline. In the latter case the fat droplets tend to coalesce and form large masses in the cell.

In co-operation with Dr. D. L. MacLean a histological and chemical investigation was made of the effect of the A.P.P. on the weight and fat content of the kidney in relation to the corresponding changes in the liver. In this experiment, groups of fasting female guinea-pigs were injected daily for two days with 8.4 and 3.3 mg of A.P.P. per 100 g. In addition to the controls injected with saline a group was injected with 8.4 mg per 100 g of brain extract prepared in the same way as the A.P.P. The brain extract produced a slight increase in weight and fat content of the liver over the control values. The changes were small in relation to those produced by the corresponding dose of A.P.P. The brain extract had no effect on kidney fat. The A.P.P. produced increases in kidney weight and kidney fat. The changes were proportional to the amount of A.P.P. injected, but were slight in comparison with the increases in liver weight and fat.

[A table of analytical data showing the above relationships has been eliminated.]

The histological observations, in general, supported the chemical findings, namely, that the brain extract produced a slight increase in liver fat and the A.P.P. a great increase in liver fat. The fat was distributed in fine droplets through the protoplasm of the liver cells. The anterior pituitary extracts also produced a fatty infiltration of the kidney, which was slight in relation to the fatty changes in the liver. The fat in the kidney varies in its distribution. It is usually seen in the loops of Henle and occasionally in the proximal convoluted tubules. In comparing the kidneys and livers of the individual animals, whether in the control (fasting) group or in the groups which received A.P.P., it was seen that where a particularly fatty liver was encountered, the kidney was correspondingly fatty.

It is apparent that anterior pituitary extracts can increase kidney weight and kidney fat and that these changes may be a reflection, though much reduced, of the corresponding changes in the liver.

Effect on Body Fat

As in previous studies [78], we found that the A.P.P. caused a fall in the body fat of rats. A group of fifteen female rats was fasted and injected daily for three days with 85 mg of A.P.P. per 100 g of body weight. The group of eight control animals was injected with an equal volume of saline (3.0 cc) at the same times. The carcass fat (body less liver) in the experimental group was 4.99 g per 100 g of body weight and in the control group was 5.65 g. The liver fats of these animals were 458 mg per 100 g of body weight and 131 mg respectively. The decrease in body fat due to the anterior pituitary injections was therefore 660 mg and the increase in liver fat was 327 mg. About half of the fat lost from the depots may, therefore, be accounted for by that found in the liver under these conditions.[1]

[1]The results of experiments with deuterium-containing fats made in co-operation with Dr. Hugh Barrett and Miss Jessie Ridout indicate that all the liver fat comes from the body reserves under these conditions.

The problem of the effect of the anterior pituitary injections on body fat was also attacked using fed guinea-pigs which received daily injections of extract during a 9-day period. The animals were fed a commercial ration and the daily consumption of food was measured. The ration given to the control animals (1 day later) was adjusted so that their food consumption was approximately equal to that of the experimental animals. One cc of extract, equivalent to 10 mg of A.P.P., was given daily to the experimental animals, while the controls received 1 cc of saline.

After a period of nine days the liver fat, intestinal fat, and fat in the carcass was determined. The fat content of the intestines was found to make no appreciable difference in the results, so it has been included under depot fat (Table 39.VIII). Two such experiments were done and in one of

TABLE 39.VIII

FEMALE GUINEA-PIGS

Series	No. of Animals	Initial Weight (g)	Change in Weight (g)	Daily Food Intake (g)	Body Fat per 100 g Body Minus Liver (g)	Liver Fat per 100 g Initial Weight (mg)	Liver Fat (%)
a	20	287	3	13.5	6.00	146	4.08
b	20	268	−15	13.5	4.01	164	3.95
c	18	201	22	14.0	5.00	129	3.34
d	18	227	0	16.6	3.53	117	2.79

Series a, c. Injected once daily with 1 cc saline for nine days.
Series b, d. Injected once daily with 10 mg A.P.P. per pig for nine days.
Fed a mixed diet.
(The experiment of series a and b was repeated with series c and d.)

them (series c and d) the controls did not receive as much food as the animals to which the anterior pituitary injections were given. Despite this the body fat in the latter group fell below the control value. In series a and b there is a fall in body fat due to the anterior pituitary injections. The animals receiving extract also lost weight in relation to the controls.

It is noticeable that a daily dose of 10 mg of A.P.P. for nine days to fed guinea-pigs produced no increase in liver fat, but in fasting guinea-pigs receiving extract for three days a great increase in liver fat occurs (Figure 73).

DISCUSSION

The results of a single injection of the anterior pituitary extract in rats suggest that the intensity of action is definitely less at 48 hrs after administration than at 24 hrs. This interpretation is not necessarily correct since it involves the assumption that the only action of the substance is to transfer fat from the depots to the liver. The rate of utilization of fat in the liver may have increased and this, rather than a decreased rate of mobilization from the depots, might cause a fall in the amount of fat in the liver. When the injections are repeated at daily intervals the findings suggest that the level of liver fat reaches its highest point on the third day. In guinea-pigs the peak is attained somewhat earlier. These time relationships might be affected by such factors as dosage of the extract, the reserves of depot fat, etc. We cannot explain at present the falling off in liver fat while the injections are continued. This might be due to depletion of "easily mobilizable" fat, but there are still appreciable amounts of glycerides present in the depots when the decrease in liver fat occurs.

When three daily doses of A.P.P. were given to rats the increase in liver fat noted on the third day was apparently directly proportional to the dose used (Table 39.III, Figure 72).

A comparison of the data in Table 39.II with that in Figure 73 shows that female guinea-pigs are much more susceptible to the A.P.P. than female rats. In guinea-pigs a daily dose of 3.8 mg per 100 g produced in two days an increase in liver fat above the initial level of approximately 940 mg per 100 g of initial body weight. In rats a dose of 75 mg produced an increase of liver fat, calculated on the same basis, of 420 mg. The results on mice cannot be compared directly with those obtained in other species since the response in mice is much more rapid and, if observations are made after two or three days, the findings are extremely erratic. There is no doubt, however, that mice are as susceptible as guinea-pigs to the A.P.P. and because of their rapid response they are preferable for testing purposes.

In the present investigation the amount of fat in the liver of rats, which were fasted but not injected with A.P.P., tended to remain at the original level or to decrease. The ketone body excretion did not exhibit an appreciable increase during fasting. Other workers have found rats very resistant to ketogenesis (e.g. Levine and Smith [498]), but in certain cases a fasting ketogenesis has been noted in this species (Cori and Cori [230]). The extent depended on the season at which the observations were made. Dible [251] also observed an increase in the excretion of ketone bodies in the fasting rat and a slight increase in liver fat. Mottram found that a great increase in liver fat occurred in fasting rabbits and guinea-pigs. This increase exhibited a periodicity which we have not observed. In our experience there is a steady and progressive increase in liver fat up to the end of three days fasting in guinea-pigs. In mice kept at 0° C for from two to 4 hrs, Lánczos [480] has reported an increase in liver fat during fasting. In the present investigation it is quite apparent that an increase in liver fat can occur in fasting mice to an even greater extent than that found in guinea-pigs. In mice or guinea-pigs in which the liver fat increases during fasting, after the initial definite fall in liver weight, an increase in weight occurs. In rats, on the other hand, after the initial fall the liver weight continues to decrease slowly. The values of the ratio

$$\frac{\text{increase in liver weight}}{\text{increase in liver fat (fatty acids)}}$$

during fasting in guinea-pigs and in guinea-pigs and rats receiving A.P.P. are of the same order (average of 3.5 in fasting guinea-pigs, 2.6 in fasting guinea-pigs receiving A.P.P., and 3.2 in fasting rats receiving A.P.P.). These values are those observed 24 hrs after the beginning of fasting or after administration of A.P.P.

The increase in the liver weight of fasting rats receiving anterior pituitary extract for short periods is due chiefly to an influx of fat and water (Table 39.IV). In the livers of fasting rats 24 hrs after a single injection of extract, 51.3 per cent of the increase in liver weight was due to fat, 43.8 per cent to water, and only 4.9 per cent to non-fatty solids. The protein nitrogen and non-protein nitrogen were increased slightly in amount by the injections, but due to the influx of fat and water the percentage of these values fell. It has been pointed out that if the injections of anterior pituitary extract are continued for longer than three days, or if the injections are stopped so that the liver fat decreases, the ratio

$$\frac{\text{increase in liver weight}}{\text{increase in liver fat}}$$

will increase. Under these conditions it is indicated that the nitrogen content of the livers will increase out of proportion to the fat content. Effkemann and Herold [279] found that in rats and pigeons anterior pituitary extracts and "unspecific organ extracts" produced increases in liver weight due to increases in nitrogen and water content and not to increases in fat or glycogen. Their experimental animals were, however, fed. It may be pointed out that in previous experiments [78], and in the experiments reported here, any increases in liver weight produced by extracts of liver, pancreas, or brain have not been nearly as great as those produced by similar doses of anterior pituitary extract. Schaffer and Lee [669] observed that short periods (10–18 hrs) of treatment with a growth hormone preparation produced in fasting rats a decrease in the percentage of non-protein nitrogen in the liver. We have confirmed this observation but found, as mentioned above, that the absolute amount of non-protein nitrogen in the liver showed a slight increase. This relation was caused by the increase in liver weight due chiefly to the accumulation of fat and water.

In the rather controversial subject of water storage in the liver with the various other constituents it is usually assumed that little or no water accompanies the deposition of fat. Kaplan and Chaikoff [437] have presented strong evidence to show that in dogs under various experimental conditions liver water is directly proportional to a liver fraction the chief constituent of which is protein, and that water does not accompany liver fat or glycogen in appreciable amounts. They do not exclude the possibility, however, that water in small amounts may accompany liver fat or glycogen. The average value of the ratio of water to protein in dogs was found to be 4.3 by these workers. If the nitrogen content of the alcohol-insoluble liver fraction in rats be considered to represent protein (Table 39.IV and 39.V), the ratio of water to protein was 3.09 in the controls and 3.55 after the injection of A.P.P. The proportion of water to protein, therefore, apparently increased slightly after the injection of the A.P.P. and it would appear also from the absolute increases in water and protein that there was not a strict relationship between them. It appears, however, that liver water is much more closely associated with protein than with fat.

The results of the present study on ketosis show, in confirmation and extension of the findings of Butts and Deuel [160], that female animals excrete more ketone bodies than males. In Table 39.VI this difference may be observed both in the fasted guinea-pigs and in those which received A.P.P. This sex difference is also seen in the deposition of fat in the livers of mice and guinea-pigs to which A.P.P. has been administered. The results in the latter species are given in Table 39.VII, while those in mice will appear in a subsequent publication by one of us (J.C.).

When the liver fat is increased in guinea-pigs by fasting or injection of A.P.P. there may be only an insignificant rise in ketonuria (Table 39.VII). In rats, on the other hand, a smaller increase in liver fat after injection of A.P.P. is accompanied by a rather intense ketonuria. It will be remembered, however, that the amount of A.P.P. required to produce similar increases in liver fat is much greater in the rat than in the guinea-pig.

It would appear probable that the rise in liver fat precedes the increase in ketonuria. While the data in Tables 39.II and 39.VI support this view the results in other experiments are by no means as definite. To make a decision on this point large groups of animals would have to be studied at short intervals after treatment with A.P.P.

It may be pointed out that the effects of the A.P.P. are in some respects analogous to those of fasting alone. The evidence for this view has already been mentioned but may be summarized as follows. The increase in liver fat and ketogenesis produced by the A.P.P. are inhibited by feeding and are therefore best shown when the effects of the A.P.P. are superimposed on those of fasting. The increase in liver fat (due to fasting alone or to fasting with the administration of A.P.P.) is greater in mice and guinea-pigs than in rats. During fasting, female guinea-pigs respond more readily than males with an increase in liver fat and ketonuria, and this is also true of the responses to the A.P.P. The administration of A.P.P. produces a fall in body fat. It therefore appears that the mobilization of fat produced by fasting is intensified by the injection of A.P.P.

The significance of the slight but definite increase in kidney fat when the A.P.P. is administered is not clear. Further studies of this problem could profitably be made.

SUMMARY

1. In fasting animals the anterior pituitary preparation causes a much greater increase in liver fat in guinea-pigs and mice than in rats. Fasting alone produces a pronounced increase in liver fat in guinea-pigs and mice. This is greater in the latter species. The amount of fat in the liver of the rat is frequently decreased by short periods of fasting.

2. Female guinea-pigs exhibit a greater increase in liver fat than males during or after the administration of the anterior pituitary preparation. The ketogenesis produced by the injections is also greater in females than in males (confirming Deuel). The ketogenesis produced in female guinea-pigs is not nearly as great as that produced in female rats when the liver fat rises to similar levels.

3. The fat which accumulates in the liver of the fasting rat after anterior pituitary injections rapidly disappears on stopping the injections. Despite continued daily injections of the preparation to fasting rats or guinea-pigs, a decrease in liver fat occurs after several days.

4. Associated with the increase in liver fat in guinea-pigs, due to administration of anterior pituitary preparation, there is an increase in kidney fat.

5. In fasting rats or in fed guinea-pigs the preparation causes a fall in body fat.

6. The preparation produces an increase in liver weight which is due chiefly to deposition of fat and water. A slight increase in non-fatty solid material also occurs.

40. A Study of the Source of Liver Fat Using Deuterium as an Indicator

H. M. BARRETT

C. H. BEST

JESSIE H. RIDOUT

One of the many problems arising out of the recent researches carried out in the Department of Physiology and in this department is the source of the fat which accumulates in the liver when animals are maintained on a diet poor in lipotropic factors and when certain extracts of the anterior pituitary gland are administered. This problem may be attacked by the use of "labelled" fatty acids. While there are several methods of preparing these "ear-marked" molecules, none of these possesses all the advantages which may be secured by the use of deuterium.

This communication consists of two parts. In the first a micro-density method for the determination of deuterium oxide, elaborated by one of us (H.M.B.), is described. In the second part the results of the application of this method to certain problems of fat mobilization are presented and discussed.

PART I. A MICRO-DENSITY METHOD FOR THE DETERMINATION OF DEUTERIUM OXIDE

Rittenberg and Schoenheimer [646] have described methods for the use of deuterium-containing molecules in studies of intermediary metabolism. To determine the deuterium content of water arising from the combustion of organic material, they utilized both the interferometer method of Crist *et al.* [233] and the Richards [637] density float. The first of these methods requires costly equipment, the second is unnecessarily sensitive for most of the analyses encountered in our investigations. For these reasons a new procedure was developed.

Originally appeared in the *Journal of Physiology*, XCIII (1938), 367–81. From the School of Hygiene, University of Toronto.

[A condensation of Part I follows. For technical details consult the original.

The water obtained from the combustion of deuterium-containing material was collected, after final purification by distillation from alkaline potassium permanganate and phosphorus pentoxide, and was weighed in a pycnometer on a Kuhlmann microbalance. . . . It was found that repeated fillings could be duplicated within $\pm 15\gamma$ which was about the accuracy with which duplicate weighings on the empty bulb could be made. (A second bulb of approximately the same shape and size was used as a counterweight.) These weighings were tedious and time-consuming and a microbalance of a different design was found to be preferable.

A Torsion Microbalance

The balance to be described is similar to one first constructed some years ago for use in adsorption measurements in the Department of Chemistry of this University. Grateful acknowledgement is made to Professor F. B. Kenrick of that Department, under whose direction the original balance was constructed. Weights are constructed by cutting 6.0 cm lengths of tungsten wire. Several determinations of the weight of 25.0 cm lengths of this wire showed it to be remarkably uniform. 25.0 cm weighed $1100 \pm 5\gamma$. One 6.0 cm length therefore weighed 264γ. Eight of these 6.0 cm lengths were placed on the basket supporting the pycnometer bulb.

The centre of gravity is adjusted so that 264γ causes a deflection of 40–50 divisions on the scale. At this sensitivity the deflection is proportional to the increase in weight for deflections of 35 divisions on either side of the position where the balance beam is parallel to the floor. This is determined by adding successive 1.0 cm lengths of the tungsten wire; at positions near the limits of swing of the balance the sensitivity becomes somewhat greater. Readings are therefore always taken within 35 divisions of the neutral position. Each of the eight weights gave deflections equal to $44 \pm \frac{1}{2}$ divisions. 1 mm deflection was therefore equal to about 6γ.

The pycnometer bulb, filled at 32.00° C with purified water is placed on the left-hand basket and an empty bulb of similar size but of somewhat greater weight on the right-hand basket. The capacity of the pycnometer bulb filled at 32.00° C with redistilled water equals 0.263450 g. 100 per cent deuterium oxide has a density 1.1078 times that of ordinary water at 32.00° C (calculated from the figure of 1.1074 25°/25° of Tronstad *et al.* [759] and Lewis and Macdonald's [500] data for the change of volume of deuterium oxide with temperature). The difference in weight between the bulb filled with 100 per cent deuterium oxide and redistilled tap water equals $0.1078 \times 263,450\gamma = 28,400\gamma$. The percentage of deuterium oxide by weight in an unknown sample is therefore

$$\frac{\Delta s}{28,400} \times \frac{(0.263450 \times 1.1078)}{(0.263450 + \Delta s)},$$

where Δs equals the difference in weight in γ between the unknown sample and redistilled ordinary water. The deflection produced by one 6 cm length of wire (44 ± ½ divisions) is equivalent to 1.02 per cent deuterium oxide. One division on the scale therefore corresponds to 0.0232 per cent deuterium oxide. Duplicate fillings of the pycnometer from the same water sample checked within ±1 division.

The effect of variation of temperature of the water in the thermos flask in which the pycnometer was immersed amounts to 13 divisions per 1.00° C change. This observed change is identical with the change calculated from the alteration in density of water with temperature corrected for the cubical expansion of the pycnometer bulb. As this temperature is maintained at 32.00 ± 0.02° C the error from this cause amounts to less than ½ division.]

TABLE 40.I

SOLUTIONS OF DEUTERIUM OXIDE AND WATER PREPARED FROM 99.6 PER CENT DEUTERIUM OXIDE

Prepared Concentration D_2O %	Concentration Found D_2O %
6.31	6.31
2.98	3.00–2.94*
2.61	2.53
1.47	1.48
1.11	1.11
0.98	0.94–0.96*
0.52	0.47–0.48*
0.29	0.29–0.27*
0.08	0.07

*Duplicate analyses.

Table 40.I shows the results of a series of analyses carried out on prepared dilutions of 99.6 per cent deuterium oxide with redistilled ordinary water. Duplicate determinations on the same sample have an error no greater than ±0.03 per cent deuterium oxide. As the sample used for analysis is less than 0.3 g this accuracy compares favourably with that attainable with the interferometer using a sample of similar size.

The procedures necessary for the analysis, with the exception of the weighing, can be carried out in approximately 15 min.

PART II. THE SOURCE OF THE EXCESS FAT WHICH
ACCUMULATES IN THE LIVER[1]

Experimental Methods

In the experiments to be described the procedure consisted in feeding large groups of female mice on the following diet: meat powder 20 per cent by weight, brown bread 37 per cent, linseed oil (containing from 5 to 7 atoms per cent of deuterium introduced by means of a palladium catalyst) 15 per cent, "purina" (commercial mixed diet) 10 per cent, sucrose 10 per cent, yeast 4 per cent, and salt mixture (McCollum's No. 185) 4 per cent. Vitamins A and D were added and 25 mg of choline for each 4 g of food were provided. In some experiments the diet included 20 per cent of linseed oil containing deuterium and only 15 per cent of meat powder. The feeding periods varied from 9 to 14 days as indicated in the tables. The average food consumption was approximately 3 g per mouse per day. The mice were kept in individual cages in a room in which the temperature was maintained at approximately 28° C. At the end of the feeding period on the above diet, groups of mice were killed to secure control values. The livers from seven to ten mice were pooled for an analysis. Fatty acids were estimated by the direct saponification procedure. In the experiments in which neutral fat and phospholipin fractions were separated, fatty acid determinations were made on the ether-soluble fractions by the method described previously [80]. After discarding the gastrointestinal tract, the carcasses were treated in a similar manner. From 0.3 to 0.4 g of fat from each sample was analysed for its deuterium content following Rittenberg and Schoenheimer's [646] procedure for combustion and purification and utilizing the density determination method already described for the final analysis. The same procedure was applied to the livers and carcasses of the test mice which, after the control period, had been subjected to various experimental procedures such as starvation, maintenance on a high-carbohydrate or a high-protein diet, injection of anterior pituitary extract or exposure to carbon tetrachloride vapour. Comparison of the deuterium content of the fat from the livers and depots of these animals with the corresponding values from the control groups indicated the source of the excess fat in the liver.

When sufficient fat was available, duplicate saponifications were carried out. Estimations of the deuterium content of the fats were made in duplicate or triplicate. The agreement among determinations was excellent

---

[1]A preliminary note on this subject appeared in the *Proceedings of the American Society of Biological Chemists* (*J. Biol. Chem.*, CXXIII, iii [1938]).

and only average values have, for the most part, been recorded in the tables. The deuterium content of the body water was always determined (Schoenheimer and Rittenberg [677]) as this gave some indication of the amount of deuterium-containing fat being utilized by the animal at that particular time.

Since it was known that the increase in fat that occurs in the livers of animals is, under many conditions, largely neutral fat, it was important to determine the distribution of deuterium between the phospholipin and neutral fat fractions. In a number of groups of animals separation of these components of the depot fat was therefore effected. This procedure could not readily be extended to the livers in the experiments on mice as insufficient fat was available.

Experimental Results and Comments

The source of increase in liver fat in starvation. The results of four experiments in which mice were starved for various periods are summarized in Table 40.II.

In Exp. 1, for an unknown reason, the expected accumulation of fat did not occur in the livers of the mice starved either for 24 or 32 hrs. The deuterium content of the liver fat of the group starved for 32 hrs became essentially the same as that of the depot fat, providing evidence that there is an interchange of fat between the liver and depots under these conditions. Since there is so much more fat present in the depots than in the liver, transport of liver fat with its somewhat higher deuterium content to the depots would not be detected by an increase in percentage of deuterium in depot fat. Equilibrium between the deuterium content of liver and depot fat is taken as conclusive evidence of an interchange of fat between these two sites.

In Exp. 2 the amount of deuterium in the liver fat of the control animals at the conclusion of nine days feeding is almost the same as that found in the liver fat of the control group of Exp. 1. The deuterium content of the depot fat of these animals is, however, significantly lower than in the first experiment; this is undoubtedly due, in part, to the shorter feeding period. After 48 hrs starvation the liver fat has nearly tripled in amount, at the same time the percentage of deuterium in the liver fat has decreased. It is still, however, considerably above that of the depots. Since there is such a great difference between the deuterium content of liver fat and depot fat in the control animals, no conclusions as to the source of fat increase in the starved animals can be reached from this experiment. As it has already been shown that an interchange of fat between liver and depots

TABLE 40.II

FASTING MICE

Exp.	Group	No. of Animals	Liver Fat (%)	Weight of Liver Fat per Mouse (g)	D₂ in Liver Fat atoms%	Weight of Depot Fat per Mouse (g)	D₂ in Depot Fat atoms%	Av. D₂ in Depot Fat — Neutral Fat atoms%	Phospholipin atoms%	D₂O in Body Water (%)
1	Controls fed 13 days on diet with 15% linseed oil containing 5.90 atoms% deuterium	9	4.5	0.051	2.67	2.6	1.88, 1.94	1.78	2.10	0.43
		10	4.7	0.058	2.43					
	Fasted 24 hr	10	5.5	0.046	2.17	2.7	1.84, 1.82	1.85	1.93	0.54
	Fasted 32 hr	10	4.6	0.046	2.06	2.5	2.04, 2.09	2.08	1.96	0.37
	Injection of anterior pituitary extract. Killed after 7 hr fasting	10	10.8	0.153	2.06	2.9	1.98, 1.98	2.01	1.79	0.38
		10	9.5	0.131	2.02					
2	Controls fed 9 days on diet with 15% linseed oil containing 5.90 atoms% deuterium	15	2.9	0.037	2.38, 2.38	2.8	1.05, 1.04			0.11
3	Fasted 48 hr	15	9.9	0.092	1.25, 1.22	2.3	0.92, 0.92			0.10
	Controls fed 14 days on diet with 20% linseed oil containing 6.51 atoms% deuterium	8	4.4	0.036	3.92	4.5	2.91			0.54
		7	4.3	0.037	3.67	5.3	2.69			0.43
4	Fasted 52 hr	8	12.7	0.091	2.74	3.8	2.67, 2.71			0.62
		7	12.8	0.096	2.65	3.4	2.40, 2.47			0.66
	Controls fed 14 days on diet with 15% linseed oil containing 4.90 atoms% deuterium	8	5.8	0.061	2.06	6.2	2.03			0.23
		7	5.0	0.049	2.10	5.7	2.06			0.18
	Fasted 7 days	8	17.7	0.125	2.05	2.6	2.17			0.25
		7	17.2	0.115	2.04	2.3	2.13			0.27

occurs on starvation, irrespective of any increase in total liver fat, it is not possible to decide how much of the decrease in deuterium percentage in the liver fat of the starved animals is due to this cause.

In Exp. 3 much more of the dietary fat was stored in the depots. The liver fat in the starved animals has again nearly tripled in amount. The deuterium content of the liver fat although lower than that of the control animals is almost the same as that of the depot fat. It is apparent that the increase in total fat in the livers of the starved animals must have arisen largely from a deuterium-containing source, that is, by transport of fat from the depots to the liver.

Exp. 4 in which the mice were starved seven days confirms this result. Here no significant change occurred in the deuterium content of the liver fat of the starved animals although a tremendous increase in total fat resulted from the seven days' starvation. This was the only experiment in the present investigation in which the deuterium content of the liver fat of the control animals was not significantly greater than that of the depot fat at the beginning of the fasting period. This result could be explained on the assumption that the control animals had not eaten for some time before they were killed. It will be remembered that the results of Exp. 1 showed that the depot fat and liver fat may become equal in deuterium content during starvation with no change in total liver fat.

The results of the deuterium analyses of the phospholipin and neutral fat fractions of the depot fat from the animals in Exp. 1 show considerable variation. No significant difference, however, in deuterium content appears to exist.

Injection of extract of the anterior pituitary gland. Twenty-nine mice were given a subcutaneous injection of 15 mg of extract prepared from the anterior lobes of ox pituitary glands [78]. These animals were fasted for seven hrs after the injection and were then killed. The results are shown in Table 40.II, Exp. 1. The injection of the extract has caused an extensive increase in liver fat. Although the deuterium level of the liver fat of these animals has fallen below that of the control group, it is equal to that of the depot fat. It is apparent that the increase in liver fat resulted largely from a transport of fat from the depots.

Carbohydrate feeding. Mice maintained on a high-carbohydrate diet poor in lipotropic factors develop fatty livers. Following the initial feeding period in which fat containing deuterium was provided, groups of mice were fed on the following diet: sucrose 76 per cent, agar 15 per cent, meat powder 5 per cent, salt mixture 4 per cent, and vitamins A, D, and B_1. The experimental results are summarized in Table 40.III. Since one group of

TABLE 40.III

CARBOHYDRATE DIET

Exp.	Group	No. of Animals	Liver Fat (%)	Weight of Liver Fat per Mouse (g)	D$_2$ in Liver Fat Atoms%	Weight of Depot Fat per Mouse (g)	D$_2$ in Depot Fat Atoms%	D$_2$O in Body Water (%)
3	Controls fed 14 days on diet with 20% linseed oil containing 6.51 atoms% deuterium	8	4.4	0.036	3.92	4.5	2.91	0.54
		7	4.3	0.037	3.67	5.3	2.69	0.43
	Carbohydrate diet 52 hr	10	5.7	0.048	2.32	5.3	2.87, 2.87	—
	Carbohydrate diet 7 days	8	11.5	0.096	1.10, 1.12	3.5	2.38	0.07
		6	9.9	0.090	1.20	4.0	2.54	0.14
5	Controls fed 14 days on diet with 15% linseed oil containing 6.65 atoms% deuterium	8	lost	—	—	5.2	2.51	0.25
		7	,,	—	—	4.8	2.58	0.23
	Carbohydrate diet 7 days	8	9.2	0.093	1.15	3.2	2.47	0.20
		7	8.4	0.085	0.92	3.5	2.20	0.18
6	Controls fed 14 days on diet with 20% linseed oil containing 6.69 atoms% deuterium	8	5.6	0.074	3.10	3.7	2.46	0.30
		7	4.4	0.063	3.11	4.2	2.55	
	Carbohydrate diet 7 days	8	7.4	0.096	1.10	4.8	2.03	0.06
		7	6.9	0.093	1.05	3.5	1.85	
	Carbohydrate diet 7 days followed by 52 hr fasting	7	13.8	0.174	1.49, 1.47	1.3	1.73	0.15
		7	15.9	0.214	1.98, 1.96	3.0	2.23	0.15

animals served frequently as controls for several experiments of different types, some control figures have been retabulated for convenience in both this and in subsequent tables.

In Exp. 3 after 52 hrs on the carbohydrate diet there has been a slight increase in total liver fat. The deuterium content of the liver fat has dropped markedly below that of the liver fat of the control mice and is, furthermore, significantly less than that of the depot fat. After seven days on the carbohydrate diet the total liver fat has doubled in amount, and its deuterium content has dropped to 1.15 atoms per cent. Only a slight drop in the deuterium content of the depot fat was observed.

In Exp. 5 the liver fat of the control animals was unfortunately lost. The remaining figures for liver fat and depot fat are, however, in excellent agreement with those found in Exp. 3. Similar results were obtained in Exp. 6, although here there was a somewhat larger drop in the deuterium content of the depot fat after seven days on the carbohydrate diet.

The fact that the deuterium content of the liver fat of the animals fed seven days on the carbohydrate diet was so far below that of the depots indicates strongly that the increase in fat came from a non-deuterium-containing source, that is, possibly from conversion of carbohydrate to fat. This conversion may have taken place entirely in the liver as little decrease in the deuterium content of depot fat occurred. The small drop in the level of depot deuterium is probably due to the storage of fat that has been formed from carbohydrate. Schoenheimer and Rittenberg [678], on the other hand, found that the deuterium in the depot fat of mice fed a brown bread diet for six days almost entirely disappeared. In a later paper Rittenberg and Schoenheimer [647] conclude that the rate of disappearance may be somewhat slower than they originally thought. Their results interpreted in the light of the present work suggest as one possibility the presence of some factor in their diets or experimental procedure which caused the transfer of large amounts of fat (presumably made from carbohydrate) from the liver to the depots.

The fact that seven days feeding of a carbohydrate diet to mice lowered the deuterium content of the liver fat far below that of the depots made it possible to check the conclusions drawn from the starvation experiments. Attention is drawn to the results shown in Table 40.III, Exp. 6, obtained by starving a group of mice for 52 hrs after they had been maintained on the carbohydrate diet for seven days. Starvation resulted in a marked increase in total liver fat; at the same time a decided increase in the deuterium content of the liver fat occurred. The increase was greatest in the group of animals which showed the higher level of deuterium in their depot fat. This experiment provides even more conclusive evidence that the increase in liver fat that occurs in mice following starvation results from a transport of fat from the depots to the liver.

In both Exp. 3 and Exp. 6 there was a marked fall in the percentage of deuterium oxide in the body water after maintenance of the animals for seven days on the carbohydrate diet. This decrease was much less in Exp. 5. The decrease that occurred in Exp. 6 was followed by a significant rise when the animals were starved. The amount of deuterium oxide in the body water is an indication of the amount of deuterium-containing fat that is being oxidized. The results of determinations of this value made after seven days on the carbohydrate diet suggest that little depot fat is being burned. The marked increase that occurs on starvation suggests utilization of depot fat.

Protein feeding. The small but significant decrease that occurred in the deuterium content of the depot fat of mice fed a carbohydrate diet could have been due to a breakdown and resynthesis of fat in the depots with a consequent loss of deuterium. This explanation is improbable in view of the fact that no change occurred in the deuterium content of the depot fat of mice that had been starved for seven days (see Table 40.II). The following experiments supply further evidence that the most probable explanation of the drop in deuterium percentage in depot fat which occurred in the mice when transferred to the carbohydrate diet is storage of fat formed from carbohydrate.

Groups of mice were fed a diet similar to that used in the carbohydrate feeding experiments with the exception that the 76 per cent of sucrose was replaced by an equal quantity of meat powder. The results are shown in Table 40.IV. After seven days on this diet no change occurred in the deuterium content of the depot fat and it is doubtful if even after 14 days a significant decrease has taken place. Since both after a long period of starvation and after feeding a protein diet no drop occurred in the deuterium content of depot fat, it is concluded that the deuterium in the fat is stable under these conditions in the animal's body and, further, that no breakdown and resynthesis of fat occur in the depots. In view of these considerations, storage of fat formed from carbohydrate appears to be the most logical explanation of any decrease occurring in the deuterium content of depot fat of mice fed a carbohydrate diet.

The deuterium content of the liver fat of the protein-fed mice shows a marked decrease. There is no significant increase in the total fat of the liver. Several explanations of this result are possible: (1) selective removal of deuterium from liver fat, (2) a difference between the deuterium content of different fractions of liver fat with removal of those of high

TABLE 40.IV
PROTEIN DIET

Exp.	Group	No. of Animals	Liver Fat (%)	Weight of Liver Fat per Mouse (g)	D₂ in Liver Fat Atoms%	Weight of Depot Fat per Mouse (g)	D₂ in Depot Fat Atoms%	D₂O in Body Water (%)
6	Controls fed 14 days on diet with 20% linseed oil containing 6.69 atoms% deuterium	8	5.6	0.074	3.10	3.7	2.46	0.30
		7	4.4	0.063	3.11	4.2	2.55	
	Protein diet 3 days	9	3.6	0.056	1.91, 1.89	3.8	2.45	0.15
	Protein diet 7 days	7	2.7	0.041	1.52	4.5	2.54	0.00
		8	2.6	0.040	1.46	3.3	2.56	
4	Controls fed 14 days on diet with 15% linseed oil containing 4.90 atoms% deuterium	8	5.8	0.061	2.06	6.2	2.03	0.23
		7	5.0	0.049	2.10	5.7	2.06	0.18
	Protein diet 3 days	5	5.8	0.054	1.52	5.0	2.19	0.17
		5	4.7	0.046	1.49	4.8	2.13	
	Protein diet 14 days	8	4.1	0.044	0.89	3.8	1.86	0.00
		7	4.9	0.053	0.69	3.6	1.90	
	Protein diet 3 days with exposure to carbon tetrachloride	8	13.9	0.199	1.90	3.7	2.12	0.42
		7	14.7	0.257	1.97	4.2	2.10	0.33

deuterium content, (3) conversion of protein to fat, (4) saturation or desaturation of liver fat with consequent loss of deuterium, (5) breakdown of deuterium fat with resynthesis, resulting in a disappearance of deuterium.

Selective removal of deuterium from liver fat is improbable in view of the evidence available indicating that the animal does not distinguish between protium and deuterium.

To find if a difference between the deuterium content of different fractions of liver fat existed, the following experiment was carried out. Twenty rats were fed for three days on the usual diet containing 20 per cent linseed oil (deuterium content of oil was 6.29 atoms per cent). A separation of the depot and liver fat into phospholipin and neutral fat fractions was effected. Sinclair's [706] method was employed. The experimental results are shown in Table 40.V. Although there is a significant

TABLE 40.V

DISTRIBUTION OF DEUTERIUM IN PHOSPHOLIPIN AND NEUTRAL FAT

20 rats fed for 3 days on diet containing 20 per cent linseed oil
(D_2 content of linseed oil = 6.29 atoms%)

	Total Fatty Acids	Neutral Fat (fatty acid)	Phospholipin (fatty acid)
Livers	3.11, 3.18	2.59, 2.61	3.58, 3.52
Bodies	1.20, 1.19	1.15	1.24, 1.22
	1.16*	1.16*	1.29*, 1.25*

*Duplicate saponifications.

difference between the deuterium content of the liver neutral fat and phospholipin fractions, it is not sufficiently great to account for the low deuterium value of liver fat obtained in the protein feeding experiments even if one considered it possible that all of the phospholipin could be selectively removed. In agreement with the results obtained using mice there was no significant difference in the deuterium content of the phospholipin and neutral fat fractions of the depots.

The present data are insufficient definitely to show which of the other explanations of the decrease in deuterium content of liver fat is correct. It is evident that no appreciable interchange between liver and depot fat was taking place since no change in the amount of deuterium in the depot fat occurred.

The fact that no detectable amount of deuterium was present in the body water even after seven days on the protein diet suggests that little deuterium-containing fat was being oxidized. Protein must have supplied a large part of the energy for metabolic processes. On the other hand, the fact that a decrease in total depot fat had occurred after 14 days on the protein diet (see Table 40.IV, Exp. 4) showed that some depot fat had been utilized during this period.

Exposure of mice to carbon tetrachloride vapour. Following the initial period of feeding the diet which contained deuterium fat, two groups of mice were maintained for three days on the high-protein diet. One group was exposed for 6 hrs daily to 5200 parts per million of carbon tetrachloride vapour in an exposure chamber that has been described elsewhere (Barrett *et al.* [54]). The second group served as controls (Table 40.IV, Exp. 4). Exposure to carbon tetrachloride vapour has resulted in a tremendous accumulation of fat in the liver. The deuterium content of the liver fat in the exposed group was 1.94 atoms per cent compared with 1.51 atoms per cent in the unexposed animals. The increase in liver fat came therefore, in large part, from a deuterium-containing source, that is, from the depots.

Stability of the deuterium-containing fats. In conclusion, some data are presented to indicate that no appreciable interchange between deuterium and protium was taking place in these experiments. Since fat transport and conversion were being studied, it was important to show that significant amounts of deuterium were not entering into combination with other constituents of the body. With regard to the first point, duplicate saponifications of the fat were carried out in many instances. As unstable deuterium interchanges with water and sodium hydroxide, the close agreement of the deuterium analyses in these experiments is excellent evidence that the deuterium being measured was stable.

Determinations were carried out on protein fractions separated from rat and mouse bodies and livers by precipitation with trichloracetic acid. After careful drying the protein was combusted. Owing to the presence of volatile oxides of nitrogen, the purification of the water resulting from combustion was modified in the following way. It was *intimately* mixed with about 0.05 g of potassium hydroxide and transferred to a clean tube before the final distillation was carried out. No chromium trioxide was added to the sample, otherwise the procedure was the same as that used for the fats. Satisfactory purification was indicated by the results of a colorimetric pH determination.

Glycogen fractions were separated from the livers and depots of rats that had been fed for four days on a 20 per cent fat diet (fat contained 6.69 atoms per cent deuterium). The results of the analyses of these constituents are summarized in Table 40.VI. The amount of deuterium in tissues other than fat is not more than a fraction of the deuterium content of the body water. This is in agreement with the findings of Smith *et al.* [714]. These experiments show that the deuterium is a stable label when used for

TABLE 40.VI

DISTRIBUTION OF DEUTERIUM IN ANIMAL TISSUES

Animals	Percentage of Deuterium-containing Linseed Oil in Diet	D_2O in Body Water (%)	Protein		Fat		Glycogen	
			body	liver	body	liver	body	liver
15 mice	15% for 9 days,* atoms% D_2 = 5.90	0.10	0.00	—	0.92	1.24	—	—
15 mice	20% for 14 days, atoms% D_2 = 6.20	0.42	0.06	—	2.25	3.51	—	—
20 rats	20% for 3 days, atoms% D_2 = 6.29	0.06	0.01	0.05	1.20	3.17	—	—
10 rats	20% for 4 days, atoms% D_2 = 6.69	0.10	—	—	2.62	2.86	0.00	0.04

*In this experiment the mice were fasted 48 hrs before being killed.

studies in fat metabolism. The remarkably constant level of deuterium maintained by depot fat in the animals which were starved and in those which were fed a protein diet appears to be conclusive evidence of the stability of deuterium-containing fats *in vivo*.

SUMMARY AND CONCLUSIONS

1. A method for analysing the deuterium content of solutions of deuterium oxide and water has been described. The method involves the use of a small pycnometer and a torsion microbalance of original design. The sensitivity of the balance was such that 6γ produced 1 mm deflection of the pointer. An analysis made on a sample of 0.3 g is accurate to ±0.03 per cent deuterium oxide.

2. In confirmation of the results of previous investigators who have used other methods of labelling fatty acids the findings in these deuterium studies indicate that the principal, if not the only, source of the excess fat which accumulates in the liver during fasting is the body depots.

3. The results indicate that the fat which accumulates in the liver when certain extracts of the anterior pituitary gland are administered is also derived from this source.

4. When mice are exposed to carbon tetrachloride vapour the increase in liver fat apparently comes in large part, if not entirely, from the depots.

5. When fat containing deuterium is deposited in the body reserves and the animals are then placed on a diet low in protein and other lipotropic factors but rich in carbohydrate, the fat which accumulates in the liver is not derived from the depots. The most probable source of this fat is the carbohydrate of the diet.

6. When diets rich in protein are given to animals whose depot fat contains deuterium, there is no transfer of fat from depot to liver. Furthermore, the deuterium content of the depot fat remains surprisingly constant for periods up to 14 days. No final explanation can at present be given for the interesting decrease in deuterium content of liver fat under these conditions.

7. Further evidence of the stability of fats containing deuterium both *in vitro* and *in vivo* has been secured.

Acknowledgment

It is a pleasure to acknowledge the helpful co-operation of our colleague, Dr. James Campbell, in certain of these experiments.

41. The Lipotropic Action of Methionine

C. H. BEST

JESSIE H. RIDOUT

In 1937 Tucker and Eckstein [760] demonstrated that methionine exerts a lipotropic effect. This has been confirmed in our laboratory[1] and by Channon, Manifold, and Platt [189]. The latter workers have shown that methionine, under the conditions of their experiments, exerted very little effect upon the deposition of fat in the liver unless the basal diet was such that large amounts of fat were deposited in the livers of the control animals. We have been interested in the lipotropic effects of *d*- and *l*-methionine and in the failure of large doses of the racemic mixture to produce greater effects than small doses under certain experimental conditions.

METHODS

White rats of the Wistar strain, av. wt. 200 g, were used. The liver fat was estimated by direct saponification and the results are expressed as total fatty acids plus unsaponifiable matter per 100 g fresh tissue. Animals of the same sex were used throughout an experiment and the figures given in the tables are the average values from groups of fifteen animals. The constituents of the diets are listed in Table 41.I. The diets were all supplemented by adequate amounts of crystalline vitamin B_1 and vitamins A and D in the form of cod-liver oil concentrate. The substance to be tested was added to the basal diet and a corresponding decrease in the amount of sucrose was made. The experimental period was 21 days. Daily records of the food consumption were made and from these the actual intake of the supplement was calculated.

RESULTS

The results of the first experiment are summarized in Table 41.II. They demonstrate that under these experimental conditions the lipotropic effect

Originally appeared in the *Journal of Physiology*, XCVII (1940), 489–94. From the Department of Physiological Hygiene, University of Toronto.

[1]The findings were reported to the Fourth Annual Meeting of the Canadian Physiological Society at McGill University, Montreal, on May 23, 1938.

TABLE 41.I

COMPOSITION OF DIETS

	Basal (%)	1 (%)	2 (%)	3 (%)
Meat powder*	5	5	5	5
Casein†	—	30	—	—
Cystine	—	—	—	0.10
dl-Methionine	—	—	—	0.96
Beef dripping	40	40	40	40
Sucrose	48	18	47.85	46.94
Agar	2	2	2	2
Salt mixture‡	5	5	5	5
Choline	—	—	0.15	—
Cod-liver oil concentrate	+	+	+	+
Vitamin B$_1$	+	+	+	+

*For preparation, see D. L. MacLean, J. H. Ridout, and C. H. Best [533].
†Fat-free and vitamin-free, obtained from British Drug Houses.
‡See E. V. McCollum and N. J. Simmonds [525].

TABLE 41.II

LIPOTROPIC EFFECT OF METHIONINE

Diet	Av. Daily Food Intake (g)	Av. Daily Intake of Supplement	Av. Change in Wt. (%)	Liver Fat g per 100 g rat (calc.)	(%)
Basal	9.2	—	−10	0.58	15.2
+0.125% dl-methionine	9.5	11.9 mg	−6	0.47	11.6
+0.25% "	9.7	24.2 "	−5	0.42	10.0
+0.50% "	9.4	47.0 "	−4	0.37	9.4
+1.00% "	9.7	97.0 "	−9	0.44	10.5
+8.0% casein	9.5	0.76 g	+3	0.62	14.2
+16.0% "	9.6	1.54 "	+9	0.42	9.6
+32.0% "	9.0	2.88 "	+3	0.25	6.2

of a diet containing 1 per cent dl-methionine is not significantly greater than that of one with 0.125 per cent.

Dietary casein, which contains approximately 3.2 per cent of methionine (Baernstein [35]), has previously been shown to exert a definite lipotropic action. In this experiment 47 mg of methionine daily exerted about the same effect as the diet containing 16 per cent casein which provided approximately 49 mg of this amino-acid. On the other hand, at lower or higher levels of intake of the two substances, the effects were by no means identical.

As mentioned above, Channon and his collaborators showed that the lipotropic effect of methionine was much greater when the basal diet produced a high level of liver fat in the control animals. The results in Table 41.III show that the absence of additional effects with larger doses of methionine can still be demonstrated when the control value of liver fat

TABLE 41.III

COMPARISON OF THE LIPOTROPIC EFFECTS OF METHIONINE, CASEIN, AND CHOLINE

Diet	Av. Daily Food Intake (g)	Av. Daily Intake of Supplement	Av. Change in Wt. (%)	Liver Fat	
				g per 100 g rat (calc.)	(%)
Basal	9.2	—	−6	0.89	20.5
+0.50% dl-methionine	9.3	46.5 mg	−1	0.55	13.3
+1.00% ''	9.4	94.0 ''	−6	0.64	15.5
+2.00% ''	9.5	190.0 ''	−11	0.68	16.5
+16% casein	9.0	1.44 g	+2	0.30	8.5
+32% ''	8.6	2.76 ''	+4	0.23	7.0
+0.08% choline	9.9	7.9 mg	−6	0.30	8.3
+0.16% ''	9.3	14.9 ''	−5	0.24	6.6

is high. The diet containing 2 per cent dl-methionine did not lower the liver fat as much as the one with 0.5 per cent. In this experiment the diet containing 16 per cent casein caused a greater decrease in liver fat than could be attributed to its methionine content. The choline equivalent of the dietary casein was about 5 mg per g casein. This value is the same as that previously determined.

In the third experiment (Table 41.IV) the effects of d- and l-methionine

TABLE 41.IV

COMPARISON OF THE LIPOTROPIC ACTION OF RACEMIC METHIONINE AND THE DEXTRO- AND LEVO-ROTATORY FORMS

Diet	Av. Daily Food Intake (g)	Av. Daily Intake of Supplement (mg)	Av. Change in Wt. (%)	Liver Fat	
				g per 100 g rat (calc.)	(%)
Basal	8.0	—	−11	1.06	25.7
+0.06% dl-methionine	8.7	5.2	−5	0.82	18.0
+0.50% ''	8.3	41.5	−3	0.57	13.4
+0.06% d-methionine	9.2	5.5	0	0.94	19.7
+0.50% ''	8.6	43.0	−4	0.44	10.9
+0.06% l-methionine	8.9	5.3	−4	0.69	16.0
+0.08% choline	8.3	6.6	−6	0.21	5.9
+0.02% ''	8.1	1.6	−10	0.58	16.3
+0.01% ''	8.9	0.9	−14	0.71	17.7
Basal	9.5	—	−10	0.77	18.3
+0.06% dl-methionine	9.3	5.6	−8	0.56	14.3
+0.06% d-methionine	8.5	5.1	−8	0.60	14.3
+0.06% l-methionine	9.5	5.7	−8	0.57	14.3
Basal	8.8	—	−6	0.73	18.6
+0.15% dl-methionine	9.3	13.9	−4	0.73	16.7
+0.25% ''	9.1	22.7	−4	0.63	16.0
+0.15% d-methionine	8.8	13.2	−4	0.60	15.6
+0.25% ''	8.7	21.7	−5	0.49	13.7
+0.15% l-methionine	8.7	13.0	−5	0.57	14.7
+0.25% ''	9.1	22.7	−5	0.57	14.9

are compared with that of the racemic mixture and with various doses of choline. The results indicate that both *d*- and *l*-methionine are active and that their effects are essentially similar to that of the mixture.

In the last experiment (Table 41.V) cystine, which has been shown to

TABLE 41.V

LIPOTROPIC ACTIVITY OF CASEIN COMPARED WITH THAT OF AN EQUIVALENT
SUPPLEMENT OF METHIONINE

Diet	Av. Daily Food Intake (g)	Av. Daily Intake of Supplement	Av. Change in Wt. (%)	Liver Fat	
				g per 100 g rat (calc.)	(%)
Basal	9.5	—	−6	0.73	18.6
(1) +30% casein	8.5	2.55 g	+3	0.25	7.1
(2) +0.15% choline	8.7	13.0 mg	−5	0.24	7.8
(3) +0.10% cystine	8.4	84.0 "	−5	0.71	16.8
+0.96% *dl*-methionine		80.7 "			

increase liver fat (Curtis and Newburgh [235]; Beeston and Channon [58]), and methionine were both added to the basal diet in amounts equivalent to those provided by a diet containing 30 per cent casein (Tucker and Eckstein [760]). The effect of this diet was then compared with one containing 30 per cent casein and also with one in which choline was added to the basal diet in an amount equal to the choline equivalent of the casein. The results in Table 41.V show that the mixture of the cystine and methionine exerts an insignificant effect in comparison with the casein diet which provided the same amounts of these amino-acids. The composition of the basal diet and of the others referred to in Table 41.V is described in Table 41.I.

DISCUSSION

Our results confirm and extend those reported by Tucker and Eckstein [760] and by Channon *et al.* [189]. There does not appear to be a quantitative relationship between the amount of methionine ingested and the deposition of fat in the liver. The lipotropic activity of the diet containing 2 per cent methionine was no greater than the one with 0.5 per cent. However, if the amount of methionine is reduced to 0.06 per cent, as in the experiments recorded in Table 41.IV, the falling off in lipotropic effect is very definite.

Channon, Loach, Loizides, Manifold, and Soliman [188] demonstrated that the lipotropic activity of protein supplements varied with the nature and amount of the basal protein. In the experiments reported in this paper, meat powder was used as the basal protein. It is possible that an increase in the dose of methionine might produce a further decrease in liver fat if a different protein were used in the basal diet.

Tucker and Eckstein [760] at one time suggested that the lipotropic effect of a diet containing 30 per cent casein as the only source of dietary protein was due to the opposing influences of its cystine and methionine contents. The results of their more recent experiments and of those we are now reporting do not support this interpretation. If 30 per cent casein is added to a diet containing 5 per cent meat powder as the basal protein, a definite decrease in liver fat occurs. If cystine and methionine are added to the basal diet in amounts corresponding to those supplied by the diet containing 30 per cent casein, there is little or no decrease in liver fat. Furthermore, the amount of liver fat is decreased when the amount of dietary casein is increased, but when additional quantities of methionine are added to the basal diet the lipotropic activity does not increase beyond a certain limit. This limit is reached under our experimental conditions when there are still large amounts of fat in the liver. If the lipotropic action of certain proteins is due to their constituent amino-acids, the results of these experiments suggest that other amino-acids are involved in the lipotropic activity of dietary casein. Tucker and Eckstein [761] did not obtain an increase in liver fat when cystine was added to a diet which contained 5 per cent gliadin as the basal protein, and they suggest that other amino-acids may exert the same effects as cystine or methionine. Our findings are therefore in agreement with those of Channon *et al.* [188; 189] and of Tucker and Eckstein [761] who have emphasized the probability that other factors in addition to cystine and methionine may be involved in the explanation of the lipotropic effect of protein. Some light may be thrown on the problem by the further developments of the investigations of du Vigneaud, Chandler, Moyer, and Keppel [769] and of Channon *et al.* [188; 189]. The effect of homocystine and related substances on fat metabolism is being studied by both these groups.

Summary

1. Methionine exerts a definite lipotropic action (confirming Tucker and Eckstein).

2. The activities of *d*-methionine, *l*-methionine, and the racemic mixture are of the same order under our experimental conditions.

3. In experiments in which relatively small doses of methionine have produced a significant fall in liver fat, increase in the dose has not caused a further decrease in spite of the fact that large amounts of fat were still present in the liver.

4. Our results support the conclusion of other workers in this field that factors other than cystine and methionine are involved in the explanation of the lipotropic effect of dietary protein.

Acknowledgment

We are indebted to Professor W. E. Rose and to Dr. Madelyn Womack for the preparation of *d*- and *l*-methionine.

42. The Mode of Action of Lipotropic Agents: Proof of the *in Vivo* Incorporation of Triethyl-β-hydroxy-ethyl-ammonium Hydroxide into the Phospholipid Molecule

C. S. McARTHUR

C. C. LUCAS

C. H. BEST

Several theories have been proposed to account for the lipotropic action of choline, betaine, methionine, inositol, and other compounds which exert similar effects on the deposition of lipids in the liver. The discovery (Hershey [387]; Hershey and Soskin [388]) reported from the laboratory of one of us (C. H. B.) that lecithin prevents the accumulation of excessive amounts of fat in the liver of depancreatized dogs seemed to offer support for the hypothesis, originally advanced by Leathes, that fatty acid transport involves incorporation of these compounds into the phospholipid molecule. The demonstration by Best and Huntsman [94] that choline is the lipotropically active constituent of the lecithin molecule did not alter the main concept. If choline cannot be synthesized by mammals, or if its rate of synthesis is not equal to all requirements, the amount available would probably be the limiting factor in the formation of new lecithin molecules. Thus the viewpoint has been adopted that ingested choline exerts its lipotropic effect, in part at least, by stimulating synthesis of lecithin. Using radioactive phosphorus as a tracer element, a more rapid turnover of liver phospholipids was shown to follow ingestion of choline (Perlman and Chaikoff [617]) and the relatively rapid incorporation of dietary choline into the phospholipid molecule has been established (Stetten [738]). Welch and Landau [786] have shown that arsenocholine (an analogue of choline

Originally appeared in the *Biochemical Journal*, XLI (1947), 612–18.

containing arsenic in place of nitrogen), which is lipotropic, also enters the lecithin molecule. The fact that inositol, which possesses lipotropic properties (Gavin and McHenry [317]), is also a constituent of phospholipids (Anderson [13]; Folch and Woolley [302]) is of considerable interest to those who adopt the viewpoint that a lipotropic agent exerts its effect by virtue of promoting phospholipid synthesis. Methionine and betaine probably act by supplying labile methyl groups for choline synthesis.

About 10 years ago, before tracer elements were available, Channon and Smith [193] first proposed testing the hypothesis that choline exerts its lipotropic action through promoting synthesis of lecithin. They wrote: "Light should be thrown on this question if a base could be found which possessed an action on liver fat similar to that of choline and which could be shown to be present in the liver . . . by isolation of a suitably characteristic derivative. Such a base might be found to have been incorporated in a new phosphatide molecule in which it had replaced the choline of lecithin." Channon and Smith [193] described the synthesis of the ethyl homologue of choline (triethyl-β-hydroxyethylammonium hydroxide) and discovered its strong lipotropic activity. The subsequent attempt by Channon, Platt, Loach, and Smith [192] to detect the compound in liver phospholipids, after feeding it to rats for 20 days, was unsuccessful. They utilized the lesser solubility of the chloroaurate of the triethyl homologue in their search for it in the hydrolyzed liver phospholipids. Channon et al. [192] stated at the end of an experimental paragraph, "The absence of triethyl choline chloroaurate was thus established." This wording was unfortunate since all that was actually proven was that the compound sought for was either absent or present in amounts too small to be detected by the procedure used. This failure to establish the presence of the triethyl homologue in the liver phospholipids has acted as an impediment to the general acceptance of the hypothesis that the lipotropic action of choline involves reactions which utilize the intact molecule.

The writers of this communication felt, as did Channon et al., that ". . . it is a particularly attractive hypothesis . . . that choline should exercise its action by enabling lecithin synthesis to occur" and in view of the work of Welch and Landau it was considered desirable to reinvestigate the ingenious attempt of Channon and his colleagues to use the triethyl homologue of choline as a tracer substance. The procedure used by Channon et al. [192], which would not disclose the presence of less than 20 per cent of the homologue when mixed with choline, did not seem to us adequate for the task in hand. We were thus led to reinvestigate the problem with new analytical and fractionation procedures.

When it was shown (McArthur, Lang, and Lucas [523]) that the *cholineless* mutant (34486) of the bread mould *Neurospora crassa* was unable to utilize the triethyl homologue of choline (cf. Horowitz, Bonner, and Houlahan [397]), and that there was a significant difference between the enneaiodide assay for choline (Erickson, Avrin, Teague and Williams, [291]) and the value obtained by microbiological assay (Horowitz and Beadle [396]), we were encouraged to search for an improved fractionation procedure which would clearly differentiate the trimethyl and triethyl homologues. After many preliminary trials it was found that the tertiary amines obtained by oxidative degradation of the "choline fraction" [505; 506] could be separated out by fractional "micro-distillation." The trimethylamine and triethylamine were identified as chloroaurates.

Since the correct chemical name of the compound (triethyl-β-hydroxy-ethylammonium hydroxide) is a lengthy one and since there are serious objections to the use of the chemically incorrect name "triethyl choline" we propose, for the sake of brevity, to refer to the free base as TE (i.e., the triethyl homologue) and to its chloride as TE.Cl.

It has been possible to establish unequivocally that the triethyl homologue of choline is incorporated in appreciable amounts in the liver phospholipids of rats ingesting this substance (McArthur [522]). The fact that this unnatural quaternary ammonium base, which possesses lipotropic activity, is utilized in the formation of liver "lecithin," may be taken as support for the view that the lipotropic action of choline is dependent upon the intact choline molecule and that the natural substance acts in part at least by favouring lecithin synthesis.

Experimental

Four groups of rats were fed a diet containing 1.125 per cent of TE.Cl for periods of 10, 20, 30, and 40 days, respectively. Each group consisted of 10 males and 10 females (100–170 g). The diet had the following composition: beef dripping 25; corn oil (Mazola) 5; casein 8; gelatin 12; salts (McCollum 185) 5; agar 2; sucrose 39.9; "vitamin powder" 2; cod-liver oil concentrate (Ayerst, McKenna and Harrison) 0.010. The "vitamin powder" was a mixture in powdered sucrose of such a composition that at a food intake of 8 g/day the rats would receive 30 μg aneurin hydrochloride, 25 μg riboflavin, 20 μg pyridoxin hydrochloride, 100 μg calcium pantothenate, and 100 μg nicotinic acid. The diets, freshly prepared about every five days, were stored in tightly covered tin canisters in the refrigerator. The rats, housed in individual cages with false bottoms of coarse wire screen, were supplied daily with fresh water (*ad lib.*) and food (8.0 g). Leftover food averaged 1.7–2.0 g daily. From the individual food consumption the average daily intake of TE.Cl per rat for each group was calculated to be: 10-day group, 71 mg; 20-day group, 68 mg; 30-day group, 69 mg; 40-day group, 69 mg. Thus the average daily intake of the substance, calculated as the base (69 mg $\times$ 163.3/181.7 = 62.1 mg) was nearly six times that of the rats in the experiment of Channon et al. [192] (11.5 mg). The average loss of weight of rats fed this diet for 10 days was 11.2 per cent, for 20 days 9.2 per cent, for 30 days 14.5 per cent and for 40 days was only 9.1 per cent.

The animals were stunned, the livers were removed, weighed and disintegrated immediately in a Waring blendor, under acetone, and extracted repeatedly with boiling absolute ethanol. The combined extracts were taken to dryness *in vacuo*, under N_2, at a bath temperature below 45°. The oily residue was dehydrated by repeated evaporation *in vacuo* of 50 ml portions of benzene-absolute ethanol (4:1 v/v) which were added to the flask. The dry lipid material was taken up in light petroleum (b.p. 30–60°) and made up to volume (500 ml) at about 3–4°. The solutions were kept in a refrigerated room and all samples were removed there. The analytical procedures applied to these lipids have been described recently (Best et al. [102]). Certain of the results are presented in Table 42.I.

Isolation of Liver Phospholipids

The solvent was evaporated from the main portion of the light petroleum solution of the total lipid and the residue was redissolved in a small volume (10 ml) of ether. To this solution 20 vol. of anhydrous acetone were added. The precipitation of the phospholipids was enhanced by a small addition (1.2 ml) of saturated ethanolic $MgCl_2$ solution. The mixture, after standing overnight, was centrifuged and the supernatant solution was set aside. The phospholipid, reprecipitated from ethereal solution with acetone and $MgCl_2$, was dissolved in moist ether and a small amount of ether-insoluble matter was removed. Both the ethereal solution of the phospholipids and the pooled acetone mother liquors were analysed for lipid P and choline. About 3–5 per cent of the P and about 10 per cent of the choline (enneaiodide determination) escaped precipitation.

The remainder of the phospholipid solution was evaporated to dryness and hydrolysed as described below (p. 467). Choline was determined in the hydrolysate by the enneaiodide procedure and also by microbiological assay. One minor modification was found advisable in the enneaiodide procedure of Erickson et al. [291], viz. to use a more concentrated oxidizing reagent: 1 ml bromine in 100 ml glacial acetic acid containing 10 per cent potassium acetate. On known solutions and hydrolysates of normal liver phospholipids the results obtained by the two methods were in excellent agreement.

TABLE 42.1

Effect of Feeding Triethyl-β-Hydroxyethylammonium Chloride

(20 rats (10 ♂, 10 ♀, average weight 138 g/group) fed test diets for periods shown. Average daily intake of TE.Cl 69 mg. Average weight loss of 9 per cent after 40 days on diet.)

Duration of Feeding TE.Cl (days)	No. of Survivors	Wet Weight of Livers (g)	Total Lipids (g)	Total Lipid P (mg)	Total* Choline (enneaiodide) (m.equiv.)	True* Choline (N. crassa) (m.equiv.)	TE* (mg)
10	18	117.5	7.135	153.1	2.45	2.11	55.5
20	20	118.9	11.66	187.5	2.62	2.37	40.9
30	18	112.9	9.38	173.5	2.60	2.08	84.9
40	19	115.6	13.36	154.2	2.54	1.91	103.0

*"Total choline" was determined by precipitation with KI-I₂ and titration of the enneaiodide (i.e., true choline plus any other quaternary bases precipitated by this reagent), and expressed as milliequivalents. True choline, estimated by microbiological assay with the *cholineless* mutant (34486) of *Neurospora crassa*, was similarly expressed. The difference (assumed to be due to TE) was multiplied by the m.equiv. weight of TE (163.3) to give the figures in the last column. The liver fat of animals receiving no TE (i.e., basal group or groups receiving choline supplements) showed no appreciable difference (±2 per cent) between choline assays determined chemically (enneaiodide) and microbiologically.

Preliminary Chemical Investigation of Choline Homologues

A search of the literature and some preliminary investigations in this laboratory failed to reveal a suitable method of separating choline from its mono-, di-, or triethyl homologues. Finally, resort was made to permanganate oxidation of these compounds to form tertiary amines which were found to be separable by distillation and then identifiable as their chloroaurates. All boiling-points and melting-points reported in this paper have been corrected.

Source of Compounds Required

(*a*) Trimethylamine hydrochloride (Hoffmann-LaRoche) was used without further purification.

(*b*) Triethylamine (Eastman Kodak) was dried over solid KOH and fractionally distilled to yield a product boiling at 88–89°.

(*c*) Dimethylethylamine and methyldiethylamine were prepared from ethylamine and diethylamine (Eastman Kodak), respectively, by methylation with paraformaldehyde and formic acid according to the procedure of Clarke, Gillespie and Weisshaus [204] (cf. Sommelet and Ferrand [724]). The products thus obtained were dried over solid KOH and fractionated in a Widmer column. The dimethylethylamine (b.p. 36–37°) yielded a chloroaurate m.p. 212°. The methyldiethylamine (b.p. 65.5°) formed a chloroaurate melting at 151–152°.

(*d*) Ethylene chlorohydrin (British Drug Houses) was fractionally distilled to give a product boiling at 127–128°.

(*e*) Triethyl-β-hydroxyethylammonium chloride was prepared by heating equimolecular proportions of ethylene chlorohydrin and triethylamine in sealed tubes at 120° for 24 hrs. The reaction mixture was dissolved in warm absolute ethanol (0.5 vol.) and the crystalline quaternary ammonium salt precipitated by the addition of 1 vol. of acetone and 5 vol. of dry ether. After several recrystallizations from mixtures of absolute ethanol, acetone, and ether a small portion of the product was converted to the chloroaurate, which had a satisfactory m.p. (230°).

(*f*) The other homologues of choline were prepared from the corresponding tertiary amines in a similar manner.

Oxidative Degradation of Choline Homologues

Preliminary quantitative experiments, one of which is reported here, on the alkaline permanganate oxidation of triethyl-β-hydroxyethylammonium hydroxide and collection of the resulting triethylamine showed that the procedure is applicable to TE.

To 50 ml of an aqueous solution containing 62.08 mg TE.Cl in a 250 ml Lintzel flask, 20 g of solid NaOH were added. A slow stream of air, washed by dilute H_2SO_4, was drawn through the apparatus into a tube containing 10.26 ml of 0.100N-H_2SO_4 and two drops of 0.02 per cent methyl red in 60 per cent ethanol. The strongly alkaline solution was heated to boiling and aqueous $KMnO_4$ (0.5 per cent) was added carefully from the thistle-tube at such a rate that no green colour, due to excess manganate, persisted in the reaction mixture until the oxidation had been completed. The heating and aeration were continued for a further 45 min. At the end of this period the flask and its contents were allowed to cool while being very slowly aerated. The contents of the receiving tube required 6.84 ml 0.100N-NaOH for back titration. The recovery of volatile base, subsequently shown to be triethylamine, was 100.1 per cent of theory.

Since it had been established that the trimethyl and triethyl compounds behave identically as far as the oxidative degradation is concerned, it was assumed that the mono- and diethyl homologues would behave similarly.

Separation of Tertiary Amines by "Distillation"

In view of the great difference in the boiling-points of trimethylamine and triethylamine, 3.5° and 89°, respectively, it seemed feasible to separate small amounts of these by fractional distillation. Several small stills of various designs were made and tested. The most suitable of these had the form and specifications shown in Figure 75.

The amine or mixture of amines, converted to the hydrogen sulphates or hydrochlorides, is transferred to the distilling flask (A) in methanolic solution and the solvent is driven off by warming the flask while a slow stream of nitrogen is passed through tube (E). The receiver (C) is charged with 10 ml of neutral methanol containing two drops of 0.02 per cent methyl red indicator. The distilling flask (A), the U-tube (B), and the delivery tube (H) are joined through the ground-glass joints (F) and (G). The U-tube is cooled in a bath of ethanol and solid carbon dioxide and a boiling water-bath is placed around (A) so that not only the flask but also the side arm is kept at 100°. Through the stopcock (K), 2 ml of aqueous NaOH (saturated at 35°) are run into (A) from the cup (D). The stopcock is now turned to close the opening from (D) and to connect (E) with (A) so that a slow stream of nitrogen may be passed through (A) to carry the amine into the U-tube condenser. After sweeping for 10 min the boiling water-bath is removed from (A) and the ethanol-carbon dioxide bath around (B) is replaced by a cold water-bath which is maintained at a uniform temperature of 4° by mechanical stirring and occasional additions of small pieces of ice. As the flask (A) cools, it is necessary to allow nitrogen to flow through the stopcock to prevent the methanol from being drawn

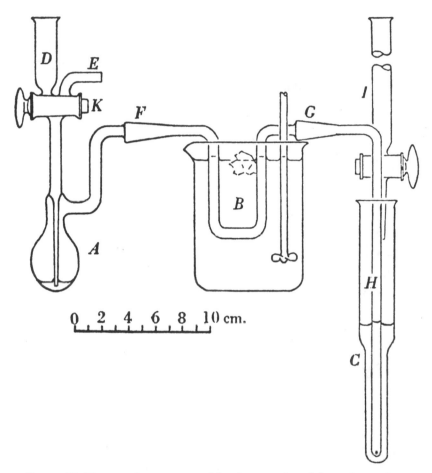

FIGURE 75. Diagram of apparatus used for the separation of the tertiary amines.

over into (B). When (A) has reached room temperature, (E) is connected to a gasometer which is arranged to deliver a slow, constant flow of nitrogen (about 3 ml/min). Sufficient standard acid is added from the burette (I) to keep this solution (C) distinctly acidic and (K) is turned to admit nitrogen from the gasometer. When the portion of acid added initially to (C) has been neutralized, further known increments of the standard acid are added from the burette and the time intervals required for the neutralization of these by the amine carried over are recorded.

Typical curves obtained with the four possible tertiary amines, viz. trimethylamine, dimethylethylamine, methyldiethylamine, and triethylamine, and a known mixture of the first compound with the last, are shown in Figure 76. Curve 1 shows that trimethylamine (80.0 mg) "distils" at 4° with great rapidity, the bulk of it going over in about 3 min. The relatively

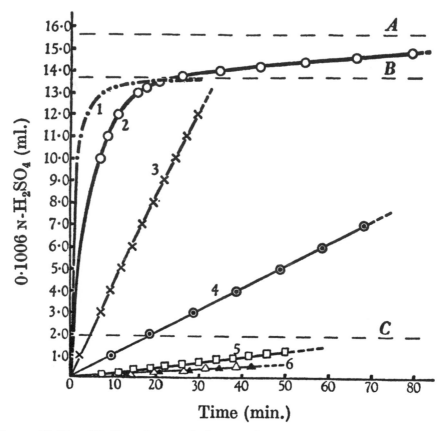

FIGURE 76. Time-"distillation" curves for known substances at 4°. Sweeping rate 3.1 ml/min for curves 1–5, 1.8 ml/min for curve 6. Curve 1, 80 mg trymethylamine; curve 2, a mixture of 80 mg of trimethylamine and 20 mg triethylamine; curve 3, 101.5 mg dimethylethylamine; curve 4, 118.4 mg methyldiethylamine; curve 5, 20 mg triethylamine; curve 6, △–△ 40 mg triethylamine, ▲–▲ 80 mg triethylamine. Lines A, B, and C cut the vertical axis at points representing the calculated titration values for the mixture of 80 mg trimethyl- and 20 mg of triethylamine, 80 mg of trimethylamine alone, and 20 mg triethylamine alone, respectively.

slow evolution of triethylamine (20.0 mg) is apparent in curve 5, while curves 3 and 4 indicate the rates of evaporation of dimethylethylamine (101.5 mg) and methyldiethylamine (118.4 mg) respectively, under the same conditions. If the rate of sweeping is kept constant from one experiment to another, the amount of triethylamine present does not affect the rate of evolution, as is shown in curve 6, which represents the rate of evaporation of 40 and 80 mg of triethylamine with slower aeration (1.8 ml N_2/min.) than that used in obtaining curve 5. Curve 2 represents the behaviour of a mixture of 80 mg of trimethylamine and 20 mg of triethylamine under the standard conditions (3.1 ml N_2/min) used to obtain curves 1 and 5 and in all subsequent work. Since the slope of the curve for evaporation of triethylamine is constant with a constant sweeping rate, projection of the upper linear part of curve 2 should cut the vertical axis at a point representing the volume of standard acid required to neutralize the trimethylamine. The difference between this value and that of the total titration should, therefore, represent the amount of acid consumed by triethylamine. The agreement between theory and practice is satisfactory (see also Figure 78).

Examination of the Rat Liver Phospholipids

Hydrolysis. The phospholipid fractions from each of the four groups of animals were treated separately. Each was dissolved in 10 ml of warm ethanol and emulsified by forcing the solution in a thin stream into 100 ml of 5 per cent (v/v) aqueous H_2SO_4. The mixture was refluxed for 8 hrs. After removal of the fatty acids by shaking several times with ether and precipitation of the bulk of the sulphuric acid with baryta the hydrolysate was neutralized to phenol red by the addition of 0.1 N-NaOH and made up to a volume of 500 ml.

Choline determinations in the hydrolysates. Portions of each of the four hydrolysates obtained from the acetone-insoluble phospholipids were analysed in replicate for choline by the chemical (enneaiodide) and microbiological (*Neurospora crassa, cholineless*) methods. The results are tabulated in Table 42.II.

TABLE 42.II

CHOLINE CONTENT OF HYDROLYSATES OF ISOLATED LIVER PHOSPHOLIPIDS

(Results expressed as mg/500 ml of hydrolysate.)

Days of Feeding	Chemical Procedure (calculated as choline)	Microbiological Procedure (calculated as choline)	Difference (calculated as TE)	TE (as % "total choline")
10	249	216	44.4	17.1
20	263	242	28.3	10.5
30	246	202	59.3	22.7
40	254	194	80.8	29.4

Since the chemical procedure estimates total quaternary ammonium base while the microbiological method responds only to choline (and to a very much smaller extent to the methyldiethyl and dimethylethyl homologues of choline), any difference in assay was tentatively attributed to the presence of the triethyl homologue.

Oxidative Degradation of Phospholipid Hydrolysates

40-day group. The portion (350 ml) of the hydrolysate which remained after removal of samples for analytical purposes was oxidized directly with alkaline permanganate in the Lintzel apparatus as described above except that just sufficient standard H_2SO_4 was added to the receiver during the oxidation to keep the distillate acidic to methyl red. Because of the limited capacity of the reaction flask, the operation was performed on three separate portions. To the combined distillates containing the tertiary amines another volume of standard H_2SO_4, equal to that required for neutralization, was added and the acidic solution was set aside for further investigation.

30-day group. Because oxidation of the unfractionated hydrolysate (above) gave rise to ammonia (from hydrolytic products of cephalins) as well as tertiary amines and further because the volume of permanganate solution required was so great, it was deemed advisable to isolate the quaternary bases for oxidation. The remainder of this hydrolysate (470 ml), made alkaline to phenol red, was concentrated *in vacuo* to about 140 ml (bath temperature 60–70°). No volatile base was detectable in the distillate proving that the isolated phospholipid did not contain any free tertiary amine. From the concentrated hydrolysate, again made slightly acidic to phenol red, the quaternary ammonium bases were precipitated in centrifuge pots at 0° as enneaiodides. After centrifuging, the precipitate was washed once in the pots with cold potassium triiodide reagent diluted to the same concentration as was used for precipitation. The precipitate was transferred to a distillation flask with 100 ml of water and 5 ml N-H_2SO_4. The elemental iodine was removed by distillation under reduced pressure. Ionic iodine was precipitated with an excess of Ag_2SO_4 and the excess silver ions were removed by H_2S. The filtrate from the silver sulphide, concentrated to a volume of 30 ml, was oxidized in the Lintzel apparatus. After the addition of a second equivalent of standard H_2SO_4 to the distillate, it was set aside.

Combined 10- and 20-day groups. The remaining portions of the phospholipid hydrolysates from the 10- and 20-day groups of animals, each 450 ml in volume, were combined and concentrated to a volume of 200 ml. The quaternary ammonium bases were isolated as described above, except that the enneaiodide was washed twice by dispersing the precipitate in diluted potassium triiodide reagent. The isolated base in aqueous solution was made up to a volume of 100 ml and 98 ml of this was converted to tertiary amines.

Separation of the Tertiary Amines

40-day group. The aqueous solution obtained by titration of the volatile base formed by oxidation of the hydrolysed phospholipids was concentrated *in vacuo.* The residue was dehydrated by repeated distillation of 5 ml portions of absolute ethanol which were added to the distillation flask. Two 5 ml portions of absolute ethanol were used to extract the amine salts from the contaminating $(NH_4)_2SO_4$. The ethanolic extracts were taken to dryness in the microdistillation flask.

The amines, liberated and "redistilled" as previously described to obtain the time-"distillation" curve, required a total of 12.95 ml of $0.1006N$-H_2SO_4. The slope of the upper linear part of the curve indicated the presence of triethylamine. The acid required by this compound corresponded to 29.0 mg of the base. (This value agrees moderately well with that calculated from the difference between the two choline analyses, 26.6 mg.) In order to obtain a sample of this material contaminated with as little trimethylamine as possible, the contents of the receiver were fractionally "distilled" under the same conditions. The point at which to change the receiver was determined by inspection of the time-"distillation" curve. The cut was not made until the slow constant evolution of the higher boiling amine was evident. Momentarily, the flow of nitrogen was stopped while the receiver was replaced by another containing 15 ml of $0.1N$-methanolic HCl. Hot water baths were placed around the distillation flask and the U-tube and sweeping was resumed at a gradually increasing rate (4–8 ml/min). Complete transfer required about 2 hrs.

The mean molecular weight of the amine mixture was determined upon the crystalline residue obtained by evaporating the acidic absorbing liquid to dryness. The residue, washed with absolute ether and desiccated (21.5 mg), was returned to the micro-still. The volatile amines required 16.00 ml of $0.0100N$-H_2SO_4 (methyl red indicator). The mean molecular weight (134.4) suggested that the mixture consisted of 92.4 per cent triethylammonium chloride and 7.6 per cent trimethylammonium chloride.

The crude triethylamine, "redistilled" into an excess of HCl to free it from indicator, was converted to the chloroaurate in 0.5 ml of N-HCl. The precipitate, filtered and washed twice with 0.12 ml portions of cold dilute HCl, when dried *in vacuo* over P_2O_5 weighed 16.8 mg, m.p. 86–87°. Analysis: C, 16.5; H, 3.68; Au, 44.2 per cent. The compositions and m.p. of the possible trialkylammonium chloroaurates are tabulated below:

Formula	m.p.	C (%)	H (%)	Au (%)
$(C_2H_5)_3N \cdot HCl \cdot AuCl_3$	89°	16.35	3.66	44.7
$(C_2H_5)_2CH_3N \cdot HCl \cdot AuCl_3$	151–152°	14.06	3.30	46.2
$C_2H_5(CH_3)_2N \cdot HCl \cdot AuCl_3$	212°	11.63	2.93	47.7
$(CH_3)_3N \cdot HCl \cdot AuCl_3$	234–235°	9.03	2.53	49.4

30-day group. The acidified distillate obtained by Lintzel oxidation of the isolated choline was evaporated to dryness and the residue was transferred to the still. The time-"distillation" curve shown in Figure 77 indicated the

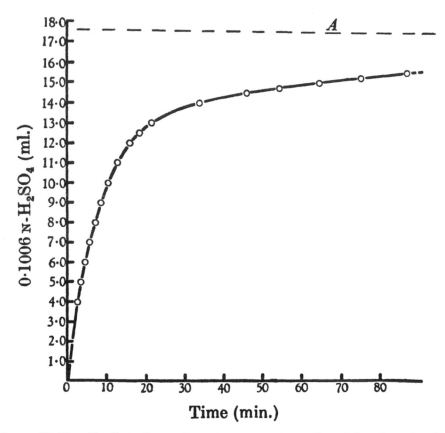

FIGURE 77. Time-"distillation" curve for tertiary amine mixture derived from liver phospholipids of 30-day group. Aeration rate 3.1 ml/min. The line A cuts the vertical axis at a point representing the total titration.

presence of triethylamine. From the amine mixture, fractionated as described in the previous section, the higher boiling fraction was separated. It was converted to the chloroaurate (81 mg) m.p. 87°. Mixed with triethylammonium chloroaurate, m.p. 89°.

Combined 10- and 20-day groups. All operations upon the combined material from these two groups were conducted with quantitative care in order to compare the recoveries obtained by oxidative degradation and fractional "distillation" with the results of the choline analyses on the bases isolated as enneaiodides. The tertiary ammonium salts were transferred to the micro-distillation apparatus. Since the amount of trimethylamine derivable from the choline in the mixture was large (30.2 ml 0.1006N-acid, calculated from the results of the microbiological choline assay), the U-tube was kept at a temperature of 4° for 1 hr without aeration to avoid too rapid transfer and possible incomplete absorption of trimethylamine. During this time amine equivalent to 13.35 ml of the standard acid was collected in the receiver, which then was replaced by a second receiver. "Distillation" and titration of the remaining part of the amine mixture were carried out in the manner previously described. Figure 78 shows the "distillation" curve obtained. The total titration amounted to 32.85 ml of the standard acid (calculated requirement from the results of the chemical analyses, 32.30 ml). The curve (Fig. 78) indicates that the mixture consisted of 3.05 m.equiv. of trimethylamine and 0.25 m.equiv. of triethylamine; by calculation (from the results of the microbiological and chemical choline assays), the values were 3.03 m.equiv. and 0.19 m.equiv. respectively.

After drying, the residue from the second receiver was transferred to the micro-apparatus for fractionation. The "distillation" was carried out with sweeping until 17.0 ml of 0.1006N-acid had been consumed. At this point the receiver was exchanged for one containing 20 ml of methanol and 0.2 ml of conc. HCl, into which the remainder of the amine was swept. The residue remaining after the removal of the methanol was converted to the chloroaurate in dilute HCl (1.9 ml). The yellow crystalline precipitate, washed with three 1 ml portions of cold dilute HCl and dried (33.4 mg) melted at 89°, mixed with methyldiethylammonium chloroaurate, m.p. 124°; mixed with authentic triethylammonium chloroaurate, m.p. 89°. A further quantity (23.5 mg, m.p. 87–89°) was obtained by concentration of the mother liquors.

DISCUSSION

Although the lipotropic effect of choline is well established and generally accepted, its mode of action has not yet been completely elucidated. Some authorities believe that the lipotropic effect may be explained by the observation that choline accelerates the turnover of the phosphorus in liver phospholipids. The assumption has been made that choline similarly promotes an accelerated turnover of all constituents of the phospholipid molecule. Experimental evidence for any increased rate of turnover of fatty acids in liver phospholipids under the influence of dietary choline, is not yet available, however, and hence a completely satisfactory explanation of lipotropic action must await further investigation.

There seems to be some confusion in the minds of certain recent writers on the subject of lipotropic action as to whether the labile methyl groups or choline *per se* is the ultimate lipotropic factor. The evidence is accumulating that the intact choline molecule is the effective lipotropic substance. Compounds such as betaine and methionine appear to exert their lipo-

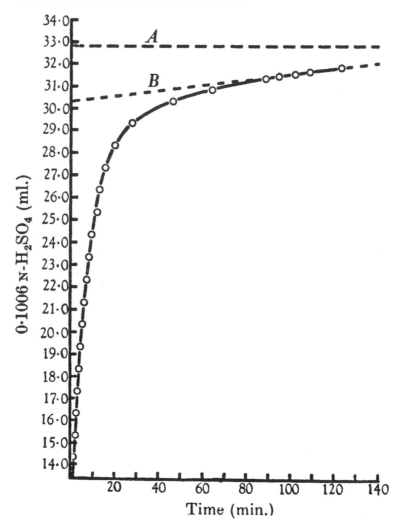

FIGURE 78. Time-"distillation" curve of tertiary amines derived from liver phospholipids (10- and 20-day groups). The choline fractions from the two groups were combined for oxidative degradation and fractionation of the tertiary amines. Intercept of line A on the vertical axis represents the total titration of the amine mixture, of line B (a projection of the upper linear portion of the curve) represents the titration value for trimethylamine; the difference represents the titration value for triethylamine.

tropic effect by contributing labile methyl groups either for the synthesis or the sparing of choline. The experiments of Welch and Landau [786] have established that arsenocholine, which is lipotropic and does not possess labile methyl groups, when fed, is incorporated *in toto* into the phospholipid molecule. In the case of this choline analogue, it is the intact molecule and not a labile methyl group which exerts the biological effect.

The present experiments with the triethyl homologue of choline, which also is lipotropic and lacks labile methyl groups, supply another example of a lipotropically active substance which is utilized intact in the synthesis of new phospholipid molecules. The arguments advanced by Welch and Landau in support of the hypothesis that the intact choline molecule is the active lipotropic substance are substantiated by the findings reported above.

Several explanations may be offered for the failure of Channon *et al.* [192] to detect the triethyl homologue of choline in the liver phospholipids of their experimental animals. The basal diet fed by them was so low in protein (5 per cent casein) that it probably did not permit metabolic processes to function normally. At this low protein intake, the quaternary ammonium chloride may have exerted a more toxic action than it did in the present experiments. Whatever the explanation, it has been possible to feed six times the daily dose used by them, and to give it for twice as long a period of time, without any greater weight loss or mortality than they observed. Furthermore, improvements in micro-analytical methods during the past ten years have probably contributed to the present successful accomplishment of the project initiated by Channon and his colleagues. The establishment of the fact that the lipotropically active triethyl homologue of choline is biologically incorporated into the molecule of liver phospholipids, removes one of the impediments to general acceptance of the hypothesis that the lipotropic action of choline involves reactions which utilize the intact molecule.

Summary

1. A significant difference between the microchemical and microbiological assays for choline in the hydrolysates of the phospholipids isolated from the livers of rats fed triethyl-β-hydroxyethylammonium chloride, suggested that appreciable amounts of an unnatural base had been incorporated into the liver of the phospholipids. Fractionation procedures were devised which led to chemical proof that the triethyl homologue of choline had been incorporated into the phospholipids.

2. This finding provides further proof that the lipotropic effect of choline is associated with the intact molecule rather than its methyl groups.

Acknowledgments

We are indebted to Dr. J. H. Ridout for the extraction of the liver lipids and some of the preliminary chemical analyses and to Miss J. M. Lang who performed the microbiological assays. The expenses of this investigation were defrayed, in part, by a grant from the Banting Research Foundation.

43. Hypertension of Renal Origin in Rats Following less than One Week of Choline Deficiency in Early Life

W. STANLEY HARTROFT, M.D.

CHARLES H. BEST, C.B.E., M.D., F.R.S.

The production of arterial hypertension by dietary deficiency alone has not previously been demonstrated. Since the report by Griffith and Wade [335] it has been well established that choline deficiency produces severe renal lesions in young rats (György and Goldblatt [342]; Engel and Salmon [289]; Handler [352]; and others). A careful study of the blood pressures of rats maintained for long periods on diets low in choline has been made by Sobin and Landis [718], who found no evidence of hypertension. The results of earlier studies by Honorato and Vadillo [395] apparently support this same conclusion. Stimulated in part by these papers, by discussions with Professor Eugene Landis, and by the early studies of choline deficiency in our laboratories (Best and Huntsman [94]), we decided to produce a severe renal lesion by this dietary means and then to study the blood pressures of the surviving animals maintained on full diets. Under these conditions, in our present series of observations all animals with severe residual renal damage developed hypertension. The average figure for ten animals in this group was 195 mm Hg. This is the mean pressure recorded by arterial cannulation. The comparable figure for 36 control animals was 118 mm Hg.

METHODS

Weanling albino rats of the Wistar strain weighing 35–42 g were fed a diet low in choline (T45) as described by our colleagues Lucas and

Originally appeared in the *British Medical Journal*, I (1949), 423–6. These histological studies were aided by a grant from the National Research Council of Canada, 1948, and the nutritional aspects of the work were financed in part by the Nutrition Foundation in New York.

Ridout.[1] The object was to produce the greatest degree of renal damage compatible with life. The animals were fed the choline-deficient diets for varying lengths of time. Most of the rats received the ration for five to six days. In the more recent experiments the animals were fed the choline-deficient diet for four five-day periods separated by two-day intervals during which the diet was supplemented with 0.35 per cent choline chloride. All the animals received a stock diet for the remainder of the experiment. In the early studies the rats were sacrificed at the age of three to four months, but it was subsequently discovered that a higher percentage developed hypertension if allowed to live for six or seven months. Control animals were pair-fed with those receiving the choline-deficient diet. These controls received the T45 diet supplemented with 0.35 per cent choline chloride. They were given the stock diet *ad libitum* at the same time as the experimental groups, and were maintained on this until sacrificed.

Indirect blood-pressure determinations according to the method of Sobin [717] were made at intervals on all rats in order to follow the progress of the experiment. At the end of the period of observation blood-pressure determinations were made by the direct procedure. The animals were anaesthetized with 90 mg of sodium amytal per kilogram of body weight, administered intraperitoneally as a freshly prepared 10 per cent solution in distilled water. The femoral artery was exposed and cannulated with a 24-gauge needle. Drops of 1 per cent aqueous solution of procaine hydrochloride were placed on the artery during dissection to prevent spasm. The needle was attached to a fine-bore mercury manometer, and the system filled with Ringer's solution. Owing to the inertia of the system the readings obtained represented the mean of systolic and diastolic levels of blood pressure, and all direct blood-pressure measurements reported in this paper refer to this mean value rather than to systolic levels. The animals were killed by exsanguination. This procedure effectively emptied the hearts, which were weighed to the nearest $1/100$ g, and these figures are expressed in the tables as percentages of the total body weights. In all but the earliest experiments, in order to obtain the greatest possible objectivity, the observations concerning blood pressure and heart weights were made without the observer (W.S.H.) knowing whether the animal belonged to the control or to the experimental group.

Paraffin sections of the viscera were made after fixation in either 10 per

[1]The composition of this diet was reported [516] to the Twelfth Annual Meeting of the Canadian Physiological Society, Quebec City, October 15 and 16, 1948: arachin 12, gelatin 6, casein 3, fibrin 1, cystine 0.5, salts 5, celluflour 2, sucrose 58.5, beef fat 10, corn oil 2, a cod-liver oil concentrate (Ayerst, McKenna, and Harrison) 0.015, and 1 per cent of a mixture in sucrose of 10 B-vitamins plus alpha-tocopheryl acetate.

cent neutral formol-saline or in Bouin's solution. Sections were treated with haematoxylin and eosin, Mallory's phosphotungstic acid haematoxylin (P.T.A.), Gomori's chromium haematoxylin and phloxine, and Masson's connective-tissue stain. In addition selected sections were stained for elastic tissue, for calcium, and for haemosiderin. Frozen sections of kidneys and large vessels were stained for fat and tested for cholesterol (Schultz reaction). Several sections from both kidneys of each animal were surveyed and the amount of renal damage classified as severe, moderate, or slight.

Observations were made on 62 rats surviving varying degrees of the renal haemorrhagic syndrome and on 36 control animals of similar age and weight.

RESULTS

The findings were arranged in three groups according to the degree of residual renal damage noted microscopically. Group 1 is made up of the 10 survivors of the haemorrhagic renal syndrome which had *severe* persistent kidney damage. All these animals had definite arterial hypertension. The average blood pressure was 195 mm Hg and the average weight of their hearts was nearly double the normal value. Group 2 comprises the 13 survivors of the acute period of choline deficiency with *moderate* residual renal damage. Of these, 85 per cent (11 of 13) had blood pressures of 150 mm Hg or over. The average blood pressure for this group was 165 mm Hg, and the average heart weight was one-third greater than that of the normal controls. In the remaining 39 survivors (Group 3) only *slight* renal damage was found. There is little evidence that a significant degree of hypertension developed in the members of this group. Of 36 *control* animals of similar age and weight, only one had a blood pressure greater than 140 mm Hg, and the average for the group was 118 mm Hg. [Tables I to IV of the original have been eliminated and replaced by the following condensation, Table 43.I.]

The kidney lesions took the form of tubular destruction combined with marked distension of other nephrons, many of which contained large amounts of eosinophilic colloid, particularly in the medulla. There was obvious reduction in the number of glomeruli in the severely damaged kidneys, and the remaining glomeruli showed severe degrees of thickening of the basement membranes throughout the capillary loops, while others were converted into little more than spheres of hyaline material.

[Ten figures have been omitted showing different degrees of kidney damage caused by the brief period of choline deficiency in early life.]

The vascular lesions varied from early cellular proliferation of the media

TABLE 43.I

CONDENSATION OF DATA IN ORIGINAL TABLES I TO IV

Original Table no. and Group no.	No. Animals	Residual Kidney Damage	Heart Wt. as % of Body Wt.		Blood Pressure Mean of Systolic and Diastolic (mm Hg)	
			Range and Median	Mean ±s.d.	Range and Median	Mean ± s.d.
I	10	severe	0.44–0.88 (0.65)	0.55±0.15	150–230 (200)	195±21
II	13	moderate	0.31–0.41 (0.37)	0.37±0.04	130–200 (170)	165±19
III	39	slight	0.28–0.41 (0.32)	0.33±0.03	90–185 (130)	136±17
IV	36	none (normal)	0.25–0.35 (0.30)	0.30±0.03	80–170 (120)	118±18

and adventitia of the arterioles in animals with only slight kidney damage and slight evidence of hypertension, to intimal hyalinization and fibrinoid necrosis in those with severe degrees of kidney damage and elevated blood pressure. Determinations of the non-protein nitrogen levels in the blood of two such animals showed values over 350 mg per 100 ml. No gross or microscopical evidence of atheromatous deposits was found in the larger arteries, nor could elastosis (Boyd [145]) be demonstrated in these. Small deposits of cholesterol (Schultz-positive) in some of the hyalinized glomeruli were demonstrated in frozen sections of the most severely damaged kidneys. No evidence of inflammatory disease was found in any of the sections of hearts of the hypertensive animals.

DISCUSSION

Reduction of the glomerular capillary bed incident to the kidney damage resulting from the deficiency of choline appears to be the significant factor determining the degree of hypertension eventually produced. As these renal lesions are primarily tubular (Christensen [202]; Hartroft [364]) it may at first appear paradoxical that glomerular damage is such a prominent feature of the lesions in the surviving animals. However, these authors and others have pointed out that in severe cases of haemorrhagic kidney the glomeruli are secondarily involved in the later stages of the syndrome. When appreciable numbers of glomeruli are destroyed a train of events is apparently started leading to elevation of blood pressure. The hypertension in turn produces thickening of both the glomerular loops and the arterioles. It is likely that the mechanism producing hypertension in our animals is similar to that operating in rats after subtotal nephrectomy (Chanutin and

Ferris [195]). In the present experiments the factor responsible for reducing the amount of functioning renal tissue is dietary deficiency rather than surgery. The basic mechanisms by which hypertension is initiated are probably similar to those demonstrated by Goldblatt *et al.* [324]. The effects of massive amounts of vitamin D in producing evidences of hypertension (Ham [350]) are presumably exerted through similar pathways.

It is well known that there is great variation among the members of any group of young rats in the extent of renal damage resulting from choline deficiency. A small percentage of such animals never develop advanced renal lesions even if fed the diet for many weeks. In the early stages of the experiments here reported large numbers of weanlings were left on the choline-deficient diet for periods as long as 7 to 10 days. The mortality rates in these groups were high (over 80 per cent). The small number of survivors were then given full diets, but appreciable residual renal damage was not present at necropsy several months later, and blood-pressure values during life were not significantly higher than normal levels. This finding indicated to us that a prolongation of the period of dietary deficiency had eliminated those animals most susceptible to this type of kidney damage. However, if these animals had lived they would presumably have been the ones most likely to develop hypertension. For this reason, in later experiments the young rats were not deprived of dietary choline for unbroken periods of more than five or six days. Accordingly, greater numbers survived this stage, and these included many in which a severe degree of kidney damage had been produced by choline deficiency.

In the experiments of Sobin and Landis rats were maintained on the choline-deficient diet for a period of months. During the initial period of acute deficiency 66 per cent of the males and 20 per cent of the females died. The growth of the surviving animals was distinctly slower than that of the controls, and the difference in weights at five months was conspicuous. Our experience in similar investigations confirmed the findings of these workers. The absence of hypertension in any of the animals maintained for prolonged periods on these deficient diets might be explained in either or both of two ways. Those animals most susceptible to the lack of choline may not have survived the initial period of acute deficiency. A second possibility is that the retarded growth of the surviving rats may have prevented the developments of hypertension. In our present series, animals surviving the initial period of dietary deficiency were transferred to full diets, and growth from then on approached that of the normal controls. The higher growth rates may have made greater demands on the cardiovascular–renal systems of these animals with residual kidney damage, and thus have initiated the development of hypertension.

The clinical significance of our results is not apparent. Attempts to produce the haemorrhagic renal syndrome in any species other than the rat have not yet been successful. In this laboratory further investigations are being undertaken to increase the percentage of those rats surviving "haemorrhagic kidney" which have severe degrees of residual renal damage. If this can be accomplished we will have at our disposal a useful method for the production of experimental hypertension in rats in addition to those which involve surgical intervention or the injection of hormones or of nephrotoxic agents. The problem is to determine how long to deprive the young animals of dietary choline to produce consistently the maximal amount of irreversible renal damage compatible with life.

We may suggest that the wider application of the principle of subjecting young animals to acute deficiencies of one or more essential food factors, followed by periods of growth approaching or exceeding the normal in rate, may reveal other and hitherto unsuspected effects of the initial deficiency. We hope to explore some of these possibilities.

Summary and Conclusions

In this series of observations all the rats in which a severe degree of residual renal damage was produced by a short period of choline deficiency during early life later developed a definite hypertension.

The average blood pressure of this test series was 195 mm Hg as determined by arterial cannulization, while that of the controls was 118 mm Hg.

The average weight of the hearts of the hypertensive animals was almost double that of the controls. The histological picture of the arterioles of these animals was characteristic of advanced hypertension.

When only a moderate degree of residual kidney damage was produced by choline deficiency the hypertension, cardiac hypertrophy, and other pathological changes were correspondingly less.

There is no apparent immediate clinical application of these findings. Our results suggest that further work may provide a simple way of consistently producing hypertension in an experimental animal by dietary means.

Acknowledgments

The kindly interest of Professor William Boyd is gratefully acknowledged. We are also indebted to our colleagues Dr. J. H. Ridout and Dr. C. C. Lucas for their help, and to William Wilson for technical assistance. The photomicrographs were made by one of us (W.S.H.).

44. Liver Damage Produced by Feeding Alcohol or Sugar and its Prevention by Choline

C. H. BEST, M.D., F.R.S.

W. STANLEY HARTROFT, M.D.

C. C. LUCAS, PH.D.

JESSIE H. RIDOUT, PH.D.

One of the first suggestions that over-indulgence in alcoholic beverages may damage the liver was made in 1836 by Thomas Addison [6] physician to Guy's Hospital, London. He wrote: "With respect to the causes of this fatty degeneration of the liver, very little, or absolutely nothing, is known. In most of the cases which I have met with, there has been either positive or strong presumptive evidence that the individual had indulged in spirit-drinking; and indeed the most exquisite case I ever saw in a young subject occurred in a female who had for some time subsisted almost exclusively on ardent spirits. On the other hand, the extreme frequency of the degeneration in France, where the people are but little given to such indulgence, throws considerable doubt upon such an origin of the complaint."

A few years later, in 1849, Rokitansky [649], pathologist to the Imperial Royal General Hospital in Vienna, reached a similar conclusion concerning the responsibility of alcohol for at least one type of fatty liver. Rokitansky noted the frequent occurrence of cirrhosis of the liver in drunkards. He was possibly the first to suggest that cirrhosis follows fatty changes in the liver.

The earliest references to experimental studies of the effects of alcohol were concerned with its effect on the brain (Dahlström, mentioned by Magnus Huss [411]; Duchek, [267]). Kremiansky [474], in the course of similar investigations, noted that one of four dogs receiving increasing doses of alcohol up to 6 oz (170 ml) daily for three months developed fatty

Originally appeared in the *British Medical Journal*, II (1949), 1001–17. A very brief account of this work was presented at the Detroit Meeting of the American Physiological Society, 1949.

changes of the liver and heart and a catarrhal condition of the kidneys. However, Ruge [656], in 1870, seems to have been the first to show clearly that an accumulation of fat occurs in the livers of dogs given increasing daily doses of alcohol by stomach-tube. He noted incidentally that the nature of the diet influenced the amount of fat found in the liver.

Moon [577], in his comprehensive and critical review of the experimental work on alcoholic cirrhosis, concluded in 1934 that none of the experimental procedures had been successful in producing cirrhosis in animals, other than rabbits, by alcohol alone. He pointed out that many of the so-called "positive" results with rabbits must be discounted owing to the presence of intercurrent liver infections (coccidiosis, etc.) or to a chronic periportal inflammation which is common among adult untreated rabbits. Moon concluded: "Without minimizing the contributory or predisposing influence which alcohol may exert, it must be concluded that experimental evidence has not substantiated the belief that alcohol is a direct cause of cirrhosis."

Experimental evidence that long-continued presence of abnormal amounts of fat in the liver does give rise to cirrhosis was supplied in 1938 by Chaikoff, Connor, and Biskind [181] using depancreatized dogs which had been maintained with insulin for periods up to five years. Production of cirrhosis in normal dogs by feeding alcohol to animals in which a fatty liver had previously been established by dietary means was reported by Connor and Chaikoff [219], but the relationship of the alcohol to the cirrhosis became questionable when Chaikoff and Connor in 1940 [180] produced a cirrhosis in normal dogs by dietary means alone (high fat and low protein). A series of papers from the National Institute of Health, Bethesda, Maryland, by Daft, Sebrell, Lillie, and their associates, reported that the consumption of alcohol by rats increased the severity of dietary cirrhosis and that supplements of choline chloride or of methionine (or an increase in the dietary casein) prevented the development of cirrhosis and were beneficial in its treatment [236; 503; 504; 513; 515].

More recently, however, Ashworth [28] concluded that alcohol exerts a toxic effect even when the diet is adequate. Rats on high-casein diets and others on low-casein diets were given 1.5 ml of 25 per cent alcohol per 100 g body weight by stomach-tube daily for two months, and 10 per cent alcohol was supplied in place of drinking-water; control groups without alcohol were "pair-fed" the same basal diets. Since all the rats lost weight, whether alcohol was present or not, it is questionable whether the basal diets were adequate. Interpretation of the data is therefore difficult (see "Discussion").

Although Ashworth pair-fed his rats, the calorie intake of those consuming alcohol was considerably in excess of those drinking water. To determine what effect calorie imbalance might have upon the results, we have performed experiments in which, for the first time in a study of the effects of alcohol, isocaloric pair-feeding has been used. Groups of rats not receiving alcohol were isocalorically pair-fed with those ingesting alcohol. The extra calories (equivalent to those supplied by the alcohol) were provided as finely powdered sucrose.

The effects of various lipotropic supplements added to the diets of the rats consuming alcohol were studied. The pathological changes in the liver produced in these experiments are attributed to an imbalance of calories and vitamins, particularly to an induced inadequacy of lipotropic factors consequent upon the increased calorie intake. Adequate amounts of choline chloride, methionine, or casein always protected the liver. Under these particular experimental conditions there is no more evidence of a toxic effect of pure ethyl alcohol upon the liver cells than there is of a poisonous action of an amount of sucrose which supplies the same calorie intake. In fact, there is no suggestion that either alcohol or sucrose exerts a direct hepatotoxic effect. The fatty and fibrotic changes are due to a deficiency of the lipotropic factors.

EXPERIMENTAL

A total of 188 male rats (150 to 200 g) were divided among 12 groups unequal in numbers but with comparable weight distribution (see Table 44.I). The animals were housed in individual all-metal cages provided with a false bottom of coarse wire screen. A 15 per cent (by volume) aqueous solution of purified ethyl alcohol was given in place of drinking-

TABLE 44.I

LIVER LIPIDS AND FIBROSIS

Supplement	Diet Alone *ad lib.*	Diet *ad lib.* + Alcohol	Diet Alone (pair-fed)	Diet Pair-fed + Sugar (isocaloric)
None	*0* (10) 10% 0/6	*2* (20) 18% 7/15	3 (32) 10% 2/28	*4* (12) 26% 7/9
Choline chloride 0.5%	*1* (6) 6% 0/6	*5* (20) 7% 0/18		*6* (12) 6% 0/12
Methionine 0.5%		*8* (20) 7% 0/18		*7* (12) 7% 0/10
Casein 17%	*9* (12) 7% 0/10	*10* (20) 8% 0/18		*11* (12) 7% 0/11

Average daily food consumption (without alcohol), 14 to 15 g.
Average daily food consumption (with alcohol), 11 g.
Alcohol supplied 18 per cent total calories in Groups 2, 5, 8, and 10.
Group numbers in italic face type and original number of rats per group in parentheses. Average total liver lipids as percentage of fresh liver weight is shown below group number; number of livers showing fibrosis is given as numerator of a fraction in which denominator is the number of livers carefully examined after rats had eaten diets for six months.

water to four groups of rats throughout the whole experimental period, which lasted 177 days. These groups (2, 5, 8, and 10) were offered their respective diets and the alcoholic solution *ad libitum*, and the amounts of each consumed were recorded daily. Four other groups of rats (4, 6, 7, and 11) started four days later were fed the same amount and kind of diet consumed by Groups 2, 5, 8, and 10, respectively. An attempt to achieve calorie equivalence was made by adding enough powdered sucrose to each of the former diets to supply the calories provided by the alcohol consumed by the corresponding group. These groups of rats and the remaining ones were given tap-water *ad libitum*. To assess the effects of the extra calories provided by the alcohol (or sucrose supplement) it is necessary to know the effects of the amount of basal diet consumed by the rats of Groups 2 and 4. The rats of Group 3 (started four days later than those of Group 2) were therefore "group pair-fed" on a diet-weight basis with those of Group 2. Only 12 rats were available for this group when the main experiment was started (June 24, 1948); 20 rats (referred to as Group 3A) were started one month later under identical dietary conditions. The rats of Group 0 were included to observe the effects of the basal diet alone when offered *ad libitum*, and those of Groups 1 and 9 were used to study the effects of the lipotropic supplements (choline and protein, respectively) when added to the basal diet and fed *ad libitum*. Further experimental conditions will be described in detail in the following paragraphs.

The Diet

A basal ration was desired which would be as nearly adequate as possible in all its dietary components except the lipotropic factors. However, it was considered inadvisable to permit an excessive accumulation of liver fat, since any effect attributable to alcohol alone would be difficult to assess if superimposed on a liver made excessively fatty by the basal diet. The small amount of choline chloride (0.05 per cent) added to the basal ration was determined by preliminary experiments to be just sufficient to maintain the total liver lipids at about 10 per cent, which was arbitrarily considered to be a satisfactory basal level for these particular studies.

The basal diet had the following composition, in percentages: casein 10, gelatin 5, zein 3, cystine 0.3, salts (Beveridge and Lucas [120]) 5, cellu-flour 2, sucrose 41.7, starch 10, dextrin 10, beef fat 10, corn oil 2, "vitamin powder" 1, cod-liver oil concentrate[1] 0.015, α-tocopherol acetate 0.01, choline chloride 0.05. The "vitamin powder" contained thiamin hydrochloride 0.5 g, riboflavin 0.25 g, pyridoxin hydrochloride 0.2 g, calcium

---

[1]This concentrate (Ayerst, McKenna, and Harrison, Ltd., Montreal, Canada) contained 200,000 i.u. vitamin A and 50,000 i.u. vitamin D per g.

pantothenate 1 g, nicotinic acid 1 g, folic acid 0.05 g, 2-methyl-1-4-naphtho-quinone 0.1 g, para-amino benzoic acid 10 g, and inositol 50 g, made up with finely powdered sucrose to 1,000 g. Rats consuming 10 g of diet daily received 50 μg of thiamin hydrochloride and corresponding amounts of the other vitamins.

The methionine content of the diet was estimated to be 420 mg and the cystine content (with the supplement) was 380 mg per 100 g. Using calorie values per g of 4 for protein, 4 for carbohydrate, and 9.3 for fat, the energy content of the basal diet was calculated to be 4.35 Calories per g, of which 58 per cent was contributed by the carbohydrate. The diets were freshly prepared at least once a week and were kept in tightly closed tinned cans in a refrigerator at about 4° C until required for use.

Alcoholic beverages and commercial ethyl alcohol contain compounds other than ethanol. To what extent the other components (in some cases unknown) contribute to the effects of alcohol upon the liver cannot be stated. Since the effects of ingesting alcohol may be due to the contaminants, the ethanol, or the ratio of dietary calories to the adequacy of other nutriments, it was considered important to eliminate the contaminants as completely as possible. Freshly prepared silver oxide (about 10 g per litre) was added to so-called pure 95 per cent ethyl alcohol. The mixture, shaken frequently, was left at room temperature for at least 24 hours. The alcohol was then decanted, made just alkaline with sodium hydroxide, and distilled through a packed fractionating column running at a reflux ratio of about 10 to 1. The first 20 per cent of distillate was rejected, about 50 per cent was collected, and the remainder was discarded. A 15 per cent (by volume) aqueous solution of this material replaced the drinking-water of four groups (2, 5, 8, and 10) of rats. Fresh liquid was supplied twice a week. It was dispensed to the rats from 6-oz (170-ml) medicine bottles through a short piece of curved glass tubing with a tip slightly constricted in the flame so that liquid would not run out unless the rat lapped it. Sudden movements of the cage door were avoided to minimize leakage, since it was found that jarring the bottle permitted loss of a few drops of liquid. Losses due to evaporation were shown to be negligible (less than 0.3 ml per day). Whenever, for any reason, abnormally large amounts of liquid seemed to have been consumed, leakage was suspected; the average consumption of alcohol during the previous week was then used to calculate the calories thus obtained by the rat.

TECHNIQUE OF FEEDING

The animals in Groups 2 and 4 were pair-fed on an isocaloric basis. The technique used in this isocaloric pair-feeding (which applies also to Groups

5 and 6, 8 and 7, 10 and 11) will be described in detail. The rats of Group 2 consumed the basal diet *ad libitum*, with 15 per cent alcohol to drink; the total calorie intake was determined from the average consumption of food and alcohol over three-day periods. The rats in Group 4 (started four days later) were offered the basal diet in an amount equal to the average value noted for those in Group 2, and enough finely powdered sucrose was added to this food (with thorough mixing) to supply the calories contained in the average amount of alcohol consumed by the rats of Group 2. The calculation of the amount of sucrose required was made on a somewhat arbitrary basis. Mitchell and Curzon [572], in a review dealing with the food value of ethyl alcohol, stated that "for reasons at present unknown the energy of alcohol is not as well utilized in metabolism as is the energy of glucose." Mitchell [571] estimated that the energy of alcohol is only about three-fourths as available for physiological purposes as that of sucrose. He stated that its growth-promoting power is definitely less than that produced by a sucrose supplement. In the absence of more specific information we assumed that calories from alcohol were only three-quarters as effective in causing gains in weight as were those of the sucrose supplements. Since 1 ml of absolute ethyl alcohol weighs 0.79 g and the calorie value is given as 7.1 Cal. per g, then 1 ml contains 5.6 Cal., or 1 ml of 95 per cent alcohol corresponds to 5.3 Cal. One ml of a 15 per cent by volume dilution of the 95 per cent alcohol would supply 0.8 Cal.: finally, if only three-quarters of this is available for promoting gains in weight, then 1 ml is equivalent to 0.6 Cal., or approximately to 0.15 g of sucrose.[2]

The rats were maintained on these dietary regimens for 177 days. Pairs of rats chosen at random from Groups 0, 2, 4, 5, 7, 8, 9, and 10 were killed at three weeks to determine to what extent deposition of liver lipids was taking place; again after 12 weeks pairs of rats from Group 2 and 3 were sacrificed. All rats were anaesthetized with sodium amytal (90 mg per kg body weight, intraperitoneally). The animals were exsanguinated and the livers were removed and weighed immediately. Portions of right and left lobes were taken for histological examination; the remainder was re-weighed and the total liver lipids were determined (Best, Lucas, Patterson, and Ridout [102]). Blocks of liver, kidney, and certain other tissues were fixed in Heidenhain's SUSA mixture for 24 to 48 hours. Paraffin sections were stained with haematoxylin and eosin, and, to demonstrate

[2]A more recent study by Gillespie and Lucas [320] has shown that all the energy of ethanol released upon combustion in a calorimeter is available for metabolic purposes, confirming the earlier work of Atwater and Benedict [29]. Thus in the present study, the isocaloric feeding of Groups 4, 6, 7, and 11 versus Groups 2, 5, 8, and 10, respectively, is slightly in error, but this does not affect the conclusions reached. (The alcohol-drinkers actually ingested more calories from ethanol than we had calculated.)

connective tissue, with azocarmine, aniline blue, and orange G. The degree of fatty vacuolation of the liver cells was recorded as 0, +, ++, +++, or ++++. These histological data were in agreement with the results of chemical determinations, and therefore only the latter are included in Table 44.I. Numerous sections from each liver were examined carefully for signs of fibrous-tissue proliferation.

RESULTS

No abnormalities were detected on gross, microscopical, or chemical examination of the livers of any of the animals receiving the diets containing the lipotropic supplements, whether or not alcohol (or extra sugar, isocaloric with the alcohol) had been consumed. The rats maintained on the basal diet alone (Group 0) grew well and (with the exception of one rat which showed some pancreatic disease) the total liver lipids ranged from 7.7 per cent to 12.8 per cent with an average of 9.3 per cent, and no liver fibrosis was observed. The average daily food consumption of the rats allowed to eat this diet *ad libitum* was reasonably constant at about 14 to 15 g, as was that of other rats not consuming alcohol and eating *ad libitum* (Groups 1 and 9). All the rats consuming alcohol (Groups 2, 5, 8, and 10) ate less—only about 11 g daily. The rats in the pair-fed groups (3, 4, 6, 7, and 11) were therefore offered 11 g of the corresponding diets daily. The rats of Group 3 gained less weight because of this restricted food intake, but their livers showed essentially the same chemical and histological picture as those of the rats of Group 0.

The rats consuming alcohol without adequate lipotropic factors in the diet (Group 2) developed fatty livers with an average total lipid content (20 per cent) about double that of the rats consuming the same amount of diet without alcohol (Group 3). One-half of the surviving rats drinking alcohol and eating the basal diet (Group 2) exhibited hepatic fibrosis, while in those without alcohol (Group 3) fibrosis could be detected in only two out of 28 survivors, and in one of these the fibrosis was minimal. The rats fed sugar isocalorically—i.e., those of Group 4—had on the average more fat (26 per cent) in their livers and a somewhat higher incidence of fibrosis (7 out of 9 survivors) than those receiving the alcohol (Group 2). However, in none of the livers of either Group 2 or Group 4 had the fibrosis advanced sufficiently to be considered frank cirrhosis. The greater production of fibrosis in the rats of Group 4 (sucrose) than in those of Group 2 (alcohol) probably may be explained by our failure to achieve an exact equivalence in calories between the rats of these two groups. Some evidence for this is apparent in Figure 79, in which it will be noted

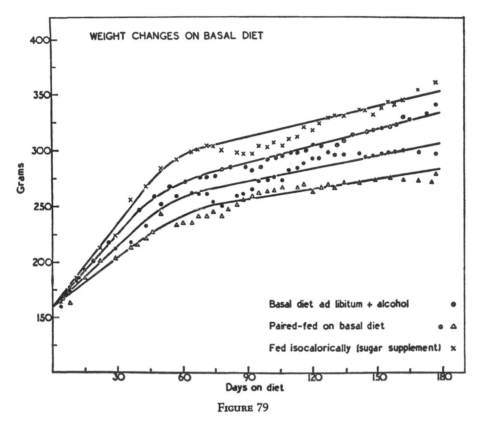

WEIGHT CHANGES ON BASAL DIET

Basal diet ad libitum + alcohol   •

Paired-fed on basal diet   • △

Fed isocalorically (sugar supplement)   x

Days on diet

Grams

FIGURE 79

that the average final weight of the rats receiving the sugar supplement exceeded by about 16 g that of the rats consuming alcohol. This is a rather small discrepancy in weight at the end of a test period of six months, but the difference it represents in calorie intake may be sufficient to account for the slightly greater liver damage. Figure 80 indicates a more successful attempt at pair-feeding in the rats receiving choline. The curves require no further comment except that the dips seen in all of them at about 80 to 90 days are related to a period of exceedingly hot weather, during which the air-conditioning equipment failed to function properly. Since the growth curves of the animals given supplements of methionine or casein (Groups 7, 8, 10, and 11) are essentially the same as those in Figure 80, they will not be presented. The rats of Group 0 (basal diet *ad libitum*) grew most rapidly, those of Groups 1 and 9 only slightly less well. The rats of Group 0 consuming 14.9 g of food per day (65 Calories) gained on the average 262 g. Those of Group 3 consuming 11.2 g (49 Calories) of the same diet gained only 137 g. Rats of Group 2 eating essentially the same amount (11.4 g) of diet but obtaining also 11 Calories

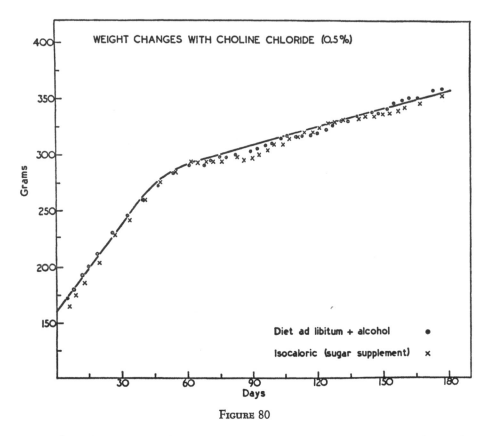

FIGURE 80

from alcohol—i.e., a total of 61 Calories per day, 18 per cent of which came from alcohol—gained 182 g. Rats of Group 4 ate 11.2 g of diet daily and were given an average sugar supplement of 2.7 g (total Calories 60, of which 18 per cent was supplied by the sucrose supplement); they gained 198 g. Thus rats of Group 0 eating 3.5 g more food per day than those of Group 2 gained 80 g more than did the latter; in spite of the calories obtained by the rats of Group 2 from the alcohol, they were still getting from 4 to 5 Calories per day less than those eating the basal diet *ad libitum*. The stunting of growth frequently attributed to the toxic action of alcohol is in these experiments due mainly to decreased food intake, unless one is willing to make the highly improbable assumption that sucrose exerts the same toxic effect as alcohol.

[Two figures, eliminated for brevity, showed identical histological fatty changes in the livers of rats of Group 2 (fed basal diet and given 15 per cent alcohol), and in Group 4 (basal diet and isocaloric sugar).]

Plate V (*b*) and (*c*), illustrates the distribution of fibrous tissue (when present) in the livers of the two groups. After careful study of many sections from all the livers these two examples were selected as representative of the two groups. The similarity in fat deposition and in the nature and extent of the fibrosis in the livers of the two groups is remarkable. Equally striking is the absence of abnormalities in the livers of the animals receiving adequate lipotropic supplements, as has already been mentioned.

DISCUSSION

Clinicians in North America and Europe have tended for many years to associate chronic alcoholism and cirrhosis. In parts of Asia and Africa, however, cirrhosis is common although alcoholism is rare. In these regions it has been noted that cirrhosis occurs most often in persons subsisting on deficient diets. Thus a consideration of the incidence of cirrhosis throughout the world reveals a correlation with malnutrition. This situation may be obscured in some areas by a high incidence of cirrhotic changes following various forms of hepatitis. Within recent years it has been recognized that the chronic alcoholic, like other malnourished individuals, often shows signs of various dietary deficiencies: the intakes of good proteins and of vitamins of the B complex are generally low.

We are not considering in this paper the effects of alcohol on tissues other than the liver. Whether or not alcoholic beverages *per se* directly injure the liver has been a subject of controversy. Even if it could be proved that these beverages do exert a toxic effect upon the liver it would still have to be shown whether the effects were due to pure ethanol, to associated toxic contaminants, to a general malnutrition, or to one or more specific dietary deficiencies.

The present series of experiments does not supply any information whatever on the possible effects of toxic agents which may occur as natural contaminants of alcoholic beverages available in commerce. However, fatty infiltration and consequent fibrosis, which closely resemble the lesions in the chronic alcoholic, have been seen in these experimental animals consuming a purified alcohol. One is therefore tempted to assume that the hypothetical toxic contaminants may be of minor importance in causing the liver lesions seen in the human alcoholic.

The above experiments show that a carefully purified sample of ethanol can cause an excessive accumulation of fat in the liver and subsequent development of fibrosis when the diet lacks adequate amounts of the lipotropic factors. Since, however, pure sugar caused lesions of a similar nature and extent, and since these, as well as those due to alcohol, were entirely prevented by dietary choline or its precursors (methionine or casein), the idea of a specific toxic effect of alcohol upon the liver cells receives no support. While the effects of general malnutrition should not be minimized, the experimental evidence establishes the fact that a specific dietary deficiency—viz., of choline—is involved in the production of the liver damage which we have observed.

Many of the older experiments, as well as some of the more recent ones in which the role of alcohol in the aetiology of liver damage was studied, were poorly controlled. When dogs, cats, rats, or other small animals are given such large doses of alcohol by stomach-tube that they are in a comatose condition during most of the time, the food consumption is inevitably low. Stunting of growth or loss of weight could be thus explained, and possibly also certain types of liver damage. In some other studies that have been reported the experimental animals were offered diets which were inadequate in many respects. To what extent multiple dietary deficiencies have influenced the effects of alcohol in these experiments cannot be determined. The diet used in our investigation has been designed to be adequate (in terms of present knowledge) with regard to all the essential amino-acids, all available vitamins, minerals, and essential fatty acids. In other words, the diet is believed to be satisfactory in all respects except in the amount of lipotropic factors. When this basal diet was adequately supplemented with choline chloride good growth (slightly better than 3 g per day) occurred. Further, the diet was designed to avoid an excessive accumulation of fat in the liver, since, as was mentioned earlier, it would be impossible to assess the effects of alcohol upon liver fat if they were superimposed on a liver made excessively fatty by the basal diet. The failure of some investigators to observe this precaution makes it difficult to interpret their data.

We do not agree that Ashworth's findings indicate that alcohol exerts a specific toxic action on liver cells. He reported that rats consuming high-casein diets showed fatty changes in the liver when given alcohol and that pair-fed controls did not. It may be noted that both groups of his rats lost weight. In the control rats this weight loss was probably due to their food intake being restricted to that of the rats given alcohol. It should be noted, however, that part of the weight loss might be explained by the absence from the diet of some of the B vitamins. It is now well known that the requirement for lipotropic agents diminishes as food intake is restricted, whether this restriction is imposed deliberately or whether it results from a deficiency of one or more vitamins. Thus it is not surprising that the livers of his control rats consuming the high-casein diet were not fatty. However, the rats given alcohol received more calories and lost less weight, but obtained no more dietary lipotropic factors than did the pair-fed controls.

The increased requirement for lipotropic substances in this group is shown by the fatty changes in the liver which were found in all these animals. Thus, it is unnecessary to invoke any specific effect of alcohol to account for these results. They are presumably due to a relative deficiency of the lipotropic factors.

In the present experiments the character and distribution of the pre-cirrhotic lesion found in the rats ingesting alcohol differed in no way from that seen in the animals which received isocaloric amounts of sugar. Chaikoff and Connor [180] stated that the diffuse character of the hepatic fibrosis produced in dogs by dietary means differed in type from that which they had previously described [219] in dogs receiving alcohol. The photomicrographs published by them suggest to us that they may have been comparing different stages of the same type of lesion in their two groups of dogs. We agree with Lowry, Daft, Sebrell, Ashburn, and Lillie [515] that alcohol aggravates dietary cirrhosis without altering the type or distribution of the fibrous tissue.

The importance of dietary factors in the prevention and treatment of liver cirrhosis has been discussed by many writers in recent years. The views expressed recently by Patek [612] and Himsworth [392] are supported and extended by the experimental studies which are here reported.

It is obvious that choline and other essentials should be supplied as naturally occurring components of a well-balanced diet, but the dietary faddist, alcoholic, or "soft-drink" addict does not consume this normal diet. One possibility, therefore, is to add choline or one of its precursors to alcoholic or saccharine[3] beverages which some individuals use to provide a large part of their calorie intake. As indicated above, the diet of the alcoholic is usually deficient not only in the lipotropic substances but also in other vitamins, and indeed in all essential food factors. The proposed fortification of these beverages with choline (or precursors), while protecting the liver against cirrhosis, would doubtless aggravate lesions due to deficiencies of other vitamins. This suggestion raises scientific, moral, financial, and gustatory problems which are far beyond the scope of this communication. Some preliminary studies of the effect of the lipotropic agents on the taste of various beverages have already been made, but we do not contemplate carrying out a comprehensive investigation of this matter. The necessary researches on the gustatory problems are relatively simple and do not lack interesting features.

[3]The word used here, "saccharine," it may be unnecessary to note, is the English adjective meaning sweet; it should not be confused with the trade name "Saccharin" applied to the sweet-tasting aromatic compound o-sulphobenzimide.

Summary and Conclusions

In these experiments on white rats there is no more evidence of a specific toxic effect of pure ethyl alcohol upon liver cells than there is for one due to sugar. This conclusion is based upon the observation that dietary supplements of sucrose cause hepatic lesions (fatty changes and fibrosis) so similar in character and extent to those produced by an isocaloric amount of alcohol that they are indistinguishable.

The results suggest that an imbalance between calorie intake and supply of accessory food factors is the cause of the liver lesions: the extra calorie intake induces a specific deficiency when the basal diet is marginal with respect to any one vitamin. Alcohol or sugar, when taken in excess, supplants choline-containing foodstuffs and at the same time, by increasing the calorie intake, augments the demand for the lipotropic agents.

A mildly hypolipotropic diet is described which allows good growth of young adult male rats and maintains the total liver lipids at about 10 per cent of the fresh tissue weight. This permits the study of the effects of alcohol upon the liver without complications due to multiple dietary deficiencies or to excessive deposition of liver fat resulting from the basal diet alone.

Rats eating this diet *ad libitum* and consuming 15 per cent (v/v) solution of pure ethyl alcohol in place of drinking-water for six months develop fatty livers, and about one-half of them show pre-cirrhotic fibrosis.

An adequate supply of dietary choline or its precursor methionine (either free or in casein) protects the liver; neither excessive deposition of lipids nor fibrosis could be detected in any of the rats receiving lipotropic supplements.

Since the usual vitamins are present in the basal diet in more than adequate amount, and since the lesions are prevented by extra choline, the conclusion may be drawn that the hepatic changes associated with the ingestion of pure ethyl alcohol in this experiment are due to an induced choline deficiency.

Problems connected with the proposal to supplement alcoholic beverages and saccharine aerated water ("soft drinks") with choline or its precursors are mentioned.

Our findings are, of course, not necessarily applicable to alcoholism in human subjects. If they should prove to be so, it is increasingly obvious that individuals who habitually consume large amounts of alcohol or sugar lack adequate amounts of the lipotropic agents as well as of other dietary essentials.

The classical hepatic lesions (fatty changes and fibrosis) associated with alcoholism in human subjects, the first descriptions of which are mentioned in our introduction, may prove to be due specifically to a lack of the lipotropic agents.

Acknowledgments

This work has been supported by the Nutrition Foundation of New York and the Banting Research Foundation, Toronto. We are indebted to our colleague Dr. Jean Patterson for her invaluable help. The photomicrographs were prepared by one of the authors (W. S. H.) with the technical assistance of Mrs. K. M. Robertson.

45. Effects of Dietary Protein, Lipotropic Factors, and Re-alimentation on Total Hepatic Lipids and Their Distribution

C. H. BEST, M.D., F.R.S.

W. S. HARTROFT, M.D., PH.D.

C. C. LUCAS, PH.D.

JESSIE H. RIDOUT, PH.D.

Interest in the distribution of fat within the liver lobule has been stimulated by the observation that in the widespread disease kwashiorkor the stainable fat is found predominantly in the periportal regions. This subject has recently been reviewed by Brock [149]. It is, of course, a long step from the distribution of fat in the liver of the human infant to that seen in the rat, even when an attempt is made to utilize diets similar to those that produce the characteristic lesions in the human liver. The initial distribution of fat under standardized experimental conditions may not be the same as that which is seen at a later stage. Our lack of knowledge of the anatomy and physiology of the liver lobule prevents us from explaining the mechanisms which determine the localization of fat even when this is sharply defined and consistently reproducible. However, experimental work is steadily revealing new facts that are contributing to the solution of these problems.

In choline deficiency in the rat the first appearance of stainable fat is in the area around the central veins (Lillie, Ashburn, Sebrell, Daft, and Lowry [503]; Glynn, Himsworth, and Lindan [322]; Hartroft [365]). In fasted rats given anterior pituitary extract the initial distribution of the fat is definitely periportal (Best and Campbell [78]; Best, Hartroft, and Sellers [88]). Some years ago Dible reported that in rats and rabbits during starva-

Originally appeared in the *British Medical Journal*, I (1955), 1439–45. (A preliminary account of some of these findings was read at the 37th Annual Conference of the Chemical Institute of Canada, Toronto, June 21 to 23, 1954.)

tion the distribution of fat is sometimes mainly periportal [251; 252]. Shils and Stewart [699] have drawn attention to the periportal distribution of fat in the livers of rats fed corn-meal diets and remarked upon the similarity of the lesion to that described by many clinicians in children suffering from kwashiorkor. A similar distribution has been noted in rats consuming other plant materials, such as rice, cassava, and wheat flour (Shils, Friedland, and Stewart [697]).

Several reports of fatty livers not responding to the usual supplements of choline or its precursors have appeared recently (Wang, Hegsted, Lapi, Zamcheck, and Black [778]; Litwack, Hankes, and Elvehjem [507]; Sauberlich [668]; Singal, Hazan, Sydenstricker, and Littlejohn [707]; Harper, et al. [361; 362; 808]). The basal diets fed to the rats in which this condition has been encountered have usually been low in protein. Under these conditions choline has often failed to maintain the liver fat within the normal range, although it has generally prevented any great increase in total liver lipids.

We wish to report some effects of varying the nature and amount of protein in the diet on the total lipids and distribution of stainable fat in the livers of rats and on the lipotropic effect of choline in these diets. Histological studies suggest that the abnormal lipid whose accumulation is not prevented by choline has a different distribution from that seen when the deficiency involves choline or its precursors. It was also noted, during a study of the accumulation and removal of stainable fat in periportal regions, that re-alimentation after diminished food intake due to dietary (protein) deficiency resulted in a transitory fatty liver, the demonstrable fat being exclusively periportal in distribution.

METHODS

Five separate experiments will be reported involving some 300 albino (Wistar) rats. The animals were kept in individual cages with a false bottom of coarse wire screen. Fresh food and water were supplied each day; food intake was recorded daily and rats were weighed weekly. Unless otherwise stated, the animals were fed the diets *ad libitum* for three weeks and were then killed by stunning and exsanguination. Livers were removed at once and weighed. Portions were taken for histological examination, and the remainder of the tissue was analysed for total lipids (extraction with hot alcohol, rectification of the lipid residue with a mixture of petroleum ether and chloroform 3:1 v/v). The percentage composition of the variable components of the basal diets fed in each experiment is shown in Table 45.I.

TABLE 45.I

PERCENTAGE OF VARIABLE COMPONENTS IN BASAL DIETS

(All diets contained celluflour 2, salts 3, sucrose-vitamin-B mixture 1, cod-liver oil concentrate 0.010, alpha-tocopheryl acetate 0.010, and sucrose to 100 per cent.)

Group no.		Casein	Fibrin	Soy Protein	Peanut Meal*	Methionine	Corn Oil
I	a	3				0.45	5
	b	6				0.36	5
	c	9				0.27	5
	d	18				—	5
II	a		—	9		0.45	5
	b		9	—		0.33	5
	c		3	6		0.41	5
	d		6	12		0.28	5
	e		6	12		—	5
III	a	3		—	—	—	2(+10)†
	b	3		10	10	—	2(+10)†
IV				2	2	(0.27)‡	(20)§
V	a||	3				0.45	2(+10)†
	b||	18				—	2(+10)†

*Defatted (solvent process) peanut meal, washed with 50 per cent ethanol to remove free and bound choline.
†In these diets 10 per cent beef fat was added as well as 2 per cent corn oil.
‡This supplement of organic sulphur was provided as cystine.
§Diet IV contained 20 per cent Primex (hydrogenated vegetable oil) and extra tocopheryl acetate (total 0.035 per cent).
||Diets Va and Vb contained 0.50 per cent choline chloride.

It should be noted that in these studies vitamin B_{12} (300 μg per 100 g) was added to the vitamin mixture described by Ridout, Lucas, Patterson, and Best [643], thus providing 3 μg per 100 g of ration. Basal diets are identified by the numerical suffix -0.

HISTOLOGICAL EXAMINATION

The distribution of demonstrable fat in the livers was studied in frozen sections (5 μ) of formalin-fixed tissues using Wilson's trichrome—oil red 0 technique. Paraffin sections (5 μ) of Bouin-fixed tissues were stained with haematoxylin and eosin.

The sections were examined under a code number by one of us (W.S.H.). The amount of demonstrable lipid was graded from 0 to ++++. [Eight photomicrographs illustrating the histological distribution of the stainable lipid have been omitted.] Although in Tables 45.II, 45.III, and 45.IV the distribution of the lipid is recorded merely as periportal or centrolobular, the degree of localization varied considerably. The term "periportal" was applied not only when the fat-containing cells were restricted to regions immediately surrounding the portal vein and hepatic artery alone, but also when this distribution extended much farther towards the central vein but did not envelop it. In almost all cases, however, the lobular distribution of the lipid was remarkably clear and well defined. Often there was evidence of increased glycogen deposition, especially in the periportal regions (cf. Ramalingaswami, Sriramachari, and Patwardhan [627]).

DIETARY CONDITIONS

In Experiment I the lipotropic effect of choline was compared in diets containing different amounts of protein (casein). In these diets (Ia, Ib, Ic, and Id, Table 45.I) the total methionine was kept constant at 0.54 per cent by adding sufficient supplementary DL-methionine. This amount of methionine is equal to that present in the last diet, which contains 18 per cent casein. Groups of six male rats (weighing 70 to 90 g) were fed these basal diets supplemented with choline chloride as shown in Table 45.II.

In Experiment II the rats were fed an animal protein (fibrin), a vegetable protein (soya bean), and mixtures of the two (Table 45.I). Again, in this experiment enough DL-methionine was added to all diets (except IIe) to bring the total to 0.54 per cent. Groups of eight male rats (65 to 80 g) were fed these basal diets supplemented with choline chloride as shown in Table 45.II.

Experiment III permits comparison of the effect on the distribution of stainable fat in the livers of feeding a low-protein diet (3 per cent casein) without supplementary methionine (Diet IIIa) and with supplementary methionine (Diet Ia). A similar comparison was made in high-protein diets containing less than half as much methionine (250 mg) as does 18 per cent casein (Diets IIIb and Id respectively). Groups of ten female rats (65 to 90 g) were fed the basal diets IIIa-0 and IIIb-0 (Table 45.I), alone or supplemented with choline chloride (0.5 per cent), as shown in Table 45.III. Four groups were fed *ad libitum*; rats of the fifth group (IIIb-0 p.f.) were fed the same average amounts of food each day as were consumed by those in Group IIIa-0.

In Experiment IV the effect was studied of prolonged consumption of a diet very low in vegetable protein (soya protein 2 per cent plus peanut protein 1 per cent). This ration (IVa-0, Table 45.I), which contains only 32 mg methionine per 100 g of mixture, was variously supplemented with choline chloride (0, 0.36 per cent, and 1 per cent, Table 45.III) and fed *ad libitum* for 85 days to male rats (180 to 200 g).

Experiment V was planned to supply data on the time relationships of both the accumulation of periportal liver lipids in rats on a low-protein diet and their removal when the animals were transferred to a "curative"

TABLE 45.II

Effect of the Nature and Amount of Dietary Protein on the Lipotropic Potency of Choline

(Sufficient DL-methionine added to keep total constant at 0.54% in all diets except IIe-0. Male rats [65 to 90 g] fed rations for three weeks.)

Experiment and Diet no.	Choline Chloride (%)	Average Daily Food Intake (g)	Average Change in Wt. (g)	Total Lipids (% Liver Wt.)	Portal Range	Portal Mode	Central Range	Central Mode
Ia-0 (6)*	0	5.6	−8	12.5	+/+++	+++	0/+	f.tr.
Ia-1 (6)	0.12	4.6	−9	16.0	+/+++	+++	0/±	f.tr.
Ia-2 (6)	0.36	4.9	−10	9.9	±/+++	+	0/tr.	0
Ib-0 (6)	0	5.9	+5	9.8	±/+++	+	0	0
Ib-1 (6)	0.12	7.1	+15	11.3	+/+++	+	0/±	0
Ic-0 (6)	0	9.6	+54	10.7	+/+++	±±	0/±	f.tr.
Ic-1 (6)	0.12	10.5	+61	9.1	+/+++	++	0/f.tr.	0
Ic-2 (6)	0.36	10.2	+61	6.8	+/++	+	0/±	0
Id-0 (6)	0	11.9	+93	8.9	f.tr./±	f.tr.	0/±	±
Id-1 (6)	0.12	12.1	+105	6.6	0/±	0	0/tr.	0
Id-2 (6)	0.36	11.8	+100	5.8	0/±		0/tr.	0
IIa-0 (6)	0	6.7	+10	9.0	+++/+++	+++	0/+	tr.
IIa-1 (8)	0.12	6.7	+10	8.7	+/+++	+±	0/+	tr.
IIa-2 (6)	0.36	7.0	+12	7.7	±/+++	+++	0/tr.	0
IIb-0 (8)	0	9.7	+55	6.7	tr./+±	+	0/±	tr.
IIb-1 (8)	0.12	10.4	+63	5.8	f.tr./+±		0/±	0
IIb-2 (6)	0.36	10.4	+58	5.8	+/++++	+++	0/+	0
IIc-0 (6)	0	11.0	+49	10.7	+/++++	+++	0/++	±
IIc-1 (8)	0.12	11.4	+52	9.3	±/++++	+++	0/v.f.tr.	tr.
IIc-2 (6)	0.36	10.1	+46	8.4	tr./++++		v.f.tr./tr.	0
IId-0 (8)	0	13.7	+102	7.9	v.f.tr./±	tr.	0/v.f.tr.	v.f.tr.
IId-1 (8)	0.12	13.0	+109	6.0	f.tr./tr.	tr.	0/v.f.tr.	v.f.tr.
IId-2 (8)	0.36	14.0	+119	5.5	tr./±	tr.	v.f.tr./f.tr.	v.f.tr.
IIe-0 (8)†	0	9.9	+55	27.2	+/+++	+(?)	+++/++/+++	+++
IIe-1 (8)	0.12	12.0	+67	6.5	0	f.tr.	±/+	±±

*The figures in parentheses are the number of rats used in the experiment.

†Six out of the eight rats in this group, which were fed the basal diet *unsupplemented* with methionine, died with kidney lesions and fatty livers.

f.tr. and v.f.tr. = faint and very faint trace.

TABLE 45.III

Effects of Choline in Diets Inadequate or More Adequate with Respect to Protein

(Diets IIIa and IIIb contained 3% and 18% respectively, of casein. Diet IV contained 3% protein [2% soya protein plus 1% peanut protein supplied as defatted meal].)

Experiment and Diet no.	Choline Chloride (%)	No. of Rats	Average Daily Food Intake (g)	Average Change in Weight (g)	Total Lipids (% Liver Wt.)	Lobular Distribution of Stainable Fat	
						Portal	Central
IIIa-0	0	10*	5.7	−12	19.9	+ to ++	++ to +++
IIIa-1	0.50	10*	5.1	−13	5.8	++	±
IIIb-0	0	10*	10.3	+45	23.1	++	++ to +++
IIIb-Opf†	0.50	10*	6.0	+8	14.3	+ to ++	++ to +++
IIIb-1	0.50	10*	11.1	+60	5.2	±	v.f.tr.
IVa-0	0	10‡	7.0	−75	26.1	+ (?)	+++ to ++++
IVa-1	0.36	15‡	6.3	−74	7.3	±	0
IVa-2	1.0	15‡	6.6	−76	5.8	±	0

*Female rats (65 to 90 g).
†Pair-fed with rats in IIIa-0.
‡Male rats (180 to 200 g).

diet high in protein (Table 45.I, Diets Va and Vb respectively). Forty female rats (65 to 80 g) were fed the low-protein diet (Va-0, 3 per cent casein), which was supplemented with methionine to make it equivalent in that respect to the "curative" diet containing 18 per cent casein; both diets contained 0.5 per cent choline chloride. Pairs of rats were killed after being fed the low-protein diet for 2, 4, 8, and 16 days, respectively. The remaining 32 rats were transferred to the "curative" diet (Vb containing 18 per cent casein). Groups of eight rats were killed after consuming the "curative" diet for 3, 7, 14, and 21 days, respectively. In addition 25 similar rats were fed a commercial stock ration ("master fox chow," Toronto Elevators, Ltd.). During the first 16 days these rats were pair-fed with those given the low-protein diet. Five rats were killed at the end of this time, and the remainder were then allowed to eat the chow *ad libitum*; groups of five rats were killed after 3, 7, 14, and 21 days, respectively.

RESULTS

Livers from many normal rats of our colony have been examined during past years. The livers were subjected to chemical analysis and sections treated with oil red 0 were scrutinized carefully. Normal values for total liver lipids by our methods of extraction and rectification range from 5 to 8 per cent, the mean and standard error being 6.62 ± 0.09. The values for 20 male rats were 5.19 to 7.48, mean 6.31 ± 0.14; and for 38 females, 5.9 to 8.03, mean 6.79 ± 0.10. No histologically demonstrable fat could be seen in most livers. Recently, since the above experiments were completed, we have been reinvestigating the "normal" rats of our colony and have found a more frequent appearance of fat in at least some hepatic parenchymal cells. This fat often occurs only as a few to many fine droplets per cell, but occasionally some cells (2 to 12 per high-power field) are seen to be filled with fat. These latter cells appear to be distributed at random within the hepatic lobules. This increased frequency of appearance of cells containing stainable fat is being investigated further.

Experiment 1

Most of the stainable fat in the livers of rats consuming the basal diets low in casein (Ia-0, Ib-0, and Ic-0) was in periportal regions, with only a trace in centrolobular areas (see Table 45.II). It should be noted that these diets contained considerable methionine. We believe that adequacy of this choline precursor in these basal diets has been important in keeping the centrolobular areas clear. Even with 0.36 per cent of choline chloride the amount of fat in periportal regions was not significantly reduced. As the amount of protein in the diet was increased, less total lipid and periportal fat was observed; only traces of periportal fat could be detected when the diet contained 18 per cent casein (Id-0). The lipotropic effect of a given amount of choline (as estimated by chemical analysis of liver tissue) improved as the protein content of the diet increased, but even large doses of choline were unable to prevent some deposition of abnormal fat so long as the protein in the diet was low.

Experiment II

The limited effectiveness of choline chloride in maintaining normal liver lipids is seen in other diets low in protein—for example, soya protein and a mixture of soya protein with fibrin. Diet IIa-0 (9 per cent soya protein) gave total liver lipids of 9.0 per cent; even 0.36 per cent choline chloride failed to reduce the value significantly. As in Experiment I, the deposition of centrolobular fat was prevented by choline, but the stainable fat in periportal regions was much less affected. Fibrin at 9 per cent (Diet IIb-0) produced lower total lipids (by chemical analysis 6.7 per cent) and considerably less stainable fat in periportal regions than did the soya protein, but the livers were not normal. Addition of choline chloride did not appreciably alter the findings. A mixture of these two proteins at a total protein level of 9 per cent (Diet IIc-0) also permitted the deposition of considerable periportal fat that was not affected by choline, although some prevention of lipid deposition could be shown analytically. Twice as much of the same protein mixture (that is, soya protein 12 per cent plus fibrin 6 per cent, Diet IId-0) resulted in a more nearly normal liver: only a trace of stainable fat could be detected in periportal regions and only a faint trace in the centrolobular area. Choline reduced the total lipid, but did not alter appreciably that seen in periportal regions.

The results when rats were fed Diet IIe-0 are of particular interest. This ration was the same as Diet IId-0 except that the supplementary methionine was omitted. In the absence of this choline precursor the liver became very fatty (27 per cent total lipids), the bulk of the stainable fat appearing in centrolobular position (+++ to ++++). Since the distribution of fat was diffuse throughout the lobule the amount in periportal regions was difficult to estimate, but it was recorded as +. A small supplement of choline chloride (0.12 per cent) reduced the total lipids to 6.5 per cent— that is, within the normal range—but a small amount of stainable fat could still be seen around the central vein as well as in the periportal region. Had more choline been given, this centrolobular fat would probably have been eliminated.

Experiment III

The well-established fact that choline deficiency leads to an accumulation of fat in the centrolobular region was confirmed, as was the newer observation that stainable fat in the periportal region is connected with protein inadequacy. The ration containing 3 per cent of casein without supplementary methionine (Diet IIIa-0) was not eaten well; it caused a moderate loss in weight and resulted in the development of a fatty liver. The total lipids reached 19.9 per cent; there was considerable fat in periportal regions, with even more in centrolobular areas. A similar ration containing 0.5 per cent choline chloride resulted in a liver almost free from centrolobular fat but with considerable fat remaining in periportal regions. The total lipids were, however, only 5.8 per cent. Diet Ia-0, a similar ration but with added methionine, was eaten in almost identical amounts and resulted in much lower liver lipids (compare 12.5 per cent with 19.9 per cent), the difference being mainly due to absence of fat from the central areas, as might have been predicted. Diet IIIb-0, methionine-poor but containing 18 per cent of protein, was eaten more freely, permitted a fair gain in weight, and caused a fatty liver, with the abnormal lipids mainly centrolobular, as was anticipated. Paired feeding reduced the total lipids somewhat, but did not change the distribution of stainable fat appreciably. Inclusion of choline chloride (Diet IIIb-1) improved slightly both food intake and gain in weight, and almost completely prevented any stainable fat from appearing in the centrolobular region; a little remained in portal areas.

Experiment IV

Prolonged consumption of a diet low in protein and free from choline produced a very fatty liver, some of the lipid appearing in periportal areas, but most of the abnormal fat being centrolobular (Table 45.III). The centrolobular deposition of stainable lipids was prevented by choline. Thus the effects of a low-protein diet on stainable liver lipids were essentially the same whether the rats were fed for three weeks or three months.

Experiment V

Development of a fatty liver upon realimentation has been noted frequently (for example, MacFarland and McHenry [527]; Best, Lucas, Patterson, and Ridout [103]), but the distribution of stainable fat in the present experiment proved interesting, being exclusively periportal. The low-protein diet (3 per cent casein) resulted in a decreasing food intake (Table 45.IV), in spite of adequate vitamins (including choline) and methionine. Despite the diminishing caloric intake and consequent loss of

TABLE 45.IV

RATE OF APPEARANCE OF STAINABLE LIPIDS IN PERIPORTAL AREAS AND EFFECT ON LIVER LIPIDS OF REALIMENTATION WITH AN
ADEQUATE DIET AFTER A PERIOD ON A SIMILAR RATION LOW IN PROTEIN

(Forty female rats, 65 to 80 g, fed Diet Va-0 containing 3% casein; pairs of rats killed after periods shown. After 16 days the remaining rats were fed Diet Vb-0, containing 18% casein, for periods shown. Both rations contained 0.54% total methionine and 0.5% choline chloride.)

Experiment and Diet no.	No. of Rats	Period Fed (days)	Average Daily Food Intake (g)	Average Change in Weight (g)	Total Lipids (% Liver Wt.)	Lobular Distribution of Stainable Fat	
						Portal	Central
Va-0	2	2	7.1	−2	5.4	+	0 to f.tr.
	2	4	5.6	−10	6.2	0 to +	0
	2	8	5.0	−9	7.1	+ to ++	0
	2	16	4.8	−16	9.1	++	0
Vb-0	8	3	9.6	+19	18.0	+++	0
	8	7	9.3	+38	11.0	++	0
	8	14	10.0	+64	6.3	0 to +	0
	8	21	10.8	+91	5.1	f.tr.	0

weight, the livers became increasingly fatty, the deposition of fat occurring in periportal regions. When the rats were transferred to a similar diet in which the protein was made more adequate (casein 18 per cent) they ate twice as much and began to gain weight. Coincident with this sudden increase in food consumption during the first three days on the "curative" ration there was a dramatic increase in the total liver lipids (to 18 per cent), all of it occurring in periportal regions. With continued intake of about the same amount of food, however, the abnormal fat soon disappeared, the liver appearing normal both histologically and chemically at the end of three weeks. No such increase in liver lipids occurred following realimentation in rats pair-fed a commercial ration throughout both the period of decreasing food intake and of realimentation.

DISCUSSION

The data presented above show that protein inadequacy leads to the prompt appearance of stainable fat in periportal regions of the liver. It is a well-established fact that choline deficiency results in a rapid accumulation of abnormal lipids, mainly glyceride in nature, in centrolobular areas; the present data confirm this. The essential difference in the lesions can best be recognized when the deficiency is of mild degree and of brief duration; more severe or more prolonged deficiencies lead to a more generalized distribution of stainable fat, often obscuring the original site of appearance of the lipid.

For complete protection of the hepatic cells in the portal region the amount of protein necessary depends upon its nature, fibrin being much more effective than casein, which is better than soya protein. The deleterious effect of diets low in protein on the cells in the portal region may be related to some inadequacy of essential amino-acids (cf. Lucas and Ridout [517]). The effect of protein on hepatic cells around the central veins appears to be attributable largely, if not solely, to its content of the choline precursor methionine. Protein inadequacy in regard to protection of the liver appears to begin at about 12 per cent in the diet when casein is fed, and below 6 per cent in the case of fibrin (cf. data of Winje et al. [808]); choline inadequacy begins at about 0.12 per cent (expressed as chloride). It should be emphasized that these values may vary considerably, depending upon the strain, age, and sex of the rat, upon the adequacy of the diet with respect to other essential nutrients, upon environmental temperatures, and on other factors less well understood.

These observations may help to resolve two anomalies in the literature—namely, the occasional discrepancy between the chemical and histological estimations of liver fat and the lack of response of certain types of dietary fatty livers to the lipotropic agents. The term "fatty liver" has somewhat different connotations according to the viewpoint of the user. To the pathologist who is concerned with the appearance of the organ the liver is described as fatty if fat is evident microscopically in suitably stained sections. Not every cell need contain stainable fat. Cells in certain regions only may be affected, yet the organ would be referred to as a "fatty" liver. The biochemist, on the other hand, is concerned with the results of the chemical analysis—that is, with the quantity of lipids extractable from the tissue. Only when the analytical figure is increased appreciably above the normal range of values for the species would the chemist describe the liver as "fatty." The pathologist may see stainable fat, sometimes in considerable amount, before there is any significant increase in the extractable lipids. An erroneous impression of the magnitude of the increase above normal may be obtained unless attention is paid to the extraction procedure used, and especially to the base to which the analytical data are calculated, whether it be to fresh tissue, dry tissue, fat-free tissue, or dry, fat-free tissue. We have discussed elsewhere the merits and disadvantages of each of these (Ridout et al. [642]). There are situations—for example, in protein depletion—where the values might better be expressed as percentages of body weight, or, better still, referred to the desoxypentosenucleic acid (D.N.A.) content of the liver. Campbell and Kosterlitz [166; 167; 168] found that, although ribonucleic acid and phospholipid are lost from the liver in protein deficiency, the D.N.A. content of the liver of the adult rat varies linearly with body weight and is not affected by the protein content of the diet. Where effects of variations in dietary protein are under study, and particularly where a considerable change in the number of functional liver cells is apparent (as in necrosis or cirrhosis), the D.N.A. content of the liver should prove a useful basis for comparing changes in lipids and other hepatic components. However, at present in our laboratory the common practice is followed of referring the data to the fresh weight basis. All values are also calculated to the dry, fat-free basis, as this sometimes permits more useful comparisons, but these data are not always reported.

In choline deficiency hepatic lipid values of 15 to 40 per cent of fresh liver weight are commonly observed. Figures of 25 to 45 per cent reported in rats fed diets low in protein (for example, Harper, Benton, et al. [359]) are expressed as percentages of dry liver weight. When referred to the fresh weight the total hepatic lipids are no more than about 8 to 18 per cent (usually below 14 per cent). These are certainly fatty livers, but quantitatively they are of mild degree as compared with those seen in choline deficiency. A considerable amount of stainable fat may appear in periportal areas with minimal elevation of total lipids as determined chemically. It has been suggested (Lucas and Ridout [517]) that this unmasking of normal structural lipids (fat phanerosis)[1] may be caused by improper formation of lipoproteins due to protein deficiency. Protein deficiency may seriously interfere with the formation of many vital factors which the lack of choline might not affect to the same extent (cf. Campbell and Kosterlitz [166; 167; 168]). While fibrosis or cirrhosis has not yet been produced in our rats by protein deficiency in the presence of abundant choline, even after a year, it is possible that these lesions may appear in more prolonged experiments, as Ramalingaswami has suggested (personal communication).

With regard to the second anomaly, our findings confirm and supplement those from other laboratories that fatty livers due to diets low in protein do not respond to lipotropic substances. However, it is not surprising that a fatty liver due to protein deficiency is not cured by giving supplements of choline or its precursors.

In our opinion it has been obvious for many years that the clinical use of choline and methionine to repair the liver damage produced by multiple deficiencies—that is, of protein, minerals, vitamins, etc.—is doomed to failure because most hospital diets supply an abundance of the lipotropic agents. This does not decrease in any way the potential clinical significance of experimental work on the lipotropic factors; it merely means that in the laboratory it is possible to make choline the limiting factor by the design of the experiment. The clinician rarely encounters so simple a situation. If he supplied the missing amino-acids other than methionine and made good the other deficiencies except that of choline, this substance would be the limiting factor in the clinical situation.

The importance of the balance of amino-acids in the diet in the study of fatty livers was noted in this laboratory 10 years ago by Beveridge, Lucas, and O'Grady [121; 122], who pointed out that the lipotropic activity of a protein is determined not only by its content of methionine but also by the nature and quantity of the other amino-acids present. While studying changes in liver composition during protein depletion Wang et al. [778] fed protein-free rations to rats and observed a fatty liver not completely preventable by choline (at the dosage used, which was high— 0.50 per cent choline chloride in the diet). Dick, Hall, Sydenstricker, McCollum, and Bowles [253] suggested that some fatty livers may result from failure of certain cell functions when protein anabolism is reduced—

[1]This is not the place to attempt a full discussion of the vigorously debated subject of lipophanerosis. Modern biochemical and physicochemical studies of the lipoproteins have revealed the possibility of dissociation of these compounds to give free lipids, but the conditions governing this process are not well understood.

that is, they may represent a non-specific effect of protein deficiency rather than a specific lack of any one essential amino-acid. When Harper, Benton, et al. [359] observed an anti-lipotropic effect of methionine in rats fed threonine-deficient diets containing choline, they too concluded that the extent of fat deposition in the liver depends on the balance as well as on the absolute amounts of amino-acids in the ration. The fatty livers caused by diets deficient in threonine and lysine (Dick et al. [253]; Singal et al. [707]; Harper et al. [361]), even with moderate amounts of choline in the food, are examples of fatty livers of non-specific origin—that is to say, due to inadequate or imbalanced protein—and the lesions would doubtless prove to be periportal in distribution. Indeed, Niño-Herrera, Harper, and Elvehjem [598], reporting upon the histological differentiation of fatty livers produced by threonine or choline deficiency, stated:

> In the livers of choline-deficient animals the fatty infiltration is diffuse and is most severe in the vicinity of the central vein. In the livers of animals receiving low-protein diets containing choline the distribution of fatty cells results in a network appearance in which zones of normal cells are interspersed among the zones of fatty cells and only occasionally is the fatty infiltration most severe around the central vein of the lobule. The magnitude of the fatty infiltration is much greater in rats fed a diet deficient in choline.[2]

Shils and Stewart [700] have observed a periportal distribution of fat in livers of rats fed diets consisting principally of corn meal, rice, or cassava, and found that lysine and tryptophan prevented this fatty liver. These observations are in agreement with our hypothesis that protein deficiency or amino-acid imbalance causes the periportal type of lesion.

Shils and Stewart [699] suspected that the periportal accumulation of lipids seen in rats fed corn meal may be due to some unique property of corn proteins. Since the lesion was later seen in rats fed corn, rice, wheat, or cassava, Shils, Friedland, and Stewart [697] believed that it is typical of plant products. Our finding of this periportal type of distribution whenever the amount of dietary protein is low, regardless of the source of the protein fed, confirms and extends their results but alters the conclusions.

Shils and Stewart [698] reported observing a sex difference in the distribution of stainable fat in the liver lobule: in male rats the total concentration of hepatic lipids was higher than in females and the lipid appeared first in periportal areas; in females the fat was found first in

[2]The literature concerning the site of lipid accumulation in threonine deficiency is contradictory, however. Dick and his associates reported that it occurs in the cells around the central veins. Unfortunately the histological techniques used by Niño-Herrera et al. were unsuitable for lipid studies. Using histochemical methods, Kerbel and Casselman in this laboratory have repeated the experiments relating directly to threonine deficiency and have found that the distribution of fat is clearly periportal.

central areas. Female rats responded somewhat to threonine; males did not (Shils and Stewart [700]). In our experiments, admittedly with different proteins, we have not noticed any significant difference in the distribution of stainable fat in the livers of male and female rats.

In a personal communication Ramalingaswami, who with his colleagues has published several thoughtful and stimulating papers on liver injury in protein malnutrition (for example, Sriramachari and Ramalingaswami [730]; Ramalingaswami et al. [627]), has informed us that the fat content of diets low in protein and choline may influence the localization of the fatty deposits in the hepatic lobule. After rats were fed for about three months on a low-fat, low-protein, choline-deficient diet he observed that the microscopical appearance of the livers presented a striking similarity to the picture in kwashiorkor.

In our present study the observation that may be of greatest practical significance concerns the abrupt increase in total liver lipids associated with a sudden improvement in the quality and quantity of food intake, even when the "curative" ration is adequate in protein and rich in choline (Experiment V). Liver fat increased within three days from 9 to 18 per cent, all stainable fat being present in periportal regions. This is the largest amount of extractable lipid ever observed by us when the stainable fat was present in periportal regions exclusively. A similar increase in liver fat was not observed in other rats pair-fed a commercial stock ration, suggesting that an unidentified factor prevents the sudden but transient increase in liver lipids confined to the periportal regions. These experiments, which may have their clinical counterparts in the treatment of alcoholic subjects with certain "good" diets, reveal the presence of factors in addition to protein and choline that may be concerned in the deposition and localization of fat in the liver.

SUMMARY

In rats fed diets containing a moderate amount of fat and 9 per cent or less of protein, supplementary choline failed to prevent completely the accumulation of fat in periportal regions of the liver.

Lack of adequate protein resulted in the appearance of fat in the periportal areas, while deficiency of choline (or precursors) caused an accumulation of fat in the cells bordering on the central vein. Protein inadequacy has not produced the massive accumulation of hepatic lipids seen in choline deficiency.

When rats were transferred to an "adequate" diet (containing 18 per cent casein and 0.5 per cent choline chloride) after a period on a low-protein ration (3 per cent casein) there was a dramatic appearance of a transient fatty liver (total lipids 18 per cent), the fat appearing in periportal positions only. During three weeks on the same ration the hepatic lipids returned to normal. Other rats pair-fed the same amounts of a commercial ration did not develop fatty livers, so that the transient appearance of periportal fat is not entirely due to the increased food intake. Certain points of potential clinical interest have been discussed briefly.

ACKNOWLEDGMENTS

The expenses of this study were defrayed in part by a grant to the Department from the Banting Research Foundation. Our thanks are due to Mr. Gwyn Hughes, of the Charles Albert Smith Co. Ltd., Toronto, and to Distillation Products Industries, Rochester, N.Y., U.S.A., for a generous donation of pure α-tocopheryl acetate.

We wish to thank Dr. W. G. Bruce Casselman and Dr. Jean M. Patterson for the exceptional amount of help they have given us in this study.

46. Lipotropic Dose-Response Studies in Rats: Comparisons of Choline, Betaine and Methionine

R. J. YOUNG

C. C. LUCAS

JEAN M. PATTERSON

C. H. BEST

INTRODUCTION

Some years ago a comparison of the potency of the lipotropic agents was made by Best, Lucas, Ridout, and Patterson [105]. The basal diet fed to their rats is now known to have been deficient in the newer B vitamins. Moreover, the protein mixture adopted was purposely designed so that the rats would merely maintain their weight. This was done because Griffith and his co-workers [333; 583] and Beveridge, Lucas, and O'Grady [122] had noted that factors which affect appetite and rate of growth influence the choline requirement of an animal. The effect of calorie intake on the requirement was noted by Best *et al.* [86]. Since the results of Best *et al.* [105] cannot be applied to growing animals, we have conducted comparative studies of the lipotropic potency of choline, betaine, and methionine with young rats fed several basal hypolipotropic diets which support optimal growth when adequately supplemented with methionine and choline. After considerable study one of these has been adopted for further studies in this field.

EXPERIMENTAL

White male rats (Wistar strain, weighing from 70–90 g) were kept in individual cages with floors of coarse wire screen. Fresh food and water were offered *ad libitum* and unless otherwise stated, the rats were fed the

Originally appeared in the *Canadian Journal of Biochemistry and Physiology*, XXXIV (1956), 713–20. Contribution from the Banting and Best Department of Medical Research, University of Toronto, Toronto, Canada. This work was supported in part by grants from the Banting Research Foundation and the National Research Council of Canada Consolidated Grant.

diets for 21 days. Individual rats were weighed twice weekly and their food consumption was recorded daily. At the end of the experiment surviving animals were anaesthetized with ether and decapitated. The livers were removed immediately, wiped free from blood, and weighed. The extraction of the liver lipids with hot alcohol and their rectification with a 3:1 (v/v) mixture of petroleum ether and chloroform have been described [102]. The kidneys were examined in the gross and the incidence of haemorrhagic lesions was recorded.

The nature and amount of protein used in the basal hypolipotropic diet was determined in preliminary experiments. On the basis of previous experience by one of us (C.C.L.) with a number of different hypolipotropic diets that had received varying amounts of study, a dietary mixture (Basal A, Table 46.I) was adopted to which equal increments of alcohol-extracted

TABLE 46.I

PERCENTAGE COMPOSITION OF THE BASAL DIETS

	Basal A	Basal B
Alcohol-extracted peanut meal*	8	12
Washed soya protein†	4	8
Casein (vitamin-free)	1	1
L(+)Histidine HCl	0.14	—
L(+)Lysine HCl	0.3	—
DL-Threonine	0.1	—
DL-Methionine	0.4	—
L(−) Cystine	0.2	0.2
Salt mixture‡	3.0	3.0
Celluflour	1.0	1.0
Corn starch	10.0	10.0
Dextrin	10.0	10.0
Sucrose	45.84	38.8
Hydrogenated fat (Primex)	10.0	10.0
Corn oil	5.0	5.0
Sucrose-vitamin mixture‡	1.0	1.0
Cod-liver oil concentrate‡	0.01	0.01
d-α-Tocopheryl acetate	0.01	0.01

*Solvent-process peanut meal extracted with hot ethanol (50 per cent, 70 per cent, and 90 per cent).
†Glidden's "Alpha Protein" washed three times in cold water.
‡J. H. Ridout, C. C. Lucas, J. M. Patterson, and C. H. Best, [643] Vitamin B_{12} (3 mg per kg) was added to the vitamin mixture described.

peanut meal (50 per cent protein) and "Alpha" (soya) protein were added at the expense of sucrose. This gave a series of test diets of increasing protein content (Table 46.II) which enabled us to determine the protein requirement of young male rats fed this type of diet. The amino acids histidine, lysine, threonine, methionine, and cystine were included in Basal Diet A (Table 46.I) in amounts necessary to bring the essential amino acids of the diet containing 15 per cent protein up to the levels suggested by Rose and his co-workers [652]. Weanling rats were fed these test diets for 20 days. Optimal growth occurred with the mixture containing 15 per cent protein (Table 46.II) supplied as 12 per cent extracted peanut meal, 8 per cent soya protein, and 1 per cent casein.

TABLE 46.II

EFFECT OF DIETARY PROTEIN LEVEL ON RATE OF GAIN

Diet no.	Peanut meal* (%)	Alpha soya protein* (%)	Total protein (%)	Average daily gain (7th to 20th days) (g)
A0	0	0	9	2.3
A1	1	1	10.5	3.5
A2	2	2	12	3.9
A3	3	3	13.5	4.8
A4	4	4	15	5.4
A5	6	6	18	5.5

*Alcohol-extracted peanut meal and water-washed "Alpha Protein" were used.

By calculation, the amounts of lysine and threonine in the unsupplemented 15 per cent protein mixture (Basal B) appeared to be borderline. This mixture of dietary protein was therefore tested to see whether it might be deficient in any essential amino acids other than methionine. Growth rates were observed in rats fed Diet B (Table 46.I) plus 0.4 per cent methionine and 0.3 per cent choline Cl, and in similar diets supplemented (a) with 0.3 per cent L(+)lysine HCl alone, and (b) with 0.3 per cent L(+)lysine HCl plus 0.1 per cent DL-threonine. No differences in rate of gain or in feed efficiency were observed. These results suggest that the mixture of proteins used in the hypolipotropic diet (Basal B, Table 46.I) is adequate for the rat, since this ration, when supplemented with the lipotropic factors, produced good growth. This diet is much lower in methionine than was that fed by Best et al. [105] (190 mg versus 360 mg per 100 g of diet), but is more adequate in all other respects. It was adopted for the present study. Varying levels of choline, betaine, and methionine were added to this basal diet at the expense of sucrose, as shown in Tables 46.III and 46.V.

RESULTS AND DISCUSSION

The effects of supplementary choline and betaine are summarized in Figure 81 and in Table 46.III. The addition of small amounts of choline chloride to the diet gave a dramatic reduction in liver lipids. The amount of choline found necessary for protection against haemorrhagic kidney lesions in young male rats consuming this type of diet was 0.04 per cent, that for

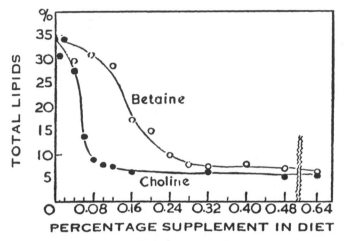

FIGURE 81. Dose-response curves showing the effect on total lipids (expressed as per cent of fresh weight) of varying amounts of choline (●) and betaine (○) when fed to rats for 21 days.

maximum growth was 0.10 per cent, and for maintenance of normal liver fat was 0.12 per cent to 0.16 per cent. The corresponding values for betaine under these experimental conditions were 0.20 per cent to 0.24 per cent for protection against haemorrhagic kidneys, 0.24 per cent to 0.28 per cent for optimal growth, and 0.32 per cent for maintenance of normal liver fat. Comparing the amounts of betaine and of choline to maintain any given amount of fat in the liver, we find the average ratio of betaine to choline is about 3.0:1 at all liver fat values from normal to 27 per cent (Table 46.IV). Since the molecular weights of the lipotropic compounds are not equal, comparisons should be made on a molar basis; the data have therefore been expressed on both a weight basis and a molar basis. The molecular weights of betaine and choline being nearly equal (117 and 121 respectively) the ratios were essentially the same (3.06:1 vs. 3.15:1, Table 46.IV). This average ratio is in line with the observation of Griffith and Mulford [334] that under their conditions betaine is approximately one-third as effective as choline. It should be emphasized that such comparisons are valid only when made on the steep portions of the dose-response curves. At higher dosage levels, where both choline and betaine are in excess of the amounts necessary to produce a maximal response, these two substances appear to be about equally effective.

Best *et al.* [105] obtained considerably different results: they observed a wide range of ratios of betaine to choline (varying from 3:1 to 8:1). Their data were obtained under conditions where growth was purposely kept to a minimum by means of an imbalance of essential amino acids. In

TABLE 46.III

EFFECT OF CHOLINE AND BETAINE ON FOOD INTAKE, GROWTH,
KIDNEY LESIONS, AND LIVER LIPIDS*

Expt. no.		Supplements (%)	Survivors Started	Kidney Lesion† (%)	Total Liver Lipids (% Wet Wt.)	Mean Values for Survivors Daily Food Intake (g)	Daily Gain (g)
		Choline‡					
1		0	2/10	100	34.5±1.80§	10.4	2.52±0.09§
	2	0.01	5/11	82	30.9±3.30	9.9	2.61±0.59
1		0.02	7/10	40	34.3±1.02	11.7	2.86±0.31
1		0.04	9/10	0	27.6±2.92	12.9	3.71±0.20
	2	0.06	11/11	0	13.7±1.06	11.8	3.84±0.21
1	2	0.08	21/21	0	8.9±0.59	12.0	3.70±0.21
1	2	0.10	21/21	0	7.8±0.18	12.7	4.36±0.25
	2	0.12	10/11	0	7.3±0.38	12.8	4.08±0.41
1	2	0.16	21/21	0	6.2±0.12	13.2	4.04±0.15
1		0.32	10/10	0	6.1±0.27	12.4	3.36±0.31
	2	0.48	10/10	0	5.2±0.17	13.4	4.20±0.33
	2	0.64	7/10	0	5.5±0.15	13.6	4.06±0.29
		Betaine‡					
1		0.04	3/10	90	29.6±5.90	8.8	1.38±0.38
1	2	0.08	7/21	76	30.9±3.06	10.4	2.63±0.31
	2	0.12	7/21	60	28.5±2.80	11.9	3.62±0.34
1	2	0.16	19/21	24	17.1±1.64	12.5	3.60±0.15
	2	0.20	11/11	9	14.9±1.40	11.9	3.67±0.32
	2	0.24	11/11	0	9.8±0.60	11.9	3.82±0.26
	2	0.28	11/11	0	7.8±2.80	12.6	3.95±0.39
1	2	0.32	21/21	0	7.5±0.49	13.1	3.94±0.16
	2	0.40	11/11	0	7.8±0.69	12.6	3.93±0.28
	2	0.48	10/11	0	7.0±0.62	11.9	3.89±0.39
1		0.64	10/10	0	6.2±0.53	14.0	3.98±0.30

*Young male rats (Wistar strain), 70–90 g.
†Incidence of haemorrhagic kidney lesions.
‡Choline was supplied as choline Cl in amounts 1.15 times the value shown.
  Betaine was supplied as betaine HCl in amounts 1.31 times the value shown.
§Mean ± standard error.

TABLE 46.IV

LIPOTROPIC RATIO OF BETAINE TO CHOLINE AT DIFFERENT LEVELS OF LIVER FAT

Betaine per 100 g Diet		Liver Fat (%)	Choline to Give Same Liver Fat		Betaine to Choline	
mg	millimoles		mg	millimoles	Weight ratio	Molar ratio
120	1.02	26.8	41.7	0.34	2.88	2.97
160	1.37	18.0	54	0.46	2.96	3.05
200	1.71	12.8	62	0.51	3.22	3.33
240	2.05	9.8	74	0.61	3.24	3.36
280	2.39	8.2	92	0.76	3.04	3.12
320	2.73	7.5	105	0.87	3.04	3.12
360	3.07	7.3	110	0.91	(3.27)*	(3.38)*
400	3.42	7.2	118	0.98	(3.39)*	(3.69)*
480	4.10	7.0	120	0.99	(4.00)*	(4.13)*
				Average ratio	3.06	3.15

*Values shown in parenthesis are not included in the average since they were derived from data obtained in the region of maximal response, and not on the steep portion of the dose-response curve.

TABLE 46.V

EFFECTS OF DIETARY METHIONINE ON FOOD INTAKE, GROWTH, KIDNEY LESIONS,
AND LIVER LIPIDS IN THE ABSENCE OF CHOLINE

| Supplements* (%) | Survivors | | Incidence of Kidney Lesions | Total Liver Lipids (% Wet Wt.) | Mean Values for Survivors | |
| | | | | | Daily food intake (g) | Daily gain (g) |
	Started					
Methionine in absence of added cystine						
0	7/8		4/8	28.2±2.55†	11.5	1.86±0.20†
0.08	6/8		4/8	28.8±2.91	11.7	2.90±0.22
0.16	8/8		0	21.2±1.68	11.9	3.22±0.21
0.24	8/8		0	13.8±1.91	12.9	3.50±0.30
0.28	8/8		0	13.3±0.74	12.9	3.85±0.27
0.32	8/8		0	12.1±0.92	13.4	3.84±0.33
0.40	8/8		0	11.8±0.88	14.3	4.29±0.29
0.48	6/8		0	9.8±0.51	13.7	3.87±0.28
Methionine with 0.2% cystine added to basal diet						
0	3/8		8/8	31.0±5.08	9.6	1.87±0.29
0.08	5/8		3/8	34.1±0.58	11.3	2.77±0.59
0.16	7/8		1/8	18.8±2.76	12.9	3.56±0.24
0.24	5/8‡		0	11.9±2.03	11.6	3.61±0.39
0.28	7/8‡		0	11.8±1.25	12.3	3.55±0.28
0.32	8/8		0	9.8±0.75	12.9	3.55±0.22
0.40	8/8		0	8.1±0.43	11.6	3.13±0.32
0.48	7/8‡		0	8.3±0.68	11.9	3.28±0.24

*Total methionine content of the basal diet 0.19 per cent, cystine content 0.12 per cent.
†Mean ± standard error.
‡Mortality due to pneumonia.

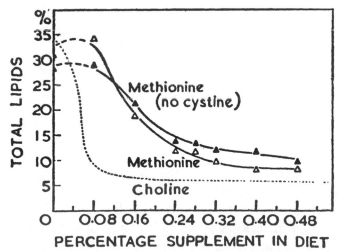

FIGURE 82. Dose-response curves showing the effect on total liver
lipids (expressed as per cent wet weight) of varying amounts of
methionine when fed to rats with (△) and without (▲) supplementary cystine (0.2 per cent).

addition the diet was deficient in folic acid and in vitamin B_{12} which were not then available. The difference in the findings emphasizes the importance of the nature of the basal diet in such studies.

The difficulties attendant upon attempts to measure the lipotropic activity of methionine have been discussed elsewhere [71; 122; 753; 755]. The results of another endeavour in this direction using Basal Diet B (with and without added cystine) are summarized in Table 46.V and Figure 82. Under these conditions methionine was not as effective as betaine, when compared on a weight basis, in preventing the accumulation of fat in the liver, either in the presence or absence of cystine. When the comparison was made on a molar basis (Table 46.VI) the potency of methionine was

TABLE 46.VI

RATIO OF METHIONINE TO CHOLINE TO PRODUCE VARIOUS AMOUNTS OF LIVER FAT

Added Methionine per 100 g Diet		Liver Fat (%)	Choline to Give Same Liver Fat		Methionine to Choline	
mg	millimoles		mg	millimoles	Weight ratio	Molar ratio
(a) No cystine added to basal diet*						
80	0.54	28.8	36	0.30	2.22	1.80
120	0.81	26.5	42	0.35	2.86	2.56
160	1.07	21.2	51	0.42	3.13	2.54
200	1.34	16.7	56	0.46	3.57	2.89
240	1.61	14.0	59.5	0.49	4.04	3.28
280	1.88	12.8	61	0.50	4.59	3.72
320	2.14	12.3	63	0.52	5.08	4.12
360	2.42	11.8	65	0.54	5.53	4.49
400	2.68	11.5	66	0.55	6.08	5.00
(b) Cystine (0.2%) added to the basal diet*						
80	0.54	34.1	20	0.17	4.00	3.25
120	0.81	28.8	36	0.30	3.34	2.71
160	1.07	19.5	53	0.44	3.02	2.46
200	1.34	14.6	59	0.49	3.39	2.74
240	1.61	11.8	65	0.54	3.69	2.99
280	1.88	10.2	72	0.60	3.88	3.14
320	2.14	9.5	76	0.63	4.22	3.43
360	2.42	9.2	79	0.65	4.55	3.69
400	2.68	8.8	82	0.68	4.88	3.95

*Basal diet contains 190 mg methionine and 120 mg cystine per 100 g of diet.

more comparable with that of betaine. However, unlike the case of betaine, the lipotropic potency decreases as the methionine content of the diet increases. This decrease in lipotropic efficiency of methionine is a linear function occurring in both the presence and absence of added cystine. In this experiment the inefficiency of the higher levels of methionine to reduce the liver fat to the normal range was more evident in the absence of dietary cystine (Table 46.V and Figure 82). However, rats fed the diet containing the higher levels of supplementary methionine in the absence of added cystine ate more ration and gained in weight more rapidly than rats receiving comparable methionine with cystine. This increased food consumption and concomitant gain in weight probably tended to increase the deposition of liver fat. However, in similar unpublished experiments the greater gain was not always observed in the absence of added cystine.

In these experiments higher values were obtained for liver fat at the suboptimal levels of choline or betaine than in the experiments reported by Best *et al.* [105]. It is believed that the more adequate diet used in the present study permitted greater growth with the result that more of the limited supply of methionine and choline were utilized for growth, leaving less available for lipotropic purposes. In addition, we know now that the diet used by Best *et al.* was deficient in folic acid and vitamin B_{12}. These vitamins have since been shown to be involved in the metabolism of the lipotropic compounds (*vide* [787]). The lower choline requirement and the high betaine-to-choline ratios found at that time were probably due to the higher methionine content of the basal diet coupled with poorer growth.

Summary

A hypolipotropic basal diet is described that contains a minimal amount of protein for optimal growth of rats when supplemented with methionine and choline. Dose–response curves are given showing the lipotropic effects of graded supplements of dietary choline, betaine, and methionine.

The average lipotropic ratio of betaine-to-choline over a range in liver fat from normal to 27 per cent is 3.06:1 when compared on a weight basis and 3.15:1 when compared on a molar basis. The lipotropic ratios (molar) of methionine-to-choline in the absence of cystine increased from 1.8 to 5.0 and in the presence of added cystine varied from 2.5 to 4.0. Methionine was as effective as betaine (molar) only at the lower dosages. At the higher levels methionine was less effective. Even the highest dose failed to maintain the liver fat within the normal range.

THE EFFECT OF PROLONGED CHOLINE deficiency in primates has thus far received very little attention. When our experiments were undertaken, no data on the effects of choline deficiency in primates were available, with the exception of one preliminary report from Professor Stare's laboratory at Harvard University. The paper to follow gives some of the preliminary findings in such a study but the complete picture will not be available until the investigation is completed, perhaps several years hence.

Four monkeys have now been maintained for over five years on a purified diet free from choline but with sufficient protein (and methionine) to permit slow growth. Liver biopsies have been obtained each year. All four monkeys on the choline-deficient diet had developed very fatty livers by the end of the first year and control animals fed the same diet supplemented with choline had not.

The distribution of fat, mainly periportal, seen in the first sections examined resembles that seen in kwashiorkor. However when further sections were cut, more recently, from the paraffin blocks prepared by Dr. Wilgram from the earlier biopsy material, areas have been noted in which the lesion in the choline-deficient monkey resembles that in the rat more closely than we had originally recognized. There were many areas in which the deposition of fat was around the central vein. There were other regions in which the lipid distribution was predominantly periportal but the picture was a mixed one from which different observers might draw different conclusions.

Though the development of cirrhosis in these monkeys has been much slower than in rats fed exactly the same diet, the hepatic lesions now resemble to a remarkable degree those seen in the rat and those seen in the human alcoholic.

In a way the production of cirrhosis in the primate on a choline-deficient diet, if confirmed, is the culmination of over thirty years of work on one aspect of the study of lipotropic phenomena.

47. Kwashiorkor Type of Fatty Liver in Primates

GEORGE F. WILGRAM, M.D.

COLIN C. LUCAS, PH.D.

CHARLES H. BEST, M.D.

Kwashiorkor is today one of the most serious and widespread diseases of infancy in the world. The nutritional basis for the disease is generally accepted but debate continues as to whether the malady is due primarily to a disproportion between total protein and caloric intake, whether an imbalance of amino acids is involved, or whether a deficiency of some unidentified food factor contributes to the problem. Clinical studies are being conducted in many centres but with the exception of one preliminary report [549] no experimental investigations using primates are known to us.

One of the characteristic features of kwashiorkor is an accumulation of stainable lipid in the liver. This fat occurs throughout the liver lobule in advanced cases but is seen first, and later predominantly, in the periportal areas [248]. The condition of the patient is improved markedly by feeding skim milk powder, and recent publications by Brock [150; 151] suggest that the important ingredient is the improved supply of amino acids.

Members of this Department have long been interested in fatty livers of dietary origin. Shortly after the lipotropic action of choline and betaine had been established [94], an effect of dietary protein on this phenomenon was noted [79; 95; 188; 194]. This led to the discovery that methionine possesses a strong lipotropic activity [760], which appeared at first to account for the effects of dietary protein [113; 191]. Later Beveridge et al. [121; 122] reported that the balance of essential amino acids as well as the supply of lipotropic factors affects the fat content of hepatic cells in the rat. Others have elaborated upon this phase of the problem [361; 362; 707; 708]. Lack of choline had long been known to result in a centrilobular

Originally appeared in the *Journal of Experimental Medicine*, CVIII (1958), 361–70. A preliminary description of this work was reported at the Federation of American Societies for Experimental Biology, Philadelphia, March, 1958. This work was supported in part by the Life Insurance Medical Research Fund, New York, and the Nutrition Foundation, Inc.

distribution of the newly deposited hepatic lipids in rats. More recently protein deficiency has been shown to cause the stainable lipid to appear in periportal areas of the livers of rats [87; 517].

The present study deals with findings in primates. Monkeys have been fed purified diets free from choline and betaine and low in methionine, but believed to be adequate in other respects. (When choline was present the monkeys gained in weight; one female had a baby and suckled it.)

Biopsy specimens of liver revealed that after one year on the choline-free diet considerable amounts of stainable fat were present. Fat appeared predominantly in periportal areas. The type and site of lipid accumulation in these experimental animals had a close resemblance to that seen in certain stages of kwashiorkor. The livers of the choline-supplemented animals appeared perfectly normal.

METHODS

Four male *Cebus* monkeys weighing between 1.5 and 2 kg and four *Rhesus* monkeys (two males, two females) weighing between 3.5 and 4 kg were acclimated to their new environment after arrival in our colony. All animals proved to be healthy and free of infectious diseases. They gained weight on nutritious, mixed, natural foodstuffs. After six months of acclimatization the animals were given the purified rations.

Two *Cebus* and two *Rhesus* monkeys were given a choline-deficient diet the composition of which follows. Two *Cebus* and two *Rhesus* monkeys received the same diet supplemented with choline chloride (0.3 per cent).

[Two tables, giving the composition of the diets, and details of the preparation of the food, have been omitted. A condensation follows. The percentage composition of the choline-deficient diet (MK-2) was: peanut meal (extracted with 50, 75, and 95 per cent ethanol to remove choline compounds) 10, soya protein 10, sugar 33, starch 13, dextrin 13, lard 18, salts 3. The dry ingredients were blended thoroughly in a Hobart Food Mixer. To each kilogram of dry mixture, 55 ml. of water was added and the pasty mixture was baked on a biscuit sheet in an oven at 180° for 20 minutes. After cooling for 10 minutes, 20 g of a corn oil solution of vitamins A, D, and E (500 i.u. vitamin D, 2000 i.u. vitamin A and 0.01 g alpha-tocopheryl acetate per g of oil) was poured over the cake and 20 g of a mixture of water-soluble vitamins in sucrose was sprinkled from a salt shaker over the surface. The salts and sucrose-vitamin mixture were similar to those commonly used in this department [643], with the inclusion in the latter of 0.12 μg of vitamin B_{12} and 20 mg ascorbic acid per g. The cake was cut into biscuits weighing about 20 g each. To ensure freshness, a batch was baked about every five days.]

The monkeys were housed in individual units in a room which was thermostatically controlled at 30° C and in which an automatic switch provided light for half a day. The cages were roomy enough to allow for moderate activity, but in addition, all animals were given an opportunity daily to exercise vigorously in a special compartment adjacent to the cages.

Both groups of animals were fed their diets *ad libitum* for a period of about one year, at the end of which time liver biopsies were taken by laparotomy under general (nembutal) anaesthesia. Lipids were determined on about 5 g of biopsy material (Table 47.I). Blood was withdrawn at regular intervals from the animals by venipuncture and analysed for total lipids, total phospholipids, and total cholesterol (Table 47.II). Total liver lipids were extracted with hot alcohol (3 times, 5 ml per g each time) after grinding the biopsy specimen in a Waring blendor and treating the minced tissue with 5 volumes of redistilled acetone. The combined acetone and alcohol extracts were taken to dryness *in vacuo* (water bath 45°); lipids in the residue were taken up in 3:1 (*v/v*) petroleum ether (b.p. 40–60°)–chloroform. Values for blood lipids were obtained by a slight modification of Bloor's alcohol-ether extraction method [131]. Cholesterol was determined on aliquots of the petroleum ether-chloroform solutions by the method of Sperry and Webb [729]. Phospholipid P was determined by King's method [453] and phospholipid was calculated using the factor 25.0 × P. Total lipids were determined gravimetrically.

TABLE 47.I

LIVER LIPIDS

Monkey no. and Sex	Dietary Choline Chloride (%)	Liver dffr.* % w. wt.†	Total Lipids		Phospholipids		Free Cholesterol		Total Cholesterol	
			% w. wt.†	% dffr.*	% w. wt.†	% dffr.*	% w. wt.†	% dffr.*	% w. wt.†	% dffr.*
(a) *Cebus* monkeys										
1 M	—	20.78	12.50	60.1	2.88	13.86	0.265	1.27	0.392	1.89
2 M	0.3	19.31	6.11	31.7	2.98	15.44	0.266	1.38	0.358	1.85
3 M	—	19.95	21.78	109.4	2.16	10.86	0.218	1.09	0.322	1.62
4 M	0.3	23.01	8.61	37.4	2.87	12.47	0.219	0.95	0.306	1.33
(b) *Rhesus* monkeys										
5 F	—	20.03	13.65	68.1	2.93	14.63	0.255	1.27	0.345	1.72
6 F	0.3	20.32	5.92	29.1	3.62	17.82	0.255	1.26	0.316	1.56
7 M	—	20.89	19.50	93.3	2.87	13.73	0.254	1.22	0.443	2.12
8 M	0.3	23.66	7.26	30.7	3.49	14.75	0.244	1.03	0.384	1.62

*dffr. = dry, fat-free residue.
†w. wt. = wet weight.

Histological sections were done on small pieces of biopsy material and stained with hematoxylin-eosin. Histochemical tests were performed to detect the presence of reticulin fibres and connective tissue in paraffin sections. Fat was stained with oil red O in frozen sections [806].

TABLE 47.II
SERUM LIPIDS

Monkey no. and Sex	Dietary Choline Chloride (%)	Amount per 100 ml Serum					
		Mos. after institution of diet			Mos. after institution of diet		
		6	9	12	6	9	12
		serum total cholesterol			serum total phospholipids		
		mg	mg	mg	mg	mg	mg
Cebus							
1 M	—	171	142	109	250	229	169
2 M	0.3	220	154	168	315	269	259
3 M	—	158	136	153	204	139	187
4 M	0.3	238	154	203	338	206	313
Rhesus							
5 F	—	159	133	36	269	233	61
6 F	0.3	229	250	135	300	238	152
7 M	—	138	100	110	225	168	140
8 M	0.3	180	175	160	304	256	269

RESULTS

(a) Weight Changes

The choline-deficient *Cebus* monkeys kept their weight throughout an experimental period of fourteen months; the *Rhesus* monkeys increased in weight by about 30 per cent over the same period. The choline-supplemented *Cebus* and *Rhesus* monkeys increased in weight by about 22 per cent and 65 per cent, respectively, over the same period.

(b) Biochemical Findings

It can be seen from Table 47.I that there was a two- to threefold increase in extractable lipids in the livers of the choline-deficient animals. In contrast, there was a decrease in all fractions of the blood lipids in the choline-deficient monkeys (Table 47.II). These biochemical findings are consistent with those obtained in other species.

(c) Pathology and Histology

Upon laparotomy no serous fluid was detectable in the abdominal cavity in any of the animals. The gross inspection of spleen, intestine, pancreas, and kidneys did not reveal any abnormality. The great vessels of the abdominal cavity showed no sign of pathological changes. The only visible finding in the deficient monkeys was a slightly enlarged, firm, yellowish liver whose capsule was smooth and shiny without any adhesions. The livers of the supplemented animals, however, appeared perfectly normal.

Histological examination of the choline-deficient livers with fat stains revealed fine lipid droplets throughout the entire liver lobule, but the main site of fat accumulation was the periportal area. Here lipid appeared frequently in huge coalescing globules that squeezed the remaining cytoplasm to a narrow rim. The nucleus in these lipid-laden hepatic cells often was displaced into a corner of the liver cell. Sometimes numerous smaller droplets were discernible instead of one large globule. The Kupffer and sinus cells as well as the biliary system appeared normal. No abnormal reticulin or collagenous fibres were observed in these animals after one year on the choline-deficient diet. Also, no fatty cysts were discernible, nor were there any signs that the lipid-laden cells had ruptured.

The livers of the choline-supplemented monkeys did not exhibit any stainable lipid and appeared perfectly normal in every respect.

[Four photomicrographs have been omitted showing the distribution of fat in the livers of the choline-deficient monkeys and the normal appearance when the diet was supplemented with choline.]

Discussion

The essential amino acid requirements of monkeys are not known to us. Even the choline requirement is still not known.

The appearance of stainable lipid in the periportal areas of the liver lobules of *rats* is generally considered to indicate that some protein deficiency or amino acid imbalance exists in the ration. The periportal accumulation of lipid in our *monkeys* fed the diet deficient in choline raised suspicion that the food was inadequate in protein. While this conclusion would be the correct one in rats it appears unwarranted in primates under our experimental conditions, for the following reasons. When choline (0.3 per cent, as chloride) was included, good growth was obtained and perfectly normal livers were observed. One female on the choline-supplemented diet became pregnant and gave birth to a normal offspring that she suckled and raised in good health. The essentially satisfactory nature of the basal ration is indicated by the fact that even the animals fed the choline-free diet did not lose weight, and some actually gained, in spite of a fatty liver. The methionine content of the diet (about 160 mg per 100 g) would be considered very low for a species with a rapid rate of growth (*e.g.* the rat) but it was apparently reasonably adequate for the slower growing monkeys, when choline was present.

When the choline content of the diet is insufficient, methionine may act as precursor for the biosynthesis of choline. When dietary methionine is limited, the evidence is strong that it is preferentially used for growth and maintenance [122; 754; 755]. This hypothesis is supported by the observation that the monkeys fed the choline-deficient diet grew to a limited extent and had moderately fatty livers. Inclusion of choline in the diet eliminates the need for the body to divert any significant amount of methionine for lipotropic purposes—practically all is available for growth or maintenance. This would explain why the choline-supplemented monkeys grew well and had normal livers.

Attempts to estimate the food consumption of the monkeys were defeated by their wasteful behaviour. We were forced to use *ad libitum* feeding. With further experience we hope to achieve a reasonable degree of accuracy in paired feeding.

The pathological finding of a fatty liver raises the question as to what caused the abnormality. The fatty liver in these monkeys obviously was due to some nutritional factor. With a diet of the type fed here three factors come to mind: (*a*) lack of choline, (*b*) insufficient methionine, and (*c*) general deficiency of protein. The fact that supplementary choline prevented the development of fatty livers might seem to justify the conclusion that the first condition, *viz.* lack of choline, was responsible. However, a further analysis of the situation reveals other possibilities. The basal diet was designed to be free from both choline and betaine and low in methionine, which is a biological precursor of choline. Part, or all, of the hepatic lesion might be attributed to the low methionine content in the protein mixture used.

The biological value of a protein depends on its amino acid composition. When one essential amino acid is present in short supply, the other dietary amino acids are available for synthesis of body protein only in amounts proportional to that of the limiting amino acid [171; 650]. If one accepts this concept, one has to conclude that restriction of dietary methionine will limit the extent to which the body can utilize the other amino acids supplied in the diet. In other words, the diet low in methionine is probably also unsatisfactory with respect to other amino acids in spite of the amount of protein supplied. Therefore, a decision as to the primary dietary etiological factor in the production of the fatty liver is not easily reached. The improvement brought about by choline supplementation could be due in part to sparing methionine and consequent improvement in the availability of the other essential amino acids in the dietary protein.

Summary

Fatty livers resembling those seen in the early stages of kwashiorkor have been produced in primates. Monkeys were fed, for about one year, purified diets free from choline and betaine and low in methionine. Supplementation with choline slightly improved food consumption and gain in weight. Choline prevented the appearance of any stainable lipid in the liver of the control animals. The extent to which the slightly greater intake of protein, including methionine, in the choline-supplemented animals contributed to the prevention of the periportal accumulation of fat in the liver is being determined.

ACKNOWLEDGMENTS

The authors wish to acknowledge the guidance of Dr. Gertrude van Wagenen in establishing a monkey colony. The authors are similarly indebted to Dr. Frederick Stare and his associates for having provided advice in the handling and feeding of primates.

The help of Mr. Norman Edwards in the care of the animals and of Dr. A. M. Rappaport in the skilful performance of the laparotomies is gratefully acknowledged.

We wish also to thank Dr. Jean M. Patterson for the chemical analyses.

48. The Lipotropic Agents in the Protection of the Liver, Kidney, Heart, and Other Organs of Experimental Animals

CHARLES H. BEST, F.R.S.

The award of the Croonian Lectureship has given me exceptional pleasure and a sense of great responsibility. In selecting a title I have considered the principal subjects in which I have endeavoured to keep abreast, and the choice has thus been narrowed to insulin and experimental diabetes, heparin and thrombosis, and the dietary factor choline and its precursors, which we have termed the lipotropic agents. Certain of the effects of these three substances might be discussed in a single lecture, since they all affect either the formation, distribution, or the state of fat in the body. The action of a lipokinetic constituent of the anterior pituitary, first clearly demonstrated in our laboratory in 1936 (Best and Campbell [78]) which increases the rate of mobilization of depot fat to the liver (Barrett, Best, and Ridout [53]; Stetten and Salcedo [739]), might also have been included. The fat-mobilizing effect of anterior pituitary extracts may be due to Evans' somatotropin, to the adrenocorticotropic hormone, to a more specific but as yet unidentified substance or, of course, to more than one of these. The four factors, insulin, choline, heparin, and "adipokinin" (Weil and Stetten [784]) have given us a measure of control over fat metabolism which our predecessors did not enjoy. There are, of course, other dietary and hormonal agents affecting these processes which one would have to discuss in a comprehensive treatment of the field. I shall not even list these and, indeed, after a very brief consideration of insulin and heparin, particularly in relation to fat metabolism, I shall limit my discussion to "the lipotropic agents."

Originally appeared in the *Proceedings of the Royal Society*, B, CXLV (1956), 151–69. Delivered June 16, 1955.

The attack on the problem of pancreatic diabetes which Banting initiated and which he and I made in 1921 was, as you know, a frontal one. Our essential working hypothesis was that an internal secretion of the pancreas existed. Professor J. J. R. Macleod was one of the great authorities on carbohydrate metabolism who did *not* believe that all the evidence pointed to an internal secretion of the pancreas, and in his stimulating and very critical lectures to us, his senior students and junior research workers, in 1920, he insisted that there was no more convincing evidence for an internal secretion than for a detoxifying action of the islands of Langerhans. During the summer and autumn of 1921 Banting and I followed in seventy-five separate successful tests the definite and in many cases the dramatic and characteristic fall in blood sugar in our depancreatized dogs after the administration of insulin-containing extracts. When we had succeeded in preparing uniformly potent extracts from commercially available ox pancreas, by alcoholic extraction and subsequent chemical removal of fatty substances, many programmes of research were revealed and made readily possible. In one particular study we administered our partially purified extract for 70 days to a completely depancreatized dog with consistent antidiabetic effects and without signs of general toxicity, except hypoglycaemia which our frequent blood-sugar determinations enabled us to detect and correct. We were eager to proceed with the further chemical fractionation and purification of our product, with the extension of our preliminary findings on carbohydrate, protein, and fat metabolism, and with the clinical application of our results. The problems were legion and selection was our main difficulty. The situation was complicated by the fact that no junior workers or technical assistants were available, and many of the most promising studies required day and night supervision of our animals. In the long list of suggestions which we mailed to Professor Macleod in the early autumn of 1921 there were some which were particularly attractive, and which have been of abiding interest, to me.

Our attention had been repeatedly focused on the effects of insulin on fat metabolism by the frequently observed suppression of diabetic ketonuria, by the prevention of the well-known diabetic fatty infiltration of the liver, and by the obvious increase in body fat which some of our insulin-treated depancreatized animals exhibited. All of these effects were recorded in our first notebooks, and the observations were later extended and established in collaboration with Professor Macleod, Professor J. B. Collip and others, during the development phase of the insulin investigations. The discovery of the lipotropic agents was a direct outgrowth of the isolation of insulin, and the effects of this hormone on fat metabolism are intimately connected with those of the dietary factors.

Heparin was discovered by McLean in 1916 in Howell's laboratory and named by Howell and Holt in 1918. During those years McLean, Howell, and others must have had very much the same hope and objective as we did when the work on the distribution and purification of this material was initiated in Toronto in 1929. Up to this time the only source of heparin had been the liver of the dog; such extracts contained toxic products introduced by the method of preparation and were of low potency. A recent graduate in chemistry, Mr. Arthur Charles, came to work with me on this problem in the Department of Physiology, and my colleague Dr. D. A. Scott, in what was then my Division of the Connaught Laboratories, joined the group. This work soon revealed that a commercially available tissue, beef lung, is an excellent source of heparin, and it provided us, and interested scientists in all other countries, with a method for the preparation of a potent, highly purified product with which to study the prevention of thrombosis and clotting, and other phenomena. (Professor Donald Y. Solandt, my close friend and colleague in that phase of the heparin work [719; 721] which had to do with the first use of an anticoagulant in the prevention of coronary and intramural thrombosis in dogs, died at the age of 48 on March 30 of this year, in Toronto). It may be recorded that Dr. J. McLean, after the death of Professor Howell, requested us to act as custodians of the original records of the discovery and early development of heparin. These documents are in the library of our Institute. We have been interested in the lipaemia-clearing and fat-mobilizing effects of heparin since my former colleague Professor Beecher Weld, who first confirmed and extended the original observation of Hahn [344], drew this to our attention [791]. This subject was discussed by Sir Howard Florey in the Croonian Lecture for 1954, with brief references to the work of his own laboratory, and many other very important papers have recently appeared in this rapidly developing field which promises a great deal of physiological interest in relation to fat metabolism.

There was an urgency about the work on insulin and on heparin, perhaps because the obvious clinical applications emphasized the necessity of making available a safe and satisfactory product, although knowledge of the chemical structure of these substances was in an elementary state. This pressure has not been prominent in the development of the choline field although there have been many exciting phases. The chemistry of the key substances has been well known for many years. The diets of people in well-developed countries contain an abundance of the lipotropic factors and in other parts of the world specific deficiencies are obscured. The mild frustration, if any at all has existed, has had more to do with the natural reluctance of good clinicians to deprive even the confirmed alcoholic of

choline and methionine, with continuance, of course, of alcoholic suste-
nance and of dietary essentials apart from the lipotropic factors. Studies of
this type have not been conducted for a sufficient time to permit a decision
on the extent to which the work on experimental animals is applicable to
man. While there has been no lack of potential applications, as we shall
see, this work in our laboratories has followed a wide variety of pathways
which have been selected for us, in large part, by changing interests and
the training of our co-workers and students. It has been fascinating to
watch this pool of knowledge gradually fill until it has touched many
aspects of physiology, biochemistry and experimental pathology. I have
described recently, and in some detail, the historical development of this
field which had its origin in the prolonged treatment of depancreatized
dogs with insulin in Professor Macleod's department [73]. It was reported
by two graduate students from my department (Hershey and Soskin [388])
that degenerative changes in the liver could be prevented by including
crude lecithin in the diet, i.e., that the lecithin preparation had the same
effect as beef pancreas in the prevention of hepatic lesions. A little later,
using rats as test animals, my colleagues and I were able to identify choline
as the active component of lecithin [90]. Since that time we have written
several reviews describing advances in the knowledge of the role of choline
and its precursors as dietary factors [100; 101; 104].

The Fatty Liver

The central feature of deficiency of the lipotropic agents is the fatty
liver which has been observed in the dog [84; 97; 180], rat [94], mouse
[97; 789], rabbit [135], guinea-pig [176], hamster [354], calf [430], pig
[596], monkey [549], and duckling [64]. In much less than 24 hours after
a choline-deficient diet has been substituted for a normal one, an excess of
stainable fat appears in the liver of the rat. The amount of extractable fat
rapidly increases until at the end of one week it is perhaps six times the
normal value. The increase is in the glyceride fraction and in cholesteryl
esters, and there is an interesting relationship between them (Best, Lucas,
Patterson, and Ridout [102]). During this period of rapid hepatic deposition
of fat, produced by the dietary deficiency of choline, there is no perceptible
decrease in the total choline of the body or of the liver (Best, Channon,
and Ridout [80]; Jacobi, Baumann, and Meek [420]; Jacobi and Baumann [419]). Free choline is difficult to measure, and the amount found
in blood has grown less and less with each improvement in the method of
preserving the bound choline intact. Some day it may well be established
that the level of free choline in blood and other tissues is one of the best

indices of the rate at which the lipotropic agents are being supplied and utilized. The necessity of an almost constant flow of dietary choline or its precursors to the liver and other tissues to maintain normal conditions adds great interest to these studies. (See Plate XI *a, b.*)

Some of the very early morphological changes which affect the liver when choline is removed from the diet were reported in 1934 by MacLean and Best [532]. We saw and described the intracellular storage of fat. Our photomicrographs showed definite evidence of the extracellular phase of fat storage, but the development of fatty cysts was not recognized until Dr. W. S. Hartroft, who has made during the past eight years many fine contributions to the work of our department, published his descriptions. Hartroft's observations have shown how the rapidly enlarging fat globules break the cell membranes in such a way that a pool of fat becomes enclosed by the remnants of the cytoplasm of the parent group of cells. This fat does not lie freely in the liver tissue but is contained within a simple epithelial cyst. Fatty cysts may fuse one with another or with single fat-laden cells. The cysts rupture and the remnants of the emptied structures condense into fibrotic trabeculae which are very characteristics of the early stages of experimental dietary cirrhosis in the rats [369]. (Plate XII.)

The Cirrhosis of Choline Deficiency

In 1934 MacLean and I [532] presented evidence of early fibrosis in the liver of dogs which were fed on a diet deficient in choline. We stated that in some areas of the liver the number of fibroblasts and leucocytes were abnormally large, and that the liver cords were separated by dilated capillaries and *by areas of beginning fibrosis*. While these reports marked the beginning of work on the hepatic fibrosis of choline deficiency, it was some five years later when György and Goldblatt in rats [341] and Chaikoff and Connor in dogs [180] noted the development of a definite cirrhosis in animals maintained on diets low in choline. There has been a considerable difference of opinion about the distribution of the fibrous tissue which appears in choline deficiency, but I must not attempt a detailed discussion here. (Plate XI *c.*)

Lillie, Ashburn, Sebrell, Daft, and Lowry [503], Glynn, Himsworth, and Lindan [322], and Hartroft [365] have made an excellent case for the non-portal origin of hepatic fibrosis and cirrhosis in the choline-deficient rats. Hartroft [367] has described intratrabecular fatty cysts in many human cases with a history of alcoholism or of other conditions which are characterized by large fatty livers, and this finding suggests that the mechanism by which some types of clinical cirrhosis are produced may be similar to that which can be studied, stage by stage, in the experimental animals.

We have conducted studies for the past six years on the fatty liver and fibrosis produced in rats by the substitution of dilute alcohol for drinking water [86]. With non-intoxicating doses which supply about 30 per cent of the total calories, all our findings support the conclusion that there is no specific toxic effect on liver cells *at this dosage* and that the damage *in this species* is completely prevented by an adequate diet. The characteristic lesions appear when the lipotropic factors alone are deficient and are seen at the same time and to the same extent when equicaloric amounts of pure sugar or pure alcohol are ingested. Small amounts of choline or methionine completely prevent the pathological changes in both the alcoholics and the "sucrotics."

The clinical pathologist frequently finds it difficult to interpret and to apply the findings of the experimentalist, but we all agree that a significant part of the clinical advance has followed this route. He has not accepted without some reserve the recent experimental findings in dietary cirrhosis. The experimentalist can plough his lonely furrow and preserve the purity and independence of his subject, but he has a fine opportunity in this field to create in animals by reproducible procedures the counterparts of several classical clinical lesions and to convince the clinician that these *may* be produced by a certain sequence of events.

THE CURE OF HEPATIC CIRRHOSIS IN EXPERIMENTAL ANIMALS

There have been several attempts to cure hepatic cirrhosis of dietary origin by returning choline or its precursors to the diets [343; 423; 514; 515; 622]. In all of these experiments cirrhosis was produced by feeding hypolipotropic diets low in protein for periods of about five months. The incidence and severity of the hepatic lesions were estimated in some cases by autopsy of animals selected at random and in others by inspection at laparotomy or by study of biopsy material.

Everyone agrees that choline rapidly removes the excess of fat. Lowry and his associates [515] concluded that the lipotropic substances had no effect on the diffuse fibrosis, but György and Goldblatt [343] felt that their findings indicated real regression of the cirrhotic process when the latter was not too advanced.

During recent years our group has been accumulating data on the cure of dietary cirrhosis. A laparotomy was performed on every rat and the degree of cirrhosis was estimated by inspection. A biopsy specimen was removed from every fourth animal. The findings indicate, in confirmation of previous workers, that when the cirrhosis is mild or moderate, choline causes a striking improvement in the gross appearance of the livers, a definite regeneration of new tissue, and an apparent regression of the fibrosis (Plate XIII (*a*) and (*b*). In an attempt to determine if fibrous tissue is actually reduced in amount, samples are being analysed for hydroxyproline. This amino acid is a major constituent of connective tissues and is essentially absent from the proteins of other structures. Our results are in agreement with others that in very severe cirrhosis the effect of the lipotropic supplements on fibrous tissue has been negligible even when treatment has been prolonged.

MULTIPLE-FAT EMBOLI FROM RUPTURED CYSTS

It has been shown that the fatty cysts may rupture into the bile canaliculi or into the hepatic sinusoids (Hartroft and Ridout [373]; Hartroft and Sellers [375]). With the return of choline to the diet a third route of removal is apparently available for the excess fat. There is abundant evidence that this fat within the normal liver cells disappears with great rapidity, and there are strong indications that some time later the accumulations within the fatty cysts may be called upon and presumably restored to the normal intracellular route of metabolism.

The study of the fate of the fat which is discharged into the liver sinusoids has provided many interesting findings. Lesions are produced in lungs by the intracapillary accumulation of fatty particles. It is possible that the blocking of the lung capillaries may lead to conditions in the rat somewhat similar to the pulmonary complications which some alcoholic patients exhibit. The experimental findings stimulated the successful search for pulmonary fat emboli in human alcoholics (Durlacher, Meier, Fisher, and Lovitt [274]). In the rats which have been subjected to prolonged choline deficiency, embolic fat and later calcified areas appear in the heart. In the kidneys there is also embolic fat, and a condition similar to the Kimmelstiel–Wilson syndrome in diabetic patients is produced by blocking of capillaries with fat presumably from the ruptured hepatic cysts. We have not suggested that these experimental findings throw any light on the clinical condition. Details of these pathological changes are given by Hartroft [366; 367; 368].

[Twelve coloured photomicrographs, showing various effects of choline deficiency, have been omitted.]

CARDIOVASCULAR LESIONS

Several years ago lesions of the aorta, carotid and coronary arteries in rats kept on a choline-deficient diet for some 200 days were reported

(Hartroft, Ridout, Sellers, and Best [374]). We had also been interested in the cardiac necrosis of choline deficiency by the report of Kesten, Salcedo, and Stetten [450] who found interstitial myocarditis in young rats fed choline-deficient diets containing 30 to 40 per cent of ethyl laurate but who did not mention fat deposition. More recently, using a diet with a high content of *naturally occurring fats* and very low in choline we have observed cardiac necrosis in 90 per cent of our test rats [800]. Coronary arteries showed lesions in three-quarters of these animals, but the incidence of aortic changes was much lower and did not exceed 15 per cent [801].

In the heart, fat rapidly accumulates within the cardiac fibres, and very large amounts may be present within two weeks. The lesions are best seen in young animals on severely choline-deficient diets. In coronary arteries there is an infiltration of fat into the intima, but mainly into the media, and sometimes even the adventitia is involved. Fatty endothelial cells may eventually undergo hyperplasia and the media may thicken. In the aorta intimal hyperplasia of fatty endothelial cells may develop, but most frequently fat appears first in the spaces between the elastic laminae of the media. Later on this is followed by necrosis, fibrosis, and sclerosis with calcification of the involved areas. This gives the aorta a typical bamboo stick appearance. Interference with the nutrition of the elasto-muscular tissue in the aorta which lacks vasa vasorum in the rat, may prove to be an important mechanism by which aortic sclerosis is produced in choline deficiency. Another factor may be a disturbance of the electrolyte equilibrium caused by the renal damage. In our experimental animals a mechanism similar to that of the clinical syndrome known as secondary hyperparathyroidism which is caused by the failure of damaged kidneys to excrete calcium and phosphorus, may play an important role. The participation of the kidney in the aetiology of fatty changes in heart and coronary vessels in choline deficiency is strongly emphasized by the fact that cardiovascular changes occur only rarely without concomitant kidney damage. The possibility still remains, however, that the primary factor in the production of heart and coronary lesions is choline deficiency and that kidney damage may be an important but secondary factor [799].

Female rats are less prone than males to develop the ill effects of choline deficiency, but cardiovascular lesions in females have been observed when somatotropin and androgens were given at the same time [797]. Large supplements of cholesterol in young female rats and smaller ones in males have increased the rather low incidence of cardiovascular lesions produced in these particular studies by choline deficiency alone. Cholesterol given in the same amounts to control animals receiving the same amounts of the diet, but with added choline, have exhibited no cardiovascular lesions in these short-term experiments [798].

This is not the place to attempt any clarification of the rapidly advancing, urgently needed, but confused knowledge of the field of experimental sclerosis and atherosclerosis (Katz and Stamler [439]). We have been *primarily* interested in *choline deficiency* and not in atherosclerosis. I must emphasize that the lesions which we have produced directly or indirectly in rats by this deficiency are characterized by infiltration of fat by medial sclerosis of the Moenckeberg type. There is no true atheroma formation. The lesions are not associated with high levels of plasma cholesterol and, indeed, in rats the level of cholesterol in blood is decreased when there is deficiency of dietary choline [177; 353; 644]. In the studies of other investigators in which atheromatous changes were observed in experimental animals consuming food containing cholesterol, the presence of choline in the diet may be one of the necessary factors to ensure sufficient intake of cholesterol to permit its atherogenic effects to be exhibited [549; 608; 811]. While in the rat the provision of adequate choline prevents damage produced by certain doses of cholesterol in short-term experiments [798], it is highly probable in this species, as is certainly true for the rabbit and perhaps for other animals, that at higher levels of cholesterol intake in long-term experiments [549; 608; 811], the effect of the sterol will not be counteracted by that of the nitrogenous base. The interplay of anatomical, physiological, and nutritional factors, and species differences in the response to these require further study.

Other Primary and Secondary Lesions in Choline Deficiency

The acute haemorrhagic kidney produced by choline deficiency in young rats (Griffith and Wade [335]) has now been studied by György and Goldblatt [342], Engel and Salmon [289], Christensen [202], and in many other laboratories. The first lesion appears to be deposition of fatty particles in the cells of the proximal convoluted tubules (Hartroft and Best [371]). The damage progresses rapidly and a high proportion of animals succumb to uraemia within 10 days. With the use of more severe diets older animals also show the acute renal lesions. A more chronic type of injury may also be produced in mature animals, and here the search for counterparts of clinical lesions will not go unrewarded (Hartroft [364]).

Passing reference must suffice to the extensive intraocular haemorrhages seen in weanling rats deprived of dietary choline (Griffith and Wade [355]; Bellows and Chinn [61]; Burns and Hartroft [159]). These lesions of the hyaloid arterial system are apparently secondary to renal damage. The delayed disappearance of the neuro-muscular response after nerve section in choline-deficient rats is probably related to renal injury [93]. Similar findings are obtained after removal of both kidneys (Keeler and

Best, unpublished). Several reports have been published on the production of hypertension which results from a very short period of choline deficiency during early life. The rats are maintained on completely adequate diets both before and after the five or six days of choline deprivation during which the renal injury is produced [355; 372; 579]. While this is, I think, the only established example of hypertension due to dietary deficiency, the mechanism of production may well be essentially similar to that resulting from renal ischaemia (Page and Corcoran [609]). The clinical application is certainly not apparent, but the lesson to be learned is clear—a few days of dietary neglect during early life initiates a reaction which, in one species, may lead to a fatal hypertension.

Many years ago Solandt and Best [720] found some indications that severe choline deficiency may interfere with acetylcholine production. These findings could not be obtained consistently and considerable doubt of their significance has remained (Li [502]). Recently, Hove and Copeland [403] have reported the production of a muscular dystrophy in rabbits by choline deprivation and dramatic improvement following the return of choline to the diet. These results revive the hope that a connection between neurohumour production and the lipotropic factors can be established, and we have in progress a new study of cardiac vagal action in rabbits on choline-deficient diets. I may state that a part of the pleasure which I would get from exploration of this borderland, if it should prove to exist, between dietary factors and neurohumours, would derive from my close association with Sir Henry Dale since 1922 and more recently with Professor Otto Loewi.

Several reports from the Alabama Polytechnic Institute have described the occurrence of malignant hepatomata in rats kept on a choline-deficient diet (Copeland and Salmon [220]; Engel, Copeland, and Salmon [288]; Salmon and Copeland [659]). Wilson [804] has seen similar lesions in mice. In some of these studies bentonite, which interferes with the absorption of choline and other dietary factors, was given [805]. György [340], who has also observed the formation of tumours, has suggested that there may be some toxic factor present in the choline- and protein-deficient diets. Buckley and Hartroft [155] in our laboratory have reported metastasizing liver tumours in choline-deficient mice. I am not aware of any other dietary deficiency which results, even indirectly, in new growth.

Sellers and You [691; 693] have studied the effect of cold on fat deposition in liver. Diets which in the warmth (22° C) produce on the average a five-fold increase in liver fat, cause a barely significant change in the cold (1.5° C). Some of these experiments have lasted five months, and the animals kept in the cold have been completely free of cirrhosis. This choline-sparing effect of cold is presumably related to the increased metabolic rate necessary for the survival of the animals, but the mechanism of the effect is as unexplained as is the insulin-sparing effect of exercise.

Interesting modifications of the effects of choline deficiency can be produced by depriving the animal of insulin, by altering thyroid function, and by giving growth hormone. Thyroidectomy or propylthiouracil reduces the number of fatty cysts without decreasing the fat content of the liver. Administration of thyroid substance lowers the fat content but leaves large cysts in the central vein area (Sellers and You [692]). In unpublished studies Dr. James Salter has found that growth hormone injected daily may double the increase in liver fat produced by choline deficiency alone. Best, Huntsman, and Young [98] recorded the huge depositions of liver fat which may be produced by deficiency of both insulin and choline in the same dog.

DIETARY PROTEIN AND LIVER FAT

Every aspect of the dietary properties of protein is of interest in our world today. The first indication that the protein content of the diet affects the deposition of excess fat in the liver was made 20 years ago when Best and Huntsman [95] observed that casein added to a diet low in choline exerted a choline-like action. We indulged in some speculation about the possible formation, during protein metabolism, of betaine which, as we had previously shown, has a lipotropic action. The lipotropic effect of protein was confirmed and extended by Channon and Wilkinson [194]; certain phases of this work were discussed by Best and Channon [79]. Two years later Tucker and Eckstein [760] showed that methionine is the principal lipotropic constituent of protein. There is some difference of opinion whether or not methionine accounts for all this activity [113; 190; 278; 761; 762]. Beveridge, Lucas, and O'Grady [122] emphasized the importance of the amino-acid balance in the protein of the diet in which the effects of various lipotropic agents are assessed. In the early investigations we, like others, had used diets low in protein, but after realizing the importance of the adequacy of dietary protein, we utilized hypolipotropic diets low in methionine but adequate in other amino-acids. Several groups of investigators and their associates have continued studies with low protein diets and have found that, under certain circumstances, some deposition of fat occurred in the liver despite the presence of adequate amounts of choline [360; 668; 707]. Lucas and Ridout [516] have recently provided evidence that these fatty livers are attributable to the low protein content of the diet. Best, Hartroft, Lucas, and Ridout [87] have extended these findings and have emphasized particularly the distribution of the fat within the liver lobule. A periportal distribution of fat in the livers of rats fed corn meal, rice, or cassava has been observed (Shils and Stewart [699; 700]; Shils, Friedland, and Stewart [697]). These observations support the view that protein deficiency and amino-acid imbalance are responsible for this particular periportal lesion.

THE LOCALIZATION OF FAT AND THE ARCHITECTURE OF THE LIVER

It has been well established for many years that in choline deficiency in rats the first appearance of the fat is around the central vein area of the lobule (e.g., Lillie et al. [503]; Glynn et al. [322]; Hartroft [365]). In starvation or in the increased mobilization of fat which may be produced by the injection of anterior pituitary extract into fasted animals, the distribution of fat is periportal. The most dramatic accumulation of fat in periportal regions which we have observed occurred when food intake rose abruptly as a result of increasing the amount of protein in a previously inadequate diet [87]. In an experiment of this type the average content of liver fat in eight animals rose from 8 to 18 per cent in three days, and the distribution of the newly formed or deposited lipid was entirely periportal. The physiological mechanisms governing the location of newly deposited fat within the liver lobule of the rat are most intriguing.

We have profited from the recent findings of the members of our staff who have been studying the architecture of the liver. Dr. A. M. Rappaport has been interested for several years in this field, and his work has been considered by authorities in this and many other countries as a noteworthy contribution. We have especially appreciated the friendly interest of Sir Harold Himsworth. I shall not discuss these investigations in detail, but Rappaport has obtained considerable new evidence that the unit of structure and function in the liver is the acinus. The name was first used in this connection by Malpighi (1666) to describe the tissue adhering to the smallest branches of the portal vein. The afferent blood supply to the acini is, as we all know, the hepatic artery, and the portal vein and the efferent blood vessels are presumably small venules collecting the blood from the glomus of sinusoids and draining it into the collecting channel, the central vein. The starting point of Rappaport's investigations was the proof first provided by Markowitz, Rappaport, and Scott [552] and by Markowitz and Rappaport [551] that the use of antibiotics saves the lives of dogs after complete ligation of the hepatic artery. Skilful use of these findings enabled Rappaport and Lotto to produce acute hepatic necrosis and, for the first time, experimental hepatic coma. Interestingly enough the fatty changes in the surviving cells can be promptly relieved by perfusion of the liver with oxygenated blood from the animal's own femoral artery, delivered with the help of an extracorporeal pump into the portal vein (Rappaport [629]). These same techniques have been used in combination with pathological and histochemical studies to elucidate the structure and function of the liver. Rappaport's new conceptions permit logical explanations of several puzzling clinical lesions such as, for example, paracentral necrosis (Smetana, Keller, and Dubin [713] and personal communication to Dr. Rappaport). The outline of the liver acini may be revealed by the production of hepatic ischaemia (Rappaport, Borowy, Lougheed, and Lotto [630] or by the periportal accumulation of lipid after realimentation (Best *et al.* [87]) or in the early stage of fat deposition in choline deficiency (Hartroft [365]). When these initial "pericentral" or, better, peripheral acinar depositions of fat in choline deficiency are replaced by fatty cysts and later by fibrous tissue, pseudolobulation in cirrhosis occurs. This pseudolobulation was so called because it was thought to introduce a new lobulation in addition to the time-honoured hexagonal one, but it is, in fact, a true outline of a single acinus [630] or groups of acini (Rappaport and Hiraki, unpublished).

The initial deposition of fat around the periportal area when the fat comes from the depots as in starvation or in the fasted animal given growth hormone may well be related to the fact that this is the first hepatic area in which the arterial blood could deposit its load of fat. An explanation of the deposition of fat in the periportal area in protein deficiency, as distinct from methionine and choline deficiency, is not easy to find. It may be that here a part of the explanation is the revealing of fat which was already there—perhaps combined with protein as lipoprotein. In the absence of adequate protein in the diet the lipoprotein complex may break down, as my colleagues Lucas and Ridout [517] have suggested, and thus permit the fat which normally does not take the usual stains to be detected. This suggestion will not explain, however, the large depositions of fat in periportal areas seen in realimentation when adequate amounts of protein are available. This fat appears coincidentally with the suddenly increased food intake and may represent the deposition of fat from, in this case, the portal vein blood in the first hepatic cells to be supplied. These suggestions merely indicate avenues for further exploration.

The appearance of fat within a few hours of the beginning of choline deficiency in the "pericentral" region of the lobule, to use the perhaps outmoded nomenclature, strongly suggests that the effects of this nutritional deficiency first appear, as do those of oxygen lack, at the periphery of the hepatic acini.

TRANSMETHYLATION, ACTIVE METHIONINE, VITAMIN B12, AND FOLIC ACID

In the same year (1937) in which methionine was recognized as a lipotropic factor it was shown to be an essential amino-acid. When testing the ability of demethylated methionine, i.e., the "unnatural" amino-acid homocystine, to replace methionine as a growth factor, du Vigneaud, Dyer, and Kies [771] and Rose and Rice [651] secured opposite results. Du Vigneaud observed no growth with homocystine. In his first report on this subject in Toronto in 1939 he referred to the lead given by the basic work in the lipotropic field; the appearance of fatty livers in these rats suggested a lack of choline. The addition of choline to the diet produced both growth and disappearance of the fat. Du Vigneaud, Chandler, Moyer, and Keppel [770] envisaged the transfer of a methyl group from choline to homocystine to form methionine. This was an important new biochemical concept—the process of transmethylation—which subsequent studies with isotopically labelled methyl groups have amply confirmed and extended.

Studies with labelled and sometimes doubly labelled methyl groups have shown that two types of methylation occur in the body: (1) transfer of an intact methyl group, or (2) reduction of some one-carbon fragment to form a new methyl group [19; 287; 443; 530; 658; 702; and many others]. The one-carbon fragment that acts as the immediate precursor appears to be either formate or some active unit containing the formyl radical. The most important source of carbon atoms for the new methyl groups appears to be the β-carbon atom of the amino-acid serine (Arnstein and Neuberger [20]; Elwyn, Weissbach, Henry, and Sprinson [286]). It is sometimes difficult to decide whether the experimental data supply evidence in favour of transmethylation or biosynthesis of new methyl groups. A fascinating account of the development of this field up to 1951 has been written by du Vigneaud [768].

Until recently it appeared that all compounds serving as methyl donors were methylated onium compounds, i.e., choline, betaine, and certain thetins. Methionine was a notable exception. The studies of Borsook and Dubnoff [142], and more recently of Cantoni [172; 173], have shown that methionine is first converted to an active form by the presence of adenosine triphosphate. Active methionine has now been identified as an S-adenosyl addition product, making it, like all the other donors of methyl groups, an onium compound (Figure 83).

The first evidence for the synthesis of methyl groups *de novo* was obtained by Toennies, Bennett, and Medes [752]. They obtained slow growth in rats fed diets containing homocystine but no known source of methyl groups. This observation suggested and subsequent studies con-

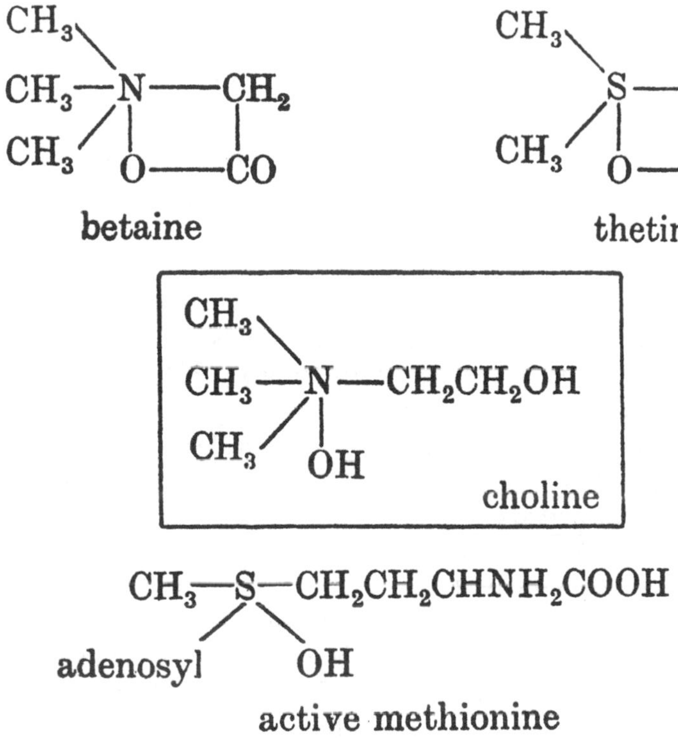

$$CH_3—N—CH_2$$

betaine

thetin

choline

active methionine

FIGURE 83

firmed that the rat possesses a limited ability to make methyl groups by a synthetic process. The efficiency with which this occurs depends on the adequacy of the diet in other respects and is particularly affected by vitamin B_{12}. (I remember with what keen interest Banting and I received the word in 1922 that Dr. George Minot had responded well to insulin and had returned to clinical investigation. The attention of all medical scientists was later focused on his work with Murphy which resulted in the discovery of the liver treatment of pernicious anaemia.) It is interesting that the haematopoietic principle in liver, now identified as vitamin B_{12}, is, under certain conditions, an active lipotropic agent supplementing the choline supply by biosynthesis of methyl groups. It is apparently not necessary for transmethylation (Arnstein and Neuberger [20]; Stekol, Weiss, Smith, and Weiss [735]). Folic acid, the other vitamin so important in haematopoiesis, also plays a part in lipotropic phenomena and, although the finer details are not yet clear, it is apparently involved in the metabolism of the one-carbon fragment [736]. Excellent surveys of recent progress in this field may be found in reviews by Welch and Nichol [787]; by my former pupil Jukes with Williams [435]; and by Stokstad [742].

THE MECHANISM OF THE ACTION OF CHOLINE

As a physiologist, I am even more attracted to this phase of the choline story than to the experimental pathology and biochemistry which I have just discussed. Our first thought regarding the mode of action was that choline might increase the rate of phospholipid formation. The necessary tools were not then available to investigate this, but very soon other groups of workers using isotopically labelled phosphorus (e.g., Chaikoff [179]; Entenman, Chaikoff, and Friedlander [290]), choline containing ^{15}N (e.g., Boxer and Stetten [144]), and more recently fatty acids labelled with ^{14}C (Weinman, Chaikoff, Entenman, and Dauben [785]) have shown that choline increases the turnover of choline-containing phospholipids. Since the absolute amount of these phospholipids in liver does not increase when choline is given, the fatty acid moiety of this fraction must either be utilized in the liver or be transported elsewhere.

Stetten and Salcedo [739] provided evidence that in the absence of dietary choline the extra glyceride appearing in the liver is due to impaired transport of fatty acids from the liver. Studies of blood lipids seem to support the transport hypothesis. In the absence of choline or its precursors from the diet, there is a progressive fall of total lipids, bound cholesterol and phospholipids in the serum of rats. Upon restoring choline or betaine to the diet the concentration of these blood lipids returns promptly to within the normal range (Castro-Mendoza et al. [177]; Ridout et al. [644]). In choline-deficient dogs McKibbin, Thayer, and Stare [531] observed a fall in plasma cholesterol, and in our laboratory Rosenfeld and Lang (unpublished) found a similar decrease in serum phospholipids. Wilgram, Lewis, and Blumenstein [802] have found a profound fall in low-density lipoproteins and α-lipoproteins in the serum of choline-deficient rats. These data appear to be consistent with the view that one action of choline is to favour the transport of lipids from the liver.

One of the early attempts to elucidate the action of choline was made by Welch, Irving, and Best [788] in a study of liver slices from choline-deficient and choline-supplemented animals. The oxygen consumption of the slices from the choline-deficient animals was definitely reduced, but when the figures were adjusted to ignore the gross intracellular fattiness of the choline-deficient livers, there was no significant difference between the two groups. Some doubt still remains in my mind regarding the physiological ethics of eliminating fat by arithmetic alone!

When Zilversmit, Entenman, and Chaikoff [826] showed that choline stimulates lecithin turnover in the liver but not in the plasma, they believed that the removal of liver fat under the influence of choline is effected by utilization of fat within the liver itself rather than by an increased transport to peripheral tissues via plasma phospholipids. In 1951 Artom [21] reviewed the current knowledge of the mechanism of action of lipotropic factors. Recently he has studied the effect of choline on the oxidation of labelled fatty acids in liver slices [22] and more recently in slices from heart and kidney [23]. The addition of choline *in vitro* had no effect on the production of $^{14}CO_2$, but injection of choline into the rat before it was killed caused an increased production of $^{14}CO_2$ whether the rat had been fed a choline-deficient diet or one adequately supplied with choline. These results with liver have been confirmed by Rosenfeld and Lang (unpublished). In spite of these additions to our knowledge of the role of choline in the oxidation of fatty acids the picture is obviously far from complete.[1] A suggestion has also been made that choline inhibits the rate of fat formation from labelled acetate in liver slices [24], but it appears most promising in our search for the mechanism of the lipotropic action of choline to determine as accurately as possible the rate of flow of fatty acids from the liver to the blood, depots and peripheral tissues.

Optically active glycerolphosphatides, identical with those found in nature, have been synthesized by Dr. Erich Baer and his associates in our department [32; 33; 34]. The use of such synthetic phosphatides with appropriate labels may help to solve some aspects of the action of choline.

Our successors will make more intensive use of these tools which our generation has provided. Insulin promotes the formation of fat from carbohydrate in the liver and other tissues using some of the energy it secures from the increased rate of oxidation of sugars. Heparin may help to control the size of fat particles in blood and their distribution. The pituitary adipokinetic principle promotes fat utilization and mobilization from the depots to the liver. Choline prevents abnormal accumulation of fat in the liver and other tissues. The rather barren framework which these facts serve to outline is, we trust, made of good steel, but it will be much more attractive when the bricks of future findings are in their proper places.

Acknowledgments

It is a pleasure to acknowledge my indebtedness to my colleagues and students who have helped me in many ways in the preparation of this lecture and to mention by name: Professor C. C. Lucas, Dr. Jessie H.

[1]There are two series of more recent investigations which are of great interest in relation to the action of choline. The first is that of Kennedy, who has found an important intermediary in phospholipid synthesis in the form of the choline ester of cytidine diphosphate. (See review by Kennedy [446].) The second study is that of Dianzani and his colleagues, who have shown that choline deficiency leads to a decrease in the levels of pyridine nucleotides (D.P.N.) in the liver [250].

Ridout, Professor W. S. Hartroft, Professor E. A. Sellers, Dr. Jean M. Patterson, Dr. A. M. Rappaport, Dr. Bruce Casselman, Dr. George Wilgram, Dr. B. Rosenfeld, and Dr. James Salter.

Part III: OTHER PHYSIOLOGICAL STUDIES

SIR HENRY DALE AND PROFESSOR A. V. Hill *were my not-too-stern examiners for the Doctor of Science degree of the University of London. I had two periods of work in Dale's laboratory, in 1925–26 and again in 1928. In 1928 I went to University College and conducted some preliminary experiments on respiratory physiology in Hill's laboratory. I was working in the Sir William Bayliss Memorial Laboratory which had been built and equipped with the funds awarded to him after his lawsuit with the opponents of the use of animals in medical research. I spent considerable time watching Professor E. H. Starling set up his heart–lung preparations. Professor Hill, a little later, studied the dynamics of sprint running at Cornell University at Ithaca, New York. When he left for home he gave us the apparatus which he had used in those investigations. Dr. Ruth C. Partridge, who had added a brilliant Ph.D. in Physiology to her fine training in Physics, worked with me in electrical timing experiments on the world's fastest sprinters. The records which we obtained on Percy Williams and Miss Myrtle Cook are given in the first part of Paper 49.*

In the second part are recorded the findings which I obtained at the Olympic Games at Amsterdam in 1928 on the blood sugar of Marathon runners at the finish of this gruelling race.

49. Observations on Olympic Athletes

C. H. BEST

RUTH C. PARTRIDGE

The results of the experiments of Furusawa, Hill, and Parkinson [316] at Cornell indicated that observations, by electrical timing methods, on the world's fastest sprinters, might be of considerable physiological interest. One of us (C.H.B.) had hoped to collaborate with Hill in studies of this kind at the Amsterdam Olympic Games, but it was found impossible to make the necessary arrangements. At these games the 100-metre and the 200-metre events were won by Percy Williams, who since has several times equalled the world's record for the indoor 60-yards race. The women's 400-metre relay event was won by the Canadian team, and a new world's record for the distance was established. The fastest member of this team (Miss Myrtle Cook) now claims the world's record for 100 metres; her times for the 50- and 60-yard indoor races are the fastest that have been officially recorded. It has been possible recently to conduct electrical timing experiments, using these Canadian athletes as subjects. The results of these observations and a discussion of them form the first part of this paper.

In the second part the results of a short study of the blood sugar content of "Marathon" runners at the end of the race are given. The change in the sugar content in the blood of athletes, attributable to muscular exercise, has received considerable attention. No attempt to review the subject completely will be made here. The blood sugar content is often appreciably raised by short sprints, but this is not always the case. Several reports on the low blood sugar values found in runners at the end of long distance races have appeared. In 1924 Levine, Gordon, and Derick [497] determined the blood sugar content of 11 long distance runners. The blood samples were obtained from a vein and were secured in from 2 to 30 minutes after the finish of the race. In four of these runners a blood sugar of 0.050 per cent or less was found, and in two others the value was 0.065 per cent. In three of the others the amount was within normal limits. The remaining two had higher values, presumably due to the food they consumed before the blood sample was secured.

Originally appeared in the *Proceedings of the Royal Society*, B, CV (1929), 323–32. Communicated by Prof. A. V. Hill, F.R.S. From the Department of Physiological Hygiene, University of Toronto.

Through the kindness of Professor Buytendijk, facilities were provided for blood sugar work at the stadium laboratory in Amsterdam during the Olympic Games. Estimations of blood sugar were made on 10 of the contestants immediately after the finish of the 1928 "Marathon" race.

PART I. ACCELERATION STUDIES ON ATHLETES

Method

The method used in the electrical timing of runners is identical with that developed by A. V. Hill and his collaborators [316]. The detailed description of the apparatus used by the authors has appeared in a previous paper [109]. The runner carrying a light magnet on his chest passes a series of coils set at known distances parallel to the track. As the magnet is carried past each coil, a current is induced in the coil and is transferred to a recording apparatus, which consists of a suitable galvanometer, camera, and time marker. The photographic record of the runner's rate of progress along the course is carefully measured, using a vernier microscope, and the speed between the various points is calculated. The acceleration of the runner and the maximum speed can thus be readily obtained.

This maximum speed has the value fga in the equation of motion of a runner [316]. In this equation $y = fga[t - a(1 - e^{-(t/a)})]$, y is a known distance, t is the time taken to travel this distance, a is the "viscosity" constant,[1] f is the propelling force expressed as a fraction of the body weight, and g is the acceleration due to gravity. Thus the determining factors of the maximum speed are f, the proportion of the body weight exerted, and a, the "viscosity" factor. To obtain the "viscosity" factor several methods of calculation have been used. In earlier experiments [109] the equation $y = fga(t - a)$, which is nearly true when t is large, was used. Taking a large t value and corresponding y, and knowing the maximum speed, fga, the a was calculated. The a value obtained was fitted into the equation $y = fga[t - a(1 - e^{-(t/a)})]$ and if this a value fitted the equation for all values of y, it was adopted. Since the equation from which a was derived was approximate, a slightly different value of a was sometimes found to be more suitable. In the present experiments where one object is to compare the viscosity constants of various subjects, another method is used. We are indebted to Professor John Satterly (of the Department of Physics) for suggesting this procedure. For this purpose the equation $dy/dt = fga(1 - e^{-(t/a)})$ [316] is utilised. If dy/dt is denoted by v_t and fga by v, the equation becomes

---

[1]The "viscosity" is actually proportional to the reciprocal of a; a is of the dimensions of time.

$$v_t = v(1 - e^{-(t/a)})$$

or

$$v - v_t = ve^{-(t/a)}$$

$$\log_e(v - v_t) = \log_e v - (t/a).$$

Since log v is a constant, a straight line resulted when $\log_e(v - v_t)$ was plotted against t. The slope of the straight line gives the value $1/a$ from which a is determined. While the graphical method gives an approximate value of a, it is difficult to place the line to obtain a value which can be consistently secured by different workers. Consequently the least squares method of obtaining the slope of the line has been adopted to secure the most probable value of a. In this procedure the value $\log_e(v - v_t)$ is the y value, and the time, taken from the start at the half-way distance between the coils, is the value of x. The formula used for the solution is

$$\frac{1}{a} = \frac{(\Sigma x)\,(\Sigma y) - n\Sigma\,(xy)}{(\Sigma x)^2 - n\Sigma\,(x^2)}.$$

Observations

Williams ran three times the same afternoon on an indoor dirt track, where a 70-yard straight was available. A short board track was provided for the "pull-up." On two of these occasions he began his run from a point 1 foot along the track from the centre of the first coil. The third run was started on an improvised track, some 30 yards back from the first coil, i.e., he was allowed a running start. In the first and second runs his maximum speed was 11.42 yards and 11.41 yards per second. In the third run the maximum speed was 11.41 yards per second. These results illustrate the fact that the maximum speed is very constant in reliable subjects under any one set of circumstances, and furthermore show that the shortness of the track did not interfere with the development of this subject's maximum speed. The runners were advised to decrease their speed after passing the 60-yard coil.

In his first run Williams attained his maximum speed of 11.42 yards (10.44 metres) per second between 45 and 50 yards. His speed between the 50 and 55-yard coils was 11.42, and between the 55 and 60-yard coils was 11.40 yards per second. The figures secured from the record of Williams' second run are given in Table 49.I.

The same procedure was adopted in the experiments in which Ball was the subject. His maximum speed in his second run and in his third (flying start) agreed well, viz., 10.66 and 10.65 yards per second. In his first run he apparently did not make a maximum effort.

In Table 49.II the maximum speeds, *a* and *f*, are shown for Williams, for Ball, for two good 100-yard runners (E.C.M. and J.H.R.) and for two untrained men.

TABLE 49.I
SPEEDS ATTAINED BY PERCY WILLIAMS

Distance (yards)	Time from One Coil to the Next (seconds)	Time at the Coils (taken from the start) (seconds)	Time at the half-way Distance between the Coils (taken from the start) (seconds)	Speed at the Half-Way Distance between the Coils (yards per second)
0				
	0.210		0.11	1.52
⅓		0.22		
	0.689		0.56	3.87
3		0.91		
	0.435		1.13	6.89
6		1.34		
	0.732		1.71	8.19
12		2.08		
	0.826		2.49	9.68
20		2.93		
	0.484		3.15	10.33
25		3.39		
	0.466		3.62	10.73
30		3.85		
	0.458		4.08	10.90
35		4.31		
	0.458		4.54	10.90
40		4.77		
	0.445		4.99	11.22
45		5.21		
	0.438		5.43	11.41
50		5.65		
	0.445		5.88	11.23
55		6.10		
	0.445		6.32	11.23
60		6.54		
	0.457		6.77	10.90
65		7.00		

NOTE. The centre of the first coil was placed 1 foot from the start. The first movement of the galvanometer string was taken as the actual time the runner started. As the lag of the galvanometer is constant and every time used in the calculations is the difference between the times of two galvanometer movements, no error is attributable to this lag. If it were possible to make arrangements so that the magnet would be held motionless exactly above the starting line, the first movement of the runner towards the first coil would be accurately registered by the start of the deflection of the galvanometer. In the calculations it is assumed that the start of the first deflection of the galvanometer coincides exactly with the moment the magnet moves from the starting line. It is realized that a slight error is unavoidable when this method of registering the start is used, but we have been unable, as yet, to find a more satisfactory procedure.

The experiments on the women runners were conducted on a circular track where a 50-yard straight was available. The same procedure as used with the men was followed. In Table 49.III the figures for one of Miss Cook's runs are given.

TABLE 49.II

RELATION BETWEEN MAXIMUM SPEED AND "VISCOSITY"

Subject	Maximum Speed (yards per second)	Viscosity Constant a	Viscosity Constant $e^{-1/a}$	Proportion of Weight exerted f (%)
Williams (1)	11.42	1.35	0.48	79
Williams (2)	11.41	1.34	0.48	79
Ball (1)	10.33	1.27	0.45	75
Ball (2)	10.66	1.27	0.45	78
E. C. M. (mean 2)	10.60	1.27	0.45	77
J. H. R. (mean 2)	10.59	1.27	0.45	77
E. W. McH.	7.96	1.03	0.38	72
W. S.	7.90	1.00	0.37	74

TABLE 49.III

SPEEDS ATTAINED BY MISS MYRTLE COOK

Distance (yards)	Time from One Coil to the Next (seconds)	Time at the Coils (taken from the start) (seconds)	Time at the Halfway Distance between the Coils (taken from the start) (seconds)	Speed at the Halfway Distance between the Coils (yards per second)
0				
	0.241		0.12	1.38
$\frac{1}{3}$		0.24		
	0.714		0.60	3.73
3		0.96		
	0.504		1.21	5.95
6		1.46		
	0.832		1.88	7.21
12		2.29		
	0.940		2.76	8.51
20		3.23		
	0.565		3.51	8.85
25		3.80		
	0.568		4.08	8.80
30		4.36		
	0.536		4.63	9.32
35		4.90		
	0.526		5.16	9.50
40		5.43		
	0.531		5.69	9.41
45		5.96		
	0.567		6.24	8.82
50		6.53		

In Table 49.IV the values of a and f and the maximum speed are given for the women athletes.

As Williams and Miss Cook may at present be regarded as the fastest male and female sprinters, it is interesting to compare the curves of their runs obtained by plotting speed against distance. The curves are shown in Figure 84.

TABLE 49.IV

GIRLS' OLYMPIC RELAY TEAM. RELATION BETWEEN MAXIMUM SPEED AND "VISCOSITY"

Subject	Maximum Speed (yards per second)	Viscosity Constant a	Viscosity Constant $e^{-1/a}$	Proportion of Weight Exerted f (%)
Miss Cook (1)	9.50	1.32	0.47	67
Miss Cook (2)	9.27	1.33	0.47	65
Mrs. Smith Hogarth (1)	9.45	1.28	0.45	69
Mrs. Smith Hogarth (2)	9.45	1.28	0.45	69
Miss Griffiths (1)	9.09	1.32	0.47	64
Miss Griffiths (2)	9.28	1.32	0.47	66
Miss Bell (1)	9.09	1.31	0.46	04
Miss Bell (2)	9.09	1.31	0.46	65

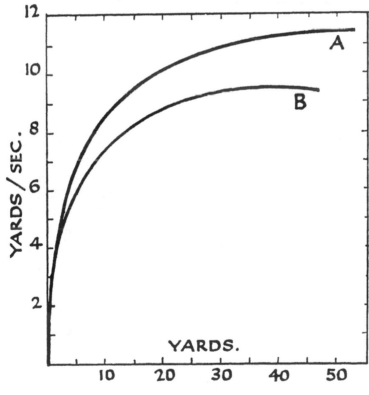

Change of speed with distance.

A.—Percy Williams.   B.—Myrtle Cook.

FIGURE 84

Discussion

The consistency with which a reliable trained runner, i.e., one who exerts himself to the utmost in every run, can repeat his performance is a very remarkable physiological fact. This fact is demonstrated by the observations of Furusawa, Hill, and Parkinson. In our previous work [109] the maximum speed of our chief subject was attained with great consistency in different runs on the same day, and the series of three observations on Williams, recorded in this paper, illustrate the same point. The records on the women athletes show that they accelerate in a more irregular manner than the men.

Williams attains his maximum speed of 11.42 yards (10.44 metres) per second (23.3 miles per hour) between the 45- and 50-yard coils. He requires approximately 5.4 seconds to reach this speed. It is quite possible that his maximum speed would be greater on an outdoor track. The use of the indoor track, however, eliminates the effect of wind on the runner's speed.

Hill calculated that a following wind of 10 miles per hour would improve a fast runner's time for the 100 yards by about 0.3 seconds. A head wind of the same velocity would increase the time by about 0.5 seconds [390].

Miss Cook reaches her maximum speed of 9.5 yards (8.69 metres) per second (19.4 miles per hour) between 30 and 40 yards. She requires approximately 5.2 seconds to reach this speed.

It is apparent from Table 49.II that Williams, like H.A.R., is superior to other runners because of the magnitude of his *a*, that is, the smallness of his "viscosity." The method of calculating the viscosity factor is such that slight differences in this value are not significant. Williams has, however, a "viscosity" slightly smaller than that of any other male runner who has been investigated, and appreciably less than that of most of them. The "viscosity" of the women runners compares very favourably with that of the best male athletes. The proportion of their body weight they are able to exert as propelling force is, however, considerably less.

PART II. BLOOD SUGAR STUDIES ON "MARATHON" RUNNERS

Methods

Before the "Marathon" race, arrangements were made with certain of the contestants that they should go to the laboratory immediately after they had finished. The first subject arrived within 5 minutes after he crossed the finishing line. The blood sample was secured immediately. Samples of blood were obtained from the others within 20 minutes of the time of their finish.

The blood samples were obtained from the ear. The Hagedorn-Jensen method was used in estimating the sugar content of the blood. The various solutions were carefully standardized and tested before use.

Observations

The results of the blood sugar estimations, and a few rough notes on the condition of the subjects at the finish, and on the food they consumed during the race, are shown in Table 49.V.

TABLE 49.V

CONDITION OF MARATHON RUNNERS AT THE CONCLUSION OF THE RACE

Country	Name	Blood Sugar at Finish (%)	Remarks on Food Taken before and during Run	Notes on Physical Condition at Finish
Holland	Van Leenen	0.085	Meal at 11.30 A.M.; nothing afterward or during run	Condition fair; no cyanosis or dyspnoea
Holland	Van der Steen	0.100	Bread and cocoa at 12 noon; one egg during run	Appeared to be in excellent condition at finish
Japan	Yamada	0.092	Rice and melon at 12.30; lemonade with added sucrose during run	Condition good; finished fourth
Japan	Isuda	0.091	Moderate meal of rice at 12 noon; lemonade with added sucrose during run	Condition good; felt very comfortable; finished sixth
Mexico	Torres	0.055	Meat and eggs at 11 A.M., cocoa during run	Inco-ordination of muscular movements; very cyanosed; profoundly exhausted; pulse very rapid; blood pressure before race 110/60, after 85/40
U.S.A.	Henigan	0.088	Meat and eggs at 11.30 A.M.; tea and grapefruit during the run	No cyanosis, slight dyspnoea; no inco-ordination of muscular movements
U.S.A.	Michelson	0.053	Meat and eggs at 11.30 A.M.; small part of one orange just after finish about 5 minutes before blood sample was taken	Moderate cyanosis; appeared very weak; pulse 85; blood pressure 105/75; finished ninth
U.S.A.	Frick	0.062	Meat and potatoes at 11.30 A.M.; tea once or twice during run	Slight cyanosis; very tired
U.S.A.	De Mar	0.099	Meat and potatoes at 11.30 A.M.; one glass of milk during run	Condition fair; very tired; finished very slowly
South Africa	Steyther	0.099	Moderate meal at 10.30 A.M.; tea at quite frequent intervals during run	Condition good; no cyanosis

Race started at 3 P.M. Distance 26 miles 600 yards (42.38 km). Time of winner, 2 hours 32 minutes and 57 seconds.

Discussion

Three of the 10 runners studied had a definite hypoglycaemia at the end of the race. One in particular (Torres) showed certain of the signs which accompany hypoglycaemia in experimental animals. As this runner was cyanosed, oxygen want must also be considered as a possible cause of these signs. One of the factors which prevents the development of hypoglycaemia at the finish of long distance races is probably the ingestion of food during the race. Dextrose should be the most efficient food. The manner in which the race is terminated may also exert some effect on the sugar content of the blood taken immediately after the finish. The sugar content of the blood might be increased by a sprint finish. On the other hand some of the runners came in very slowly and were probably recovering, during the last stages of the race, from the much more rapid expenditure of energy made during the earlier part. In this case the sugar content of the blood at the finish would probably be higher than at some earlier time. The carbohydrate reserve of the body at the start of the race is also undoubtedly important. The most important factor in the prevention of hypoglycaemia, on theoretical grounds, must be the ability of the runner's body to convert other substances into dextrose, i.e., the rate and extent of gluconeogenesis.

Summary

1. Electrical timing experiments on Olympic champion male and female sprinters, have been carried out. The male sprinter, whose performance was studied in these experiments, is superior to others who have been investigated, because of the smallness of his "viscosity." The "viscosity" of the women runners compares favourably with that of the best male athletes, but the proportion of body weight they are able to exert as propelling force is considerably less.

2. Blood sugar determinations made on 10 "Marathon" runners, immediately after the finish of the 1928 race, demonstrated the presence of definite hypoglycaemia in three of the subjects.

ACKNOWLEDGMENTS

It is a pleasure to acknowledge the helpful interest of Professor J. G. FitzGerald, Director of the School of Hygiene and of the Connaught Laboratories, in this work. We are indebted also to Dr. C. Vancaulaert for help in obtaining blood samples, to Dr. J. G. Bramwell for some of the data on the condition of the runners at the finish of the race, and to Mr. William Parkinson for assistance in the electrical timing experiments.

MY INTEREST IN HISTAMINE BEGAN
*with the news, in the summer of 1922, that H. H. Dale and H. W. Dudley
were coming soon to Toronto from London to survey the insulin situation,
on behalf of the British Medical Research Council. I read everything that
Dale and his colleagues had written on histamine and many articles by
other investigators. We talked more about insulin than histamine during
our first meeting but the assurance that there would be a place in his
laboratory for me in 1925 stimulated me to keep abreast of the literature
on histamine.*

*The details of the work on this amine, in which I played a part, were
published in a series of articles, three of which are reproduced here as
Papers 50, 51, and 52. These reports describe: (a) The isolation of histamine
for the first time from bacterially uncontaminated mammalian tissue (I was
very much the junior member of this team and learned a great deal from
my colleagues); (b) An interesting synergism between the effects of choline
and histamine on blood pressure; (c) The establishment of an enzyme
system which inactivates histamine, by the application of a quantitative
method for estimating the amine. I suggested the obvious name for this
system. This paper marked the beginning of the intensive study of the
enzymatic destruction of this amine and the eventual recognition of a
series of histaminases.*

*In the studies on insulin, choline, heparin, and glucagon in our labora-
tory the findings resulted from a direct attack on a problem. The results
obtained answered the questions asked. The original objective in the work
on the change in histamine content of tissues was to illuminate the
formation of histamine. When disappearance of naturally-occurring and
added histamine was detected the objective was promptly changed and
factors affecting destruction of the amine were investigated.*

50. The Nature of the Vaso-Dilator Constituents of Certain Tissue Extracts

C. H. BEST

H. H. DALE

H. W. DUDLEY

W. V. THORPE

It has long been known that simple watery or alcoholic extracts of various organs of the body produce a pronounced depressor action when injected intravenously, especially in the carnivora. Oliver and Schäfer [605] observed such an action with an extract of thyroid gland, Mott and Halliburton [580] with extracts of brain and nervous tissues, Vincent and Sheen [775] with extracts from liver, muscle, and various glandular organs, and other observers with a wide range of organs from different species. The suggestion that these effects were explained by the presence of choline in such extracts was shown to be inadequate by Vincent, with Osborne [607] and Sheen [775], who found that the action was but little affected by administration of atropine. Popielski [624] suggested that a common depressor agent, for which he suggested the name "vasodilatin," was present in such tissue extracts, and a hint appeared to be given as to its chemical nature when Dale and Laidlaw [242] found that the base now generally known as "histamine" produced the vascular and other characteristic effects of the hypothetical vaso-dilatin, when injected in relatively minute doses. Barger and Dale [51] soon afterwards succeeded in isolating from an extract of intestinal mucous membrane sufficient of this base for chemical as well as physiological identification. The quantity obtained, however, was small in relation to the total activity of this kind exhibited by the extract, and the nature of the raw material left it doubtful whether the histamine came from the living cells of the mucous membrane, or from the intestinal contents with which they had been in contact. For some years after this, though the correspondence in action, between the chief depressor constituent of various organ extracts and histamine, was widely recognized,

Originally appeared in the *Journal of Physiology*, LXII (1927), 397–417. From the National Institute for Medical Research, Hampstead.

the probability of their chemical identity seemed rather to be weakened. We may mention, for example, the observations of Stern and Rothlin [737], who extracted from the spleen a principle acting like histamine, but, finding that it was largely destroyed by heating with dilute alkali, concluded that it could not be histamine, which is stable to such treatment. We shall show later the need for caution in drawing such conclusions; but the balance of evidence and of opinion seemed to be unfavourable to the identification until Abel and Kubota published an important paper in 1919 [3], in which they claimed to have made probable the presence of histamine itself, or of some substance closely related to it, as the essential depressor constituent of extracts from a number of organs and tissues, and of the products of partial hydrolysis of pure proteins. In some respects their evidence failed to be completely convincing. From two tissues only—the pituitary gland and the gastro-intestinal mucous membrane—did they obtain pure salts, the picrate and chloroaurate, of histamine. The quantities so isolated were small in relation to the original depressor activity, the pituitary raw material was a commercial dried preparation of the whole gland, and the considerations mentioned above left a doubt as to the significance to be attributed to the presence of a small amount of histamine in an extract from material which included intestinal mucous membrane. In all other cases they were unable to make the final purification needed for chemical recognition. They showed that a depressor substance was present which, when dried with sodium carbonate, could be extracted with hot chloroform, and which had actions like that of histamine on the blood-pressure and on plain muscle; but such evidence could do no more than make it probable that something having similar solubilities and similar activity to those of histamine was present; it would not justify a general conclusion that histamine itself was the main depressor constituent of the tissues.

Our own renewed investigation of the chemical nature of the depressor substance has been prompted partly by a growing conviction of its physiological significance, and partly by recent claims made for the therapeutic value of depressor constituents of the liver, in particular. Papers by one of us (Dale) with Richards [244], Laidlaw [243], and Burn [158] have given grounds for, and indicated the trend of, the physiological speculations. Another of us (Best) had taken part in experiments on the production and testing of the liver extracts, used in one group of the recent observations on their therapeutic effects. Our attention was, for this reason, first directed to the identification of such vaso-dilator substances, in liver extracts, as had a clearly recognizable type of immediate action. Histamine itself, together with relatively large amounts of choline having been isolated from the liver extract, we extended the observations to another organ extract, that of lung, which exhibits a peculiarly intense histamine-like action.

The results obtained with these two tissues seem so significant that it appears desirable to publish them now, leaving for future publication the result of the investigation of other organs. It should be made quite clear at the outset, however, that our findings must not be assumed to be applicable to every case in which the intravenous injection of an extract of any organ has been found to lower the systemic arterial pressure. Evidence has long been available which forbids the attribution of some such effects to histamine or to choline, or to both acting together. As Vincent and Curtis [773] have recently pointed out, Vincent and his earlier co-workers obtained depressor effects by injecting extracts of brain matter into atropinized rabbits. Vincent and Curtis state that they have again obtained such depressor effects with organ extracts in atropinized rabbits. Since atropine annuls the action of choline, while the rabbit under ether or urethane is not sensitive to the vaso-dilator action of histamine (Dale and Laidlaw), these effects were clearly of another type. We are not here concerned with them. Our purpose has been to examine the nature of the substance producing the histamine-like action, so widely prevalent in organ extracts, and, since we found it in association with the other, of that producing the weaker, choline-like action. The physiological experiments have been carried out by Best and Dale, while Dudley and Thorpe have been responsible for the chemical side of the investigation; but the two kinds of technique have been used in close co-operation at all stages.

PHYSIOLOGICAL ANALYSIS OF THE ACTION OF LIVER EXTRACTS

The experiments under this heading formed the real starting-point of the investigation. One of us (C.H.B.) had been engaged in Toronto with D. A. Scott in the preparation and testing of liver extracts for the therapeutic investigation mentioned above. A quantity of extract was prepared here [in Britain] by a method and under conditions practically identical with those which were being used in the Connaught Laboratories, Toronto. The opportunity of having this preparation carried out on a large scale we owed to the British Drug Houses, Ltd., and especially to the friendly and expert co-operation of their technical director, Mr. F. H. Carr, and his staff. The details are given below in the chemical section. Here it need only be mentioned that the final procedure used in purifying the extract, viz. the precipitation of the depressor constituents from solution in 80 per cent alcohol by adding 3 volumes of acetone, appeared to render it highly improbable that they were simple bases like histamine and choline. Neither of these substances, in concentrations of the order indicated by the activity of the extracts, is precipitated at all from pure solution under these conditions.

Nevertheless, a few orientating experiments soon established the fact that the immediate, depressor action exhibited by such extracts, when injected intravenously into the anaesthetized cat or dog, was chiefly of the histamine type. In a cat anaesthetized with ether, by measuring the evanescent effects of small doses of the order of 0.01 cc, it was easy to balance the effects against those of small doses of the order of 0.001 mg of pure histamine.[1] The equivalents having thus been determined in terms of depressor action, the solutions were then compared for their stimulant activity on the plain muscle of the isolated uterus of the guinea-pig. Their activities in this direction showed a practically identical relation.

Exp. 1. Cat anaesthetized with ether. Vagi cut. Arterial pressure from carotid. Intravenous injection. Liver extract (L.E. No. 1) diluted 10 times compared with a solution of histamine containing 0.01 mg of the base in 1 cc. A number of trials gave a final equivalent:

$$0.1 \text{ cc diluted liver extract} = 0.12 \text{ cc histamine solution}$$
$$= 0.0012 \text{ mg histamine.}$$

∴ 1 cc L.E. No. 1 contains the depressor equivalent of *0.12 mg histamine.*

Exps. 2 and 3. Isolated uteri of virgin guinea-pigs. Equivalents were obtained indicating:

7 cc of extract No. 1 are equivalent to 1 mg histamine;
9 cc of extract No. 1 are equivalent to 1 mg histamine.

Average 8 cc of extract No. 1 are equivalent to 1 mg of histamine;
or 1 cc of extract No. 1 is equivalent to *0.125 mg histamine.*

A more specific test of the histamine-like nature of the action was afforded by the uterus of the rat, which, as Guggenheim [336] showed, is peculiar in the fact that the tone and rhythm of its plain muscle are inhibited by histamine, which must be applied in relatively large doses to produce any definite effect. In this respect again the action of the liver extract corresponded with that of histamine. The quantitative relation could not be clearly determined, and there were indications that the inhibitor, histamine-like action was complicated by the presence in the extract of something having a weak stimulant action; but the main action was clearly of the histamine type.

We further tested the action of the extract by injecting it intravenously

---

[1]The preparation used for comparison was the crystalline diphosphate, sold as "Ergamine diphosphate" by Burroughs, Wellcome, and Co.; but the solutions were made up and doses expressed in terms of histamine base.

into unanaesthetized guinea-pigs. In young guinea-pigs weighing about 200 g an injection of 0.05 mg of histamine usually, but not quite invariably, produces death from asphyxia, due to constriction of the bronchioles; 0.1 mg is an invariably fatal dose. The lethal dose may, therefore, be placed somewhere between these two limits. 0.02 mg never produces noteworthy symptoms.

Exp. 4. The extract used in this experiment (L.E. No. 2) had been assayed on a cat under ether, in comparison with histamine, small doses being used, with the result that the undiluted extract was calculated to be equivalent in depressor action to a histamine solution containing about 0.1 mg of the base per cc. Five guinea-pigs, weighing about 200 g each, were given intravenous injections, with results as follows (death indicated by †):

Dose	Result
(1) 0.1 mg histamine	† 6 minutes
(2) 0.1 mg histamine	† 3¼ minutes
(3) 0.8 cc L.E. No. 2	† 4 minutes
(4) 0.2 cc L.E. No. 2	No symptoms
(5) 0.75 cc L.E. No. 2	† 4 minutes

The signs produced by histamine and the effective doses of the extract were identical. The autopsies also showed the same picture in all the cases in which death resulted. The heart continued to beat for some minutes after complete cessation of respiratory and other movements. The lungs showed the characteristic permanent distension, and there was no other definite abnormality to suggest that any action was produced by the extract which was not identical with that of histamine. It will be seen, further, that the lethal effect on guinea-pigs corresponds with what would be expected from its depressor equivalent. A dose of extract equivalent in depressor action to 0.02 mg of histamine produces no obvious signs, while doses equivalent to 0.075 and 0.08 mg produced asphyxial death with approximately the same rapidity as 0.1 mg of histamine itself.

This evidence suggested that a substance acting like histamine not only contributed to the depressor action of the extract, as measured by the immediate, evanescent effect on the cat's blood-pressure, but was the predominant agent in its production. No indication, indeed, had thus far been obtained of the presence of any differently acting depressor substance. A further test on this point, however, could be obtained by observing the action of the extract on the artificially perfused blood vessels of the cat's leg. These vessels readily lose their vaso-dilator response to histamine under these conditions, while retaining their responsiveness to vaso-dilators of other types. We accordingly carried out a series of artificial perfusions of cat's hind legs, with defibrinated cat's blood, or, in some cases, with Locke's solution containing gum and a small proportion (1 in 10 millions) of adrenaline. The apparatus used for perfusion, and that for recording venous outflow and limb volume, were the same as those described by Burn and Dale [158]. In the early stages of the perfusion we found, as they had done, that a small dose of histamine, injected into the arterial cannula, produced a definite vaso-dilatation. Even at this stage, however, a dose of the liver extract, which had been found to produce an equal fall of arterial pressure in the anaesthetized cat, produced a definitely greater vaso-dilatation in the perfused organ, as shown both by a more pronounced acceleration of the venous outflow, and by a greater increase of the limb volume. This indication of the presence in the liver extracts of some other vaso-dilator principle became much clearer when the stage of the experiment was reached at which histamine no longer produced its vaso-dilator effect, but a simple relatively weak vaso-constriction in its place; the depressor equivalent of the liver extract still produced at each injection a vaso-dilatation, less pronounced, indeed, than that which it initially evoked, but quite definite.

This indication of the presence in the extract of another vaso-dilator agent, the effect of which persisted when that of histamine had disappeared, was obtained in every perfusion experiment made on the leg of a cat, whether with blood or with a gum-saline solution. The nature of this other principle became clear when we further added a small dose of atropine (0.2 mg) to the perfusing blood. When the vaso-dilatation, which atropine itself produces under such conditions, had subsided, and the perfusion had again become regular and the limb-volume steady, we again compared the action of histamine with that of a depressor equivalent of the liver extract. They now produced identical effects of vaso-constriction; the additional, and previously persistent, vaso-dilator action of the extract had been abolished by the atropine, and the histamine-like effect alone remained. The probability that the other vaso-dilator substance was choline became very strong, and was increased when we found it possible to make an artificial mixture of histamine and choline, with which the effect of the liver extract at every stage of a perfusion experiment could be reproduced with great precision. The particular sample of liver extract which we were then using was matched in activity by one containing *0.1 mg of histamine and 17 mg of choline per cc.*

It will be obvious that the conditions of the perfusion experiment on the cat's leg, in which the capillary-dilator effect of histamine is at best evanescent and always relatively weak, gave an undue prominence to the arterio-dilator action of the choline-like constituent. We found, indeed, that the addition of choline to a histamine solution, in the proportion above indicated, made but a trifling addition to its depressor effect on the anaesthetized cat, though it had been so effective on the perfused vessels. This contrast is readily explained, if we suppose, as a large body of evidence entitles us to do, that the vascular tone is strongest in the smallest peripheral vessels, including the capillaries, of the cat under ether, while in the perfused organ the capillaries rapidly lose their tone, so that the resistance to the flow is encountered almost entirely in the arterioles. The effects observed on the perfused vessels had made it clear, however, that the vaso-dilator effects of choline and histamine should not be simply additive. The relatively weak constrictor effect of a small dose of histamine on the arteries is, we have seen, easily outbalanced by the vaso-dilator effect of choline on the same vessels. Even in the anaesthetized animal we must suppose that the dilator effect of histamine is the resultant of a strong, peripheral dilator effect, and a weak, less peripheral constrictor effect. If choline is injected simultaneously in quantity sufficient to reverse the latter, so that vasodilatation occurs throughout the whole peripheral branching, the combined effect should be greater than a sum of the two. This deduction was put to the test of experiment in the following way. Choline in small doses, up to about 1 mg, causes no slowing or detectable weakening of the heartbeat, but apparently acts on the circulation as a pure vaso-dilator. Its depressor action is not qualitatively identical with that of histamine, the time-relations being somewhat different. Nevertheless it is not difficult to determine doses of the two substances which produce brief falls of the arterial pressure to identical minima. The ratio so determined varied rather widely from one experiment to another, and was by no means constant throughout one long experiment; with a shift in the incidence of vascular tone we should, indeed, expect it thus to change. It was sufficiently stable over short periods, however, for the comparison we had in view. Having determined the doses producing practically identical minima—say, 0.001 mg of histamine and 0.3 mg of choline—we prepared solutions containing these doses in equal volumes, and mixed the two. Of this mixture we now injected a dose containing half the previously injected dose of each substance—0.0005 mg of histamine and 0.15 mg of choline in the instance cited. The effect was regularly greater than that of the original dose of either; whereas, if the effect were simply additive, the combined half-doses should obviously have produced the equivalent of one whole dose of either constituent. The observation was repeated on several cats, and on one dog, always with the same result. Figure 85 shows a typical example of this potentiating effect.

So far the evidence was entirely compatible with the supposition that the immediate, evanescent, vaso-dilator effect which we were studying was due to the presence in the extract of two substances, one closely resembling

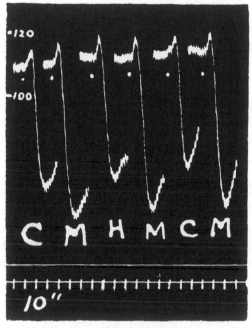

FIGURE 85. Carotid blood pressure of cat under
ether. Intravenous injections—at C, in each case,
0.3 mg choline chloride; at H 0.001 mg histamine; at M, in each case, 0.0005 mg histamine
+ 0.15 mg choline chloride.

histamine in its action, and the other as closely resembling choline. Since
a choline effect can be eliminated by atropine, while the rabbit under the
anaesthetics usually employed is not sensitive to the vaso-dilator action of
histamine, a test on this species would give further evidence as to the
completeness with which these two types of action would represent that of
the extract. On a rabbit anaesthetized with veronal, intravenous injection
of doses from 0.12 to 1 cc of the liver extract caused a relatively small, but
regular and definite fall of arterial pressure. Two mg of atropine were
then injected, and a test with a small injection of acetylcholine showed
that paralysis of response to this type of action was complete. A further
injection of the liver extract, however, caused a smaller but still definite
fall of the arterial pressure. Careful watching of the record during its
production showed that the depression was accompanied, and could probably
be accounted for, by a pronounced retardation of the heartbeat. As the
rate returned to the normal, the blood pressure returned to the original
level. This was not an effect of the type which we were investigating. We
found, further, that when the extract was purified by precipitation with
basic lead acetate, it no longer slowed the heart-rate or lowered the blood

pressure in the atropinized rabbit, but produced only such a small rise of pressure as a small injection of histamine would produce; whereas this purification left the pronounced action on the arterial pressure of the cat practically unchanged. Since we were concerned to investigate only substances lowering the blood pressure in the cat by immediate vaso-dilatation, the effects on the rabbit confirmed the view that we were dealing with associated effects of the choline and the histamine types only.

PHYSIOLOGICAL EFFECTS OF LUNG EXTRACTS

As indicated above, liver extract was chosen, in the first instance, for investigation, on account of the practical interest attributed to it at the time. So far as immediate vaso-dilator effect is concerned, however, we found that it did not exhibit any special intensity of action as compared with other organs. On the contrary, when different extracts, made by identical procedures, were compared, that from the liver was among the weaker ones in action of the type which we were studying, while that from the lung stood out above all the others so far tested, as by far the most active. In general terms it may be said that, weight for weight, lung tissue yielded about 10 times as much vaso-dilator substance as the most active of the other tissues, and about 20 times as much as liver. The work of chemical separation of the liver principles, with a view to their identification, was already in hand. It was thought desirable, therefore, to apply the same processes to lung extract, so that a comparison between the initial activities and the final yields of pure principles might eventually be made.

No such complete physiological analysis of the action was made in the case of lung as in that of liver. It was sufficiently obvious that the action was predominantly of the histamine type, atropine making no sensible difference in the depressor activity of the whole extract, as determined in comparison with pure histamine on the cat under ether. We found, further, that a dose of the lung extract equivalent in depressor action to the fatal dose of histamine, killed the unanaesthetized guinea-pig, with the typical bronchial occlusion, when injected intravenously.

ISOLATION AND IDENTIFICATION OF CHOLINE AND HISTAMINE FROM LIVER AND LUNG

Introduction

The physiological evidence having indicated the presence of principles acting like histamine and choline, we naturally tested the possibility of separating the unknown principles by the chemical methods which are used for the isolation of those bases. Choline, which had often been obtained from tissue extracts before, we expected to obtain. It was doubtful, on the other hand, whether histamine had ever been isolated in chemical purity from material under no suspicion of bacterial contamination, and, so far as we are aware, it had never been so obtained from liver or lung. It will be seen that we have isolated it in relatively large quantities, corresponding to a high proportion of the vaso-dilator activities of the original extracts.

Before we give the details of the procedures leading to their isolation, it will be useful to mention certain points in our experience of the behaviour of these bases, when present in mixtures with other constituents of an organ extract. At the successive stages of the isolation we have met with examples of their being precipitated where they ought to remain dissolved, remaining in solution in the presence of reagents which ought to precipitate them, failing to be extracted by solvents which ought to remove them, or disappearing under treatment to which they should be stable. A few examples may be given.

(1) At the outset of our work we had before us the fact that Best and Scott at the Connaught Laboratories of the University of Toronto, in preparing the liver extract, found that substances responsible for the depressor action here in question were largely precipitated, from solution in 80 per cent alcohol, by the addition of 3 volumes of acetone. This precipitate was dissolved in water to furnish the preparation used in therapeutics, and this solution was the starting point of our own investigation. When histamine and choline are dissolved in 80 per cent alcohol, in proportions yielding a much more actively depressor solution, the solution remains perfectly clear when 3 volumes of acetone are added. The conclusion might easily be drawn that the depressor action of the precipitate from the liver extract is not due to either of these bodies; but the conclusion would be wrong.

(2) If sodium carbonate in excess is added to a solution of histamine in water and the mixture evaporated to dryness, the histamine can be extracted almost quantitatively from the residue by hot chloroform. This method was extensively used by Abel and Kubota [3], who regarded any depressor substance not so extracted as not histamine. Koessler and Hanke [465] showed, and we can confirm the observation, that from a pure solution of histamine, or one containing histidine in addition, the histamine can be separated by adding excess of caustic alkali and shaking with amyl alcohol. We found that preparations, in which a histamine-like action had been concentrated into a small bulk of relatively purified solution, failed to yield any significant amount of histamine to either of the above methods of extraction, and, further, that the proportion recognizable physiologically

in the alkaline residue was in some instances only a small fraction of that originally present. We were at first inclined to regard this as definite evidence that the depressor substance was something other than histamine, until we found that histamine itself, added in known quantity to a sample of such a solution, was not extracted by these methods in larger proportion than the natural depressor agent, and that nevertheless it disappeared to varying extents in the alkaline mixtures from which its extraction was attempted. Other methods for extracting the depressor substance had to be found, and when it was extracted it proved to be wholly histamine.

(3) In connection with the experiment on lung (see below) it was found that a small, but appreciable amount of depressor material escaped precipitation with phosphotungstic acid. At first we were inclined to believe that this indicated the presence of active substances other than histamine and choline. It was discovered, however, that this assumption was false, and that the precipitation of the histamine and choline (and other bases) had been incomplete owing to the large amount of sodium acetate in the solution.

(4) The fact that histamine added to an organ extract disappears, as judged by the physiological test, on boiling with alkali, while pure histamine solutions are stable under such conditions, was observed by Dale and Dudley [240], when investigating pituitary extracts. In our early experiments with liver extract, the apparent disappearance of depressor activity on boiling with alkali might have suggested that it could not be due to histamine. Previous experience warned us against drawing such a conclusion, which would certainly have been wrong.

(5) Depressor activity of the histamine type has been concentrated in solutions which failed to give the Pauly reaction, which was strongly developed by equidepressor solutions of pure histamine. Again we were misled, until we had tested a sample of the concentrate to which histamine had been added, and again failed to obtain the colour reaction. In some instances a positive reaction was obtained when the diazobenzene-sulphonic acid was added first to the solution to be tested and the mixture was then made alkaline with sodium carbonate solution, while addition of sodium carbonate first and diazo-reagent last to the same solution had a negative result. In other histamine-containing mixtures this behaviour to the order in which the reagents were added was reversed, and finally, in other cases it was impossible to produce a typical Pauly reaction in solutions known to contain histamine, no matter in what order the reagents were used. We have been surprised and impressed by the unreliability of the Pauly reaction in the presence of other substances, and are very doubtful as to the value of quantitative methods based on it.

The literature, dealing with the depressor substances of tissue extracts, contains many examples of the deduction, from the apparent physical or chemical properties of the agent in a particular case, that it cannot be histamine. Having been ready to draw such conclusions ourselves, we have become by experience ever more doubtful of their soundness. In the case of histamine especially, and of choline in minor degree, when identity of physiological action has been proved, the evidence of chemical difference needs the closest scrutiny and control before it can be accepted as decisive.

METHODS EMPLOYED FOR THE ISOLATION OF CHOLINE AND HISTAMINE

The methods which led to the successful isolation of these two substances followed the lines of those in general use for the separation of bases. After preliminary purification with basic lead acetate, which occasioned only such loss of activity as was inevitable in dealing with bulky precipitates, the bases were precipitated as phosphotungstates, which contained practically the whole of the activity. From this precipitate the bases were regenerated and fractionated by the silver method of Kossel and Kutscher. Choline was isolated as the mercurichloride from the "lysine" fraction, and in one experiment by direct treatment of the neutralized solution of the bases, liberated from the phosphotungstate precipitate, with mercuric chloride.

As Barger and Dale had already observed, in isolating histamine from ergot [50] the histamine-like activity did not all come down in the "histidine" fraction but was spread over this and the "arginine" fraction. These two fractions were accordingly precipitated together: thus a solution containing both bases and basic acids was obtained, and success or failure in obtaining the histamine from this depended on the degree to which the unwanted constituents of the mixture were removed, before picric acid was applied to precipitate the histamine itself. It was frequently found possible to obtain further quantities of pure histamine picrate from mother liquors, which refused to yield more of the material directly, by removing the picric acid and submitting the residue to the process of fractionation again.

The first task was to devise a method for the separation of the bases from the basic acids of the "histidine-arginine" fraction. As stated above, the properties of histamine are so modified by the presence of other substances, that chloroform extraction of the residue obtained by evaporating the solution to dryness, after adding excess of sodium carbonate, was unsuccessful; and the same applies to many other modifications, based on the general principle of anchoring the acids as salts and then extracting the free bases with a solvent, in which the former are insoluble.

The method which proved, in our hands, most satisfactory was to grind up the concentrated solution with a large excess of baryta, sometimes with the addition of a little plaster of Paris, and, after thoroughly drying the mass and reducing it to powder, to extract it in a Soxhlet apparatus with absolute ethyl alcohol. Some loss of activity inevitably accompanied this procedure but from the alcoholic extract pure histamine picrate was isolated.

EXPERIMENTAL

Liver Extract

66 kg of perfectly fresh ox liver were rapidly minced and stirred into 95 per cent alcohol (2.25 l per kg tissue). After standing for 24 hours the liquid was filtered and the residue re-extracted for a further 24 hours with 60 per cent alcohol (2 l per kg original tissue). To the combined extracts 0.18 cc sulphuric acid per litre was added. This precipitated a certain amount of inactive material and reduced the frothing during concentration, which was carried out *in vacuo* below 50°. To the concentrated liquid sufficient alcohol was added to bring the content of the latter to 80 per cent. The addition of 3 volumes of acetone to this extract produced a precipitate which contained over 70 per cent of the depressor activity of the original extract.[2] The solution of the precipitate in water was neutralized with sodium hydroxide and treated with basic lead acetate until no further precipitate was produced. Lead was removed from the filtrate and washings by means of H_2S, and, after filtration, the liquid was concentrated *in vacuo* to 1050 cc. Sulphuric acid was added to give a concentration of 5 per cent and phosphotungstic acid (25 per cent in 5 per cent H_2SO_4) was then added until precipitation was complete, 5 l of the reagent being required. The precipitate was filtered off and washed with 5 per cent H_2SO_4. The filtrate, after removal of the sulphuric acid by means of baryta, had no depressor activity. The phosphotungstate was decomposed by grinding it with excess of baryta in water at 60°. From the filtrate barium was removed by means of sulphuric acid. It was concentrated *in vacuo* to 400 cc.

190 g silver nitrate in 400 cc water were then added to the solution which was faintly acid, and the precipitate formed was filtered off. This was shown physiologically to contain no depressor substances. The filtrate was then saturated with baryta, and, after standing in ice-water, the precipitate was collected and washed with saturated baryta solution.

Histamine. The precipitate was suspended in dilute sulphuric acid, a sufficient quantity being taken to render the liquid just acid to Congo red.

[2]Although this precipitation with acetone is in a sense irrational, the experience of working up a batch of 196 lb of liver in which it was omitted proved that the 30 per cent loss of activity involved was more than compensated for by the purification effected at the same time.

H$_2$S was then passed through the liquid which, after removal of silver sulphide and barium sulphate by filtration, was neutralized with baryta and concentrated *in vacuo* to 25 cc. It gave a strong Pauly reaction, and, tested physiologically, contained depressor activity equivalent to 240 mg of histamine.

25 g crystalline barium hydroxide were added to the solution, the mass was ground up and then thoroughly dried in a vacuum desiccator over sulphuric acid. It was then ground to a fine powder and extracted for 3 hours with absolute alcohol in a Soxhlet apparatus. The extract was diluted with water and neutralized with sulphuric acid; some baryta had been extracted and this was precipitated as sulphate. After removing the alcohol *in vacuo* the barium sulphate was filtered off. Physiological assay of the solution showed that it contained depressor activity equivalent to 75 mg histamine. The residue in the thimble had formed a hard non-porous mass. It was therefore ground up afresh with a little plaster of Paris and again extracted; this procedure was repeated three times. The combined extracts then displayed physiological activity corresponding to 122 mg histamine. They were concentrated *in vacuo* to 25 cc and treated with sodium picrate. 608 mg of crystalline picrate were obtained (M.P. with decomposition, 220°). After recrystallizing twice from water 431 mg of pure *histamine dipicrate* (= 86 mg base) were obtained (M.P. with decomposition, 241°). It was identified by analysis and comparison with a specimen of histamine dipicrate; mixed melting point determinations showed no depression, while crystalline form and physiological activity were identical.

Analysis. 0.0410 g picrate gave 0.0779 g nitron picrate.
Picric acid: found 80.41 per cent.
Picric acid: calculated for C$_5$H$_9$N$_3$(C$_6$H$_3$O$_7$N$_3$)$_2$ 80.48 per cent.

No attempt was made to procure the maximum possible yield of pure histamine dipicrate from this batch by reworking the mother liquors. In another experiment, which is summarized in Table 50.I, the amount of histamine dipicrate actually isolated was increased by slightly more than 35 per cent by exhaustive treatment of the residues.

Choline. From the "lysine" fraction (i.e., the filtrate from the precipitation with silver nitrate and baryta) silver and barium were removed in the usual manner and the bases reprecipitated as phosphotungstates. The precipitate was decomposed with baryta in the cold, excess Ba removed as sulphate, and the neutral liquid was then concentrated to 100 cc *in vacuo* and acidified with a small quantity of acetic acid. Hot mercuric chloride solution was added until precipitation was complete. After filtration sodium acetate was added until no further precipitate formed. The combined precipitates were dissolved in boiling water from which, after filtering off a small insoluble residue, 260 g (= 17.5 g base) of pure *choline mercurichloride* (M.P. 250°) were obtained. The identification was assured by preparing the picrate and chloroaurate from this salt. The properties of these salts coincided with those of choline; the picrate melted at 242–4° and the chloroaurate at 266–9° (with decomposition).

Analysis of chloroaurate. 0.1938 g gave 0.0855 g Au.
> Au: found   44.12 per cent.
> Au: calculated for $C_5H_{14}ON, AuCl_4$ 44.47 per cent.

Lung Extract

Histamine. 10 kg fresh ox lung were minced and extracted with alcohol as described for liver. The acetone precipitation was omitted. The extract was concentrated *in vacuo* to a small bulk, shaken out with ether to remove fat and finally reduced *in vacuo* to a volume of 2 l. It was then purified and fractionated in the same manner as the liver extract.

The physiological activity of the "histidine-arginine" fraction corresponded to that of 400 mg histamine. Alcoholic extraction of the baryta-treated material recovered activity equivalent to 300 mg histamine. From this extract 1.288 g pure histamine picrate was obtained, and on grinding up the mass in the Soxhlet thimble and re-extracting with alcohol a further quantity of 0.146 g histamine dipicrate was obtained. In all therefore 1.434 g pure histamine dipicrate (= 287 mg base) was obtained.

Analysis. 0.0406 g picrate gave 0.0773 g nitron picrate.
> Picric acid: found   80.58 per cent.
> Picric acid: calculated for $C_5H_9N_3(C_6H_3O_7N_3)_2$ 80.48 per cent.

The more soluble fractions from the recrystallization of the histamine dipicrate were freed from picric acid, and, after adding a large excess of sodium carbonate, dried and extracted with hot chloroform. A small amount of depressor substance was extracted, but it was not possible to isolate the histamine from this in a state of purity. This alkaline residue was then extracted with alcohol and 0.115 g of a non-depressor picrate (M.P. 199°) was obtained from the extract, which was identified as methylguanidine picrate.

Two curious and unexpected facts were encountered in the investigation of the lung extract. The lysine fraction contained no substances precipitable in the usual way by phosphotungstic acid and the filtrate from the first precipitation of the bases as phosphotungstates, when tested physiologically, contained depressor material of activity equivalent to 40 mg histamine.

As no such quantity had escaped precipitation in any of the previous experiments on lung and liver extracts the matter was investigated. It was found that the large amount of sodium acetate[8] in the solution was responsible for the failure of phosphotungstic acid to precipitate completely the histamine and other bases present; for, after most of this salt had been removed and the remainder converted into sulphate, the addition of phosphotungstic acid produced a copious precipitate from which choline was isolated and a mixture of the picrates of histamine and creatinine obtained. Methylguanidine too was isolated from this precipitate in considerable quantity as the picrate. No doubt remained, therefore, that the depressor activity which at first had escaped precipitation by phosphotungstic acid was, in fact, due to choline and histamine.

Appended is a table showing the physiological assays at each stage in the separation of histamine, in the two experiments given in detail above, and in two others conducted on similar lines. In the experiment with 72 kg of ox liver, 97 mg histamine (as dipicrate) were isolated directly. By reworking the residues a further quantity of 178 mg histamine dipicrate (= 36 mg histamine) were recovered.

The activities are expressed as milligrams of histamine.

TABLE 50.I

HISTAMINE CONTENT OF DIFFERENT FRACTIONS

	Original Extract	Basic Lead Acetate	Phospho-tungstic Acid	Silver Fraction	Alkaline Extraction	Pure Histamine (isolated as dipicrate)
Ox liver (66 kg)	—	250	320	240	122	86
Ox liver (72 kg)	390	195(?)	280	204	140	133
Ox lung (500 g)	22	17	16	12.5	10	3.2
Ox lung (10 kg)	750	530	460	400	300	287

It will be observed that in the experiments with liver extracts the physiological evaluation of the amounts of histamine obtained after decomposition of the phosphotungstates is somewhat higher than that after the previous stage of the fractionation. The physiological assay is based on the comparison of very small volumes (0.003–0.03 cc) of the solutions in question with amounts of histamine of the order of 0.003 mg. It is obvious, therefore, that the factor by which the result of the actual test must be multiplied is very large, and it is unreasonable to expect a high degree of accuracy. A comparison of the figures under "basic lead acetate" and "phosphotungstic acid," therefore, merely indicates that the histamine-like activity is quanti-

[8]Most of the sodium was introduced by using a solution of sodium phosphotungstate in 5 per cent H_2SO_4 for the precipitation of the bases.

tatively precipitable by the latter reagent, and recoverable without appreciable loss from the precipitate.

Throughout the fractionations all final mother liquors and discarded precipitates were tested physiologically, and in no instance was any evidence obtained which indicated the presence of any depressor substances other than histamine and choline.

It is interesting to note that, in the experiment with 66 kg ox liver, the proportions of choline and histamine actually isolated in chemically pure condition are very close to the ratio (17 mg choline to 0.1 mg histamine) determined by physiological assay of the extract by Best and Dale before the chemical investigation was commenced. It appears, therefore, that the proportional loss involved in the method of fractionation is approximately the same in the case of each base.

An outstanding quantitative fact, which has been revealed by this investigation, is the very high content of histamine in lung as compared with that in liver, and in other tissues on which work is proceeding. It will be seen that, averaging the above figures, 1.58 mg pure histamine has been isolated per kg of liver, while 27.64 mg were obtained per kg of lung. There is a reasonably good correspondence between the physiological observations on the relative depressor effects of the original extracts from the two tissues and the yields of histamine obtained from them by chemical fractionation.

Discussion

It is desirable, perhaps, still further to emphasize the limitations of our problem. We were not directly concerned with the question whether extracts prepared from liver, or other organs, produce a lowering of pathologically high blood pressure, delayed in onset and long continued in effect. We were concerned with the immediate and evanescent depressor effects shown by such extracts when injected intravenously into a cat or dog. We were aware, indeed, that this immediate action was in use for the assay of one type of liver extract, and had appeared to give an index of its activity in producing a prolonged therapeutic action. If the existence of this latter should be established by others, it may become desirable to consider whether it may be due to the slow liberation of histamine from association with the more complex constituents of a crude tissue extract—a possibility not incompatible with some of our own observations on the curious behaviour of that base. We are not, however, here concerned with such possibilities. Further, it was no part of our purpose to account for all the falls of arterial blood pressure which have been described as following the injection of various crude extracts and suspensions—effects in some of which intravascular precipitation, fibrin formation, agglutination of corpuscles, or endothelial injury might conceivably be concerned. Our object was to discover the nature of the depressor substances which occur in extracts from practically all tissues, are soluble in water and strong alcohol, and produce an effect in which a predominantly histamine-like action can be recognized. At the present stage our evidence is further limited to extracts of liver and lung. In the case of the liver extracts used by us, in the first instance, and later in that of the lung extract, though there to a much smaller degree, we found that the histamine-like depressor effect was complicated and reinforced by a choline-like action. In neither case did we detect any important depressor action which did not correspond to one of these. From these extracts we have isolated histamine and choline in quantities sufficient for complete chemical identification. A series of questions arises with regard to this identification, some of which can be met on the evidence before us, while some suggest problems rather for further investigation.

(1) We must consider whether the quantities of pure bases isolated warrant the supposition that the whole of the effect which we were studying was accounted for by their presence. In the case of the lung extract we consider that the figures which we have given render such a supposition reasonable. It is true that the original estimate, on the crude extract, indicated the presence of a physiological equivalent of 750 mg of histamine, and that slightly less than 300 mg of that base were finally isolated as the pure dipicrate. It will be seen, however, that there was no exceptional loss at any one stage of the long process of purification, such as to indicate that any part of the activity was due to much more complex substances. When we tested the purification by basic lead, or the precipitation by phosphotungstic acid or by silver, on a small scale, there was no indication of any definite loss; the activity was wholly in the filtrate, or wholly in the precipitate. On the large scale the mere bulk of the materials and the physical properties of some of the precipitates made quantitative recovery a practical impossibility, and we did not, in fact, expect to obtain it. We were left with the clear impression that, if we had actually added histamine to a large bulk of such an extract, and attempted to isolate it by the same procedure, the yield would probably have shown no higher proportion to the quantity added than the histamine which we actually isolated bore to the naturally occurring depressor agent. When it is also remembered that choline made some contribution to the "histamine equivalent" determined in the earlier stages of the purification, and that it would increase the apparent amount of "histamine" to a degree out of proportion to its own separate activity, we think we may fairly claim to have established a strong probability that the whole of the histamine-like activity of the lung extract is due to histamine itself.

In the case of the liver extract, the isolation of histamine was rendered more difficult by the fact that it was present in much smaller proportion, in a solution containing a much larger quantity of inactive constituents. It is, further, not without significance that the chemical work on the lung extract was carried out later, and therefore with the aid of additional experience. We have little doubt that we could now isolate a larger proportion of the histamine-like constituent of liver extract as histamine itself. Although, therefore, the actual quantity isolated was somewhat less in proportion to the physiological equivalent originally determined than in the case of the lung extract, we think it probable that, in the liver extract also, the histamine-like activity was due to the presence of histamine itself. The position is very similar in the case of choline. We did not follow it so systematically by physiological assay through the different stages. Since, however, the proportion between the quantities of choline and histamine finally isolated was roughly the same as the proportion determined from the physiological activities of the original extract, the loss was evidently of the same order in the two cases. We find no good reason for supposing that the excess of the choline-like action originally present, over that of the choline isolated in chemical purity, was due to any other substance than choline itself.

(2) It is of interest to inquire whether the bases are present in the tissues as such, or separated from some combination in the process of extraction. The problem in the case of choline is no new one. Choline has previously been obtained from many tissues, and much has been written in support of, or in opposition to, its claims to be the depressor substance present in such extracts. The much greater activity of histamine gives a proportionately greater interest to the question of its presence as such in the tissues. The method of extraction which we have used is of the simplest possible kind. The perfectly fresh tissue has been disintegrated as rapidly as possible and extracted immediately with cold alcohol. Some small-scale experiments, in which only a physiological estimate has been made, have been carried out with even greater care. The chest of a living animal was opened under anaesthesia; a lung was removed, dropped straight into alcohol cooled with solid CO_2, and thus frozen immediately; it was then minced while frozen and returned to the cold alcohol. The extract thus obtained showed a histamine-like activity of the same order as that obtained without these extreme precautions, and as great as that of a similar extract made from the corresponding lung, removed an hour after the animal's death. There is good reason, therefore, to believe that the histamine is present as such, at least as soon as the cells are killed by contact with the extracting alcohol. The evidence, indeed, of its presence in the cells during life may be said to be as good as that of the presence of lactic acid in a living muscle, or

even rather better, since we have found no evidence that the proportion of free histamine increases in the period immediately following the death of the animal.

(3) Histamine being either present as such in the living cell, or released therefrom at the moment of death, questions of great interest arise as to the manner in which it was held by the protoplasm during life, and prevented from producing its intense physiological action. It may be there only potentially, in the form of some inactive precursor. On the other hand, it is conceivable that histamine is present as such in the cell interior, being prevented from leaving it so long as the cell membrane is physiologically intact, and that it produces its action only if some stimulus or injury causes its escape into the extra-cellular fluids. On these points we have no evidence, and it may be very difficult to obtain it.

(4) The presence of so much histamine in a tissue, as can be extracted from the lung, can hardly be without physiological significance. 100 g of lung tissue—say, the lungs of a dog—may be expected to contain as much as 7 or 8 mg of the base—a quantity which, if suddenly released into the circulation of the animal, would have a profound, shock-like action. Merely to mention two possibilities, which can only be considered in the light of further and more direct evidence, it is conceivable either that the lung acts as an organ of internal secretion with respect to histamine, or, on the other hand, that it merely captures histamine which has escaped into the venous blood from more vigorously metabolic tissues, and holds it pending its final disposal. In the latter case the blood would not only be oxygenated, but also physiologically purified, during its passage through the lung.

Here, however, we are merely concerned with the demonstration of the fact that histamine itself is the main depressor constituent of certain tissues, and, in the case of the lung especially, a surprisingly abundant one. These facts seem to justify the expectation that this potent base will be found widely distributed in the tissues, and to reinforce the suggestion that it must have some important function in the control and adjustment of the circulation through the small blood vessels.

Summary

Histamine and choline have been isolated from alcoholic extracts of fresh liver and lung, in quantities sufficient to account for the immediate vaso-dilator activities of those extracts. Histamine is responsible for the greater part of this activity, and is present in remarkably large amount in the extract from lung. The physiological significance of its occurrence is discussed.

51. The Disappearance of Histamine from Autolysing Lung Tissue

CHARLES H. BEST

The presence of histamine in extracts of normal lung accounts for a very large proportion of the vaso-dilator activity of these extracts. The physiological significance of the occurrence of histamine in normal tissue has been discussed by Best, Dale, Dudley, and Thorpe [82]. The question of changes in the amount of histamine in lung tissue during autolysis has not previously been investigated, and it was thought that interesting information might be obtained from a study of this problem. The effect of autolysis of minced lung tissue on the naturally occurring and on added histamine is recorded in this communication. It has been found that histamine disappears during the autolysis.

METHODS

Autolysis. Perfectly fresh ox or horse lung was finely minced and the minced material was mixed by passing it several times through the mincer. Weighed samples of this material were then treated with hydrochloric acid, as will be described later, to determine the initial histamine content of the lung tissue. 20 g portions of the minced lung were then weighed out and transferred to 200 cc flasks. 100 cc of physiological saline and 15 cc of toluene were added to each flask. The flasks were placed in an incubator which was kept at 37° C. The contents of the flasks were well mixed by shaking at hourly intervals for the first five or six hours. Flasks were removed from the incubator from time to time and histamine estimations carried out.

Histamine estimation. The histamine was estimated by the following procedure which has been found by McHenry and the author in the Department of Physiological Hygiene, University of Toronto, to give consistent results and invariably to recover added histamine within the limits of the error of the physiological method used in the comparison of the final solution with a standard solution of histamine. To 20 g of tissue, or to a

Originally appeared in the *Journal of Physiology*, LXVII (1929), 256–63. From the National Institute for Medical Research, Hampstead.

suspension of this amount of tissue in saline, 50 cc of concentrated hydrochloric acid are added. The mixture is heated under a reflux condenser until the liquid boils. The heat is then slightly reduced and the temperature of the liquid kept at approximately 95° C for 30 minutes. Histamine is not lost when the solution is boiled for a much longer period with larger amounts of hydrochloric acid (Hanke and Koessler [356]). The mixture is then transferred to a round bottom flask and is concentrated *in vacuo* approximately to dryness. The residue in the flask is extracted with 200 cc of 95 per cent alcohol. The combined extracts are distilled *in vacuo*. Two or three treatments with alcohol are carried out. The residue from the extracts is then suspended in distilled water and 40 per cent sodium hydroxide added until the solution is neutral to litmus. The mixture is then filtered. The clear filtrate may contain 2 per cent sodium chloride or slightly more, but in the small amounts injected this salt does not interfere with the physiological assay. The method of assay of histamine on etherized cats was identical with that used in previous researches from this laboratory. In a fairly sensitive cat it is possible to discriminate between doses of histamine which differ from each other by 15 per cent. The histamine values are expressed in mg per 100 g of tissue. The test dose of histamine was usually approximately 1/1000 mg. As there were usually about 10 mg of histamine per 100 g in the extract at the beginning of the experiment, a slight experimental error in testing is multiplied by a large figure in the calculation of the total amount of histamine present. "Ergamine diphosphate" (Burroughs, Wellcome, and Co.) has been used as the standard and the weight of the base taken as one-third that of the salt. The standard solution of histamine was usually prepared on each test day. It has been found, however, that a solution of histamine will retain all its depressor activity for at least a month when kept in the incubator at 37° C or in the laboratory at room temperature if toluene to the extent of 10 per cent by volume is added and the container is shaken occasionally.

Rate of autolysis. In the first experiment the progress of the autolysis was followed by determining the increase of non-protein nitrogen and of amino-acids in the mixture. These determinations were carried out as follows: 30 cc of the minced lung in saline mixture were treated with sufficient trichloroacetic acid to secure a concentration of 2 per cent. The mixture was shaken and allowed to stand overnight. It was then filtered. Total nitrogen was determined in the clear protein-free filtrate by the Kjeldahl procedure. To estimate the amino-acids 10 cc of this filtrate were neutralized with 0.1 N sodium hydroxide using phenolphthalein as the indicator. Formaldehyde [727] neutralized in an identical manner was added and the acid liberated was determined by titration with 0.1 N sodium hydroxide.

Phenolphthalein was used as the indicator in all three titrations and the same faint pink tint was adopted. Non-protein and amino-acid nitrogen were determined in the first experiment only.

EXPERIMENTAL RESULTS

Natural histamine. In the first experiment two 20 g portions of minced horse lung were treated as described above to determine the histamine originally present. The solutions obtained were found to contain vaso-dilator material corresponding to 5.9 mg of histamine per 100 g of original tissue. It was not possible to detect any difference between vaso-dilator effects of equal amounts of the final solutions obtained in the duplicate determinations. Equally satisfactory agreement between duplicates was consistently found throughout this series of experiments. Two flasks each containing 20 g of the minced tissue, saline, and toluene were removed from the incubator after 2, 5, 9, 15, and 25 days at 37° C. Samples of the mixture were removed for nitrogen estimations and the vaso-dilator activity of the remaining solution was determined. Figure 86 shows the disappearance of the vaso-dilator activity during incubation. The figures show that the histamine content of the mixture is constant within the limit of experimental error after the fifth day of incubation.

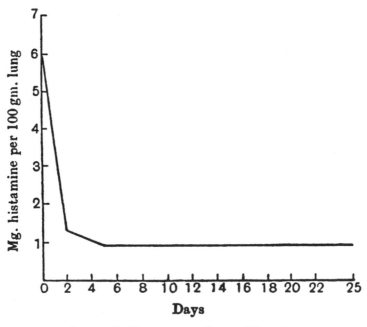

FIGURE 86. Disappearance of natural histamine.

In this experiment the non-protein nitrogen was determined at the beginning, and after 2, 5, 9, and 15 days. The values were as follows: 0.33, 0.54, 0.71, 0.82 and 1.00 g per 100 g of tissue. The figures for the amino-acid nitrogen showed a similar increase. Although the histamine content of the solution did not change appreciably after the fifth day it will be seen that the non-protein and amino-acid nitrogen continued to increase after that time.

Histamine added. When the two flasks had been removed on the fifteenth day, a second experiment was started. To the contents of each of eleven remaining flasks, which had already been incubated for 15 days, 5 mg of histamine were added. Histamine determinations were made immediately on the contents of two of the flasks. The value obtained was 5.2 mg. The determination made on similar material before the addition of the 5 mg of histamine at the fifteenth day indicated 0.16 mg. The recovery of the added histamine was therefore satisfactory. The contents of four of the flasks were heated at 90° C for 4 minutes. The nine flasks were then returned to the incubator. Determinations made two days later showed 5.25 mg in the flasks the contents of which had been heated. The unheated samples contained 3.4 mg. Six days after the histamine was added, the heated flasks showed 4.85 and the unheated 1.6 mg histamine. A determination made on the eighth day on the remaining flask showed 1.7 mg. These two experiments show that both natural and added histamine disappear during autolysis under the conditions of these experiments. Heating at 90° C for 4 minutes prevents this disappearance.

In a third experiment the histamine value fell from 10 mg at the beginning to 0.8 mg per 100 g on the ninth day of incubation; 5 mg of histamine per 100 g were present in the tissue and 5 mg were added.

Figures 87 and 88 illustrate the results of the fourth and fifth experiments. The lung used in Exp. 4 (Figure 87) was not quite as fresh as that used in the other experiments. This may explain the slower disappearance of the histamine in the unheated samples in this experiment. In the fifth experiment there is a more rapid disappearance of natural and added histamine. In both these experiments the heated samples show no detectable loss of the vaso-dilator substance.

Reaction of mixture. The pH of the liquid in which the minced lung was suspended was approximately 7.2 at the beginning of the experiments. In one experiment in which the solution was adjusted to pH 2 with hydrochloric acid, there was no disappearance of histamine during six days' incubation. The same solution at pH 7.2 showed a large decrease in histamine content during the same incubation period.

Other organs than lung. In a few preliminary experiments in which tissues other than lung were studied, it was found that minced liver or kidney also possessed the property of causing histamine to disappear. In one experiment no detectable amount of histamine disappeared from a

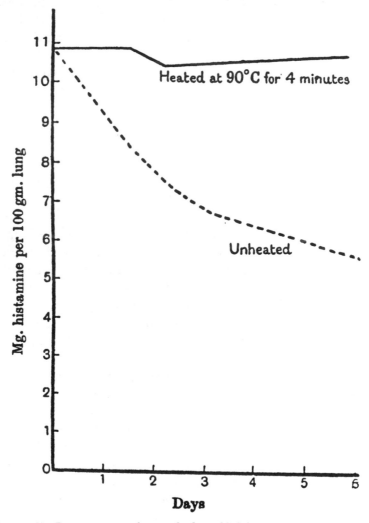

FIGURE 87. Disappearance of natural plus added histamine. 5 mg natural—6 mg added.

suspension of minced muscle during six days incubation. In the experiment with liver and kidney, 5 mg of histamine per 100 g of tissue were added. The original samples of liver and kidney contained 0.6 mg and 0.3 mg vaso-dilator activity expressed as histamine per 100 g. At the end of six days' incubation the unheated flasks contained 0.54 mg and 1.1 mg per 100 g. There was no perceptible loss of vaso-dilator activity in the control samples which had been heated at 90° C for 4 minutes after the addition of the 5 mg of histamine.

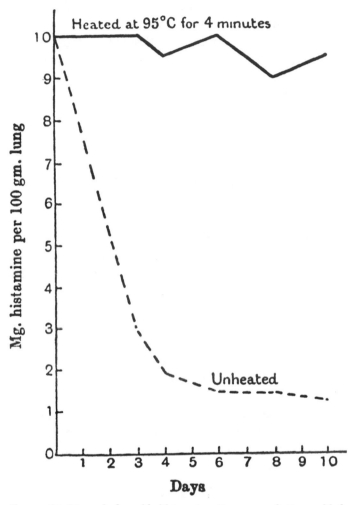

FIGURE 88. Natural plus added histamine. 5 mg natural—5 mg added.

Absence of bacteria. It has been stated by Bradley [146] and by others that micro-organisms do not multiply in a suspension of tissue containing 10 per cent toluene if the mixture is shaken every few hours during the first 24 hours of incubation at 37° C. I am indebted to Dr. P. P. Laidlaw for making cultures from several of the lung suspensions used in these experiments, and for examining stained film-preparations from similar material. The suspensions from which the cultures were taken had not been heated at 90° C and had been incubated at 37° C for 15 days. There was no growth in some of the culture tubes, while in others growth was apparent only after 24 or 48 hours. This finding was taken to indicate the absence of rapidly growing vegetative forms of bacteria. Film-preparations were made from samples of three suspensions which had been incubated for 25 days. No organisms were found.

In several experiments the findings of Best, Dale, Dudley, and Thorpe [82] that lung contains very little vaso-dilator activity which is eliminated by atropine were confirmed. The administration of atropine did not appreciably change the value for the assay of extracts made from material taken at the beginning or the end of the period of autolysis.

The faint possibility existed that some change might be produced in the histamine during the autolysis which would render it susceptible to the strong hydrochloric acid used in the preparation of the extracts for testing. Samples were therefore removed from four flasks which had been incubated for five days. The contents of two of the flasks had been heated at 90° C for 4 minutes before incubation. These samples were filtered and tested without further treatment on etherized cats. The assay on the sample from the unheated material indicated a loss of approximately 80 per cent of the original histamine content. There was no evidence of any loss of histamine in the sample which had been heated. The test of the sample from the heated material gave only such a slightly lower value for the histamine content as would be expected with the less perfect method of extraction employed. The disappearance is therefore not due to the action of the acid on histamine made more susceptible during the autolysis.

The extracts obtained in all the experiments produced a characteristic histamine-like fall in blood pressure. In no case was there any suggestion that the loss of vaso-dilator activity was due to the presence of some antagonistic, pressor material. In some cases the histamine content of extracts was below the limit of detection. There was no evidence of any vaso-constrictor substance in these extracts.

DISCUSSION

The thermolabile activity shown by lung and other tissues incubated in a saline suspension, which causes the disappearance of naturally occurring or added histamine, may prove to possess physiological significance. The experiments recorded in this paper are not concerned with a possible vital function of this action, but only with the phenomenon as seen and studied *in vitro*.

The findings (*a*) that the disappearance of the histamine is completely prevented by heating the suspension at 90° C for 4 minutes; (*b*) that the disappearance proceeds rapidly during the first period, becomes slower, and practically ceases while there is still histamine available; and (*c*) that the addition of more histamine to this mixture produces a renewed disappearance of the vaso-dilator substance, all indicate that the property of lung here investigated possesses some of the characteristics of an enzyme.

The experiments in which atropine was administered show that choline is not an important factor in these results. There is no suggestion that the presence of histamine is masked by the production of vaso-constrictor substances. The time relationships of the action of the known vaso-constrictor materials are such that the sharp fall in blood pressure and the return to the normal level produced by histamine would be changed if appreciable amounts of these substances were present. It has been shown by Kendall [445] that histamine is inactivated by formaldehyde. If a substance with an aldehyde group were produced during the autolysis, an addition compound might be formed with histamine and the vaso-dilator activity of the latter destroyed. This compound would probably be broken up by the strong acid, but whether the structure responsible for the vaso-dilator activity would then be left undisturbed is not as yet known. A more likely possibility is that the mechanism of the disappearance of histamine will be found to be oxidative, since Ewins and Laidlaw [294] have shown that tyramine is oxidized during perfusion through isolated liver. In a very interesting paper Miss Hare [358] has recently shown that this oxidation is due to a definite enzyme system. The fate of the histamine which has disappeared presents a very fascinating problem, the approach to which will be facilitated by the preparation of a much more potent histamine-inactivating material. Some progress in this direction has been made in experiments carried out recently with E. W. McHenry in Toronto.

The thorough study of the distribution in the various tissues of this histamine-inactivating property should yield interesting information. The preliminary experiments reported in this paper demonstrate that kidney and liver possess this property.

SUMMARY

It has been shown that lung and other tissues, when suspended in saline and incubated in the presence of toluene at 37° C, cause the disappearance of naturally occurring or added histamine. The substance or system producing this disappearance is thermolabile.

ACKNOWLEDGMENTS

It is a pleasure to express my deep appreciation to Dr. H. H. Dale for the hospitality of his laboratory and for his active and helpful interest in this work. I am also indebted to Dr. H. W. Dudley for help in many ways.

52. The Inactivation of Histamine

C. H. BEST

E. W. McHENRY

The transient effects produced by the intravenous or subcutaneous injection of small or moderate doses of histamine suggest that the body may possess an efficient means of elimination or inactivation of this substance. When histamine is slowly injected intravenously, relatively large amounts can be administered without the appearance of the characteristic signs which the more rapid injection of small quantities to the same animal produce. It has been reported that very little histamine is found in the urine even after the intravenous injection of large doses of the substance (Oehme [602]). The possibility that the amine may be eliminated by passage from the blood into the intestine has not been investigated.

The recent isolation of histamine from extracts of fresh normal lung, liver (Best, Dale, Dudley, and Thorpe [82]), muscle (Thorpe [751]), and spleen (Dale and Dudley [241]), suggests that the mechanisms responsible for the inactivation of the amine in the body may have considerable physiological significance.

It has been shown by one of us (Best [69]) that lung and other tissues, when suspended in saline and incubated in the presence of toluene at 37° C, cause the disappearance of the physiological activity of naturally occurring or added histamine. In this paper the results of a further study of the distribution, properties, and action of the substance or system producing this inactivation are presented.

METHOD OF ESTIMATION OF HISTAMINE

The histamine content of tissues has been determined by a method which utilizes the stability of the amine in the presence of hot HCl. Samples of the fresh tissue are weighed and 20 g are added to 150 cc of 10 per cent HCl. Heating at 95° C for one hour or less completely disintegrates the tissue. The mixture is then evaporated to dryness *in vacuo*. Two portions, 50 cc each, of 95 per cent ethyl alcohol are added separately and are re-

Originally appeared in the *Journal of Physiology*, LXX (1930), 349–72. From the Department of Physiological Hygiene, University of Toronto.

moved, with some of the acid, by distillation. The residue in the flask is suspended in water, and the remaining trace of acid is neutralized with 20 per cent NaOH. The liquid is filtered through paper, and the flask and the paper are repeatedly washed with distilled water. The histamine is then assayed by comparison of its physiological activity with that of a standard solution of histamine on the blood pressure of the etherized cat. Whenever there is a possibility that choline or a derivative is present, the unknown solutions are assayed against histamine before and after atropinization of the test animal. The accuracy of the method has been tested repeatedly during the last three years. Added histamine can invariably be recovered from tissues with an error of not more than 15 per cent. Histamine estimations have also been made by the quantitative Pauly reaction procedure (Koessler and Hanke [464]).

Distribution of the Histamine-inactivating Property

The histamine-inactivating material was first demonstrated in horse lung and, subsequently, in beef lung, liver, and kidney. It was obvious that the absolute amount of this material in various tissues could not be ascertained until the methods of extraction and assay had been thoroughly investigated. The relative distribution of the activity could, however, be determined by using samples of the various tissues removed immediately after death from an animal and incubated under exactly comparable conditions. The tissues have been obtained from healthy normal dogs which were gently anaesthetized with ether and bled out. 20 g samples of the various tissues were weighed, suspended in 100 cc of 0.9 per cent NaCl, and after a short interval the reaction of the mixture was adjusted to pH 7 with NaOH. Although in subsequent experiments an incubation period of 12 hours or less was found to be sufficient for the destruction of appreciable amounts of histamine, in these experiments 72 hours incubation at 37° C was used. It is unnecessary to report in detail the large amount of data which has accumulated from the determinations of the initial histamine content of the tissues and the amount remaining after incubation, with the necessary controls on the enzyme activity, etc. Fortunately the results have been sufficiently uniform so that the figures from the six experiments can be averaged without involving the risk of distorting the relative values. The findings are given in Table 52.I. The essential procedures can be described by reporting one experiment in more detail.

Exp. 1. The kidneys were removed from a 15 kg dog which had been bled out under ether. Weight of kidneys 85 g. The tissue was minced and three 20 g portions were weighed out and transferred to flasks. 150 cc of 10 per cent HCl were added to one flask and the initial histamine content of the tissue was determined as described above. Assays before and after atropinization of the test animal showed that the depressor activity attributable to histamine was negligible, i.e., there was not enough histamine to assay. 100 cc of 0.9 per cent NaCl were added to each of the other flasks. One flask was heated until the contents boiled. 40 mg of histamine were then added to each flask, and they were placed in an incubator at 37° C for 72 hours. Histamine determinations on these tissues showed that the heated material contained 36 mg, and the unheated material 0.3 mg. 20 g of moist kidney therefore destroyed practically 40 mg of histamine in 72 hours under these conditions.

Values for the histamine content of the various dog's tissues are also shown in Table 52.I. It is apparent that the histamine distribution is not the same in this species as in others (Dale [239]). It is perhaps significant

TABLE 52.I

DISTRIBUTION OF HISTAMINE-INACTIVATING SUBSTANCE AND OF HISTAMINE IN DOG TISSUES

Tissue	No. of Specimens of Tissue Examined	Mg Histamine Inactivated by 1 kg Tissue	Histamine, Determined by Blood Pressure Method, Expressed as mg per kg of Tissue
Blood	6	55	0.4
Muscle	4	30	7.0
Liver	6	0–10	33.0
Kidneys	10	1000	4.0
Spleen	4	35	not determined
Lung	6	35	16.5
Heart	6	0	4.0
Skin	2	0	not determined
Adrenal	2	25	"
Digestive tract			
stomach	4	0	30.0
duodenum	6	1000	35.0
jejunum	2	1000	35.0
caecum	2	1000	20.0
Bladder	1	35	not determined
Urine	2	0	0.2

that most of the previous determinations have been made on the tissues of herbivorous animals.

Comparison of the histamine-inactivating power of various beef tissues has demonstrated that the kidney is at least twelve times as active as the lung, and more active than any other tissue investigated. Beef kidney was, therefore, the obvious source of the larger amounts of the histamine-inactivating substance which were necessary for further investigation.

Preparation of a Stable Powder

Active aqueous or alcoholic extracts of beef kidney can be prepared, but the histamine-inactivating substance is unstable in these solutions. After some experimentation, a useful initial procedure was found to be the immediate extraction of the fat with acetone and ether and the rapid drying of the residue in a current of air. The dry material was finely ground and was stored in air-tight containers. The details of the preparation of one lot of this dry material will illustrate the methods. 22 kg of fresh kidney were finely minced, and the minced material was placed in a vessel containing 225 litres of 95 per cent acetone. After 12 hours extraction the acetone was removed by filtration. The residue was washed twice with small amounts of acetone and twice with small amounts of ether and was then dried in air.

When care was taken to remove all the acetone and ether, and to keep the container in which the powder was stored well sealed, no loss of histamine-inactivating power could be detected by the tests which were carried out each month for the period of a year. The potency possessed by this powder is practically the same as that of the fresh kidney from which it was prepared. Under favourable conditions 200 mg of the crude powder will inactivate 2 mg of histamine in 24 hours. If the powder is dissolved in water at pH 7 and the mixture filtered, the clear filtrate contains about half the activity of the original powder. These aqueous solutions are not stable, but glycerine extracts retain their activity for at least three weeks. The glycerine may be removed by dialysis without loss of active material. The results of preliminary experiments indicate that the histamine-inactivating substance may be considerably concentrated and purified by selective adsorption and subsequent release from an adsorbing agent, but materials obtained by these procedures were not used in the investigations reported in this paper. It may be mentioned here that the active extract can be sterilized by passage through a Berkefeld filter. Sterile histamine solution incubated under aseptic conditions with sterile kidney extract is rapidly inactivated. The faint possibility that bacterial action might be contributing to this inactivation of histamine is, therefore, eliminated.

The Properties of the Histamine-inactivating Material

Temperature

In all the investigations described in this section, the kidney powder prepared as described above was used. The effect of temperature was studied by determining the action of 200 mg of the kidney powder on 2 mg of histamine at pH 7, during 24 hours incubation. The histamine-inactivating material is inactive at 5° C, slightly active at 20° C, and the maximum activity is at approximately 37° C. At 60° C or above there is no inactivation of histamine. The histamine-inactivating material is destroyed at 60° C, as there is no inactivation of histamine during subsequent incubation of this material at 37° C.

Hydrogen-Ion Concentration

The effect of hydrogen-ion concentration has been investigated by incubating the kidney powder and histamine in various phosphate buffer mixtures. Citrate buffers could not be used because the citrate inhibits the histamine-inactivating material. Care had to be taken to keep the phosphate-ion concentration constant, since phosphate also affects the activity. The

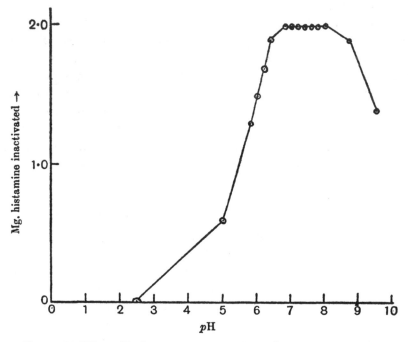

FIGURE 89. Effect of hydrogen-ion concentration on histamine inactivation.

reaction of the buffer mixtures was adjusted by HCl or NaOH. The activities of the histamine-inactivating material at hydrogen-ion concentrations from pH 2.5 to pH 9.5 are shown in Figure 89. If the material which has been incubated at pH 2.5 is adjusted to neutrality and incubated again there is no return of activity. The effects of hydrogen-ion concentrations lower than pH 9.5 have not been determined. All the buffers we have used to secure this range of pH interfere with the action of the histamine-inactivating substance. Michaelis' barbituric acid buffer (Michaelis [563]) is more satisfactory than the others we have investigated.

Time Relationships

Under this heading two series of investigations will be considered: (1) the determination of the amount of histamine destroyed in various intervals of time, when the ratio of histamine to histamine-inactivating substance is kept constant, and (2) the determination of the amount of histamine destroyed in a definite time, when the proportion of histamine to histamine-inactivating substance is varied.

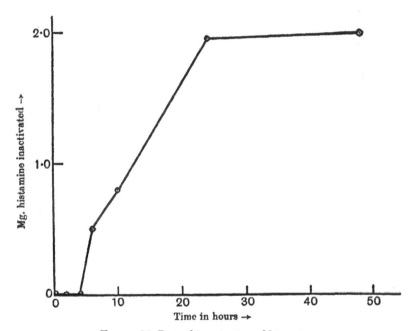

FIGURE 90. Rate of inactivation of histamine.

A curve illustrating the rate of disappearance of histamine from a mixture containing 200 mg of kidney powder and 2 mg of histamine in 100 cc of phosphate buffer solution at pH 7 is shown in Figure 90. Each point on this curve represents the average of determinations made on two solutions. The duplicate values were in every case the same within the limits of experimental error. These results show that, under these conditions, the destruction of histamine is practically complete in 24 hours. In Figure 91 the rate of disappearance of histamine, when the amount of the amine is kept constant at 0.2 mg and the amount of powder is varied from 0.2 g to 1 g, is shown. In the experiment, the results of which are illustrated in

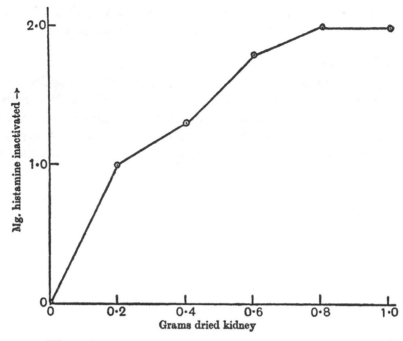

FIGURE 91. Effect of concentration of histamine-inactivating substance on histamine destruction (24 hrs).

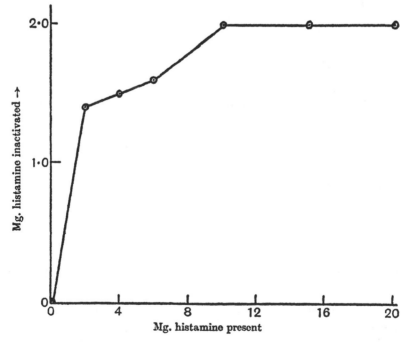

FIGURE 92. Effect of concentration of histamine upon its inactivation (24 hrs).

Figure 92, the amount of kidney powder is kept constant at 0.2 g and the quantity of histamine is varied from 2 to 20 mg. In all these experiments 100 cc of phosphate buffer solution at pH 7 were used.

The Effect of Various Ions

In this series of experiments we studied the disappearance of histamine from a mixture containing 500 mg of dried kidney, 2 mg of histamine, and 100 cc of distilled water, in which the salt of the ion under investigation was present in 0.1 molar concentration. Sodium, potassium, calcium, and ammonium chlorides, sodium sulphate, and disodium phosphate were used. The calcium chloride solution was adjusted to neutrality with a small amount of sodium hydroxide. The results showed that, of the anions, sodium and potassium were without effect. Ammonium produces a slight, and calcium a very pronounced, inhibition of histamine inactivation. The chloride ion has no effect. Sulphate inhibits the inactivation, while phosphate definitely accelerates the action of the kidney powder. In attempting to use McIlvaine's citrate buffers it was found that the citrate ion, in 0.02 molar concentration in neutral solution, prevents the inactivation of histamine.

A series of experiments in which the effects of various concentrations of cyanide were studied was carried out. 200 mg of dried kidney and 2 mg of histamine and 100 cc of distilled water were used. Potassium cyanide to secure 0.004, 0.002, 0.001 and 0.0005 molar concentrations was added. In every case there was complete inhibition of the histamine-inactivating power of the kidney powder.

The Effect of Oxygen

The results of the cyanide experiments suggest that the mechanism of this inactivation of histamine may be oxidative. To investigate the effects of oxygen, histamine and material containing the inactivating substance were incubated at 37° C in atmospheres of oxygen and of nitrogen. The procedure and the results can be presented by describing one experiment.

Exp. 2. A solution of 2 mg of histamine in 10 cc of a distilled water extract of kidney powder was placed under toluene in each of two flasks. The flasks were immersed in a water bath which was kept at 37° C. Oxygen was bubbled through one flask and nitrogen through the other for a period of 4 hours. The disappearance of histamine from the oxygen flask was 25 per cent, while the loss from the nitrogen flask was just detectable. In another experiment the results with hydrogen were the same as with nitrogen.

In Exp. 2 the histamine-inactivating material was in solution and in contact with the histamine, before the oxygen was displaced by the other gases. There may have been some oxygen uptake in this period. In another experiment the air was removed from a flask containing kidney powder and histamine in phosphate buffer solution. Nitrogen was allowed to flow in. The flask was then sealed and incubated for 24 hours. No inactivation of histamine was observed, while a control experiment, in which 2 mg of histamine were destroyed, demonstrated that the histamine-inactivating material was active.

To investigate the possibility that the change responsible for the inactivation of histamine was reversible, attempts were made to reactivate the solutions which had been incubated, by reducing agents. The solutions were treated with powdered zinc and HCl, or with sodium sulphite, and kept at various temperatures, but no reappearance of histamine could be detected.

THE SPECIFICITY OF THE HISTAMINE-INACTIVATING SUBSTANCE

The only other known enzyme-like substance or system which has the property of destroying an amine is the tyramine oxidase (Hare [358]), studied in Hopkins' laboratory by Miss Hare. Tyramine added to a solution containing the histamine-inactivating material may be roughly assayed by comparing the blood pressure raising effect of the solution with that of a solution in which is dissolved a known amount of tyramine. When tyramine is incubated with the histamine-inactivating substance, under the optimum conditions for the inactivation of histamine, there is no perceptible loss of the physiological activity of tyramine. The optimum conditions for the oxidation of tyramine by liver tissue are quite different from those under which histamine is most rapidly inactivated by the powder obtained from kidneys. Moreover, the distribution and the effect of cyanide on the activity are not the same for the two systems. These findings suggest that there is a specific substance or system in the body for the inactivation of histamine.

The properties of this substance or system, which is responsible for the disappearance of histamine, are similar to those of the better known enzymes. One or more enzymes may be responsible for the change in the histamine molecule which takes place under the conditions of our experiments. We suggest, however, that the substance, or system, which produces a change in structure responsible for the loss of physiological activity of histamine be designated histaminase. Until more is known of the reaction in which we are interested, we propose to discuss it as the histamine-histaminase reaction.

The Inactivation of Histamine by Formaldehyde

A. I. Kendall [445] has reported that the addition of small amounts of formaldehyde to a solution surrounding an isolated uterus or section of intestine will completely inhibit the contractions ordinarily produced by histamine. He assumed that formaldehyde produces a condensation product with histamine, according to the equation:

$$RNH_2 + O : CH_2 \rightarrow RN : CH_2 + H_2O.$$

One of us pointed out in a previous paper (Best [69]) that this reaction must be considered as a possible, though unlikely, explanation of the inactivation of histamine by certain tissues. With this in mind some study has been made of the inactivation of histamine by formaldehyde.

The effect of formaldehyde has been determined by adding the desired amount to tissue extracts containing histamine and to pure histamine solutions. The histamine was then assayed by the blood-pressure method. As the results were not in complete accord with those of Kendall, who used isolated smooth muscle as a test object, experiments were also made using the isolated virgin guinea-pig uterus, following the technique described by Burn and Dale [156]. In most cases the results of assay of histamine by the two methods were in good agreement.

To a muscle extract, the histamine content of which had previously been determined, formaldehyde was added to give a concentration of 0.3 per cent. Direct blood-pressure assays showed that 60 per cent of the histamine was inactivated within 30 minutes at room temperature and that, during a further period of 4 hours, no more inactivation occurred. At the end of this time the formaldehyde concentration was doubled. A further slight inactivation occurred. The injection of the same concentration of formaldehyde in saline, without histamine, has no effect upon the blood pressure of the etherized cat.

The incompleteness of disappearance of histamine activity is not due to insufficient formaldehyde. On the basis of the equation postulated by Kendall, 300 times the quantity of formaldehyde necessary for the reaction was present.

Approximately the same amounts of histamine in lung extract, and of pure histamine in solution, were inactivated by a given concentration of formaldehyde. In the case of pure histamine the inactivation was found to occur within 5 minutes, while 30 minutes were required for tissue extracts. Treatment of samples from these solutions, immediately after inactivation, with hydrochloric acid, as in the routine determination of histamine carried out in this laboratory, restored approximately two-thirds of the lost depressor activity.

The effect of temperature upon the histamine-formaldehyde reaction was determined by making up a pure histamine solution, to which was added formaldehyde to give a concentration of 0.3 per cent. This was divided into two lots, each of which was kept under a layer of toluene in a separatory funnel, one at room temperature, the other in an incubator at 37° C. Samples were removed at intervals and assayed by the blood-pressure method. Some of the samples were also assayed on the isolated uterus. The results of the two methods of assay agreed well. At room temperature there was 40 per cent inactivation of histamine in 24 hours. No further change occurred until after 12 days, when a slight loss was detected. At 37° C there was 50 per cent inactivation within 24 hours with no further detectable change during 5 days. From then on, a gradual decline in depressor activity occurred, until none was left at 33 days. Complete inhibition of the depressor effect of histamine was not secured at room temperature under the conditions of these experiments. It will be noted that there are two stages in the inactivation of histamine by formaldehyde. The first, in which about 50 per cent of the activity is lost, is immediate, and is probably due to the condensation reaction suggested by Kendall. The second stage is delayed and may be an oxidation phenomenon.

A similar immediate partial inactivation of tyramine, as indicated by a loss in pressor activity, is observed after addition of formaldehyde.

Because of the discrepancy between Kendall's results, i.e., complete inactivation, and the partial loss found when determinations were made by the blood-pressure method, the effects of formaldehyde-treated histamine on the isolated virgin guinea-pig uterus were studied. In the preliminary work with the isolated uterus, a number of solutions used for blood-pressure tests were assayed against standard histamine solutions on the isolated uterus. The results secured by the two methods were in good agreement. But it was noted that, with solutions containing the larger amounts of formaldehyde, the uterus did not respond well after the first addition of formaldehyde solution, despite thorough washing. Moreover, the initial contraction with such a solution was delayed. It seemed likely that this might be due to the effect of the formaldehyde, not upon the histamine, but upon the uterus. Four similar experiments were, therefore, performed in which increasing amounts of formaldehyde were added to the uterus bath immediately before the addition of histamine. The formaldehyde solution was carefully neutralized. A concentration of formaldehyde of about 0.12 in 100 affected the uterus so that it would no longer react to histamine, even after several washings. Concentrations of formaldehyde considerably less than this, which diminished but did not obliterate the histamine effect, did not produce a loss in sensitivity of the uterus to histamine. Kendall stated that, using concentrations of aldehyde not less than 1 in 750, he secured no results when he added histamine. It seems possible that in this concentration the formaldehyde acts on the histamine, but also poisons the uterus.

The Histamine-Histaminase Reactions

The change produced in histamine by histaminase may be physical or chemical. It is possible that a sorption compound is formed, but it seems likely that such a complex would be broken up by hydrochloric acid digestion. The possibility has already been considered that the change might be that of condensation, similar to the aldehyde-histamine reaction suggested by Kendall, but the differences between this reaction and the histaminase reaction have been pointed out. Moreover, the physiologically active amine is in part restored when the formaldehyde-histamine compound is boiled with hydrochloric acid. It seems likely that histaminase produces a more profound change in histamine. Ewins and Laidlaw [294] found that tyramine was oxidized in the organism to hydroxyphenyl-acetic acid, with a probable intermediate, alcohol stage. Guggenheim and Loeffler [338], investigating the metabolism of amines, isolated corresponding compounds as end products from several amines, but were unable to obtain iminazole-acetic acid by inactivation of histamine.

Certain features of the histaminase reaction have been mentioned. Histamine is so altered that digestion with hydrochloric acid does not restore the physiological activity. The change is oxidative, since potassium cyanide inhibits it completely, and it is accelerated by oxygen and inhibited under anaerobic conditions. If histaminase produced iminazole-acetic acid from histamine the concentration of the iminazole nucleus in the digest would be unchanged. The Koessler-Hanke modification of the Pauly reaction (Koessler and Hanke [464]), while not specific for iminazole derivatives, is useful for their estimation. Employing the Koessler-Hanke procedure, we have studied the iminazole values of histamine solutions, before and after the action of histaminase. The results of these determinations have been compared with the depressor activity of these solutions.

Preliminary experiments were carried out to determine the total histamine and iminazole values of solutions secured by incubating mixtures of the kidney powder, water, and added histamine. In the determination of iminazole values it is necessary to have solutions that are free from substances which interfere with the diazo reaction. In these earlier experiments two methods of precipitation of the proteins and interfering substances were used. These were: (1) lead acetate, with removal of lead by hydrogen sulphide or sodium phosphate; (2) Schenk's reagent (2 per cent mercuric chloride in 0.8 per cent hydrochloric acid) and removal of the mercury with hydrogen sulphide. The procedure from this point was the same in the two cases. The mixture was filtered, the filtrate evaporated to dryness on a water bath, and the residue taken up in a known volume of water for the colorimetric determinations.

In these experiments inactivation of only a part of the added histamine was secured. The diazo value of the solution of kidney powder was very large, and, when calculated as histamine, was usually several times that of the histamine added. After the incubation period the digests, one of each pair having been heated to boiling before incubation, were treated with the routine HCl procedure and subsequently with lead acetate or Schenk's reagent. The iminazole value was consistently less after Schenk's reagent than after lead acetate. The results of these preliminary experiments suggested that some of the physiological activity disappeared without a corresponding loss of the iminazole value. Unsuccessful attempts were made to separate and identify the iminazole compound which it was thought might have been formed. These experiments were complicated by the high diazo values secured. To overcome this, in the experiments outlined, it would be necessary to carry out procedures to eliminate the compounds other than histamine which give the diazo reaction. As an alternative to this tedious procedure, it was considered advisable to attempt to measure the changes in the iminazole ring of histamine when the amine was added to the fluid perfused through isolated kidneys. The technique of this perfusion is described in the following section.

TABLE 52.II

EFFECT OF PERFUSION ON HISTAMINE AND IMINAZOLE
CONTENT OF BLOOD

	Histamine (mg)	Iminazole (mg)
Before perfusion	0.02	131
After perfusion	0.04	83
Loss	—	48

Initial blood volume 1100 cc.   Final volume 1000 cc.

In a control experiment kidneys were perfused with blood without added histamine. Portions of the blood were taken before and after perfusion for determination of histamine by the depressor method, and of iminazole derivatives by the diazo reaction, after precipitation with Schenk's reagent. The results are shown in Table 52.II. In this and subsequent experiments all iminazole values are calculated as milligrams of histamine base.

The average iminazole value before perfusion, in a series of experiments, was 15 mg per 100 cc blood; after perfusion 10 mg per 100 cc.

In a similar experiment histamine was added to the blood. The results are shown in Table 52.III.

TABLE 52.III
DISAPPEARANCE DURING PERFUSION OF HISTAMINE ADDED TO BLOOD

| | Histamine (mg) | Iminazole | | |
		Total (mg)	Due to blood (mg)	Due to histamine (mg)
Before perfusion	283	386	91	295
After perfusion	108	208	61	147
Loss	175	178	30	148
Initial blood volume 840 cc. Final volume 570 cc.				

The kidneys were found to contain almost no histamine at the end of the experiment. As determined by physiological assay, two-thirds of the histamine was inactivated during perfusion. This was accompanied by a loss of iminazole of the same order. Presumably this loss was due to a disruption of the iminazole ring.

In all the above experiments the somewhat difficult and tedious methods of precipitation with Schenk's reagent or with lead acetate were used. The subsequent experiments were carried out to find a simple and more rapid method of preparation of solutions for colour determination. A histaminase solution was prepared by extracting dried kidney with water, using 1 g of dried kidney to 9 cc of water. As this extract does not retain its potency indefinitely, a fresh solution was made up for each experiment. Using this source of histaminase, test solutions were prepared by adding distilled water to the mark of a 100 cc flask containing enzyme solution and histamine. These mixtures were transferred to a 250 cc Erlenmeyer flask and toluene was added. After the desired period of incubation the toluene was removed. Determinations were made of the histamine content of the aqueous solution, without further treatment, by the blood-pressure method, and of iminazole. The physiological estimation was carried out without difficulty, but, in the diazo reaction, green colours were developed by the unheated solution and clear yellow by the control solutions. Neither colour could be matched with the Koessler-Hanke cresol-red, methyl-orange standard. Presumably there were substances present in these solutions which inhibited or masked the diazo reaction.

An attempt was made to remove these interfering substances by adsorption on Eastman's special carbon. Histamine was adsorbed and could not be removed by leaching with 1 per cent dipotassium hydrogen phosphate, 1 per cent potassium dihydrogen phosphate, or 1 per cent acetic acid. Washing with 1 per cent ammonia removed some of the histamine, but the filtrate did not give a satisfactory diazo colour.

To separate the iminazole compounds from those substances interfering with the colour reaction dialysis was tried. At first the Hanke and Koessler [357] apparatus for continuous dialysis was employed, with fish-bladder condoms as the sacs. This apparatus proved to be cumbersome and difficult to regulate. However, assays for histamine by the depressor method and for iminazole derivatives, using the diazo reaction, could be performed directly on the fluid outside the sac without further treatment. It was found that consistent results could be secured without the complicated apparatus. The material to be dialysed was placed in a fish-bladder condom, a layer of toluene added, and the sac suspended in a beaker. Water was placed in the beaker to the level of the liquid in the sac. The water was replaced by a second similar quantity at the end of two days. After four days the two lots of diffusates were combined, and the volume made up to a definite figure. The dialysis was carried out in a cold room.

TABLE 52.IV

DIFFUSIBILITY STUDIES

Histamine Initially Present	Histamine (blood-pressure assay)			Iminazole in Diffusate		
	Diffusate (mg)	Sac (mg)	Total (mg)	Total (mg)	Due to kidney solution (mg)	From the added histamine (mg)
0	0	0	0	1.4	1.4	0
0	0	0	0	1.3	1.3	0
5	0	0	0	2.2	1.4	0.8
5 (boiled control)	3.6	1.0	4.6	5.0	1.4	3.6
10	3.0	0.8	3.8	3.9	1.4	2.5
10 (boiled control)	6.9	2.0	8.9	8.1	1.4	6.7

For these dialysis experiments, mixtures of kidney extract, histamine and water under a layer of toluene were employed. These were incubated for a desired interval at 37° C, and then heated to boiling to terminate the histaminase reaction. The mixtures were then washed into the dialysis sacs. In three sets of experiments similar results were secured. The results of one series are given in Table 52.IV. The "iminazole" values are calculated as milligrams of histamine base in this and subsequent tables.

In two cases a known quantity of histamine was added to portions of the diffusate. The iminazole value of the resulting solution equalled the value of the diffusate, calculated as histamine, plus the added histamine. This eliminates the possibility that some substance may have developed during the histaminase reaction which masks the diazo reaction.

In these dialysis series, solutions in which the histamine had been inactivated gave a diffusate having a low diazo value. The results secured from the blood-pressure assay were in good agreement with those secured by the diazo method when a blank correction for iminazole contributed by the kidney solution was made. These results suggest either (1) that the change produced in histamine involved the rupture of the iminazole nucleus, or (2) that there was produced a complex non-dialysable compound. This second possibility will be discussed later.

The first suggestion is in agreement with the results secured from the perfusion experiments. The preliminary experiment reported in this section did not reveal such a change, but in this case conditions were different and only a relatively small part of the histamine had been inactivated. It occurred to us that there might be a series of progressive changes in the histamine molecule, after the first of which the physiological activity might be weakened without the iminazole ring being affected. The later steps in the reaction might lead to a disruption of the ring. With this in mind it was decided to carry out an experiment in which histamine and iminazole were determined after varying periods of incubation.

The period of incubation required for the inactivation of histamine is greatly influenced by the ratio of the amounts of histamine and histaminase. For this time series a standard preparation, consisting of 25 cc kidney solution, 5 mg histamine base, and 75 cc water, was used. Control flasks, the contents of which were boiled to destroy the enzyme, were prepared and examined after each interval. This incubation period varied from 4 to 72 hours. After incubation the solutions were heated to boiling to terminate the reaction and were then dialysed. Estimations of histamine by the blood-pressure method, and of iminazole by the diazo reaction, were made on all diffusates. The results of these are given in Table 52.V.

The iminazole values, after correction for the amount in the kidney solution, are lower than the histamine determinations, but the decrease in the iminazole parallels the loss of histamine. This is particularly noticeable in the solutions incubated for the longer periods, in which larger amounts of histamine were inactivated.

The possibility exists that a non-diffusible compound of histamine may have been produced. The contents of the sac after dialysis, in several of the above experiments, were carried through the hydrochloric acid digestion procedure. Iminazole determinations were made and the results agreed closely with the histamine values obtained by the blood-pressure method of assay. The small correction for the iminazole value of the kidney extract

TABLE 52.V

DISAPPEARANCE OF HISTAMINE DURING INCUBATION WITH A KIDNEY EXTRACT

	Histamine in Diffusate (blood pressure) (mg)	Iminazole		
Incubation Period (hr)		Total in diffusate (mg)	Due to kidney solution (mg)	From the added histamine (mg)
4	3.5	4.5	1.7	2.8
4 (control)	3.8	4.1	1.7	2.4
8	3.0	3.9	1.7	2.2
8 (control)	3.6	4.1	1.7	2.4
24	1.2	2.5	1.7	0.8
24 (control)	3.6	4.5	1.7	2.8
72	0	2.0	1.7	0.3
72 (control)	3.6	4.1	1.7	2.4

inside the sac was calculated utilizing the assumption, which has been verified for added histamine, that the iminazole is distributed in the same concentration in the fluids inside and outside the sac.

In all this experimental work, where the histamine has been almost completely inactivated by histaminase, the iminazole value has been proportionately decreased. The dialysis experiments, the results of which are more clear-cut than those secured by precipitation methods, show that the iminazole content is lowered in roughly the same ratio as the physiological activity of histamine is diminished. The estimation of iminazole by means of the diazo reaction, is, at best, unsatisfactory. We have found, as have many others, that the formation of the colour is easily inhibited or masked by interfering substances, which are difficult to remove. Moreover, the colour secured is not specific for the iminazole ring. In the dialysis experiments the iminazole value contributed by the kidney solution has been subtracted from the total, and the difference is due to the added histamine. The evidence justifies the conclusion that, under the conditions of these experiments, the iminazole ring in the histamine molecule has been broken.

A study of the mechanism of the breaking of the iminazole ring and the search for products of this change furnish opportunity for further work. The results of preliminary experiments, using the Barcroft apparatus, demonstrate that there is an uptake of gas, presumably oxygen, during the inactivation of histamine; but quantitative data, which should be very interesting, have not as yet been secured.

PERFUSION EXPERIMENTS

The results of the study of the distribution of histaminase demonstrate that in the dog the kidney contains more of this enzyme than any other tissue, with the exception of the intestine. To investigate the ability of various tissues to inactive histamine under more physiological conditions a series of perfusion experiments on isolated dog's tissues have been performed. Kidneys perfused with defibrinated blood, heparinized blood, gum-ringer solution, and Ringer's solution have been studied; also liver perfused with defibrinated blood through the hepatic artery and portal vein, isolated hind limbs perfused with defibrinated blood, and surviving isolated hearts perfused with Ringer's solution through the coronary arteries. In each experiment a known amount of histamine was added, usually very gradually, to the perfusion fluid. At the end of the experiment the perfusion fluid and the tissue were analysed for histamine.

Very little description of the perfusion apparatus or of the technique of the experiments is necessary. In most of the experiments the tissues were removed from the anaesthetized animal as soon as it had been bled out. In the experiments where artificial perfusion fluids were used the animals were not bled out. The necessary cannulae were inserted and the tissue was placed in a cabinet in which the air was kept at 37° C and saturated with water vapour. The Dale-Schuster [245] system of diaphragm pumps was used to circulate the blood, which was aerated with oxygen containing 5 per cent CO_2 in the Hooker artificial lung in the manner described by Burn and Dale [158].

The results of the kidney experiments are shown in Table 52.VI. A protocol of one experiment, in which each of the tissues studied is perfused, is given.

Exp. 3. Kidney. A dog weighing 18 kg was anaesthetized with chloroform. 40 mg of heparin were injected intravenously. 930 cc of blood were removed from the aorta and collected in a vessel containing 100 mg of heparin. The aorta and vena cava were cut, between ligatures, just distal to the origin of the renal vessels. All branches of the aorta and vena cava were ligatured for a distance of 3 cm above the renal vessels. Cannulae were placed in the aorta and vena cava, and the kidneys, with some 10 cm of each ureter attached, were removed. Weight of kidneys 93 g. Connections with the arterial and venous systems of the perfusion apparatus were made and the flow of blood was started. The rate of flow was kept constant at approximately 65 cc of blood per minute. 200 mg of histamine in 50 cc of Ringer's solution were added from a burette during the first two hours of the perfusion. Calculated amount of histamine in kidneys at beginning of experiment was less than 1 mg. Some urine was secreted during the first two hours. After four hours the perfusion was stopped. Weight of kidneys, which were oedematous, was 127 g. Histamine contained in kidneys 8 mg. Histamine contained in the perfusion fluid and washings from the apparatus 36 mg. Histamine inactivated 156 mg.

Exp. 4. Liver. Weight of dog 14 kg. Weight of liver 480 g. Volume of defibrinated blood 950 cc. Blood flow from hepatic vein 150 cc per minute. 100

TABLE 52.VI
Results of Perfusion Experiments

Organ Perfused	Weight of Organ Before (g)	Weight of Organ After (g)	Volume and Character of Perfusing Fluid (cc)	Histamine Added (mg)	Perfusion Time (hr)	Histamine in Organ after Perfusion (mg)	Histamine in Fluid after Perfusion (mg)	Total Histamine after Perfusion (mg)	Total Histamine Inactivated (mg)
Kidney	—	103	580 blood	10	3	0.4	0.2	0.6	9.4
Kidney	—	127	930 blood	20	3	0.2	0	0.2	19.8
Kidney	—	95	500 blood +	100	3	1.2	6.6	7.8	92.2
Kidney	90	186	300 gum ringer + 610 blood + 100 saline	300	4	42	108	150	150
Kidney	149	207	950 blood	150	5	2.9	1.6	4.5	145.5
Kidney	137	178	800 blood	200 slowly	4½	2.9	2.2	5.1	194.9
Kidney	52	173	430 blood + 170 gum ringer	200 slowly	4½	0.7	0.1	0.8	199.2
Kidney	150	202	1100 blood	200 slowly	5½	9.5	1.1	10.6	189.4
Kidney	99	157	840 blood	None control	4	0.3	0.4	0.7	—
None control	—	—	610 blood	10	4	—	9.6	9.6	0.4
Liver	—	758	950 blood + 400 gum ringer	100	3	70	25	95	5
Liver	—	728	620 blood + 600 gum ringer	100	3	66	24	90	10
Liver	—	748	940 blood	200 slowly	4	112	30	142	58

mg of histamine added slowly during the first half-hour of perfusion. Calculated amount of histamine in liver at beginning of experiment 17 mg. Liver increased considerably in bulk. Weight after four hours 720 g. Histamine contained in liver 68 mg. Histamine contained in perfusion fluid and washings 25 mg. Histamine inactivated 24 mg. In two other similar experiments the liver inactivated 26 mg and 21 mg of histamine.

Exp. 5. Isolated limbs. Isolated limbs from a dog weighing 7 kg were perfused with 500 cc defibrinated blood at the rate of 130 cc per minute. 100 mg of histamine added slowly during the first hour: four hours perfusion. Histamine in muscles and skin 41 mg. Histamine in perfusion fluid 12 mg. These figures suggest that about 47 mg of histamine were inactivated, but some may have been retained in the bone marrow.

Exp. 6. Heart. The heart was removed from a 10 kg dog under ether, and was perfused through the coronary arteries in the usual manner. 25 mg of histamine were added slowly to the perfusion fluid. The heart beat grew progressively weaker. At the end of three hours the perfusion fluid contained 18 mg of histamine and the heart 5 mg. In none of these experiments was there any evidence of inactivation of histamine or formation of any depressor substance. In control experiments the isolated heart beat well for at least three hours. In the experiments where histamine was added the duration was usually three hours. The beat was usually not satisfactory for that period.

Perfusion Fluid

In several experiments the amount of histamine inactivated by the oxygenated perfusion fluid alone was determined. Histamine does not disappear from oxygenated Ringer's solution under the conditions of our experiments. The amount inactivated by 600 cc of oxygenated defibrinated blood in four hours was never greater than 2 mg. It may be mentioned here that blood added to kidney powder accelerates the inactivation of histamine, but relatively large amounts of blood are necessary (200 cc of blood to 200 mg of kidney powder). We have not found any histaminase activity in the six samples of normal human blood (50 cc samples) which have been studied.

Discussion

The studies reported in this paper demonstrate that the properties of the histamine-inactivating material under investigation are those which are characteristic of enzymes, and the name histaminase is suggested for the system or substance which is responsible for this loss of the physiological activity of histamine. The optimum conditions for the action of this enzyme are quite different from those of the tyramine oxidase. The physiological activity of tyramine is not destroyed by histaminase. The distribution of histaminase in the body is not the same as that of the tyramine oxidase.

A study of the distribution of histaminase in dog's tissues shows that, in this species, the kidney and intestine are the richest sources of the enzyme. It is not difficult to suggest a reason for the presence of relatively large amounts of the histamine-inactivating material in the wall of the intestine, since it has been shown that the amine is destroyed during passage from the lumen of the gut into the blood (Koessler and Hanke [466]). If it should be shown that some, as yet undetermined, product of the histamine-histaminase reaction is needed in the body, an adequate explanation of the presence of histaminase in such amounts in renal tissue might be forthcoming. It is possible that the kidney is particularly sensitive to histamine, and that the high concentration of histaminase exerts a protective action. The absence of the enzyme from heart muscle is an interesting point. In a number of experiments with heart muscle an increased depressor value, which was not demonstrable in the atropinized animal, was noted after incubation. As this finding was not invariably obtained, further study is needed before its significance can be discussed. The distribution of histaminase in the intestine is worthy of further investigation. The results thus far obtained indicate that the substance is present in very small amounts, if at all, in the dog's stomach, and they suggest that there is no very significant variation in the concentration in various parts of the intestine. A more detailed study may show that this latter finding is only relatively true. Skeletal muscle, liver, and spleen apparently contain very little histaminase. Lung and blood contain moderate amounts of the enzyme. It will be interesting to study the histaminase content of the tissues of animals which are more or less susceptible to histamine than the dog. A convenient unit of histaminase would be the activity necessary to destroy 1 mg of histamine during 24 hours incubation at 37° C, in a phosphate buffer solution at pH 7.

The figures in Table 52.I show that the lungs of the dog do not possess as high a concentration of histamine as the liver or intestine. In unpublished work we have found that the histamine content of normal cat's lungs is approximately 10 mg per kg of tissue. Beef or horse lung may contain 60 to 90 mg per kg, which is appreciably greater than the amount found in other tissues of the same species. Investigations to determine the significance of the high concentration of histamine in lung tissue should, therefore, be carried out, using these, or perhaps other herbivorous animals, rather than the dog or cat.

The study of the properties of histaminase has been facilitated by the preparation of a stable powder from fresh beef kidneys. The optimum conditions for the activity of histaminase and the effects of change in the ratio of the amounts of enzyme and substrate are very similar to those of many other enzymes. The inhibiting effect of citrate and of calcium, and the favouring influence of phosphate ions, are interesting points. The complete inhibition of histaminase by small amounts of cyanide and by the lack of oxygen indicate that the change produced in histamine is oxidative. Preliminary experiments show that there is an uptake of oxygen during the inactivation of histamine, but it has been decided to postpone a comprehensive study of this subject until a more concentrated preparation of histaminase is available. Attempts to recover histamine by treating the histamine-histaminase mixtures after incubation with reducing agents have been unsuccessful. Although considerable time has been expended in studying the histamine-histaminase reaction, little is known as yet about the mechanism. Under certain conditions, which are described above, the iminazole ring is broken during the reaction, and the loss of iminazole is roughly parallel to the decrease in histamine content of the solutions. We have not proven that histaminase cannot produce some loss of the physiological activity of histamine without a breaking of the iminazole ring. A short study of the inactivation of histamine by formaldehyde is included in this paper, since the results demonstrate some differences between the mechanism of this type of inactivation and that of histaminase. Formaldehyde produces an immediate effect upon histamine as judged by the loss of physiological activity, which is decreased by about one-half. The condensation product presumably formed is decomposed by boiling with hydrochloric acid and two-thirds of the lost activity may be restored. Histamine loses all its activity when it is incubated for some time with formaldehyde. Amounts of formaldehyde greatly in excess of that theoretically required to combine with histamine cause only a partial loss of activity within a limited time. Large concentrations of formaldehyde affect an isolated uterus, so that it no longer responds to histamine. This is probably due to a poisoning effect upon the uterine muscle and not to a reaction with histamine.

The results of the experiments on the distribution of histaminase suggest that the kidneys may be particularly adapted for the inactivation of histamine in the body. The perfusion experiments can be regarded as a step in the direction of a study of the physiological significance of histaminase. The conditions under which the kidneys were perfused were not as satisfactory as those used in the investigation of urine formation (Verney and Starling [767]). A few minutes elapsed from the time of death of the animal and the start of the perfusion. No difficulty in obtaining the moderate blood flow provided in these experiments was encountered under these conditions. The kidneys appeared normal during control experiments, and when the histamine was added slowly the tissue was not conspicuously oedematous for the first hour or more of the perfusion. Extreme oedema was usually present at the end of the experiment. In the experiments with kidneys very little histamine was found in the tissue at the end of 4 hours. When liver was perfused, relatively little histamine disappeared in spite of the much greater amount of tissue and a more rapid blood flow. A large amount of histamine was found in the liver at the end of the experiment. Meakins and Harington were led to suggest, by the results of their experiments on the absorption of histamine, that the liver might act as a trap for the amine. The results of these liver experiments are in accord with the findings of Dale and Laidlaw [242], and Guggenheim and Loeffler [338], who were unable to demonstrate the inactivation of more than very small amounts of histamine under similar conditions. The very rapid inactivation of histamine by the perfused kidneys gives support to the suggestion that the kidneys may perform the same function in the intact organism. In the kidney-perfusion experiments, as would probably be the case in the living animal, small quantities of histamine are presented to large amounts of histaminase and the conditions are, in so far as the relative concentration of the two factors is concerned, favourable for the rapid inactivation of the amine. The results of the perfusion experiments in general support the findings of the distribution study and, in addition, suggest that further investigation of the physiological significance of histaminase will be profitable.

Since it has not been established that histamine is the causative agent in any pathological condition there would be no obvious clinical application of histaminase, even if it should be established that the ability of an organism to inactivate histamine can be increased by administration of the enzyme. It is hoped that histaminase may prove a useful tool in the study of the physiological significance of histamine.

Summary and Conclusions

1. The properties of the histamine-inactivating substance are those characteristic of enzymes, and the name histaminase is suggested for the active material which, under the conditions of our experiments, produces the change in structure of the histamine molecule that is responsible for the loss of the physiological activity of the amine.

2. A study of the distribution of histaminase in the dog indicates that kidney and intestine are the richest sources of the enzyme in this species.

3. In the dog the histamine concentration in the lungs is not as high as that in certain other tissues.

4. The histamine-histaminase reaction is inhibited by lack of oxygen and by small amounts of cyanide. Under certain conditions the decrease in the iminazole content of the solutions is roughly parallel to the loss of histamine. This finding suggests that histaminase produces a rupture of the iminazole ring in the histamine molecule. A short study of the action of formaldehyde on histamine has revealed certain differences in the mechanism of action of the aldehyde and of histaminase.

5. Perfusion experiments have been carried out using kidneys, liver, heart and hind limbs of the dog. The results show that the isolated kidneys inactivate histamine much more rapidly than the other tissues investigated.

6. The significance of the results of this study of the inactivation of histamine is discussed, and the direction that further work will take is indicated.

ACKNOWLEDGMENT

It is a pleasure to express our thanks to Miss Gertrude Gavin, M.A., for the expert assistance she has given us in certain aspects of this work.

PROBABLY MY INTEREST IN ANTI-
*coagulants dates from experiments performed as an undergraduate on turtles
in 1920. The great protective phenomenon of blood clotting, which obviously saves our lives so frequently, was a nuisance when it blocked the
cannula which we used for recording blood pressure. It was not until
1928 that I seriously considered working on this problem. The assays of
histamine and choline which I was conducting in Sir Henry Dale's
laboratory were complicated by the blood clots which sometimes formed. I
decided then that we must attempt to concentrate and purify the anticoagulant, heparin, which was available in a crude form from normal animal
tissue.*

*A further introduction to the experimental papers is provided by using
parts of two reviews I have written on anticoagulants.[1]*

*I wish to focus your attention for a time on anticoagulants which have,
at least experimentally, been shown to prevent thrombosis. I will begin
with the one I first used and which was generally available in physiological laboratories forty years ago, i.e., hirudin.*

I

The date of the first use of venesection in human patients would be difficult
to establish. Leeches were employed to replace venesection probably a thousand
years ago and their use was widespread until the turn of the century and
continues in some countries to this day. My father had them available but I
never saw him use them in his medical practice. The druggist or chemist kept
leeches in water in glass jars with a bit of sand in the bottom. They were
not fed for months at a time but the water was changed. In the eighteenth

---

[1]The first excerpt is taken from "A Short Essay on the History of Anticoagulants"
which appeared originally in *Anticoagulants and Fibrinolysins*, ed. R. L. MacMillan
and J. F. Mustard (Toronto: Macmillan, 1961). The second excerpt is from *Essays
in Surgery* (Toronto: University of Toronto Press, 1950).

century leeches were exported from Bavaria and Bohemia to France by special large "diligences"—the "leech express"! Dr. Erik Jorpes tells us that for many years in Sweden and many other European countries, apothecaries were forced, by law, to keep jars of leeches on their shelves [432]. In 1884 John B. Haycraft [380], working in England and also in Strasbourg, reported that blood flow from a leech bite was not easily arrested. He noted that the blood within the body of the leech (Hirudo medicinalis) remained fluid indefinitely and when ejected it did not coagulate. Various experiments were undertaken to determine the source and action of the anticoagulant factor. The conclusion was reached that the leech secretes from its mouth a fluid which destroys the "blood ferment." An extract of leech heads was effective in preventing clotting of dog's or rabbit's blood but not that of Crustacea. It had no action on the curdling of milk, the clotting of myosin or in hastening rigor mortis.

Krüger in Dorpat [610], Dickinson [254] in England, and Erich Schultze [679] of Greifswald in Germany, purified the extract of leech heads and attempted unsuccessfully to isolate the active substance. In 1902 Franz in Jacoby's laboratory in Göttingen [310] attacked the problem. Jacoby was interested in transfusions of blood and suggested to Franz that he should assay the leech extracts under standard conditions on rabbit blood and that he should then use the test as a guide in the purification of the active material. The potency of the leech extract was preserved with thymol and large quantities of stable active material were made available. A method of preparation was evolved which consisted of extracting leech heads in saline for two hours at 60° C. The liquid was centrifuged and the precipitate discarded. The clear supernatant was dried in a desiccator over sulphuric acid. A solution of the dry powder was readily made in distilled water. The active substance was not dialysable and the results of salt precipitations suggested a protein-like structure. In 1903 Professor Jacoby [422] suggested the name "Hirudin."

In 1909 my friend, the late Professor John Mellanby [560], studied the mechanism of action of hirudin and while it is frequently not profitable to attempt the interpretation of older experiments in terms of modern knowledge, it would appear from his results that hirudin contained an antithrombokinase and also an antithrombin. Since Mellanby's thrombin may well have been contaminated with kinase, some of his procedures—even in his careful and experienced hands—gave results which could be interpreted in more than one way. In addition to obtaining strong evidence that hirudin was both an antithrombin and an antikinase, Mellanby showed that fibrinogen removed hirudin from the scene of action. An earlier worker, Bodong [136], had concluded, erroneously it appears, that fibrinogen had been chemically changed by hirudin so that its potential for fibrin formation was decreased.

Interest in hirudin has continued almost to the present time. In 1929 Waldschmidt-Leitz, Stadler, and Steigerwaldt [777] showed that the anticoagulant action of hirudin was lost during tryptic digestion. In 1957, F. Markwardt [554], of the Pharmacological Institute in Greifswald, isolated hirudin in crystalline form. It is a protein with a low molecular weight of about 16,000 as determined by osmotic pressure measurements. Chromatographic and electrophoretic studies indicate a single substance. Fifteen amino acids have been identified. There are relatively large amounts of cystine, asparagine, and glutamic acid. The substance is a potent antithrombin and has been assigned an activity of 8500 antithrombin units per mg. This would be based on the equivalent number of International Units of thrombin inactivated. The prevention of thrombosis by hirudin has not been studied and the substance has not been used in the treatment of human patients. To complete this picture the exact arrangement of the amino acids in hirudin should be determined, the protein should be synthetized and the actions of the pure product should be subjected to a comprehensive investigation by the most modern and well-established methods.

I must confine my remarks about heparin strictly to the historical aspects because we expect plenty of good-natured differences of opinion about the mechanisms of its various actions and its place in therapeutics or in the prevention of disease. There is controversy about almost all important discoveries. Many people almost made each of these advances. In some cases the claims are false; the scientific world is not convinced by others; exceptionally, the discovery is clear-cut and has been overlooked.

II

The clinical use of purified heparin was accelerated and facilitated by the interdepartmental co-operation suggested by Professor W. E. Gallie soon after he became Head of the Department of Surgery in his Alma Mater. Dr. Gallie came to my office in the Department of Physiology and suggested that a research in which both Surgery and Physiology could participate might be productive of new knowledge and that the joint effort would be beneficial to both departments. After giving his proposal some consideration I asked him if he would be interested in having a member of his staff collaborate with workers in my department who were investigating the effect of heparin in the prevention of experimental thrombosis. Dr. Gallie felt that this problem would provide an excellent opportunity for co-operation and he nominated Dr. Gordon Murray as the representative of his department. Dr. Murray had previously been interested and active in several researches on vascular problems.

One of the results of the co-operative work arising from Dr. Gallie's proposal was that purified heparin, which could be given safely to human subjects, was first used on the surgical wards of the Toronto General Hospital in the treatment of patients in whom thrombus formation was feared. In addition to the new scientific knowledge which was obtained, the heparin researches won for the Department of Surgery a second Hunterian Professorship of the Royal College of Surgeons. The first was held by Dr. Gallie in 1924 and the second by Dr. Gordon Murray in 1938.

Dr. Murray's Hunterian lecture carried the title "Heparin in Thrombosis and Embolism" [585]. Dr. Murray graciously acknowledged his indebtedness to the members of our group in Physiology and in the Connaught Laboratories and to Professor Gallie, Head of the Department of Surgery.

Paper 53, which now follows, formed a part of a symposium which was planned to honour Dr. Jay McLean who discovered heparin in 1916, while still a medical student, working in Professor Howell's laboratory at Johns Hopkins University. He had hoped to participate in the symposium but died on November 14, 1957.

53. Preparation of Heparin and its Use in the First Clinical Cases

CHARLES H. BEST, c.b.e., m.d., d.sc., ll.d., f.r.s.

Many of us who were friends of the late Dr. Jay McLean, had looked forward with great pleasure to seeing him again at this time and to discussing the problems which occupied so much of his attention. We all join Dr. Wright in paying tribute to Dr. McLean, the discoverer of heparin, and to Professor W. H. Howell and his colleagues, who extended this work and focused our attention on many of the most important problems in this field. A number of years ago Dr. McLean wrote to me and asked if we would take the responsibility for his collection of notes and reprints and other documents relating to heparin. I was honoured and extremely pleased to accept this invitation.

It is almost always true that a very careful search of the literature will reveal papers which anticipate, to varying degrees, the discovery of a signal advance in medical or other sciences. In 1912, Doyon [261] published a paper in which he described an attempt to isolate and characterize an anticoagulant released by the injection of peptone in a dog. This work was interrupted by World War I. There are a number of other intriguing findings in the literature, for example that of Schmidt [674] in 1892, but their significance could only be appreciated after the discovery of heparin by Dr. McLean [535] in 1916.

On November 14, 1940, Dr. Jay McLean wrote me a long letter describing the whole history of his work on heparin, and a great deal about his subsequent researches. I will quote parts of this letter.

You may, however, be interested to know that the first presentation of the anticoagulant at a scientific society was made February 19, 1916, before the Society of the Normal and Pathological Physiology at the University of Pennsylvania. A. N. Richards, the Secretary was then Professor of Pharmacology, and is now Vice-President of the University for Medical Sciences. These talks were not published although the secretary may have a record in the minutes of the Society. . . . Concerning the lack of articles on heparin in the literature by me, you may be interested in the following. When I wrote the paper on "The thromboplastic action of cephalin," Doctor Howell did not think that I should

Originally appeared in *Circulation*, XIX (1959), 79–86.

include anything about the discovery of the anticoagulant. He felt that this should be studied more thoroughly and a paper written about it later. I argued, however, that I had made this finding during that academic year's work in 1915–1916, and felt that it should be included as a record of the work done during that period. I felt this more strongly because I had already accepted a Fellowship in the Department of Research Medicine at the University of Pennsylvania under Dr. Richard Pearce for the following academic year, 1916–1917 and therefore could not continue the work in Baltimore. He finally agreed to permit its inclusion in the body of the paper.

. . . At first, Doctor Howell was very skeptical that I had found a true anticoagulant. You know that from my method of preparation, I was using very weak heparin and therefore its anticoagulating action was not noticed with the suddenness and brilliancy of an exploding bomb. Furthermore, you will recall that I was searching for coagulants, not an anticoagulant, and that the end point of my experiments was a clot such as is promptly and solidly formed by cephalin. It was only through very careful records, the systematic saving of the little tubes in which I tested the substances, and then repeating the experiments with the same lot of material and finally making new preparations that I gradually became aware that I had an anticoagulant. Naturally I regard the statements in the literature that I discovered this "accidentally" as not correct. It was discovered "incidentally" in the course of the problem but not "accidentally."

. . . You will find in the beginning of my laboratory note-book, which I am sending you, the extent of the problem Doctor Howell outlined in his own handwriting, namely, "The preparation of pure cephalin." In looking over this note-book, will you tolerantly excuse its lack of neatness?

. . . As regards the earlier studies with the anticoagulant, you might be interested in the following: one author calls my attention to the fourth sentence in the first paragraph of my 1916 paper, which would give one the impression that Doctor Howell suggested that I study cuorin and heparphosphatid for their thromboplastic action. The facts are that the problem Howell originally gave me was simply to make cephalin as pure as possible from the brain and to test each fraction I separated out in the phosphatid group for its thromboplastic action. I finished most of this work between October 15 and January 1916. . . . I first prepared cuorin in January 1916, and it was in January, February and March that I established definitely its anticoagulating action, first of cuorin and then heparphosphatid. It was not until later that Doctor Howell became actively associated in work with the anticoagulant by intravascular injections and mechanism of action in vitro.

I can't think of any other material I have that might be of interest to you. May I, however, offer a suggestion which you may or may not deem worthy of mentioning in your lecture. Doctor Howell has always been perfectly clear and fair in his statements about the discovery of the anticoagulant. As the years go by, more authors credit him with the discovery, apparently disregarding my 1916 publication and the statements he made in his 1917 and 1918 publications. In his Harvey Lecture, he definitely states that this work was done by me, and in his 1918 paper you will note that he says "In the course of *his* (*that is Jay McLean's*) work, the anticoagulating action was discovered."

Doctor Howell has always simply stated that he and Holt "first described" heparin.

Dr. McLean attempted several times to return to active experimental work in the heparin field but was engaged in clinical practice.

It was apparent from correspondence which I had with Dr. McLean that he had been trying to interest the United States Public Health Service and institutions in various other countries in doing something about the preservation of his notes, reprints, and other heparin memorabilia. He finally decided to send all of these historical documents to us in the Department of Physiology and the Banting and Best Department of Medical Research. The documents are now stored in the Library of the Charles H. Best Institute.

I had many friendly letters from Dr. McLean. He was most generous in his appreciation of the contribution of our group in Toronto. On May 6, 1940, the discoverer of heparin wrote, "I regard you and the work you stimulated in Toronto to have brought about the debut of heparin for clinical use." My colleagues, Arthur Charles, David Scott, Gordon Murray, Louis Jaques, and T. S. Perrett, deserve a very large share of this praise.

In 1918, Howell and Holt [408] proceeded with the extension of McLean's work. They state, "Attention was first called to this substance during some work done in this laboratory by Jay McLean," that is, to the substance heparin. Howell and Holt go on to say that they varied the methods in many different ways, and finally selected one which yielded a reliable preparation of heparin. In the copies of these articles in the McLean files, there are many interesting marginal comments; for example, Dr. McLean has pointed out that this description of his work by Professor Howell and Dr. Holt was really the first published announcement of the discovery of heparin. There are many interesting points also in Howell and Holt's paper. They introduced, for the first time, the word "heparin"; McLean had referred to these compounds carrying the anticoagulant activity as "phosphatids from heart or liver." They found that heparin could be prepared from lymph glands as well as from heart and liver, as originally shown by McLean. The antagonism between cephalin and heparin on the clotting system was described in the Howell and Holt paper. It has been questioned whether the material that Howell and Holt had was actually heparin, since it was soluble in the crude form in ether. It is now considered that it probably was heparin, since it became insoluble in ether after repeated alcohol precipitations. In 1922 and 1925 Howell [405; 406] described the preparation of heparin in more purified form and in 1928 he [407] published a detailed report on its chemical and physiologic reactions.

In 1924 Mason [557] showed that heparin would prevent the intravascular clot produced in rabbits and dogs by the injection of thromboplastin from tissue extracts. These were true clots and not platelet thrombi. In 1925 my close friend C. I. Reed [632] found that heparin was an effective anticoagulant in dogs and was well tolerated. In 1927, Shionoya [701] reported that the administration of heparin did not prevent the agglutination of platelets when blood was made to pass through a collodion tube. Thus it seemed that heparin might be an anticoagulant but not an antithrombotic agent.

Professor Howell undoubtedly anticipated many of the developments which took place in the future. He expressed the hope that heparin would find a suitable application in experimental work and possibly in the therapeutic treatment of disorders of coagulation. Professor Howell thought it not improbable that this substance might be of physiologic significance, and in discussions on coagulation of the blood he often referred to heparin as a "physiological anticoagulant."

While working in Dale's laboratory in London in 1928 I had decided to organize a group, on my return to Toronto, to study the chemistry and physiology of heparin. Later that year, Dr. E. W. McHenry and I, eager to use an effective anticoagulant in our histaminase work, found it possible to prepare active fractions from ox liver by Howell's method. A little later I made a comprehensive study of the literature and it became apparent that very little work indeed was being done in this field. A potent anticoagulant, that could be used for long continued administration in animals, was not available. No anticoagulant preparation was safe for clinical work and none was being used. In the Connaught Laboratories I had been intimately concerned with the preparation of insulin and of liver extract for administration to human patients and I visualized a similar advance in the heparin field. Progress was, apparently, also inhibited by the lack of convincing evidence that heparin inhibited platelet agglutination as well as coagulation.

It was obvious that further chemical work on the purification of heparin must precede physiologic and clinical studies. In 1929 I was able to interest a young organic chemist, Mr. Arthur Charles, in this problem, and he made some preliminary studies with me in the Department of Physiology and then joined forces with my colleague of long standing, Dr. D. A. Scott. From that time on the chemical work on heparin was conducted in the Connaught Laboratories, of which I was then an Assistant Director.

On November 10, 1931, I wrote to Professor W. H. Howell:

I would very much appreciate your opinion with regard to several questions in connection with heparin. During the last few years we have been using great amounts of this material in physiological and bacteriological work. Quite recently, one of the junior members of the Connaught Laboratories, which, as you know, are a department in the University, has interested himself, at my suggestion, in the preparation of heparin from beef liver. He is now in a position to make fairly large amounts of the material which is at least as potent as that distributed by Hynson, Westcott, and Dunning. One half gram of this material is being forwarded to you under separate cover. Would you have any objection if this material should be sold by the Connaught Laboratories? (*Now the Connaught Medical Research Laboratories whose objectives are the support of research by the sale of biological products at the lowest possible price.*) I believe that the price would be much more reasonable. As you know, there is a very high tariff on biological products going into the United States so there is very little likelihood of any interference with the American business of Hynson, Westcott, and Dunning.

On November 14, 1931, I received the following reply from Professor W. H. Howell in his own handwriting.

I am interested and pleased to know that you have got a usable preparation of heparin out of beef liver. I never could make that source give a decent preparation. As to your selling it, there can be no objection to that, of course. I have feared, at times, that the Hynson, Westcott, and Dunning firm would give up its production, as they always claimed that it was a losing proposition to them, so it may be well to have another source. I have been very anxious for them to market a purified heparin, potency 1 to 50 or 100, but the method I gave to them makes their product too expensive, they think.

The work on heparin in the University of Toronto was the product of activity in three departments—Physiology, the Connaught Laboratories, and the Department of Surgery.

Dr. David Scott and Dr. Arthur Charles [198; 199; 200; 684] were extremely successful in their chemical work during the years 1933 to 1936. The most important and novel steps in the preparation and purification of heparin which they introduced were (1) the finding that autolysis of tissue resulted in a much higher yield of heparin, (2) the discovery that beef lung yielded almost as much heparin as liver—this made it possible to use a much cheaper source of raw material, (3) the finding that the destruction of protein by trypsin in the crude protein-heparin complex, was an extremely important factor in the further purification of the anticoagulant, (4) the preparation of a crystalline material as the barium salt—they found that this purified material was of uniform composition and potency. The Danish workers, Schmitz and Fischer [676], had isolated in 1933 the anticoagulant material from dog's liver as the brucine salt. Neither the brucine salt nor the barium salt lent itself to any large-scale production. Somewhat later Charles and Scott were able to convert the crystalline barium salt of heparin into the sodium salt.

The labels on the bottles of heparin prepared by Hynson, Westcott, and Dunning from dog's liver by Howell's procedure, stated "1 mg. will prevent the coagulation of 5 cc. of cats' blood in the cold." Charles and Scott used this preparation as a reference standard and assigned it a potency of 5 units per mg. In terms of this material the potency of the crystalline barium salt was 110 units per mg but for simplicity in calculation Charles and Scott decided to assign the figure of 100 units per mg. The material provided for the international standard of heparin was the sodium salt prepared from the crystalline barium salt. The potency of the international standard [594] of heparin was defined as 130 units per mg, that is, there are 130 arbitrary units of heparin per mg of the international yardstick. It is calculated that the potency of the international standard is 28 times that of the early Hynson, Westcott, and Dunning preparation. The Connaught Laboratories in Toronto have made two international biological standards—the one for insulin and the one for heparin.

In addition to obtaining heparin in a highly purified form I thought that another point should be settled before the anticoagulant should be submitted for clinical trial. This was the ability or inability of heparin to prevent the agglutination of platelets, which is the first step in the formation of a thrombus as distinguished from a clot.

In 1929, the year after we started our work on heparin, Professor W. E. Gallie, Head of the Department of Surgery in Toronto, nominated Dr. Gordon Murray to collaborate with workers in my department, who were investigating the effects of heparin in the prevention of experimental thrombosis. I was fortunate in having in my department at that time, Dr. T. S. Perrett, a Fellow from the Department of Surgery. I was also fortunate in having a pupil who was taking his doctor's degree in physiology. This student soon became a colleague in the heparin work and a very close friend. He was, as you know, Dr. Louis Jaques, who later became the Head of the Department of Physiology at the University of Saskatchewan and an international authority on many aspects of blood clotting and thrombosis. Dr. Jaques, among the other services which he rendered to our department, sent me one of his own pupils, Dr. Frank Monkhouse, who received his Ph.D. in Physiology from my department in 1952. Dr. Monkhouse is, therefore, my scientific grandson and he, in his turn, has become an authority on different aspects of the great field of blood coagulation and thrombus formation.

The work on the effect of heparin on experimental thrombosis begun in 1929, was pushed forward by Dr. Murray, Dr. Jaques, Dr. Perrett, and myself. We [589] found that the incidence of obstruction of peripheral veins in dogs by thrombi formed as a result of mechanical or chemical injuries to the intimal surfaces of the blood vessels was definitely decreased when solutions of purified heparin were administered before and for long periods following the injury. These results were obtained in studies of some 300 veins. Thrombi were not observed even after very severe chemical injury while the animal was well heparinized. We found that the intimal surfaces of veins removed from heparinized animals several days after the injection of heparin had been discontinued appeared, on microscopic examination, to have recovered completely from the injury. The microscopic examinations revealed, in some cases, minute masses of platelets, filling small crevices in the intima. Healing was, however, complete as judged by the absence of thrombus formation after discontinuing the anticoagulant.

The experimental evidence of the prevention of thrombus formation initiated by platelet agglutination, was completely satisfactory before attempts were made to apply solutions of purified heparin to clinical problems.

At various stages in the purification of heparin attempts had been made to use the material as an anticoagulant in transfusing human patients. In 1924 Mason [558] used crude material and obtained reactions which varied from slight chills to severe headache and high fever and nausea. In 1928 Howell [407] used somewhat purer heparin and reported a slight reaction in 2 of 10 transfusions carried out on six patients. Godlowski [323] in 1933 reported on the use of heparin in human patients, and although he found low levels of toxicity, the preparation he used was extremely crude and of low potency. In 1936 Hedenius and Wilander [381] studied coagulation times of healthy human subjects. They found that heparin produced no ill effects when the material was given intravenously. This heparin was obtained from Dr. Erik Jorpes and was made by the Charles and Scott procedure.

The work on heparin in Toronto, begun in 1928, proceeded steadily. With each advance in purification we, Murray, Jaques, Perrett, and Best, studied the effect on experimental thrombosis and Dr. Gordon Murray made clinical trials beginning in May 1935. When the crystalline sodium salt became available it proved to be safe and effective for the heparinization of patients.

On May 8, 1935, Dr. Jorpes wrote to me from Stockholm in his own hand.

I am sending you a copy of the preliminary report about heparin, and would like to use this opportunity to thank you for all the hospitality shown to me and to Mr. Bjurling during our visit in Toronto in 1929. We have greatly benefited from your experience in the manufacture of insulin.

The heparin work has been a very hard task. For a very long time I believed that my preparations were only impurities as compared with those of Charles and Scott. I greatly admire their working capacity. They have opened this field, which before them was quite hopeless.

On May 28, 1935, I answered.

I have been interested in some physiological work on heparin recently; as a matter of fact, we have been administering some to human subjects. I hope that we will see you at the Physiological Congress in Russia this summer.

Up to the time of this letter there had been no published reference to the use of highly purified heparin in clinical cases but as Dr. Jorpes has written, the idea of using heparin to prevent the formation of thrombi was in the minds of all who came in close touch with the problem. Its realization merely depended on the availability of a satisfactory preparation of heparin. The clinical problem was attacked in Toronto and in Stockholm, as soon as pure heparin was obtainable. The studies by Crafoord [231] and later by other workers in Sweden, were proceeding at the same time as those of Dr. Gordon Murray [590] in the Toronto General Hospital. The results obtained clearly indicated that certain types of clinical thrombosis could be prevented by the treatment with purified heparin. These findings were made possible by the preparation of pure heparin from beef liver or lung. The word pure is used here to indicate a uniform preparation, of standard potency, and free from toxic components rather than in the true chemical sense.

Dr. Jorpes and his colleagues have made a very large number of fine contributions to the heparin field. The cellular origin of the anticoagulant, the chemistry, the mechanism of action, the clinical use in a great variety of conditions, and many other subjects have been illuminated by the work of this group, which is well summarized by Dr. Jorpes [431; 432] in his monographs. I have had the pleasure of knowing a number of the Swedish "anticoagulationists" in addition to Dr. Jorpes. Dr. Per Hedenius and the late Dr. Hjalmar Holmgren have been particularly close friends.

Our present knowledge of the chemistry of heparin has been summarized by Dr. Arthur Charles (personal communication) as follows: "Heparin is a complex polysaccharide. The carbohydrate moieties are glucuronic acid and glucosamine which are present in the molecular ratio of 1:1. The carbohydrate is highly sulphated. The amino group is not free and does not appear to be acetylated as in mucoitin or chondroitin sulphate. Evidence has been presented which indicates that the nitrogen is sulphated."

The availability of well-standardized heparin not only made possible the clinical work but also a very great deal of experimental study. Without this potent heparin the exchange transfusion experiments, carried out by

Thalhimer [748], and Thalhimer, Solandt, and myself [750] would not have been possible. The dramatic use of the artificial kidney by Kolff and Berk [467; 468] in Holland and by Dr. Gordon Murray in Toronto [587; 588] also depended on purified heparin. I will not attempt to make a complete list of the advances which the availability of potent purified heparin has facilitated.

There will obviously not be time to follow in detail the many lines of interest which developed in the middle 1930's. Members of our own group were interested in the source of heparin and its appearance in blood in peptone and anaphylactic shock. The work on Witte's peptone goes back to the publication of Schmidt-Mülheim [675] in 1880, when it was shown that injection of the material in dogs produced shock and incoagulability of the blood. In 1909 Biedl and Kraus [124] found that the blood failed to clot in anaphylactic shock. Professor Howell [406] in 1925 and Quick [626] in 1936 had obtained anticoagulant preparations from dog's blood after injection of peptone. The subject was further advanced by Wilander [794] in 1939, who isolated heparin in amounts sufficient to explain the coagulation deficiency. Waters, Markowitz, and Jaques [780] in our laboratory, showed in 1938 that the incoagulability of the blood, both in peptone shock and in anaphylactic shock in dogs, was completely inhibited by protamine. The dramatic neutralization of the effect of heparin by protamine had been shown by Chargaff and Olsen [197] in 1937. In 1940 Jaques and Waters [426; 427] isolated a barium salt of pure heparin from the blood of sensitized dogs given serum albumin.

Another point of interest in our laboratory was the enzymatic destruction of heparin by material prepared from rabbit's liver. This was carried out by Jaques [424] in 1940 and he suggested the name "heparinase" for this system. The use of silicone in preventing clotting was introduced by Jaques, Fidlar, Feldsted, and Macdonald [425] in my laboratory in 1946. This was a great improvement over vaseline or paraffin, which, of course, had been used ever since the work of Freund [311] in 1888 and of Bordet and Gengon [139] in 1901. A very great many experiments have been facilitated by the use of silicone coating of glass tubes, needles, and other apparatus.

The experimental work which D. Y. Solandt, Reginald Nassim, and I did [722] on the prevention of coronary thrombosis and intramural thrombosis in dogs by the administration of heparin, fascinated us until problems of military medicine diverted our attention in 1939. Dr. Solandt and I [719] described a method by which gradual occlusion of coronary arteries by thrombus formation may be produced in experimental animals. The thrombus formation and the resulting cardiac infarction were in a very large part prevented by the administration of adequate amounts of highly purified heparin. In discussing the possible clinical application of our findings [70] I wrote, in 1938, "If the clinical investigation of cardiac cases should be initiated, the necessity for studying very large numbers and of heparinizing only alternate cases is obvious."

In the investigation which Dr. Solandt and I made with Dr. Nassim, we evolved a method by which cardiac mural thrombi could be produced in animals. These thrombi were formed very rapidly and there was a very dramatic and extensive fall in blood platelets during this interval. The formation of the mural thrombi could be completely prevented by the administration of adequate amounts of highly purified heparin. We [722] wrote at that time, in 1939, "Since over ten per cent of the deaths associated with coronary thrombosis in man are caused by embolic sequels of mural thrombus formation, a clinical trial of heparin is indicated."

There was an attempt, in Toronto, to apply some of these results, but no comprehensive investigation was found to be possible at that time. In 1948, Wright, Marple, and Beck [819] wrote, "The possibility of preventing the extension of coronary thromboses and the development of mural thrombi in the presence of myocardial infarction by the use of anticoagulants was suggested by Solandt, Nassim, and Best in 1938. . . . Their observations were not applied to human beings on any significant scale because of the difficulties and the risk felt to be inherent in the use of heparin clinically."

When purified heparin became available in Toronto requests for this material for experimental and clinical use came from many parts of the world. One of the earliest was from Dr. Leo Mayer who wrote on December 21, 1938, "Dr. Irving Wright of the New York Post Graduate Hospital has suggested the advisability of using heparin in this case." The patient was Mr. Arthur Schulte. I remember sending heparin to Dr. I. S. Ravdin of Philadelphia who needed it for the postoperative treatment of a brilliant young doctor who had a saddle embolus at the bifurcation of his aorta. Many surgeons and physicians came to Toronto to discuss the clinical problems with Dr. Murray, or physiologic or chemical matters with our group. I remember many of these men vividly—Dr. Essex and Dr. Priestley of the Mayo Clinic and Dr. Lahey of Boston were among those who came from this country.

The interest in heparin continues to grow. Dr. Jay McLean was undoubtedly fascinated by the effect of heparin on the clearing of lipemic plasma, first demonstrated by Hahn [344], and by the great volume of recent literature on the effects of the anticoagulant on fat mobilization.

Heparin has thus already removed many barriers to the free flow of knowledge but we are still in the early stages of appreciation of its physiologic and clinical significance.

Acknowledgment

I am indebted to Dr. Arthur Charles, Dr. Frank Monkhouse, and Dr. Jessie H. Ridout for a great deal of expert help in the preparation of this paper. The efficient secretarial assistance of Miss Linda Mahon is also deeply appreciated.

54. Heparin and the Thrombosis of Veins Following Injury

G. D. W. MURRAY, M.D.

L. B. JAQUES, M.A.

T. S. PERRETT, M.D.

C. H. BEST, M.D.

While it is well established that heparin increases the coagulation time of blood, little or no experimental work on the effect of this anticoagulant on the thrombosis of blood vessels resulting from injury to the intima has been carried out. It has been shown by Zahn [824], Eberth and Schimmelbusch [277], Welch [790], and Zurhelle [830] that thrombosis of blood vessels may be produced by the application of caustics or by mechanical injury to the intima. These procedures result in the accumulation of blood platelets on the wall of the vessel at the point of injury. Leucocytes then collect at the margin of and between the platelet masses. Fibrin is subsequently laid down. Since the methods of producing the vascular obstruction used in the experiments to be reported here are essentially similar to those employed by these previous investigators, the mechanism by which obstruction is brought about is presumably the same. We have examined the blood vessels at short intervals after injury in only a few cases and cannot, therefore, describe in detail the sequence of events leading up to the formation of a plug which caused, in most of the control experiments, cessation of blood flow in the injured veins. Since in this investigation lesions in peripheral veins in which the blood flow is sluggish were being studied, it was to be expected that the obstructing mass would be composed, in large part, of red cells and fibrin. We are informed, however, by Professor Robinson, of the Department of Pathology, and by our colleague in the School of Hygiene, Dr. D. L. MacLean, that the plugs are typical thrombi. In some sections, accumulations of platelets are clearly visible, while in others the manner in which the formed elements are laid down distinguishes the obstructing mass from a clot.

Originally appeared in *Surgery*, II (1937), 163–87. From the Department of Surgery, Department of Physiology, and the School of Hygiene, University of Toronto.

In this study, injury to the lining of the veins was produced by two procedures. The first was mechanical and the second chemical. When a solution of purified heparin was administered intravenously for an adequate period, the incidence of obstruction by thrombus was very definitely less than in the experiments in which the anticoagulant was not used.

METHODS

Normal healthy dogs, weighing from ten to fifteen kilograms, have been used as experimental animals. Ether or nembutal has been employed when anaesthesia was necessary. In the determination of the coagulation time of the blood such great variation was found that considerable effort was made to secure a method which would give a consistent end-point. The difficulties of securing uniform results may be divided into two groups; first, those associated with the removal of the blood from the veins and, second, those involved in the subsequent care and handling of the sample. In confirmation of the results of previous investigators, it was found impossible to take repeated samples of blood, using a syringe and needle from the same part of the vein without shortening the coagulation time very appreciably. The third and fourth samples would often gel before they could be placed in the recording apparatus. The same difficulty was encountered in obtaining samples from cannulas or from a sectioned artery. The differences in coagulation time are no doubt due to the release of clotting factors from the traumatized areas. These difficulties can be eliminated, to a certain extent, by drawing the blood with a very small needle if certain precautions are used. The point of the needle is directed against the flow and is inserted some distance into the blood vessel. Each subsequent sample is secured from a slightly more peripheral point on the vessel. Care must be taken that the blood flows easily into the syringe and that no air enters during the withdrawal of the plunger. Even when attention is paid to these details, variations in the clotting time occur. If they are neglected, little significance can be attached to the end-point which is secured. The subsequent handling of the blood samples presents less difficulty. After testing most of the methods which have been advocated, we decided to use a mechanical device which eliminates subjective factors. The principle of our coagulometer (Figure 93) is similar to that developed by Cannon and Mendenhall [170] and modified by Stoker [741].

Coagulometer. Two metal levers, A and B, are mounted on pinpoint bearings at X and X_1. A is parallel to, and about 2 cm above, B. At one end of each lever, weights C and C_1 are attached. These may be finely adjusted and locked at any point. At the opposite end of A is a fork which supports, between its arms, the plunger D (weight, 1.340 g). This plunger is constructed from monel metal and in shape resembles two shallow cones placed base to base. The diameter at the largest point is 8 mm. Into a hole bored through the apices is soldered a short length of monel wire. To the other end of the wire is attached a cross-piece, to serve as a means of support when the plunger is suspended from the fork.

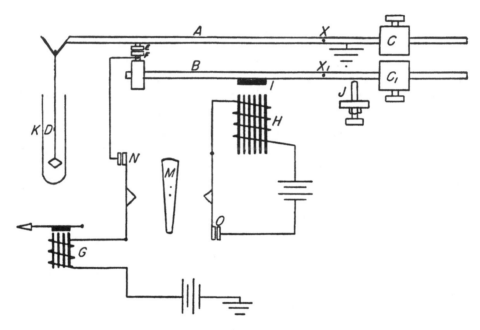

FIGURE 93. Coagulometer.

Between the fork and the fulcrum is attached a platinum point E which makes contact with a similar point F on the lever B. F is insulated from the lever B. These points are connected in series with the signal magnet G.

Under B is mounted an electromagnet H which, when charged, pulls down the lever B by means of the soft iron armature attached at I. When the circuit is broken, the lever will return to the horizontal because of the extra weight of C_1. An adjusting screw at J controls the extent of this movement. As the weight of A is greater at the forked end, the points E and F will be held in close contact and the movements of B transmitted to A through these points.

The weight C, on A, is adjusted so that the lever will just remain horizontal when D is replaced by a standard weight of 1.000 g.

In operation, 1 cc of blood is placed in the test tube K (10 mm bore by 50 mm high) and the height of the test-tube adjusted so that the plunger is just clear of the bottom when the levers are held down against H. At intervals of one minute and for a period of three seconds the magnet H is stimulated. This pulls down the lever B and permits the plunger D to sink, by its own weight, in the blood. If the blood is not coagulated, contact is made at the points E and F and the signal magnet G will record this on a kymograph. If the blood is coagulated, the plunger will be supported by the clot and no contact will be made. A record in one-minute intervals is recorded on the kymograph. This record ceases when the blood is clotted.

An ordinary household electric clock is used to control the make-and-break mechanism for the electromagnets. The second hand is replaced by a tapered arm M which once in every revolution closes the contacts N and O. The wide end of the lever M holds the points O in contact for three seconds while the narrow end closes the points N for one second. Contact at N should synchronize with the third second of contact at O. If contact is made earlier or later, a misleading record may be made. The contact points N and O should be mounted on the clock face, one a little in front of the other, and the lever M attached slightly off the right angle. If mounted in the same plane, contacts would be made at thirty-second intervals.

The apparatus in use is composed of four of the above units. One electric clock is sufficient to operate all four. The levers B are secured firmly to a shaft carried by two end-bearings. This shaft has attached to it an extra lever, carrying a weight at one end and an armature, similar to that shown on B, at the other. The weight is sufficiently heavy to balance all the levers. By this means the four units are operated by one magnet.

In an endeavour to obtain accurate checks on the blood contained in the four tubes and filled from the same sample, the test-tubes are partially immersed in a constant temperature water-bath which is kept at 37° C. The tubes are held in place by spring clamps attached to one side of the bath.

The weights of the plungers are adjusted to within 2 mg, and as the levers are balanced to the standard weight of 1.000 g, the downward pressure exerted by any plunger is equivalent to 0.340 g (weight of D [1.340 g] − 1.000 g).

Method of Producing the Injury to Veins

(a) *Mechanical means.* The blood vessels chosen for these experiments were the readily accessible radial and saphenous veins. Very little dissection was needed to free them from the surrounding tissue. The skin incision was made at some little distance to the side of the vein and the skin under-cut so that, when sewing up, the flap would fall over the vein. After about one inch of the vessel had been isolated in this way, a needle carrying a length of silk thread (size 000) was passed up through the lumen of the veins for about three-quarters of an inch so that the thread remained within the vessel wall. The vein was then crushed against the thread between the jaws of a pair of artery forceps. The forceps were clamped very tightly on the vein. The crushing was continued along the full length of the exposed vein and then repeated in at least two other planes. In later experiments, a pair of forceps with a particularly firm grip was selected and used only for the purpose of crushing. After the injury the thread was withdrawn, bleeding controlled with gauze, and the wound closed by interrupted silk sutures. The veins were left *in situ* for periods ranging from seven hours to seven days. They were then removed between ligatures, examined in the gross, and placed in formalin as the first stage in their preparation for microscopic examination.

(b) *Injury produced by injection of sodium ricinoleate (soricin)*. The second method of producing occlusion of the veins was by the injection of a solution of sodium ricinoleate. This was a commercial preparation manufactured by the Wm. S. Merrell Company, Cincinnati, U.S.A. The needle of the syringe containing the soricin is introduced through the skin into the vein. The vein is then occluded one or one and one-half inches above the needle by pressure with the finger. It is obvious that great care must be taken to use the same length of vein in all experiments of one series. Unhappily, the calibres of the veins cannot readily be measured and must be assumed to be equal. If the volumes of blood in the occluded veins are not similar, the concentrations of soricin to which the intimal surfaces are exposed will vary. If branches of the veins can be detected, these are also occluded by pressure. The sodium ricinoleate solution is then injected and prevented from escaping from the vein by pressure over the point at which the needle entered. The solution is kept in this manner in the vein for a period of three minutes. The vein is then released.

Method of Administering Heparin

In the preliminary stages of this investigation heparin was administered in a variety of ways. Certain descriptive terms have come into use in these laboratories. Local heparinization is the term used to describe the application of heparin to one particular area. This procedure was used in experiments on blood vessel surgery. Heparin was incorporated in vaselin or jelly and applied to the edges of the blood vessels about to be sutured. No significant result has been obtained by this method of administering the anticoagulant. Regional heparinization is the term used to describe the administration of heparin in such a way that the coagulation time of the blood of one limb, for example, is increased without materially affecting the blood in other parts of the body. Thus, with an infusion of heparin into the femoral artery of one limb, blood samples from the veins of the same leg show a longer clotting time than those secured at the same time from other parts of the body. This is true, however, only when small doses of heparin are administered. With larger doses more of the anticoagulant reaches the general circulation and the increase in clotting time is general. The term general heparinization describes the results of the administration of heparin into a vein or artery at such a rate that the clotting time of the blood from all parts of the body is increased. Most of the results which we are reporting in this paper were secured by general heparinization of experimental animals. The heparin was given intravenously by one of three methods. In preliminary experiments, a single injection was made by syringe. In a second series, a continuous injection of heparin dissolved in saline was made by means of a motor-driven pump. Animals receiving the anticoagulant by this procedure were maintained under nembutal anaesthesia and the injection was continued for, at most, ten hours. The third method was by a continuous injection of heparin in saline, utilizing, with slight modifications, the technique adopted by Jacobs [421], of Chicago. By this procedure it is possible to give continuous intravenous infusions to dogs for long periods of time without seriously interfering with their activity. Ether anaesthesia was used during the insertion of a cannula into the external jugular vein. The cannula was connected by a flexible metal tube to a reservoir containing the heparin solution. After recovery from the anaesthetic, the animal moved about with considerable freedom. The rate of injection was maintained at a constant level by a motor-driven pump. The injections by this method were usually continued for seventy-two hours. The parts of the apparatus which it was not feasible to sterilize by heat were thoroughly bathed with antiseptic solution before each experiment.

The Toxicity of Heparin

Since it was our hope that heparin might ultimately be safely used in human patients, the toxicity of the various preparations of this anticoagulant was a very important matter. It is evident from the literature and from our own findings that the toxicity varies greatly and, in general, inversely as the purity of the preparation.

The Howell unit of heparin is the amount which will prevent the clotting of 1 cc of cat's blood for twenty-four hours. Even when precautions are taken with regard to temperature, stirring, etc., it is impossible to estimate the potency of the solution accurately by this procedure without the use of a standard preparation. However, if a standard heparin is used and the unknown preparation compared with this, reliable results may be obtained. A standard of heparin has been set up in the Connaught Laboratories and the heparin which we have used has always been compared with this preparation.

Using heparin of a potency of 15 units per milligram, Howell and McDonald [409] injected an amount into a dog which was sufficient to render its blood incoagulable. This was approximately 0.45 mg per kilogram. This injection was repeated daily for five days. They reported no demonstrable change in the red and white blood counts or in the platelets. There was no indication of any deleterious effect on the animal. Reed [633] injected moderate quantities of heparin intravenously in normal and etherized dogs and rabbits. He found no change in temperature, no cardiovascular effect, no concentration of the blood cells, and no abnormalities in respiration. In 1924, Mason [558] reported on the use of material containing 5 units per milligram. He added from 50 to 300 mg to blood used in transfusing human patients. In about one-half the cases he observed reactions which varied from slight chills to severe headache, high fever, and nausea. Mason concluded that while the heparin used in the early part of his work was too toxic to warrant its routine clinical use in doses of 100 mg (500 units), preparations subsequently made had given encouraging results. Howell [407] reported upon the use of heparin containing 100 units per milligram in transfusions given to human subjects. He reported a slight reaction in two of the ten transfusions carried out on six patients. Godlowski [323] found no evidence of toxicity in his patients when he injected 1 mg of heparin per 10 cc of blood. This preparation contained 10 units per milligram. In our experience, the 5-unit material, which was the only preparation readily available when these experiments were started, exerted marked toxic effects when administered intravenously to dogs. Some of these dogs died and at autopsy revealed marked haemorrhages in the intestine. Later, using more highly purified heparin, 75 units per milligram, no deaths were produced in a series of some twenty dogs studied. Vomiting and pronounced muscular weakness were, however, not infrequently observed when large doses of the material were used. Recently we have employed more highly purified heparin and in some sixty dogs which received a preparation with a potency of about 250 units per milligram, for a period of seventy-two hours (500 mg; i.e., 125,000 units of heparin in all were injected), no signs of a toxic action of the anticoagulant were detected. We are indebted to Miss Winifred Chute for help in some of the early experiments.

Tests for the toxicity of this heparin containing 250 units per milligram were made upon various species of animals. Rabbits, guinea pigs, and mice were injected with sufficient of the material to render their blood incoagulable for very long periods of time. No toxic effects were produced. These findings have, however, relatively little significance in view of the fact that heparin has been much further purified by our colleagues Charles and Scott since the studies of toxicity referred to above were carried out. More recently we have had available adequate amounts of heparin of a potency of 500 units per milligram. This is dissolved in distilled water or saline and 1 cc of this solution usually contains approximately 15,000 units of the anticoagulant. The effect on human subjects will be described in more detail later, but it may be stated here that the 250-unit heparin produced definite signs of toxicity. More highly purified material, however, has been given to patients with no deleterious effects. Since adequate amounts of this relatively innocuous and very potent material are now available, it is unnecessary to describe in detail the results of toxicity tests on the cruder preparations.

EXPERIMENTAL RESULTS AND COMMENTS

Injury Produced by Mechanical Means

When the veins of a dog are crushed upon a thread inserted in the lumen, as described under Methods, thrombosis will take place in only a limited number of the veins unless considerable force is applied in the crushing process. If force is exerted and extensive damage to the veins produced, a thrombus will form, according to our experience, in approximately 80 per cent of the cases (Table 54.I). Without heparin the veins (i.e., 80 per cent of them) are found to be obstructed by thrombus when examined

TABLE 54.I

THROMBUS FORMATION IN VEINS INJURED BY CRUSHING

Method of Injury	No. of Veins	Patent	Occluded	Partially Occluded	Per cent Occluded
Crushing—moderate, no thread used	10	9	1	0	10
Crushing—moderate, thread used	10	6	4	0	40
Crushing—severe, thread used	57	8	44	5	80

forty minutes after injury. If this thrombus is left *in situ* for five or six days it is usually found, upon removal of the veins, that it entirely fills the lumen and is adherent to the vein wall.

The incidence of obstruction by thrombus formation in a vein which has been injured, as described above, is extremely small as long as the animal is maintained under the influence of heparin. An experiment of this nature was conducted in which thirteen veins were observed (Table 54.II). Following a single injection of heparin the veins were damaged, but they were removed before the effect of the heparin had worn off. All the veins of this group except three were perfectly clear on macroscopic examination. In these three, a small thrombus was present on a portion of the wall.

It was found that an adequate effect was produced upon the coagulation time of blood in dogs; i.e., the coagulation time was maintained at approximately thirty minutes, when relatively crude heparin was administered intravenously at the rate of 3.3 units per kilogram per minute.

In the next experiment to be described, heparin was given intravenously in saline solution at the same rate. The veins were traumatized and the

TABLE 54.II

EFFECT OF INJECTION WITH HEPARIN ON THROMBUS FORMATION IN INJURED VEINS

No. of Veins	Heparin mg/kg	Calculated Heparin Effect	Veins Left *in situ*	Patent	Occluded	Partially Occluded
13 { 5	60*	1½ hr	1 hr	5	0	
6	140*	3½ hr	3 hr	6	0	2 (very small thrombus)
2	180*	4½ hr	4 hr	2	0	1 (very small thrombus)
4	0.22† mg/kg/min	70 hr	70 hr	4	0	

*Single injection.   †Continuous injection.

injection continued for seventy hours. At the end of this time the veins were excised and examined. Four veins of one dog were used in this experiment. They were all perfectly clear and no trace of thrombus could be found (Table 54.II).

In the next series of experiments, thirteen veins were studied in animals which had received a single injection of heparin. The vein was traumatized immediately after the injection of heparin had been made but was left *in situ* for periods of from three and one-half to twenty-four hours. The amount of heparin injected varied in the different experiments. The results of this series are given in Table 54.III. It will be noted that of the thirteen veins one was partly occluded while the remaining twelve were completely filled with thrombus and clot.

TABLE 54.III

THROMBUS FORMATION WITH INADEQUATE HEPARIN

No. of Veins	Heparin mg/kg	Calculated Heparin Effect	Veins Left *in situ*	Patent	Occluded	Partially Occluded
1	60	1½ hr	3½ hr	0	0	1
8	100	2½ hr	4½ hr	0	8	0
4	180	4½ hr	24 hr	0	4	0

In the next series of experiments single injections of heparin (approximately 6,000 units) were given to 10-kilogram dogs. The veins were then damaged and an infusion of heparin in saline solution started immediately. This was maintained at a rate of 2.2 units per kilogram per minute for from seventy to seventy-two hours. The veins were inspected seven days after they had been injured. Nine veins were treated in this manner. Six of these showed clear lumina and a smooth, glistening intima. Three were occluded by thrombi. In one of these the obstruction was at the site of a valve to which the thrombus was attached. In the other two cases the veins were exposed for some time on the surface of an infected wound.

In the next group of experiments a vein on one side of an animal was traumatized, but no heparin was administered. This vein was examined seven to twenty-four hours later and if obstructed the corresponding vein on the other side of the animal was similarly traumatized after the injection of heparin had been started. In this group of experiments with ten control veins and ten under test, one of the controls was only partially occluded while one of the veins which had been bathed with heparin became completely plugged by thrombus. There is, perhaps, an explanation for this latter case in that the pump which was forcing the heparin into the animal stopped and the full dose of the anticoagulant was not received (Table 54.IV).

[One table in the original has been omitted.]

TABLE 54.IV

EFFECTS OF HEPARIN IN PERIPHERAL VEINS OF DOGS

(Ten animals used. Mechanical trauma. Right radial or saphenous veins, which served as controls, were examined 7 to 24 hr after injury; the left vein traumatized after heparin started; treatment with heparin continued for 72 hr; veins examined 7 days after injury.)

	Right (no heparin)	Left (heparin)
Patent	0	9
Partially occluded	1	0
Occluded	9	1*

*Pump stopped overnight, full amount of heparin not received.

In the next series 28 veins were studied. The procedure was the same as in the preceding experiment, with one exception. The control veins, i.e., those which were not bathed by heparin, instead of being examined in 7 to 24 hours, were left *in situ* for 7 days. Heparin was administered for a period of 70 hours and the test veins were left in place for 6 days after traumatization. The results of these series are shown in Table 54.V.

TABLE 54.V

EFFECTS OF HEPARIN IN VEINS INJURED MECHANICALLY

(Fourteen animals used; technique as above except that the control veins (right) were left in place for 7 days before being examined; treated veins examined 6 days after injury.)

	Right (no heparin)	Left (heparin)
Patent	4	11
Partially occluded	2	0
Occluded	8	3*

*In two of these cases there was an extensive hematoma.

It is difficult to summarize the results of these experiments in which injury to the veins had been produced by mechanical means. When no heparin had been given only 8 of 57 veins examined were, macroscopically, free of thrombus. In 37 cases in which heparin was administered for prolonged periods, 30 veins were free of thrombus on macroscopic examination, i.e., 81 per cent were patent as compared with 14 per cent when heparin was not given.

Injury Produced by Chemical Means

After some preliminary experiments had been carried out, we studied the effects of heparin on injury produced when 0.25 cc of soricin was injected into each vein. Some 204 veins were studied in this series. No useful purpose will be served by describing the experiments in great detail. The results are summarized in Table 54.VI. It will be observed

TABLE 54.VI

EFFECTS OF HEPARIN IN VEINS INJURED CHEMICALLY

(In Expt. A 0.25 cc Soricin solution was injected in all veins; in Expt. B 0.15 cc injected. Treated animals injected with 22.5 units heparin per kg body weight per hr for 66 to 73 hrs.)

	Controls (114 veins)		Heparin (90 veins)	
Expt. A				
Patent	17	(15%)	46	(53%)
Occluded	97	(85%)	44	(47%)
	Controls (12 veins)		Heparin (12 veins)	
Expt. B				
Patent	2	(17%)	12	(100%)
Occluded	10	(83%)	0	(0%)

that of the 114 veins from animals which received no heparin, 85 per cent were occluded. Of the 90 veins investigated from animals which received heparin, 47 per cent were occluded. In other words, only 15 per cent of the control veins were patent while 53 per cent of those which had received heparin were open after from 4 to 7 days. The obvious deduction from the results of this large series of experiments is that heparin in the dose used, i.e., 22.5 units per kilogram per hour, is not nearly so effective as might be desired in preventing thrombosis of veins. While a dose of 0.25 cc of soricin, under the conditions which we have described, does not produce occlusion in all cases, it was thought expedient to determine whether smaller doses might not be nearly as effective. An injection of 0.15 cc of soricin was tried in a series of 24 veins. The results in Table 54.VI show that in 83 per cent of the control series the veins were occluded by thrombi. When heparin was given in the dose which was used in most of the previous experiments, 11 of the 12 veins were completely free of thrombus. In one vein, while there was no interference with blood flow through it, there was a small thrombus firmly attached to the wall. Interestingly enough, this thrombus was composed almost entirely of platelets. These results appear to show that if a small dose of soricin is used, its effect, so far as the obstruction of veins is concerned, may be almost completely counteracted by an adequate dose of heparin administered continuously for a period of approximately 70 hours.

It may be noted here that if the veins are examined before the injection of heparin is discontinued, thrombosis is not observed in most cases even when much larger doses of soricin are used (up to 1.0 cc). Under these circumstances, thrombosis would presumably have occurred invariably soon after the effect of heparin had worn off. These higher concentrations of soricin produce almost complete destruction of the tissue with which they come in contact. Our findings also suggest that the animals should always be thoroughly heparinized before the injury to the veins is produced, if the action of the anticoagulant in preventing obstruction is to be most effective.

Regional Heparinization in Experimental Animals

A large number of experiments have been carried out in which attempts have been made to heparinize one limb of an experimental animal without affecting the blood in other parts of the body. It will be sufficient for our present purpose to describe one experiment in some detail.

A dog weighing approximately 7 kg was anaesthetized by an intravenous injection of nembutal. Both femoral arteries and veins were exposed. The clotting time of the blood from the vein of the right leg was 5 minutes, and of that from the left leg, 4 minutes. Heparin solution was then introduced from a burette through a needle into the right femoral artery. The solution contained approximately 2,200 units per cubic centimeter. Ten minutes after the injection had been started, the clotting time of the blood secured from the vein of the heparinized limb was 11 minutes, while that from the unheparinized extremity was 5 minutes. Thirty-five minutes after the start of injection, blood from the right femoral vein showed a clotting time of 11 minutes, while 15 minutes later blood secured from the unheparinized left limb showed a clotting time of 6 minutes. The heparin solution was injected at the rate of approximately 0.7 cc per minute. Four hours and thirty minutes after the start of the injection the clotting time on the heparinized side was 21 minutes, while on the other side the time was 20 minutes. The results of this experiment show that regional heparinization can be accomplished, for a time at least, when an injection of heparin solution is made intra-arterially at a fairly slow rate. After some time, however, in many of the experiments the clotting time of blood from other parts of the body showed the effects of heparin; i.e., the heparinization had become general. It is possible, of course, that if the rate of injection had been decreased regional heparinization might have been maintained.

Observations on Human Subjects

While a more detailed report will be made later on the results of the use of heparin in human subjects, a summary of the findings we have secured will be included here. The objective in these investigations was merely to determine the toxicity of the heparin preparations on human subjects and the effect on the clotting time of the blood.

The first administration of heparin to a patient on the surgical ward of the Toronto General Hospital was carried out on April 16, 1935. The brachial artery of the left arm was exposed by a small incision under local anaesthesia. A needle was inserted in the artery and the heparin solution was injected by means of a motor-driven pump. To make this solution, heparin powder with a potency of approximately 250 units per milligram was dissolved in saline solution and the mixture sterilized by passage through a Berkefeld filter. Samples of blood from the veins of the injected arm showed a rise in clotting time from the normal of 6 minutes to approximately 18 minutes. Samples of blood from other parts of the body showed, at this time, no change in clotting time. This is an example of regional heparinization in a human subject. The injection was maintained for a period of approximately 4 hours and no signs of any toxic effects were observed. Regional heparinization was carried out in several other cases.

No evidence has been obtained in experimental animals or human subjects that a negative phase, i.e., a decrease in coagulation time, develops when the injection of heparin is discontinued.

The general heparinization of the human subject was attempted on several occasions with relatively crude heparin. Toxic effects in the form of weakness, headache, and slight chills made it inadvisable to continue the injections. More recently, using heparin of a potency of 250 units per milligram, 4 of 9 clinical cases showed no toxic effects even after prolonged injection. The other 5 of these cases, however, did exhibit definite signs of toxicity and the injections of heparin had to be discontinued. The effect of a single large dose of this preparation of the anticoagulant (22,000 units) rapidly administered to a patient is illustrated in Figure 94. This patient was receiving heparin continuously at a slow rate and had been

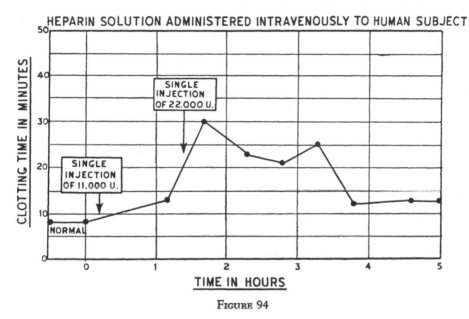

FIGURE 94

given an injection of 11,000 units one hour and ten minutes before the larger amount was administered. The rise in blood clotting time after the last injection may have been due, in part, to the effects of the previous dose.

More recently large amounts of highly purified heparin, 500 units per milligram, have been available. In the course of the purification of this substance, Charles and Scott were able to remove rather large quantities of a tarlike material which it is believed may have been responsible for the toxic properties of the cruder preparations. Seventy-six postoperative cases have now received injections of the solutions of purified heparin by the intravenous route. The period of injection has usually varied from 24 to 120 hours. An effort has been made to keep the clotting time at approximately 15 to 20 minutes, i.e., at least two or three times the usual normal range, but very high values (51 minutes) have sometimes been observed. The results on one of these cases are illustrated in Figure 95. The findings in this case are more regular than in some of the others and it has been chosen for this reason. In other cases the clotting time was frequently raised to a much higher level but, as stated above, no deleterious effects were observed. The cases which received heparin postoperatively had undergone one of the following operations: appendectomy, herniotomy —with and without living sutures—resection of colon, closure of colostomy, partial gastrectomy, drainage of empyema, bone graft of the tibia and of carpal scaphoid, or various minor operations such as excision of cysts,

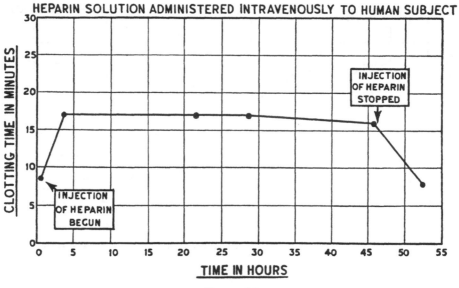

FIGURE 95

lipomata, and so on. In only one of these cases was there a haematoma at the site of operation. This was in the skin and while it may be attributed to heparin, it is also possible that it was due to inadequate haemostasis. The injections of heparin were commenced in from 2 to 3 hours after the completion of the operation.[2]

Histologic Findings

The histologic picture of veins thrombosed as a result of mechanical injury has been described by previous investigators. Our findings recorded in the tables are based on gross examination. Histologic sections were prepared of all the veins and the findings support, in general, those of the gross examination. In some cases platelet thrombi were found under the microscope in veins which had been considered on gross examination to be perfectly clear. Many of the heparinized veins, however, appeared to be completely free of thrombi, but in some of these inflammatory areas of varying sizes were present in the media or adventitia. These findings are based on examinations of several sections, but serial sections were not made.

The veins into which soricin had been injected and which subsequently became obstructed contained, on histologic examination, a mixed thrombus. If this examination was conducted twenty-four hours after the injection of the irritant, the veins were found to exhibit loss of endothelium from part

[2]A report of the earlier part of this work was presented before the Junior Inter-Urban Surgical Club of Canada in October 1935.

of the wall and substitution of this by a line of fine dark-staining granular matter. This was probably a mixture of disintegrated nuclei and soricin. The media of these veins showed varying degrees of degeneration. In some cases a large area of this layer failed to take the nuclear stains. In other cases the nuclei and fibers stained well. The former were pyknotic and broken into fine granules. The muscle fibres were separated by widely dilated capillaries and in some cases by interstitial haemorrhage. The adventitia showed changes in some cases and not in others. If any of the irritant material which was injected had leaked out of the vein, there was a marked inflammatory reaction. The thrombus examined at this stage usually filled the entire lumen and was attached over a fairly large area of the vein wall by platelets and a network of fibrin in which red and white cells were visible.

[Eight photomicrographs of cross-sections of veins showing different degrees of thrombosis have been omitted.]

The site of injection sometimes involved a valve area and in these cases the thrombus was often found attached to one of the valve leaflets.

In 72 hours after the injection, the media usually took a nuclear stain. The nuclei, however, were broken and disintegrated and the spaces between the muscle fibres were filled with phagocytic cells containing dark-staining granules and red cells. The thrombus filling the lumen appeared to be attached directly to the media in some places from which heavy fibrin threads extended outward. These were usually covered with platelets and white cells. This gave the thrombus a wavy, lacy appearance.

In the heparinized veins, sections secured 60 to 72 hours after the injection of soricin showed, in those cases where there was no obstrutcion to blood flow, a complete freedom from thrombus formation in many instances. In others a small thrombus attached to a valve or to a tiny area on the vein wall was visible under the microscope. The vessel wall, even when no thrombus was seen, showed in some areas signs of inflammatory reaction. The intima was usually normal although the nuclei seemed to be enlarged. The media usually showed an engorgement of capillaries and haemorrhage between the fibres. The nuclei of the cells of the media appeared broken or pyknotic. White blood cells were present in this layer and these were filled with dark-staining granules. The adventitia in a few cases showed signs of inflammatory reaction. The above findings were secured when the veins were removed 3 days after the injury. Six or 7 days after injury the vessel walls seemed to be largely free of inflammation but the cells of the intima were still rather hyperchromatic. In the veins where a thrombus had formed there were definite signs of organization at the end of 6 days.

DISCUSSION

The possibility that heparin might prevent thrombosis of blood vessels was appreciated by Howell and by many of the subsequent workers in this field. It has been shown by Mason [557] that heparin will prevent the intravascular clot produced by the injection of a potent solution of thrombokinase into the blood stream. Our investigations have differed from those which have preceded them in the following ways: (1) Thrombosis of veins was produced by mechanical and chemical injury to the intimal surface of the blood vessels. (2) In our more recent experiments a very highly potent and non-toxic preparation of heparin has been available in adequate quantities.

It has not previously been shown, to our knowledge, that heparin is capable of preventing the obstruction of blood vessels by thrombus and clot which form as a result of extensive injury. To accomplish this it is necessary, as we have shown, to keep the animal under the influence of heparin for prolonged periods. The heparin which was available when Mason conducted his very interesting experiments on the prevention of intravascular clotting by thrombokinase presumably had a potency of approximately 5 units per milligram. Some of our work has been conducted with heparin of a potency of 250 units per milligram, while more recently this has been of the order of 500 units per milligram. It is necessary to secure a high degree of purification if toxic products are to be eliminated. The administration of heparin of a potency of 250 units per milligram, in amounts effective in increasing the clotting time of the blood, for prolonged periods to human subjects is not a feasible procedure.

It should be appreciated that considerable care is required in conducting experiments in which the occlusion of veins is produced by mechanical injury. It is probable that if the veins of animals which were to receive heparin had been less severely injured than the controls, a large proportion of them would have failed to become occluded. In our opinion, the heparinized veins were damaged quite as severely as the controls. If there was any difference in the extent of injury, we believe that the heparinized veins received the more severe traumatization.

There would seem to be less possibility of significant variation in the procedure used to injure the veins by chemical means. The soricin was injected under rigidly uniform conditions. While it is very interesting that the heparin was not effective in preventing occlusion of a larger proportion of the veins into which 0.25 cc of the soricin was injected, it would appear that there is a very significant difference between the numbers of the veins occluded in the control and test groups. Fifteen per cent of the control veins were patent, while 53 per cent of those which received heparin offered no obstruction to blood flow at the end of the experiment.

It is quite possible that if a larger series of veins had been studied with an injection of 0.15 cc of soricin that all of the heparinized veins would not have remained patent. The results were, however, remarkably uniform in a series of 24 veins studied. There was no obvious obstruction to blood flow in any of the 12 veins removed from animals which had received heparin. The small platelet thrombus in one of the veins was not detected before the vein was opened.

Very little further comment need be made on the nature of the obstructing mass in the vein. In many of the sections the platelets were easily demonstrable. In some cases the thrombus was composed almost entirely of platelets. It would appear that if heparinization is continued for approximately 70 hours, the intimal surfaces of the veins may heal sufficiently so that there is no danger of subsequent obstruction. In many cases the veins were removed from the animals seven days after the injury had been produced. At this time, in the obstructed vessels, the thrombus was usually firmly attached to the vein wall and showed definite evidence of organization. Recanalization might subsequently have taken place. In the vessels which were patent, the intima, in the gross, appeared normal. The microscopic findings have been described above.

It has been reported by Shionoya [701] that the administration of heparin does not prevent the formation of a white thrombus when the blood is made to pass through a collodion tube. It is possible, as Howell suggested, that large amounts of more highly purified heparin might affect this process. A study of this possibility is in progress in these laboratories.

The investigations on human cases were conducted merely to determine whether regional heparinization and general heparinization were feasible procedures with the preparations which were available. It has been shown (1) that no deleterious effects were produced in several cases in which regional heparinization was carried out with moderately pure heparin and (2) that using highly purified material prolonged general heparinization would appear to be feasible.

If the general heparinization of patients postoperatively proceeds as satisfactorily as at present, it is hoped that a large group can be studied. We appreciate fully that before any deductions concerning the results of this procedure on the incidence of thrombus formation can be drawn, a series consisting of at least several hundred cases must be studied. A statistical treatment of the clinical findings at present available on the frequency of vascular obstruction by thrombus may indicate that this number is grossly inadequate. Furthermore, it may not be feasible to administer heparin in an intravenous infusion of saline solution to patients for more than four or five days after operation. So little is known about the factors which cause thrombosis that it is difficult to decide whether or not this is an adequate period. The times at which embolism most frequently occurs do not provide the required information since heparinization would be directed against the formation of the potential embolus. The procedures used at present, which are directed towards prevention of (1) tissue injury (liberation of thrombokinase), (2) infection, and (3) stagnation of blood, are based on sound physiologic principles, but the results of their application cannot, as yet, be considered satisfactory. While the findings we have reported in experimental animals justify the inference that clinical thrombosis, attributable to certain etiologic factors, might be prevented by heparin, it is usually impossible to determine what factors are in operation in a particular clinical case. It should be borne in mind also that heparin has not been proved to be of physiologic significance. While information on its distribution in the body and mechanism of action is available, no direct evidence indicating a physiologic role has been obtained.

Under these circumstances clinical research may be advantageously conducted along at least two lines: (1) attempts to determine the cases in which thrombosis is likely to occur and (2) the administration, postoperatively, for prolonged periods of a solution of highly purified heparin which increases the clotting time of the blood but produces no deleterious effects.

It is probable that attempts favourably to influence the incidence of thrombosis in postoperative cases by the administration of heparin to as many patients as possible, is not the best method of determining whether or not the anticoagulant possesses any therapeutic value. The clinical condition characterized by recurrent multiple thromboses might, for example, present a better opportunity. The use of regional or general heparinization after embolectomy in suitable cases, i.e., those in which thrombus formation would be expected at the site from which the embolus had been removed, might give decisive results. If cases are available the effectiveness of purified heparin in these conditions will be tested.

The researches on heparin in this university were initiated in 1929 by one of us (C.H.B.) with two objectives in view. The first was to make adequate amounts of more highly purified material available for physiologic work; the second was to study the effect of the anticoagulant on thrombus formation. After some preliminary experiments with E. W. McHenry, the results of which showed that beef liver as well as dog liver was a useful source of the anticoagulant, the problem of the purification of heparin and the preparation of suitable quantities was undertaken by A. F. Charles, and D. A. Scott [198; 199; 200; 684] in the Connaught Laboratories. These workers have made several reports on the results of their investigations. In their most recent paper they have described the method of preparation of a crystalline barium salt of heparin. This material consistently contains approximately 500 units per milligram. A sterile solution of this product after removal of most of the barium has been available for all of our recent investigations. We would like to acknowledge here the dependence of our work on the results obtained by Charles and Scott.

It is of great interest that Hedenius and Wilander [381], using heparin prepared by a procedure elaborated by Charles and Scott in Toronto, have reported that the material exerts no deleterious effects in human subjects when administered intravenously in amounts which raised the clotting time well above the normal value. The effect of heparin on thrombosis was not studied, but Widström and Wilander [793] believe that they have demonstrated in experimental animals an inhibiting action of the anticoagulant on the formation of fibrin in pleural exudates.

SUMMARY AND CONCLUSIONS

1. The results of our experiments indicate that the incidence of obstruction of peripheral veins in dogs by thrombi formed as a result of certain mechanical or chemical injuries to the intimal surfaces of the blood vessels is definitely decreased when solutions of purified heparin are administered before and for prolonged periods following the injury. These findings are the results of observations on some three hundred veins.

2. The findings in the experiments in which injury was produced by chemical means suggest that the effect of heparin is clearly seen only under conditions in which the extent of the injury is just sufficient to produce thrombosis in most of the veins in animals which do not receive the anticoagulant. This statement refers to the absence of thrombus formation after heparin administration is discontinued. Thrombi have not been observed even after very severe chemical injury while the animal was well heparinized.

3. While the intimal surfaces of veins, removed from heparinized animals several days after the injection of heparin has been discontinued, may appear on macroscopic examination to have recovered completely from the injury, microscopic studies may in some cases reveal minute masses of platelets filling small crevices in the intima.

4. The clotting time of the blood of the human subject may be increased by the intravenous administration of solutions of highly purified heparin. This procedure produces no deleterious effects even when the hepariniza-

tion is maintained for as long as five days. General heparinization has now been carried out in 76 patients postoperatively.

5. The clotting time of the blood in one limb of the experimental animal or human subject may be increased by the intraarterial administration of heparin without affecting to more than a slight degree the clotting time of the blood in other parts of the body. This is only true when the rate of injection of heparin is relatively slow.

6. Various aspects of these results and some of the directions along which further investigations may proceed are discussed.

ACKNOWLEDGMENTS

The Banting Foundation has generously supported this investigation by making grants at various times to two of us (G.D.W.M. and T.S.P.). The kindly interest of Professor W. E. Gallie, of the Department of Surgery, and Professor J. G. FitzGerald, of the School of Hygiene, and the help in the histologic studies of Dr. D. L. MacLean are gratefully acknowledged. We are greatly indebted to Dr. O. M. Solandt for his help in some of the early experiments with sodium ricinoleate and to Dr. F. R. Wilkinson, who has made many of the recent observations on the effect of heparin on human subjects.

The expert technical assistance of Mr. Campbell Cowan has been of the greatest value.

55. Heparin and the Formation of White Thrombi

C. H. BEST

CAMPBELL COWAN

D. L. MACLEAN

The results of a previous investigation of the action of heparin in preventing thrombosis of blood vessels in dogs (Murray et al. [589]) led us to make a further study of this problem. In this paper we wish to discuss the effects of the anticoagulant upon the formation of white thrombi, which takes place with great regularity when blood is made to pass through glass, collodion, or cellophane tubes. The only previous investigation of this aspect of the problem is that of Shionoya [701]. Rowntree and Shionoya [655], using rabbits as experimental animals, studied the accumulation of platelets when the blood flowed through a shunt made of glass and collodion tubing. Shionoya subsequently reported that heparin had no influence upon the rate of formation of white thrombi under the conditions of his experiments. We have made somewhat similar studies and find that in dogs, cats, and monkeys a definite effect of heparin can be demonstrated. Much more difficulty is encountered when rabbits are used but here also an effect can be established. The results of these experiments show that heparin exerts an effect upon the accumulation of platelets and, therefore, support the conclusions of Murray et al. who found that the frequency of the appearance of mixed thrombi, after mechanical or chemical injury to veins, was appreciably decreased when a solution of purified heparin was administered for adequate periods before and after the injury had been produced.

METHODS, EXPERIMENTAL RESULTS, AND COMMENTS

The experiments were conducted under nembutal anaesthesia. Thirty-five mg of nembutal per kg were administered intravenously to the animal approximately 30 min before the start of the experiment. Further amounts of nembutal were given as required during the course of the experiment.

Originally appeared in the *Journal of Physiology*, XCII (1938), 20–31. From the School of Hygiene, University of Toronto.

TABLE 55.I

THE EFFECT OF HEPARIN ON THE FORMATION OF WHITE THROMBI IN DOGS

Exp. no.	Control			Heparin—450 units/kg		
		Time	Observations		Time	Observations
1*	(a)	2 hr 45 min	Not occluded—white thrombi		—	—
	(b)	2 hr 30 min	" "		—	—
2	(a)	2 hr 10 min	Occluded—white thrombi		—	—
	(b)	25 min	" "		—	—
	(c)	35 min	" "			
	(d)	1 hr 30 min	" "			
3	(a)	2 hr	Not occluded—white thrombi	(c)	2 hr	Patent—no thrombus
	(b)	50 min	Occluded—white thrombi	(d)	2 hr	" "
4	(a)	2 hr	Not occluded—white thrombi	(c)	2 hr	" "
	(b)	2 hr	" "	(d)	2 hr	" "
5	(a)	2 hr	" "	(c)	2 hr	" "
	(b)	2 hr	" "	(d)	2 hr	" "
6		—	—	(a)	2 hr	" "
		—	—	(b)	2 hr	" "
				(c)	2 hr	" "
				(d)	2 hr	" "
7	(a)	3 hr	Not occluded—white thrombi	(c)	3 hr	" "
	(b)	3 hr	" "	(d)	3 hr	" "
8	(a)	3 hr 8 min	" "	(c)	3 hr	Not occluded—some platelets
	(b)	3 hr	" "	(d)	3 hr	Patent—no thrombus
9	(a)	1 hr 26 min	Occluded—white thrombi	(c)	3 hr	Not occluded—some platelets
	(b)	37 min	" "	(d)	3 hr	Patent—no thrombus
10	(a)	1 hr 54 min	Not occluded—white thrombi	(c)	3 hr 7 min	Not occluded—some platelets
	(b)	1 hr 44 min	Occluded—white thrombi	(d)	3 hr 8 min	Patent—no thrombus

*(a) indicates the right carotid artery and right jugular vein shunt; (b) the left carotid; (c) the right femoral artery and vein shunt; and (d) the left femoral.

Observations upon Dogs

The results collected in Table 55.I illustrate the very definite effect which a dose of 450 units of heparin per kg exerted upon the formation of white thrombi in dogs under nembutal anaesthesia. The shunt was composed of two glass cannulae connected by a cellophane tube 3 cm in length and of 4 mm bore. The over-all length of the shunt was 17.5 cm; the glass tubing had a bore of 2.5 mm. The diagram (Figure 96) illustrates the method of

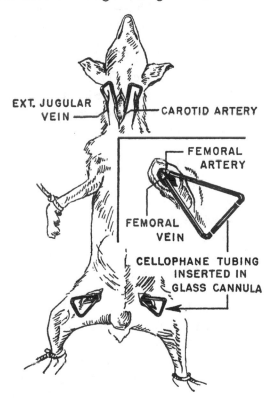

FIGURE 96. Method of installation of shunts made of glass and cellophane tubing.

installation of four of these shunts. In the twenty observations made without heparin white thrombi were observed to form and were found upon the termination of the experiment in every case. In eighteen observations in which heparin was administered the tubes were perfectly clear in sixteen cases. In two, small accumulations of platelets were observed. While these did not possess the structure of a thrombus they were, of course, the nucleus from which a thrombus might form. In every experiment a thorough search of the glass tubing and of the cellophane tube was made. The cellophane tube was examined microscopically, usually after stained sections had been prepared. The results of this series of experiments leave no doubt that, under the conditions which we have described, heparin is effective in preventing the formation of white thrombi in anaesthetized dogs.

Observations upon Cats

The effect of heparin upon the formation of white thrombi in glass and cellophane shunts was also studied in cats. Ten observations were made without heparin and ten after injection of the anticoagulant. White thrombi were observed in every case in which no heparin was administered. The tubes became plugged after varying intervals of from 11 to 44 min. In the heparin series remarkably uniform findings were secured. Large doses of heparin (2250 units/kg) were used. The loops were left *in situ* for 1 hr and formation of thrombi was not observed in any experiment.

(Three tables have been omitted dealing with the effect of heparin on the formation of white thrombi in cats, monkeys, and rabbits.)

Observations upon Monkeys (Macacus rhesus)

A series of observations were made upon monkeys using both the glass and the cellophane loops, and a cell composed entirely of glass. Without heparin, obstruction by white thrombi took place in from 6 to 34 min, with the exception of one case in which the tube was not plugged at the end of 2 hr. White thrombi were found in all instances. With heparin (2250 or 450 units/kg) the tubes did not become obstructed. In three of the eight cases no white thrombi were found. In the other five either very small accumulations of platelets or definite small thrombi were noticed. The results indicate that heparin was exerting an effect in the prevention of the formation of white thrombi in this species.

The observations, using a glass cell, were initiated because we wished to make a motion picture in colour of the formation of white thrombi. The cell is shown in Figure 97. The cannulae were made of pyrex glass and were approximately 6–7 cm in length. The cell presented to the blood a surface of about 4 sq cm. Since this was much greater than in the loop previously used, one expected that thrombi would form much more easily. The process can be watched with the naked eye or through a microscope. White thrombi formed in all cases in which heparin was not used and grew to such a size that occlusion of the glass shunt was produced in all except one instance. With heparin none of the tubes became occluded and no thrombi were observed in two of the five cases. It sometimes appears that platelets accumulate on a very rough bit of the surface and that heparin is not effective in preventing this. It is possible that when the platelets are ruptured the local concentration of some substance necessary to cause them to adhere may, in some cases, be greater than that which can be neutralized by heparin in the concentration in which it is available. These results are summarized in Table 55.II.

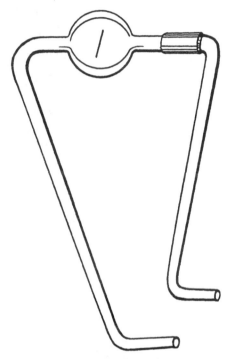

FIGURE 97. Glass cell used for studying mechanism of formation of white thrombi. The rubber tubing connects the cell with the venous cannula. Note scratch on inner surface of cell.

Observations upon Rabbits

The observations made upon rabbits were most interesting. It soon became apparent that heparin was not nearly as effective under the conditions of our experiment when rabbits were used as in the case of dogs, cats, or monkeys. Occlusion of the loops, either those of cellophane and glass, or of loops composed entirely of glass, was, however, never observed in experiments in which heparin was used. In our experience plugging of the cannulae is always produced, in large part, if not completely, by the formation of white thrombi. A red thrombus or clot subsequently forms in the stagnant or very slowly moving stream. The white thrombi may form in any part of the tube but frequently they break away and, if large enough, plug the tip of the venous cannula. In the experiments on rabbits in which heparin was used clumps of platelets were observed to form but these

TABLE 55.II

THE EFFECT OF HEPARIN ON THE FORMATION OF WHITE THROMBI IN MONKEYS

Exp. no.		Control Time	Observations	Heparin* Time	Observations
1	(a)	35 min	Occluded—white thrombi	(c) 4 hr 22 min	Not occluded—white thrombi formed within 5 min.
2	(a)	39 min	"	—	—
	(c)	9 min	"	—	—
3	(a)	5 hr 12 min	Not occluded—white thrombi	(a) 5½ hr	Not occluded—white thrombi formed within 39 min.
4	(a)	—	—	—	—
5	(a)	26 min	Occluded—white thrombi	—	—
	(b)	16 min	"	—	—
	(c)	15 min	"		
	(d)	26 min	"		
6		53 min	"	1 hr	Patent—no thrombi
7		30 min	"	1 hr	Patent when excised; one small point of white thrombus formed five times during first 20 min; nothing observed thereafter
8		35 min	"	1 hr	Patent—no thrombi

*Exp. no. 1, initial dose = 450 units/kg; second dose in 2½ hr = 1200 units; nos. 4, 6, 7, and 8, dose = 2250 units/kg.

never reached a size sufficient to produce plugging of the venous cannula. In only two cases in the rather large series of observations were the tubes found completely free of white thrombi. In both cases heparin had been used. The main point of evidence, however, that heparin influences the formation of thrombi in the experiments on rabbits, is that in no case was a thrombus formed, in a heparin experiment, which was sufficiently large to cause plugging of the tip of the venous cannula. The rabbits weighed from 1500 to 2000 g and the diameter of the cannula used was smaller than in the other species. While we believe that an effect of heparin is apparent in these experiments, it would also appear that the conditions which encourage the accumulation of platelets are operating to such an extent that it is difficult to demonstrate its influence.

Observations upon the Mechanism of Formation of White Thrombi

When an area in the glass cell, on which white thrombi always form in the absence of heparin, is watched through a microscope, the deposition of platelets can readily be studied. There would appear to be no doubt that the white thrombus is built up primarily of platelets as Bizzozero [127] originally showed. If a fresh white thrombus is pulled out of the cell by means of a fine wire and quickly dissected in saline on a slide, the individual platelets can be seen. Such a fresh thrombus must be obtained within a few minutes of its formation, otherwise the platelets become so tightly packed together that they lose their normal outlines. An early thrombus like this has a homogeneous granular character and stains uniformly a faint pink with haematoxylin and eosin staining. A thrombus that has been allowed to remain *in situ* for approximately an hour or more undergoes another change. In addition to the fusing together of the platelets one finds, in confirmation of previous workers, that they undergo a hyalinization. Staining of such thrombi indicates that a part of the platelet mass absorbs the acidophilic stains better than other portions. This results in the wavy appearance of the thrombus. More faintly staining portions of the platelet mass are frequently in close relationship to enmeshed white cells. If one wishes, however, to observe the earliest alterations in blood platelets, a study of blood films under dark field illumination must be made (Ferguson [298]).

. . . While a detailed study has not as yet been made of the mechanism of formation of thrombi under the conditions of our experiments, a great deal of evidence has already accumulated which confirms the conclusions of most pathologists that the thrombus grows distally or down-stream.

[Seven figures have been omitted showing photographic records of thrombus formation. Some of these were from a motion picture film made of the clotting process.]

In the first series of pictures the inner surface of the cell had not been scratched, but in the second series the thrombi have formed upon a scratch made upon the upper surface of the glass cell (Figure 97). There is almost no deposition of platelets up-stream from the scratch; the thrombus grows down-stream by deposition of more platelets upon those already present (see Plate X(c)). While there is a very definite deposition of platelets in the periphery of this glass cell where the blood stream is slowed, this process takes place quite as rapidly on the scratch, which is in the axial stream. The flow is rapid since the glass tubing which connects the carotid artery and the jugular vein to the cell is of approximately the same calibre as the carotid artery.

Effect of Heparin on the Circulation

Previous investigators have studied the effect of heparin upon blood pressure and heart rate and various other indices of circulatory function. The dose of heparin which we have used in these experiments produces, at most, only a transient effect upon the heart rate and blood pressure of experimental animals. In a recent experiment on a monkey in which the changes in blood pressure and heart rate were carefully noted no significant change was observed. There was no change in the electrocardiogram. The results of these observations suggest that the effect of heparin upon formation of white thrombi is not related to an action upon the circulation.

DISCUSSION

The results of the investigations which we have reported demonstrate the effect of heparin in preventing the formation of white thrombi, which is almost invariably observed in the control experiments. The findings are very definite in dogs, cats, and monkeys but more difficulty is encountered in demonstrating this effect of heparin in rabbits. Among the many possible explanations it may be suggested that the platelets of rabbit blood are more easily destroyed under our experimental conditions than those of the other species or that they liberate a more powerful "adhesive agent." While our observations suggest that the factor responsible for the clumping of the platelets is not fibrin formed from plasma fibrinogen, direct proof of the presence of an "adhesive agent" in platelets is needed to exclude the plasma fibrin theory and also others based on the physical properties of the "third blood cell."

The structure of white thrombi has interested students since the work of Virchow [776] who believed that the whitish mass, which is frequently observed in blood vessels under certain conditions, was formed by white blood cells, disintegrated fibrin and red blood corpuscles which had lost their haemoglobin. We are indebted, however, to Mantegazza [550] for the demonstration of the fact that the white thrombus does not arise by a gradual change from a red thrombus but originates in a form very similar to that in which it finally appears. Mantegazza thought the thrombus was formed of white blood corpuscles and fibrin and many of the subsequent workers had the same conception of the mode of origin. A very great advance was made in this field in 1882 by Bizzozero [127] who watched the formation of a white thrombus under the microscope. He found that when he caused slight damage to the inner surface of an arterial wall in small mammals, a thrombus was soon produced. The whitish mass was formed almost entirely by blood platelets. There were only a few white blood cells. It would appear that relatively little information has been added to that which was available in 1882. The findings of Bizzozero with regard to the origin of a thrombus have been supported by those of Eberth and Schimmelbusch [277], Zurhelle [830], and Welch [790]. Our own observations are in accord with his conclusions.

Direct evidence that white thrombi grow under the conditions of our experiments by deposition of platelets on the distal or down-stream side of the primary mass is readily obtained by observing the process in the glass cell. The proximal or up-stream side of the mass of platelets changes very little. Definite growth can be noted on the right or distal side. This phenomenon is shown even more clearly when growth of the thrombi on the scratch is watched. Observations made upon the *formation* of thrombi on the scratch and also in the narrow parts of the cannula appear to show that this process may take place without marked slowing of the blood stream. On the other hand, it is certainly true that one of the causes of thrombus formation is slowing of the stream. This, of course, has been demonstrated frequently in previous investigations and can readily be deduced from our own observations. We would like to stress the fact, however, that if there is a rough surface, such as a scratch on the glass tubing, thrombi form quickly in spite of the fact that the blood stream is moving very rapidly. It may argued with justice that growth of these thrombi is due, in part, to a deposition of platelets in the eddy formed in the stream by the first deposit of cells. Whether or not the scratch produces invisible eddy currents (certainly none can be seen until clumps of platelets are visible) and in this or some other manner produces a local slowing of the stream which is responsible for the original deposition of platelets, cannot be decided at present.

SUMMARY AND CONCLUSIONS

1. When a shunt composed of glass or cellophane tubing is inserted between an artery and a vein in anaesthetized dogs, cats, monkeys, or rabbits, large white thrombi rapidly form and, in many cases, completely obstruct the flow of blood.

2. The administration of a large dose of purified heparin usually prevents or delays the formation of these thrombi in dogs, cats, or monkeys. In rabbits growth of the thrombi is apparently inhibited, but very small clumps of platelets may form even when large doses of heparin are used.

3. The use of a transilluminated glass cell has made it possible to record the formation and growth of white thrombi on photographic film.

4. The results of this study show, in confirmation of those of previous investigators, that the thrombi usually grow down rather than up the blood stream from the original focus.

ACKNOWLEDGMENTS

We are indebted to our colleagues Dr. Arthur Charles and Dr. James Craigie for a great deal of help in these studies. The purified heparin was made by Dr. Charles in the Connaught Laboratories. Dr. Craigie has been responsible for most of the photographic work.

56. Heparin and Coronary Thrombosis in Experimental Animals

D. Y. SOLANDT, M.D., PH.D.

C. H. BEST, M.D., D.SC., F.R.S.

It has recently been shown that thrombosis of peripheral veins in dogs, produced by chemical or mechanical injury to the intimal surface, may in large part be prevented by the administration of solutions of highly purified heparin (Murray, Jaques, Perrett, and Best [590]). The accumulation of platelets which takes place in a glass shunt inserted between an artery and a vein in the monkey, dog, or cat is much reduced when the animal is adequately heparinized (Best, Cowan, and Maclean [81]).

In embarking upon a study of thrombus formation in arteries our attention was focused on the coronary vessels by the high incidence of thrombosis of these arteries in the human species. Our first problem was to perfect a technique by which a gradually occurring thrombosis of the coronary artery could consistently be produced. After an unsuccessful attempt to induce the condition by the infiltration of sodium ricinoleate around the coronary vessels, we found that the introduction of the chemical into the lumen of a section of the artery and its retention there for a few minutes resulted, in most cases, in a thrombosis of the injected vessels or one of its large branches. When the animal was heparinized before the injection of the sodium ricinoleate and during the period of observation, the formation of thrombi and the resulting infarct was, in large part, prevented.

METHODS

Dogs weighing from 8–12 kg were used. Nembutal was employed when anaesthesia was necessary. Solutions of heparin made from the crystalline material, after removal of the barium, were supplied to us by Dr. A. F. Charles of the Connaught Laboratories. The clotting time of the blood of the heparinized animals was maintained at various levels but never lower than 30 minutes. The normal range was from 4 to 7 minutes. The initial

Originally appeared in the *Lancet*, II (1938), 130–2. From the Department of Physiological Hygiene, University of Toronto.

dose of heparin given just before the injection of sodium ricinoleate was 45 units per kg, while the continuous injection, by a constant speed pump, was at the rate of 35 units per kg per hour.

The chest was opened between the fourth and fifth ribs. The pericardium was opened over the left coronary artery and the heart was lifted gently by weights attached to the cut edges of the pericardium. The epicardium was incised over the coronary artery with the point of a scapel. A section of the artery, approximately 1 cm in length, was dissected clear of the myocardium. Clips were applied at the upper and lower extremities of the section and on all the branches. The sodium ricinoleate was introduced into the lumen of the occluded section by a fine needle. The chemical was allowed to remain for from 5 to 10 minutes, when the clips were released.

In the heparinized animals stringent precautions were necessary to prevent haemorrhage. All the operative procedures were carried out by actual or electro-cautery.

One electrocardiograph lead was placed over the 6th rib adjacent to the apex-beat and the other at the angle between the 12th rib and the spinal column. Polarity was such that the normal R-wave was upright. The animal was always placed on its right side.

EXPERIMENTAL RESULTS

Tying of Left Coronary Artery

Although this procedure has been described a number of times in the literature, it was repeated to discover the effect on the electrocardiogram with the particular lead positions which we have used. The main trunk of the left coronary artery was tied in 9 dogs. In every case the R-wave of the electrocardiogram disappeared shortly after the operation. An autopsy was performed on each animal 20 to 24 hours after the operation. A sharply demarcated pale area was found covering the ventral wall of the left ventricle and extending well around the apex.

In the present report the only part of the electrocardiogram considered in relation to coronary occlusion and the resulting myocardial infarction was the R-wave. The results of these experiments which involved tying of the left coronary artery appear to indicate that, with the leads used, an absent R-wave means that a large area of the myocardium of the left ventricle is inactive.

Extravascular Injection of Sodium Ricinoleate

In each case this injection was made under the epicardium and in the region of the main bifurcation of the left coronary artery. In the 7 dogs thus treated results of electrocardiographic study showed no evidence of myocardial infarction. On autopsy no macroscopic or microscopic evidence of coronary artery thrombosis was found. Veins adjacent to the site of injection were thrombosed in the majority of cases.

Intra-arterial Injection of Sodium Ricinoleate without Heparin

The main trunk or a major left branch of the left coronary artery was injected in 13 dogs. The results are summarized in Table 56.I. The conclusions, based on a consideration of the data in columns 2, 3, and 4, appear in column 5. In each case the autopsy was performed from 20 to 24 hours after the operation. Of the 13 animals 12 showed myocardial infarction with distribution similar to that seen after tying the left coronary artery. In most cases thrombosis of the injected artery or of a large branch of this artery was found associated with the infarction. Microscopic examination of the myocardium over the pale area showed degeneration of muscle fibres and some exudation between fibres.

In most cases the electrocardiographic changes were slower in onset and development than in those where the infarction was produced by tying the artery. The R-wave usually became progressively smaller during the hours between the operation and the autopsy and in no case was this trend reversed. The state of the R-wave immediately before autopsy is given in column 4 of Table 56.I.

TABLE 56.I

SODIUM RICINOLEATE INJECTION OF CORONARY ARTERIES WITHOUT HEPARIN

Dog no.	Microscopic Evidence of Large Artery Thrombosis?	Macroscopic Evidence of Extensive Myocardial Degeneration?	Electro-cardiogram (chest lead) R-wave at End of Experiment	Coronary Artery Thrombosis Resulting in Myocardial Infarction?
1–27	yes	yes	absent	yes
2–29	,,	,,	,,	,,
3–30	,,	,,	,,	,,
4–31	partial	,,	,,	,,
5–32	yes	,,	,,	,,
6–33	no	,,	,,	,,
7–34	yes	,,	,,	,,
8–35	partial	,,	trace (1/6 normal)	,,
9–36	,,	no	reduced (1/2 normal)	no
10–37	yes	yes	,,	yes
11–38	no	,,	absent	,,
12–39	yes	,,	trace (1/6 normal)	,,
13–48	,,	,,	,,	,,

Result. 12 out of 13 dogs showed myocardial degeneration. Demonstrable thrombosis of coronary artery present in 11 out of the 13 dogs.

Apparently the injury done to the artery did not result in an immediate occlusion by thrombosis. Final blocking of the vessel was presumably, on electrocardiographic evidence, not attained until a number of hours after the vessel had been damaged. The similarity of the results in the series of dogs operated upon indicates that the method employed gives a fairly reproducible degree of injury.

Intra-arterial Injection of Sodium Ricinoleate with Heparin

The main trunk or a major left branch of the left coronary artery was injected in 12 dogs. In each case the clotting time of the blood was increased to 30 minutes or over by the administration of heparin prior to the injection of sodium ricinoleate. Continuous intravenous injection of heparin was employed to keep the blood clotting time at 30 minutes or over up to the time of the autopsy. This autopsy was performed from 20 to 24 hours after the operation.

The results are summarized in Table 56.II which is constructed similarly to Table 56.I. Only 1 of the 12 dogs showed coronary thrombosis and a resulting myocardial infarction. In some cases the R-wave of the electrocardiogram was smaller after than before the operation. In several of these the R-wave then became progressively larger up to the time of autopsy. In no case was this improvement in the electrocardiogram observed in the series with normal blood clotting time.

It was found difficult to obtain complete haemostasis at the site of operation in heparinized animals. In this series, as given in Table 56.II, 5 dogs

TABLE 56.II

SODIUM RICINOLEATE INJECTION OF CORONARY ARTERIES IN HEPARINIZED DOGS

Dog no.	Microscopic Evidence of Large Artery Thrombosis?	Macroscopic Evidence of Extensive Myocardial Degeneration?	Electro-cardiogram (chest lead) R-wave at End of Experiment	Coronary Artery Thrombosis Resulting in Myocardial Infarction?
1–53	no	no	normal	no
2–54	partial	”	”	”
3–60	”	”	”	”
4–61	no	”	”	”
5–62	”	”	”	”
6–63	”	yes	absent	yes
7–64	”	no	normal	no
8–68	yes	”	”	”
9–69	no	”	”	”
10–70	”	”	”	”
11–74	”	”	”	”
12–75	”	”	”	”

Result. Coronary artery occlusion with resulting myocardial degeneration seen in only 1 out of 12 dogs.

not listed died before the required 20 hours after the operation had elapsed. All 5 died as a result of postoperative haemorrhage. None showed macroscopic evidence of myocardial infarction.

Discussion

The results of the experiments in which sodium ricinoleate was introduced into the lumen of the coronary artery indicate that this method produces an occlusion of the vessel which may require 20 hours to become complete. It is obvious that this technique provides an excellent opportunity for a study of the earliest abnormalities associated with thrombosis of the artery. This aspect of the investigation is receiving further study.

The diagnosis of cardiac infarction was based on electrocardiographic studies and verified by macroscopic examination of the myocardium. The thrombus in the injured artery may be missed or may be pulled away by the microtome. Furthermore, thrombi formed at the site of the injury may break away and block small branches of the vessel, thus producing infarction almost as effectively as would occlusion of the main artery. The microscopic findings, for which our colleague Dr. D. L. MacLean has been responsible, will be discussed in detail in a future publication.

Very little comment on the results of the experiments in which heparin was administered is required. It is apparent that the particular type of coronary thrombosis and cardiac infarction which we have been studying is largely prevented by heparin. We have not as yet determined the duration of administration of heparin necessary to secure healing of the damaged intima, but in somewhat similar experiments on veins, heparinization for 72 hours was found to be adequate.

The availability of a potent solution of heparin which can safely be administered to human patients (Murray and Best [586]), and the proof that a thrombosis of the coronary artery in experimental animals can be prevented by its administration, makes necessary a consideration of the possibility of clinical application of these findings. The clinical and experimental conditions are, of course, by no means comparable. In the latter only one area of a coronary artery is injured. In the former there may be a sclerosis so extensive that the prevention of thrombus formation and healing of the intima at one spot would mean, at best, only a short reprieve for the patient. The great obstacle in the way of testing the action of heparin in clinical cases of coronary thrombosis is, however, the absence of premonitory signs or symptoms of the condition. It is possible that a thrombus may form with great rapidity—in experimental animals 15–20 minutes may suffice for the complete occlusion of a glass tube the size of the carotid artery. On the other hand, there is at present no method of estimating the time taken in clinical cases. Cardiologists have stated that intramural thrombi have been found in an appreciable percentage of cases of coronary thrombosis. Heparin might reduce the incidence of this complication. We hope to be able to test this possibility in experimental animals.

SUMMARY

1. A method is described by which a gradual occlusion of the coronary artery by thrombus formation may be produced in experimental animals.

2. This formation of thrombi and the resulting cardiac infarction may be prevented by the administration of adequate amounts of highly purified heparin.

3. It has been emphasized that the main difficulty standing in the way of an adequate clinical investigation of the therapeutic possibilities of heparin in acute coronary crises is the absence of premonitory signs of these conditions. This situation should stimulate both the experimental and the clinical cardiologist to further research.

ACKNOWLEDGMENTS

It is a pleasure to acknowledge the co-operation of Dr. D. L. MacLean in certain aspects of these studies. We are greatly indebted to Mr. Campbell Cowan and Mr. Jack Scattergood for expert technical assistance.

57. Experimental Exchange Transfusion Using Purified Heparin

WILLIAM THALHIMER*, M.D.

D. Y. SOLANDT, M.D.

C. H. BEST, M.D., F.R.S.

A description has already been given of experimental "exchange" transfusions between nephrectomized and normal dogs (Thalhimer [748]). Purified heparin injected intravenously as an anticoagulant prevented thrombus formation, in some experiments for many hours, and caused no toxic symptoms. The purpose of the experiments was to determine whether blood-urea could be reduced in the nephrectomized dog, and whether this non-protein nitrogenous substance which the normal dog received would be excreted rapidly. Although only a comparatively small amount of blood was exchanged in each direction, the results indicated that the study might profitably be extended, using a pump which made possible the exchange of blood at a much more rapid rate.

METHODS

Dogs (6 to 20 kg in weight) were anaesthetized with an intravenous injection of nembutal. Under aseptic conditions both kidneys were removed, utilizing either two lumbar or a single ventral incision. The exchange transfusion experiment was performed 1–5 days after the operation.

The nephrectomized dog and a normal "donor" dog were anaesthetized with nembutal given intravenously. Occasionally, when the nephrectomized dog was in coma, it was not anaesthetized until after the transfusion had started. In each dog one carotid artery and jugular vein, or one femoral artery and vein, were exposed and cannulae inserted. These were connected to a pump (Figures 98 and 99) specially designed to give a volumetrically equal exchange of blood in each direction (Solandt and Robinson [723]).

Originally appeared in the *Lancet*, II (1938), 554–6. From the School of Hygiene, University of Toronto.

*Director of the Manhattan Convalescent Serum Laboratory, New York City.

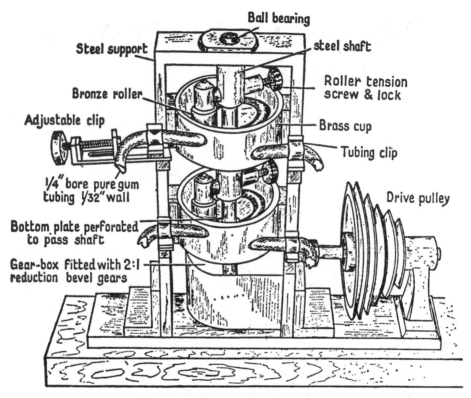

FIGURE 98. Exchange transfusion pump.

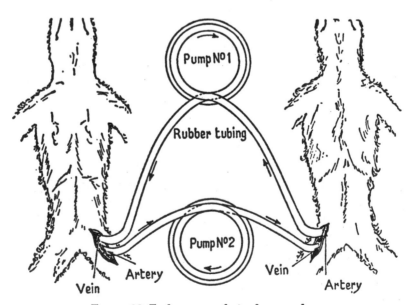

FIGURE 99. Exchange transfusion between dogs.

Samples of arterial blood were taken for analysis before starting the pump. The direction of blood flow was from the artery of each animal into the central end of the vein of the other animal. The pump was tested before each experiment to be certain that the flow was the same in both directions. Thus no change in the blood volumes of the two animals would be produced. If the pump delivered only a slight excess in either direction, one of the animals would have been exsanguinated. The first pump used delivered three litres an hour in each direction. This pump was later made to deliver six litres in each direction. With each increase in rate of exchange of blood the rate of removal of urea from the nephrectomized animal increased. Finally, a larger and somewhat modified pump, as illustrated, was constructed. This had a capacity of at least thirty litres an hour in each direction, a volume in excess of that which either the carotid or femoral artery could deliver. These arteries, in an animal weighing about 8 kg, will, however, deliver more than 12 litres of blood an hour.

Sufficient highly purified heparin (Scott and Charles [684]) was injected intravenously just before starting the pump to prevent temporarily thrombus formation. Heparin was injected subsequently either at hourly intervals or at a constant rate by means of a motor-operated piston pump. Samples of arterial blood were taken at intervals, and the urea nitrogen was determined by the method of Barrett [55]. In some experiments the urine was collected and analysed for urea nitrogen by the same method used for blood.

The nephrectomized dogs usually were killed at the end of the experiment by an overdose of nembutal. An autopsy was performed and microscopic examination of various organs was made. Some of the donor dogs were allowed to recover, to observe if they returned to a normal state, and to follow the urea-nitrogen content of their blood.

RESULTS AND DISCUSSION

After both kidneys have been removed from a dog, urea increases rapidly in the blood. In twenty-four hours it is usually in excess of 75 mg of urea nitrogen per 100 cc of blood, and in forty-eight hours may exceed 200 mg.

In the earlier work (Thalhimer [748]) even the exchange of comparatively small volumes of blood lowered the level of urea nitrogen in the blood of the nephrectomized dog, and increased it in the blood of the normal dog. The rate of removal of urea—i.e., diffusion into the tissues and excretion—in the normal animal was found to be rapid. However, only in the longer experiments, with more rapid exchange of blood, did urea in the normal dog, having reached a peak, begin to decrease. This happened even though

TABLE 57.I

RESULTS OF REPRESENTATIVE EXPERIMENTS

Experiment	Weight of Dogs (kg)		Duration of Exchange Transfusion	Rate of Exchange (litres per hour in each direction)	Blood Urea (mg/100 cc)					
	Nephrectomized	Donor			Donor			Nephrectomized		
					before exchange transfusion	at end of exchange	maximum during exchange	before nephrectomy	before exchange	at end of exchange
14	12	10	6	3	12	33	33	15	62	50
16	6	8	7	6	11	29	48	14	120	36
17	7	30	22	6	17	35	45	N	206	41
18	13	23	2	6	19	45	48	,,	105	56
19	8	12	6	6	22	29	46	,,	89	33
20	15	27	6	6	18	65	65	20	224	67
21	20	21	27	12	15	20	81	13	220	20
23	8	24	4	12	17	62	62	24	211	61
25	11	18	2	12	29	68	68	26	200	82
28	10	no. 1 21	1	12	20	52	—	11	145	72
		no. 2 18	1	12	21	44	—			57

N = normal.

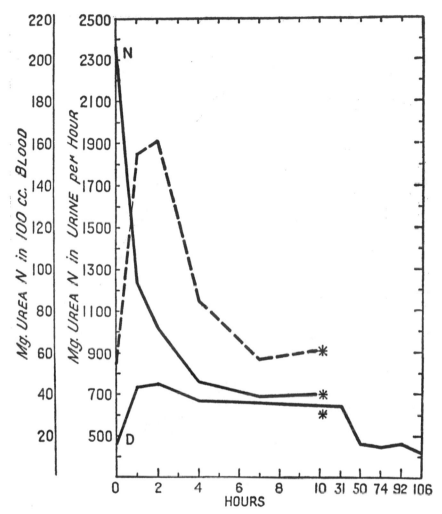

FIGURE 100. (Expt. 17.) Continuous line = blood urea; interrupted line = urine urea; N = nephrectomized dog; D = normal dog; * = end of exchange transfusion.

blood from the nephrectomized dog, high in urea, continued to be introduced into the circulation of the normal dog. Table 57.I and Figures 100–102 summarize and illustrate the results of representative experiments.

It became evident that in some experiments the lowering of urea in the nephrectomized animal's blood was not proportional to the increase of urea in the blood of the normal animal. This indicated that there must be a reservoir which supplied urea to the blood during the process of its removal. The reports of other investigators have shown that equilibrium between the tissues and the blood occurs at, or about, the blood-urea level. The existence of this reservoir is indicated in some of our experiments

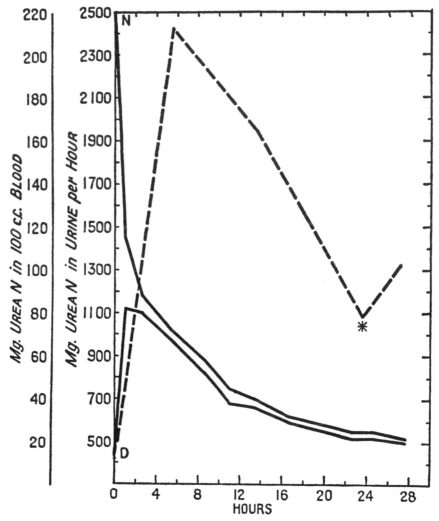

FIGURE 101. (Expt. 21.) Exchange transfusion continued over full period. Continuous line = blood urea; interrupted line = urine urea; N = nephrectomized dog; D = normal dog; * = catheter plugged.

(see no. 21) in which the donor dog excreted an amount of urea far in excess of that present in the blood of the nephrectomized dog at the beginning of the transfusion. The tissues are the obvious source of this excess. This reservoir in the donor dog must also be considered. The drop in the blood-urea of the nephrectomized dog, which occurs in the first hour of the experiment, is largely due to a dilution effect. It is probably correct to consider that, after the experiment has proceeded for a short time, the urea of the nephrectomized dog is distributed fairly evenly throughout the blood and non-osseous tissues of both animals. Once this has taken place,

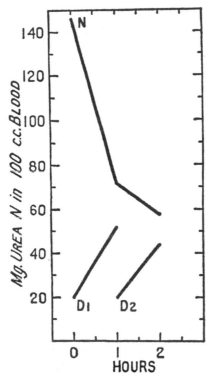

FIGURE 102. (Expt. 28) N = nephrectomized dog; D₁ = first normal dog; D₂ = second normal dog.

subsequent lowering of the urea can, of course, only be effected by excretion of this substance in the urine of the donor dog.

In some cases the exchange transfusion was started after the nephrectomized dog had become comatose. After a few minutes of transfusion it became conscious and then again lapsed into unconsciousness. This latter condition was thought to be due to the anaesthetic carried over in the blood of the donor. Before the nephrectomized dogs became comatose they sometimes exhibited signs of hyperexcitability. In this stage it was observed, in one instance by X-ray, that the left side of the diaphragm was "beating" in synchrony with the heart. Presumably a state of hyperexcitability resulted in the left phrenic nerve, which lies in direct contact with the pericardium, being excited by the myocardial action currents. It was, in effect, a rheoscopic nerve-muscle preparation.

Many of the experiments were completed with both animals in good condition, and with no signs of thrombus formation. The donor dogs usually made rapid and complete recoveries. The kidneys and other organs of most of the donor dogs which were sacrificed were found to be normal on macroscopic and microscopic examination. This is specially significant in Experiment 21, where the exchange transfusion was continued for twenty-seven consecutive hours and no abnormality of the donor was found at autopsy. In some experiments accidents occurred which were due to avoidable causes, such as thrombosis from insufficient heparin, mechanical accidents to the early models of the pump, and incompatibility of bloods.

In most of the experiments only a single donor animal was used for each transfusion. When this was so no incompatibility of the bloods of the nephrectomized and donor animals was encountered. It is well known that isoagglutinins and isohaemolysins occur in dogs, and we were on the watch for incompatibility reactions. Unlike humans, dogs do not have definite blood groups, and agglutinins and haemolysins are present in only some dogs. When they exist they usually agglutinate and haemolyse the red blood cells of many other dogs.

It was only when the experiments were extended by the use of two or three donor dogs in succession that the phenomena of blood incompatibility were encountered. Multiple donors were used in an attempt to speed up the removal of urea from the nephrectomized dog in the hope that the urea could be reduced to a normal level in two or three hours. With two compatible donors, used in succession for one hour each, as in Experiment 28, the urea was removed from the nephrectomized dogs more rapidly than when only one was used. In two experiments a third donor was used at the beginning of the third hour, but each time an accident occurred.

The only previous publication in this field is by Nyiri [601] and is entitled "Experimental Crossed Transfusions in Uraemia." Experimental exchange transfusions for other purposes have been performed by many workers but, as in Nyiri's experiments, exchange of blood was slow and no method of ensuring movement of equal volumes in each direction was used.

Nyiri described "crossed transfusions" in experimental uraemia in dogs caused by bilateral nephrectomy or by administering uranium nitrate. He did not employ an anticoagulant, but attempted to prevent thrombosis by the use of paraffin-coated cannulae. He was able to carry on several experiments for periods of two or three hours. The blood-urea nitrogen decreased in the nephrectomized dog, and increased in the donor dog, but the uraemic animal's blood-urea was not reduced below 150 mg per 100 cc from a level of 250–300 mg.

There are perhaps some circumstances which might justify the use of exchange transfusions in the human species. However, application to human subjects should be considered only after a thorough study of the technique and full appreciation of the many attendant dangers.

Summary

These experiments demonstrate that with the use of purified heparin and a specially designed pump, short-term or long-term exchange transfusions can be carried out safely between two anaesthetised dogs. The heparin does not have any toxic action. If it is used continuously and in sufficient amounts thrombosis can be prevented.

The urea which has accumulated in blood and tissues of a dog after bilateral nephrectomy is excreted rapidly in the urine of the normal donor. The excretion is sufficiently rapid to lower the urea—which for a time is greatly increased in the donor animal—to approximately normal values in 12–18 hours. When the transfusion is discontinued the donor dog may recover completely and behave in an entirely normal manner. At various intervals later, the tissues, including the kidneys, of the dogs used as donors in the successful experiments were found to be normal macroscopically and microscopically.

Acknowledgments

We would like to acknowledge help received from various colleagues both in New York and in Toronto. This work has been supported by the New York, Nathan Hofheimer, and Friedsam Foundations and by the Connaught Laboratories.

THE INITIATION AND ORGANIZATION
of the project for the preparation of dried human serum for military use
kept us very busy during most of the first year of the Second World War.
It is not possible, unfortunately, to mention the names of many in the
Canadian Red Cross Society, in the Connaught Laboratories and in the
Departments of Physiology and Physiological Hygiene of the University
of Toronto who made major contributions to the successful conduct of this
project. In addition to Dr. D. Y. Solandt and Dr. Jessie H. Ridout whose
names are on Paper 58 with mine I should like to mention Professor R. D.
Defries, Professor R. E. Haist, Professor A. L. Chute, Dr. Jack Magladery,
Mr. Roy Sproat, and Mr. Hugh Aird. Something over two million donations
of blood were secured and dried and most of this was shipped from Canada
to the depot in England. My contacts there, by letter and in person, were
primarily with my close friend, the late Sir Lionel Whitby.

I should record here also my deep indebtedness to my wife and her
sister, Miss Linda Mahon, for the immense amount of time and effort which
they gave in the initiation of the Canadian Serum Project. I thought it wise
to set a good example so I became the first blood donor but, as I have
written elsewhere, after ten donations I felt a bit anaemic and joined the
Royal Canadian Navy.

58. The Canadian Project for the Preparation of Dried Human Serum for Military Use

C. H. BEST, M.D.

D. Y. SOLANDT, M.D.

JESSIE H. RIDOUT, PH.D.

ORGANIZATION

The Canadian project for the preparation of serum for military use was initiated in the Departments of Physiology and Physiological Hygiene shortly after the outbreak of war. The expenses were secured from the research funds which were available for use in the Departments. The donors were obtained from the members of the undergraduate body of the University. As the demands of the work became greater, an application for a grant in aid was made to the Blood Storage Committee of the National Research Council of Canada. This organization provided a part of the expenses for a period of some three months, and then recommended that the Department of National Defence should take over the responsibility for the budget. Through this latter department the Canadian Red Cross Society became interested, and provided funds which defrayed some of the expenses. For the first year of the war, serum was concentrated to one-third of the volume by the Thalhimer technique.[1] After that time, the Desivac equipment was secured and since then all of the serum processed has been dried in this apparatus.

The first drying apparatus was obtained with funds made available by the Department of National Defence. The subsequent equipment and the expenses for the processing of the blood or serum in the Connaught Labora-

Originally appeared in *Blood Substitutes and Blood Transfusion*, ed. S. Mudd and W. Thalhimer (Springfield, Ill.: Charles C. Thomas, 1942), chapter XXVI. From the Departments of Physiology and Physiological Hygiene, University of Toronto. This is the published version of a lecture delivered at a meeting organized by the United States Armed Services and held in Philadelphia in 1941.

[1]We are greatly indebted to Dr. William Thalhimer and Mrs. Charles Myron for their help in the early stages of this work.

tories (a Department of the University of Toronto) have been provided by the Department of Pensions and National Health which is responsible for the health of civilians in Canada. The Canadian Red Cross Society has undertaken complete responsibility for the enlistment of donors and through their committee the serum project is being extended to include the whole of Canada. Approximately 3,500 donations per week are now being received (May, 1942).

The donations from points outside Ontario—Halifax, Nova Scotia, for example—are sent to Toronto in the form of liquid serum. All of the drying is conducted in the Connaught Laboratories. The plan, as at present organized, calls for the taking of 8,000 donations weekly throughout Canada. The material from Ontario will be sent as fresh clotted blood to the Connaught Laboratories where the serum will be made and the drying process carried out. Blood donations from other parts of Canada will be sent as serum to the Connaught Laboratories until other drying plants are made available.

The Department of National Defence has first call on all the dried serum made available, and after these demands are satisfied, the Department of Pensions and National Health will distribute the remainder. No serum is distributed directly by the Canadian Red Cross Society or by the Connaught Laboratories.

PROCEDURE

The Canadian Red Cross Society enlists the donors through appeals made in the press, over the radio, and by distribution of descriptive pamphlets. A great many organizations co-operate and supply groups of donors for the clinics. The Red Cross makes the appointment with the donor and advises him to have a very light breakfast containing no fatty material on the day on which he is to give blood. Wherever necessary, transportation to and from the clinic is provided by the Red Cross. When the donor reaches the clinic, his name, address, age, and weight are recorded and a number is assigned to him. His temperature is taken and he is given a short medical examination, and if his condition is found satisfactory he is asked to sign a form indicating his willingness to donate blood. The donors are requested to return at approximately ten week intervals.

COLLECTION OF BLOOD

The donor makes himself comfortable on a flat-topped table. The doctor selects a suitable vein and the area is cleansed with iodine and alcohol. The local anaesthetic (stocaine) is injected and a large needle, gauge 16, connected with the bleeding bottle is introduced into the vein. The doctors are assisted by a group of trained nurses who have also volunteered their services. 420 cc of blood are taken from each donor. After the donation is completed, a sterile pad is put over the needle hole and a simple bandage is placed on the arm. Donors are asked to rest for 15 minutes, or longer if necessary, and during this time are offered coffee, tea, or some cold drink. Those who really faint get a little whiskey!

APPARATUS FOR COLLECTING THE BLOOD

The blood is collected in an ordinary pint milk bottle marked at the 420 cc level. [A figure has been omitted showing the details of the collecting device.] Bleeding is done by gravity, under sterile conditions, but is facilitated when necessary by producing a slight vacuum by means of suction on the mouth-piece. When the required amount of blood has been secured, the test-tube is refitted over the needle, and a spring clamp is slipped over the upper part of both the rubber tubing connected to the mouth-piece and that connected to the needle.

PREPARATION OF SERUM

Some two to four hours after the blood has been secured, the bottle is opened, the clot rimmed, and quartered. A sample is removed at this time for typing, presumptive Kahn, and for other tests. A sterile rubber stopper is then placed in the bottle. The blood is put in a refrigerator overnight and on the following morning the serum is drawn off by means of suction into a 250 cc centrifuge cup. This serum contains some red cells which are removed by centrifuging for a half-hour. The clear serum is then drawn off.

For the first few months of the work, the sera were pooled according to the blood groups. Subsequently,[2] the sera were mixed in the same proportion as the various types occur in the population. This has been found to be as follows:

Type O—46 per cent, Type A—41 per cent, Type B—10 per cent, Type AB—3 per cent.

CONCENTRATION OF SERUM

It is unnecessary to describe in detail the Thalhimer [749] procedure which was utilized in the preparation of concentrated serum. The concentration was carried out in large cellophane cylinders, which were

[2]Investigations conducted by Dr. D. G. Gemeroy have shown that this pooling of sera in a fixed proportion by type is unnecessary when large pools are used.

suspended at room temperature in front of an electric fan. The room was air-conditioned to obtain a low humidity and an adequately high temperature.

The clinical tests on the concentrated serum at the General Hospital and others in Toronto, on a fairly large series of cases, showed no serious reactions. In Montreal, however, several severe reactions were noticed. These have been described by Rose, Weil, and Browne [653] in a recent article.

THE PREPARATION OF DRIED SERUM

The clear serum is prepared as described above. It is drawn from the centrifuge tubes by suction into a 4 litre pooling bottle. A culture is made of the bulk material, and merthiolate to secure a concentration of 1:30,000, is added. If the sample taken before the addition of merthiolate shows no contamination at the end of 7 days a large pool (48 litres) is made and the material is passed through a Seitz filter. A culture is made again, and if the test is satisfactory the serum is ready for filling into the final container. The serum is approximately one month "old" before it is dried. . . . Bottles which hold about 500 cc are approximately half filled with serum under sterile conditions in a filling cabinet fitted with a source of ultraviolet light. The bottles are then transferred to freezing racks. The room in which the freezing and drying takes place is also equipped with ultraviolet light, and the incoming air is filtered and irradiated. The workers in this room wear masks, sterile gowns, caps, and gloves. The freezing tables are designed to hold 48 bottles each. After the addition of CO_2 snow and alcohol, the bottles are rotated by hand so that the frozen serum is deposited evenly on the walls of the bottles. The temperature inside the bottle falls to from 50° to 60° below zero Centigrade. When the shelling process is complete the bottles are loaded on trays, the paper caps and air filters removed, and the trays transferred as rapidly as possible to the Desivac cabinet where the drying takes place (Greaves and Adair [331]; Flosdorf, Stokes, and Mudd [301]). The dehydration requires approximately 70 hours. At the completion the bottles are removed from the cabinet and sterile clamps are placed on the rubber tubing. This tubing is removed in the filling cabinet, and a permanent rubber cap is applied. Bacteriological cultures are made of the final product and toxicity tests are carried out routinely on rabbits and mice.

[Four figures have been omitted: one showing the bottles in which the serum was collected for freeze-drying, a second illustrating the freezing rack, a third showing the Desivac pumps and cabinet and the final one showing the finished product ready for shipment.]

The bottles are labelled, wrapped in corrugated paper, and packed in tin containers with a direction sheet. A small cloth bag containing silica gel is placed inside each tin to absorb any moisture which may be present. Tins are hermetically sealed and labelled. When the sterility and toxicity tests are found to be satisfactory, the material is released for distribution. The tins are readily opened and sterile distilled water may be added by any technique the clinician finds to be satisfactory. The dried serum dissolves very readily and may be given safely to patients of any blood type.

The clinical tests on this product in Toronto and Montreal have been completely satisfactory. We are informed that the dried serum made in England by a similar process and used in many hundreds of cases has been quite as free from reaction-producing material as plasma or whole blood.

DISCUSSION

DR. C. H. BEST, *Toronto*: The interval between the time the blood is taken and the time the serum is dried is never less than a month.

All serum has been distributed through our Department of National Defence. Some is sent to England and some is distributed to the Armed Forces in Canada. The technique for its administration is also laid down by the Department of National Defence. It is given with the ordinary type of transfusion outfit. They provide this and the sterilized water. We have nothing to do with that. It is on their instructions that the material is put out in the dried form. Water is added through the rubber cap, or in some instances, the cap is taken off and water added, as is done routinely in certain hospitals. We have insisted that the material should be used within two to three hours after reconstitution. There is in fact no reason for leaving it standing around once the water has been added. A mobile outfit would, I suppose, take the material to where the casualties were.

In reference to the size of the container, I would be happier if it held 500 cubic centimetres of serum rather than 250 cubic centimetres. However, there are some difficulties about using larger containers for the shelling. Bottles and caps are not readily available. If we do make any change, it will be in that direction. The military people feel that it is safer to have a container to which you add the water.

After careful study of some thirty-five to forty cases in Montreal and Toronto, the clinical professors of medicine at McGill and the University of Toronto gave their blessings to dried serum. Their decision was reinforced by work from England. In a great many tests they had no more reactions with dried serum than they had observed with whole blood.

In England the Medical Research Council prefers dried serum. We do not hold any brief for serum as against plasma. We believe that they are practically identical, but it was important to make a decision and then get on with it.

DR. JOHN ELLIOTT, *Salisbury, N.C.*: In any large-scale programme the transportation of citrated blood to central processing stations is important. Over a period of several years we have had more than 200 bottles of blood sent in to us. Most of the bottles contained 300 cubic centimetres of citrated blood and many of them were en route for forty-eight hours. Special refrigeration has not been used. All of the bottles of blood were received in excellent condition with little or no haemolysis. We believe that haemolysis was prevented or limited by having the bottles as nearly full as possible, so that agitation was minimized. No reactions have occurred following the administration of plasma prepared from transported blood.

PART IV: GENERAL PAPERS

59. The Division of Naval Medical Research, Royal Canadian Navy

CHARLES H. BEST

The "keel" of this Division was laid in the autumn of 1940 when it became evident, as a result of several trips to sea, that a group trained in various aspects of medical research could make valuable contributions to many operational problems confronting the Navy. This plan was discussed with the Medical Director General of the Royal Canadian Navy, Surgeon-Captain Archie McCallum, and with the Hon. Angus L. MacDonald, Minister of Naval Affairs. I well remember the evening on which Fred Banting and I went to see Angus L. The Minister and his wife gave us a warm welcome and as we "spun our yarns" he became increasingly enthusiastic about the contributions which a medical research unit might make to the Navy. He promised me his active support and was as good as his word. Fred Banting was pleased that he had been able to help me "launch a new craft." When we went back to the Chateau Laurier we talked well into the night. That proved to be the last evening that Fred and I spent together.

It is impossible to mention all the members of the Naval Staff who facilitated our ventures. Vice-Admiral Percy Nelles, Vice-Admiral G. C. Jones, Rear Admiral H. E. Reid, Rear Admiral L. W. Murray, and many others gave us invaluable support. There was also a group of younger men, most of whom later became Admirals, who facilitated our researches— Grant, DeWolf, Hibbard, Raynor, and Lay were among these.

Undoubtedly the most valuable contribution from our group arose from a study of night vision. This led to the introduction of a red lighting which eliminated, to a large extent, the loss of night vision which occurred with use of the standard lighting system then in vogue in the chartroom and on the bridge of naval vessels. The suggestion that we should work in this field came to us from Professor A. V. Hill, then British Air Attaché in Washington. He told us of some findings of Dr. R. J. Lythgoe at University College in London. Apparently Lythgoe had recommended red lighting and it had been tested in the Royal Navy but under unsuitable conditions (a moonlit night), and the results were not encouraging. Surgeon Commander D. Y. Solandt was in charge of the night vision studies. Unknown to us, the same problem was being investigated by Dr. H. K. Hartline of the Johnson Foundation at the University of Pennsylvania. Very favourable results were obtained in a laboratory in Toronto using deep red illumination of a rigidly prescribed wave-length and intensity. Solandt and I made night trials in R.C.A.F. aircraft in November and December 1940 and in January 1941 under the direction of Wing Commander T. R. Loudon and with the collaboration of the late Squadron Leader Evan Briggs. These are the first adequate service trials of red lighting on record. A report recommending the adoption of a specified form of red instrument panel illumination for aircraft was made to the National Research Council, Ottawa, and to the R.C.A.F. in January 1941. In February 1941, at the request of the United States Navy, the experimental results were presented to the United States Service authorities in Washington. Over this period Solandt and I had been making studies in Halifax using as test subjects the commanders of destroyers and corvettes. The results were so dramatically favourable that soon the skippers were loath to put to sea without installation of red lighting. Funds from private sources were used to install red lighting on the bridge of five naval vessels in Halifax. Further tests were carried out at sea in October, November, and December 1941. A detailed report including specifications for all lighting installations involved was submitted to the National Research Council and the Royal Canadian Navy in January 1942.

In November and December of 1941, Solandt and I spent some time with the Home Fleet of the Royal Navy in waters off Iceland. Admiral Sir John Tovey and Surgeon Captain Fitzroy Williams reviewed the Canadian experiments and requested that the Admiralty reopen the question. Red lighting in appropriate areas was soon adopted by the Royal Navy.

The early findings were presented at a Service Medical Research meeting in Toronto which Professor Walter Miles of Yale University attended. He was so impressed by the findings with red lighting that he moved with great speed to introduce the innovation into the United States Navy and later he developed red goggles which were widely employed in many services and which were an important addition to the red lighting. It was not long before the fighting ships of the United States Navy were equipped with red lighting.

Some years after the war an appraisal was made of the naval action against Japan and the conclusion was reached that one of the main advantages enjoyed by United States naval personnel was the ability to see the enemy before being seen. The credit for this was attributed, in large part, to red lighting. The late Dr. Lythgoe and the late Dr. Solandt deserve great credit for this development.

Solandt was responsible for other advances in our knowledge of visual problems in the Royal Canadian Navy. Surgeon Lieutenant Commander Carl G. Smith and Lieutenant John W. Dales worked very effectively with him on dark-adaptation and other studies. Lieutenant M. L. Bunker worked in co-operation with Surgeon Commander Solandt on goggles which would permit anti-aircraft personnel to follow tracer bullets. Special filters were developed which enabled an observer to see tracer bullets actually crossing the ball of the unclouded sun.

I have paid my tribute on many occasions to the memory of Donald Solandt. He was one of the best and most loyal friends I have ever had and certainly one of the most able. He suffered—from an early age—from the results of a great motivation to make a real contribution to medical knowledge. Solandt had several extensive operations for duodenal ulcer. He had a serious haemorrhage one night when we were sharing a cabin in the depot ship *Heckla* in Reykjavik Fiord, Iceland, in November 1941. But in spite of a haemoglobin of around 50 per cent, he insisted on going with me on a drifter, climbing the side of the cruiser *Sheffield* on a stormy, dark night and proceeding to England to spread the word about the results of the red lighting experiments. If he had been granted good health he would have become one of the great biophysicists of his day.

Brilliant work on the fatigue of frequency discrimination of ASDIC operators, was carried out for several years by Dr. Ruth C. Partridge, assisted by Surgeon Lieutenant Commander Harvey Hebb and Dr. Jean Fletcher.

The work on nutrition was under the direction of Lieutenant Commander James Campbell; Surgeon Lieutenant J. G. Watt, Nursing Sister E. J. Reed, Lieutenant Commander G. E. Eggleton, Lieutenant K. B. Latimer, and Sub-Lieutenant J. J. Russell worked with him. Dr. Campbell and his group were responsible for supervising improvements in the nutrition of Royal Canadian naval personnel ashore and afloat and they did their work well. The contents of the new Emergency Ration Boxes of the Royal Canadian Navy, which were based on their recommendations, withstood perfectly the severe conditions to which they were exposed in the Service and provided adequate nutrition in a highly concentrated form in emergencies.

Lieutenant Commander Campbell Cowan has left his mark on the Navy in many places. He worked with Dr. Solandt on the control of noise levels in engine-rooms and on the production of life-saving equipment.

Cowan was concerned particularly with development of the Royal Canadian Navy jacket which was given credit by many survivors for saving their lives. It not only kept them afloat but it also protected them from underwater blast.

Lieutenant Commander Cowan was at one time loaned to the Royal Navy as expert adviser on protective clothing in northern climes. He devised a suit in which the principle of a true vapour barrier was incorporated for the first time. Difficulties in procuring the correct materials in Canada prevented the early adoption of this suit by the Royal Canadian Navy.

An optical section of the Royal Canadian Navy was created. Qualified opticians and optometrists among Navy personnel were selected and assigned for duty as base opticians under the direction of an ophthalmologist. Lieutenant C. R. Shorney of the Naval Medical Research Division was the senior officer of this group of opticians. Dr. A. E. MacDonald gave invaluable services in the training of these men in special techniques. He was assisted by Lieutenant Shorney. The fitting of contact lenses by Naval opticians was undertaken. These lenses afforded protection of the eyes from wind and spray and, of course, corrected certain visual defects which had beached many an efficient officer. The Royal Canadian Navy glassless eye shield gave protection, especially when wind forces were greater than thirty miles per hour.

Two exceptionally fine officers, Surgeon Lieutenant Commander E. A. Sellers and Surgeon Lieutenant J. M. Parker, were active with other members of the group in the studies on seasickness. Surgeon Lieutenant Commander Fields and Lieutenant N. R. Stephenson assisted with these studies and later Stephenson designed the R.C.N. portable laboratory kit. Surgeon Lieutenant Commander E. J. Delorme and Surgeon Lieutenant Commander W. Locke worked on under-water physiology and later Locke and Nursing Sister (Technician) Margaret (Stock) Wright studied traumatic and burn shock. Lieutenant R. Grant, with his special knowledge of textiles, was able to give valuable help to all work relating to protective clothing and equipment.

In addition to their work on seasickness and various other problems, Surgeon Lieutenant Commander Sellers and Surgeon Lieutenant Parker took part in studies designed to assess the value of air conditioning of naval vessels. These officers were posted to H.M.C.S. *Swansea* to take part in the trials of this air-conditioned ship in the tropics. In other habitability studies, Surgeon Lieutenant Commander J. W. Scott worked with the Royal Navy Personnel Research Committee in England and on a cruiser of the Eastern Fleet studying the physiological effects of heat on naval personnel.

A brief account of this work is given in a special number of the *Journal of the Canadian Medical Services* (1946). The contributions of Dr. R. L. Noble and of Dr. Wilder Penfield, and the members of his group, are acknowledged in that publication [16].

Many people in various parts of the world facilitated the work of our Medical Research Division of the Royal Canadian Navy. Professor Beecher Weld in Halifax, many doctors and civilians in Newfoundland, personnel of the Royal Navy, of the United States Navy, and civilians in Iceland, R.C.N. and R.N. officers at the base in Greenock, Scotland, Sir Henry Dale and Sir Edward Mellanby in London, Surgeon Captain McCallum in Ottawa, all these and many others deserve our thanks. The unfailing courtesy and helpfulness of naval medical personnel in British and American ships—and ashore—made one feel that he belonged to one of the finest clubs. I should especially mention Dr. Ross MacIntyre, Surgeon General of the United States Navy and his opposite numbers in the Royal Navy. These experiences deepened a life-long conviction that Canadians are very fortunate in their association with other members of the Commonwealth and in their proximity to the friendliest neighbour that one could possibly imagine.

60. The Organization of Physiology

CHARLES H. BEST

We are all proud to work in such a vital and rewarding field, and we look back with considerable pleasure on what has been accomplished. . . . One could describe, in the fields with which he is most familiar, many advances which probably will be made in the next five years. . . . I am thinking first of research; but our subject—Physiology—will, of course, advance by good teaching, which will train our successors, quite as much as by contemporary research. Indeed the two are usually inseparable.

We should be concerned here not with the titles given to the university departments, which admittedly may be vital enough to administrators and to teaching and research staffs, but rather with the broad subject of Physiology as an independent discipline. It is inconceivable to me that knowledge of the action and interaction of the cells of the body will not advance rapidly while this most absorbing of all subjects continues to appropriate unto itself and, for its own revelation, the newest techniques of the physicists, chemists, engineers and other fundamental scientists. But we must guard our subject if we are to remain in command of it and must plan as wisely as we can for its vigorous health in the foreseeable future.

All realize that more intensive cultivation of the fields we have tilled will yield treasure which we have overlooked or failed to appreciate. This will be true even if the same simple methods and tools are used. I am quite certain that I would acquire a considerable amount of new information merely by attempting to repeat exactly many of the simplest experiments I have performed. There has been an understandable tendency to carry out the short experiments that promise quick and decisive answers, and to avoid those that are obviously more physiological but which require long periods of observation and constant meticulous care. The physicians are beginning to prescribe for patients under their usual living and working conditions—not as they exist in bed in a hospital. We in physiology must be prepared to make observations over months and years where previously we have been satisfied with minutes and hours. More pressure should be

Originally appeared in *Perspectives in Physiology*, ed. Ilza Veith (Washington: American Physiological Society, 1954). This is the published version of a paper read before an International Symposium in 1953.

exerted on us to force us to make similar observations on several different species of animals before announcing our findings. We will have to study smaller deviations from the normal and we will have to follow these for really significant periods of time. Studies extending over the full life cycles of our experimental animals will become increasingly frequent.

There has never been any conflict in my mind between Physiology as a science in its own right and as an essential and intimate part of medical teaching and research. The two are compatible and supplement each other. The same could be said of dental or veterinary physiology. The interest and obligations of teaching sometimes determine the direction research takes in a laboratory, and I suppose there are fewer conflicts between the demands of the two when this is so. On the other hand, one thinks of great investigators whose field of research has touched only very lightly on the area of knowledge demanded by his teaching schedule.

The question arises, how much teaching should we expect a promising investigator to do? It has been my experience that a little teaching does not interfere with the productivity of a research worker. There is an optimum amount for each individual which might take anywhere from 5 to 25 per cent of his time. One knows recipients of large research grants who earned the right to them while spending 80 per cent of their time on investigation, and who now devote a much smaller proportion of their day to the efficient development of the hard-won opportunity. Some of this reallocation of time is the inevitable result of accepting new administrative duties that are an integral part of the enlarged programme. I know from personal experience that many of the administrative details incident to the direction and conduct of research by a group of investigators cannot be delegated but must be dealt with by the leader of the team. The problem should, of course, be much more rapidly advanced by the availability of more skilled hands which the research grant makes possible. If the dominant interest, however, of all members of the team is the problem at hand, and if all spend 80 per cent of their working time in actual investigation or in administrative duties relating only to the research, all should be well. But in some instances this is not the case. The famous research man is sometimes diverted to administrative duties which have no direct connection with his research grant. Even this may be acceptable if the team is productive. It may mean that the head of the group is no longer the real leader but he may have opened a path which can readily be followed; or the leader in his spare time, as it were, may really provide the specific spark necessary to initiate the chain of reactions.

While increasing amounts of non-specific administrative duties may be discharged by other than research personnel, I do not believe that we will ever evolve a successful strain of directors of research who have been developed along any other route than that of extensive personal experience with the technical and scientific problems involved. The director must have experienced the thrills and disappointments himself if he is to act as the mentor and guide for successive waves of enterprising, efficient and highly motivated young people. A director should be one who really knows when a junior worker is properly motivated and otherwise equipped for a career in investigation. He should be able to recognize those who are using research merely as a stepping-stone and those, usually more senior and rather troubling people, who may be sheltering behind a forest of scientific names and complicated procedures in an obscure and little used by-way of research —or, on the other hand, may be the geniuses of the future. A director should realize, of course, that new techniques can unlock a stubborn door and reveal long clear upward trails—and that in exceptional circumstances they can produce plausible findings which may be published in long series of papers over many years before it is realized that these results are essentially meaningless and are devoid of physiological significance.

How long should a promising young investigator remain in a junior position? The answer is, of course, that he should be given his independent opportunity as soon as possible, i.e., as soon as his training, motivation, imagination, and administrative ability in research make it even faintly possible that he will accomplish more as a senior member of a team. He may well have to find another laboratory in which to develop this capacity. There are many examples of those who have remained too long and of those who have remained too brief a time as junior members.

I do not believe that a single individual can efficiently direct in research a large group of workers unless the team is broken up into small groups of a few members each who are under the direct day-to-day guidance of a leader. This means that the director is not what the name may imply, but the Chairman of a Board of Directors.

One of the great difficulties in the advance of research and in the co-ordination of facts for teaching purposes, is the breadth of the field which physiology encompasses. In many medical schools the clinical departments and sub-departments still struggle to present medical knowledge to the student and suffer more or less silently because the single physiologist, perhaps with one assistant, cannot effectively pose as an authority on all the fundamentals of medicine, surgery, obstetrics, and of ophthalmo-, oto-, rhino-, laryngology!

Even for those of us who spend a very large proportion of our time in investigation, co-ordination of advancing knowledge is difficult. . . . Only the rare leader can see all the potentialities in the approach of the expert in electronics to neurophysiology, of the superb organic chemist to endocrinology or of the nuclear physicist to metabolic interconversions of substances studied with the aid of isotopes. The best use of refrigerated rooms or of rooms capable of being maintained at high temperatures and the maximum utilization of the potentialities of the complicated measuring mechanisms now available pose other problems. A good answer must be forthcoming if physiology is to remain a comprehensible subject. One part of the answer is provided by the common ground and language which results from basic training in the fundamental sciences. A more effective co-ordination is provided by those who have extensive training in two disciplines which enables them to work in both fields and to converse in both languages. These more or less naturally occurring liaison officers provide the rebuttal to many of the suggestions of "limitations" of physiology and the time has perhaps come when universities and research councils should begin to plan more actively and deliberately to encourage the training of these essential liaison personnel. I am not unaware of the plans for the training of the new type of teacher necessary for the so-called *vertical* system of teaching and something of the same type of training, adapted to the needs of research, may help to keep physiology on its feet and marching forward at a rapid pace.

A system of liaison officers has for many years seemed to me a necessary step for the interrelation of departments in a medical faculty. In my Department we have maintained over some years a liaison between Physiology and Surgery and between Physiology and Paediatrics. These senior personnel, trained in two spheres, have decided after some years to place both feet in a single department and in our limited series the score has been two to one in favour of the clinical. . . . This suggestion of liaison, provides I believe many possibilities for success in both teaching and research fields.

Everyone who has considered our subject will have given some thought to the administrative and financial support of physiological research. In some cases a university, a business or a research council, or a government department will decide to spend some money on a new field of research. The logical first step is to secure the best possible director and let him plan, within the limitations of his budget, to accomplish as much as he can. In other cases a promising research worker develops within a university and in order to retain his services or perhaps just to make him happy, the university places funds at his disposal. But in this day few universities have funds to give their research workers and the investigator must secure support elsewhere. This comes from the government, industry, philanthropic foundations, or private donors. Many of you are familiar with the present situation in other countries and realize, as I do, the dominant position which government support has reached. I have had the opportunity to learn a lot about the organization of governmental support of research in England and in the United States, but those of us who are senior investigators in Canada have grown up, as it were, with the Medical Research Division of our Research Council, the Medical Advisory Committee of the Defence Research Board, and the Medical Grants Committee of our Dominion Health Department. I may commend particularly the Medical Division of our Research Council which, under the wise guidance of Dr. J. B. Collip and Dr. Harold Ettinger, has preserved a constancy of purpose and simplicity of organization which is very exceptional. I will be pleased to discuss these subjects in more detail later if desired but I may, for the moment, merely state that since all the people profit from the results of physiological research, support from the common pocket seems to be thoroughly justified. I will emphasize as strongly as I can that the allocation of funds should be in the hands of a judicial and broad-minded committee composed almost entirely of experienced and successful research workers each of whom has established his deep interest in the complete development of the research potential of his country.

I shall not discuss here the controversial subject of Defence Medical Research on which I admit the possession of rather definite and I think both realistic and humanitarian ideas.

We are all in favour of support from the foundations who have done so very, very much to develop Physiology and none of us would refuse an unrestricted gift from a private donor.

There remains the question of support from industry. Figures are available, I am sure, to establish the fact that there has been a dramatic increase in the last 10 to 20 years in the amount of money spent on research by industrial firms. Physiology has had its share both in research laboratories within the commercial organizations and in grants to universities. Few scientists will have any reservations about accepting financial assistance from industry provided that there is no direct or indirect exploitation of the university association by the commercial company. There are various reasons why this is less likely to happen today than in the past. The interchange of scientific personnel between university and industry has reached unprecedented levels.

The discovery of insulin, the taking out of patents by the University of Toronto, the gift of these to all countries except where a continuing service was rendered, is an interesting illustration of one way in which a research group may overcome, in part and for a time, the limitations of inadequate finances. We were offered excellent facilities in other countries but the only way which appeared to be open to us in 1922, if we wished to remain in Canada, was to accept the suggestion that a testing laboratory be set up, a royalty charged to the companies using the facilities (actually these have all been U.S.A. companies), and the surplus used for research in a manner similar to that governing the use of other research funds in the University. Since any suggestion of personal profit was eliminated, this procedure—advised by a committee set up by the University—was accepted by all of those concerned. As far as countries other than the United States and Canada go, the practical aspects of the arrangement could have caused no concern since all of these countries enjoyed as a gift the free and unrestricted use of the insulin patents. In the United States and Canada the arrangement has functioned well—perhaps in large part because of the high ethical standing of the companies concerned. From the University viewpoint the increased research activities made possible initially have helped to attract funds from many other sources both private and governmental. The insulin funds which, I believe, have been spent with very great care, have really functioned as a basic departmental budget. It would have been more satisfactory if an endowment or a firm allocation of University funds had been available.

From certain viewpoints the procedure followed by our Insulin Committee may not have been the perfect one—the precedent has certainly been abused. The Canadian National Research Council has adopted a plan under which profit from the results of research may, if desired, be divided in an equitable way between the University where the work was done and the National Research Council, with a small fraction available for the inventor if his ethics permit him to accept it. I am aware of the breadth of this small corner of our subject and will not pursue it further here.

Instead of preparing a documented lecture on our subject I have here attempted to outline my own thoughts on certain aspects of it with which I have had experience.

I predict for Physiology a continued upward progress. The limitations in many countries will be financial in nature and there has been and will be a flow of talent and a more rapid development of new workers in the countries where the investment in physiological research is greatest. This is not a new phenomenon.

I have had the opportunity during recent years of studying certain aspects of health in many countries and I may be permitted the fervent hope that the benefits of the advances of physiology will, in the future, be shared in increasing amounts by all the people of the world.

61. Convocation Address, University of Maine, August 12, 1955

CHARLES H. BEST, M.D.*

President Hauck, Members of the Faculty, Ladies and Gentlemen:

The very great honour which you have just given me is most deeply appreciated. I have always valued my intimate associations with this truly beautiful state of Maine, where my Canadian parents were living when I was born and where I spent a very happy childhood. Now, as an Honorary Alumnus of the University of Maine, I shall have an even keener interest in what goes on here, particularly, of course, in teaching and research in the biological fields.

When one is born in this country of Canadian parents, one has the option of two allegiances. I resolved this problem at a fairly early age by joining the Canadian Army. When I was discharged at the age of 19, in 1919, I had achieved the rank of Sergeant—actually Temporary Acting Sergeant-Major. (Sergeants are, of course, the backbone of any army!)

During the last war, I served as a Surgeon-Captain in the Canadian Navy. The Canadian Navy grew very rapidly in size and importance during the war. It convoyed half the total transatlantic shipping and patrolled the east coast of the U.S.A. when your ships of war were busy in the Pacific in the winter of 1941–42. On certain occasions I was the Senior Officer in a medical research team composed of both United States and Canadian Naval doctors.

This very productive interrelationship was made possible, in part, by my friendship with the physician to President Franklin Delano Roosevelt. When some years later I had the honour of acting as Public Orator of the University of London, England, and presenting the President of the United States for an Honorary Degree from the University of London at Government House in Ottawa, President Roosevelt remarked to me after the ceremony, "I remember discussing infantile paralysis with you on the beach at Herring Cove, Campobello." He knew a lot about this medical subject and his interest will be recorded as one of the factors which *will* make possible the prevention of this disease.

Originally appeared in *A D A Forecast, the Diabetics' own Magazine*, IX (1956), 1–7.
*Dr. Best delivered this address after receiving an Honorary Doctor of Science degree from the University of Maine.

After the last war I served for some six years on a Medical Committee set up by your Government in Washington. I had to fill out several forms. The first one really just asked me if I wished to serve, and the answer was "Yes." The second one wanted to know if I had any intention of going on strike against the Government of the United States. The answer was in the negative with a footnote that I do not belong to any union. The third form asked if I would take the Oath of Allegiance to the Government of the United States. My answer to this was, "I would be quite happy to do this provided I could be assured that this would not conflict in any way with my prior Oath of Allegiance to Canada." This was the last I heard of the matter and I had a pleasant time helping to spend quite a lot of your money on medical research!

My wife and I were both brought up on the shores of historic and beautiful Passamaquoddy Bay. She was born in St. Andrews-by-the-Sea, New Brunswick, which is only 15 or 20 miles as the gull flies, from West Pembroke, Maine. We met as students at the University of Toronto. Some of you may know the poem which begins:

> Sweet maiden of Passamaquoddy,
> Shall we seek for communion of souls,
> Where the distant Mississippi meanders,
> Or the distant Saskatchewan rolls?
> Ah, no! in New Brunswick we'll find it—
> A sweetly sequestrated nook—
> Where the swift gliding Skoodoowabskooksis,
> Unites with the Skoodoowabskook.
> Let others sing loudly of Saco,
> Of Passadumkeag or Miscouch,
> Of Kennebeccasis or Quaco,
> Of Miramichi or Buctouch;
> Or boast of the Tobique of Mispec,
> The Musquash or dark Memramcook;
> There's none like the Skoodoowabskooksis
> Excepting the Skoodoowabskook!

This poem was written by Professor James De Mille, who was Head of the Department of English when my wife's father attended Dalhousie University in Halifax, Nova Scotia. My father also went to Dalhousie as did my aunts and uncles and those of my wife.

Dalhousie College was founded on May 22, 1820, money for building it coming in part from the state of Maine. This was known as the Castine Fund. The money was collected by the British troops while they were in possession of the Port of Castine, Maine, from 1814, until the Treaty of Ghent, in 1815. Over 12 thousand pounds was taken in from brandy, gin, rum, sugar, molasses, and coffee. Not more than three thousand pounds, it is recorded, was used for the College.

I have taken these quotations from a book written by Mrs. W. T. Hallam, M.A., entitled: "Old Halifax." Mrs. Hallam was my father's youngest sister and I lived in her home in Toronto as a student and during the period when insulin was discovered and developed.

While this evening's Ceremony has provided my first close association with any University in Maine, there have been a number of interesting indirect contacts through my friends. Judge Harold Blackwood, one of my close friends since boyhood, is here this evening with his wife and daughter. I well remember the time when as boys we missed the train after the St. Stephen Fair and walked the 21 miles home during the night. And the time we started to row the 12 miles to Eastport, but about half way there we landed on a small island, wrestled all day and then rowed home.

Another of your graduates, Senator Styles Bridges, and I grew up together in West Pembroke and I can remember one Christmas vacation when we had an intense mutual interest in a wood lot. We must have been about 12 or 13 years old then, but we did a bit of research on the saving of labour in the production of cordwood. We cut partially through a large number of trees on the side of a steep hill and then by felling a massive one, higher up the slope, we brought the whole lot crashing down. The subsequent limbing and sawing into lengths was not nearly as interesting!

Through Ronald Bridges, the distinguished younger brother of Styles, and through Dr. and Mrs. George Anderson of Pennelville, Maine, my wife and I became even more interested than we had been in the poetry of Robert P. Tristram Coffin. One of Professor Coffin's books is dedicated to Dr. Anderson and one to Ronald Bridges.

Two years ago we spent a wonderful evening with the Andersons in Pennelville where Robert P. Tristram Coffin recited and read his own poems to us. Professor Coffin knew of my father's long and intense service as a country doctor in West Pembroke, through Ronald Bridges. Coffin's poem, "The Country Doctor," which he wrote out in his own hand and sent to me a few years ago, was originally composed with my father—and of course other country doctors—in mind.

> Under the midnight thunderheads,
> When lesser men were in their beds,
> He drove his mare by lantern light
> Of chain-lightning splitting night.
> He came to the Country's ends
> Not for fees, but for friends,
> Came like an angel fierce and fast
> He saw men first and saw them last.

The doctor's horse is mentioned twice in this poem. (The second time Coffin wrote, "He drove his old mare out of breath, Between a baby and a death.") My father was particularly proud of his horses. They were all trained to stop at railroad tracks and would do this when bringing my father home, sound asleep after long trips and difficult cases.

In the early years of this century my father brought a racing mare over from his father's farm in the Annapolis Valley, Nova Scotia. Some years ago I had the seventh generation of this stock, sired by a Hanover, shipped from Pembroke, Maine, to Toronto. "Lou Hanover" has a rather carefree life, as we don't ride or drive him much now, but I always look forward to the day when I will. I drove some of his ancestors on the race tracks when I was in my early teens. My father and I raced our horses on winter roads during the Christmas vacations and best of all, on the ice of Pennamaquan Lake! I can still hear the fascinating racing rhythm of their "Never Slip" horseshoes.

I went to Toronto at the age of 15 and it required 10 years to secure an M.A. in Physiology and an M.D. It was not surprising that the Station Master at St. Stephen, N.B., was heard to remark, "It takes that Best boy a long time to get educated."

But I should be talking to you on more serious subjects and I would like to say a little bit of what you should expect from the Profession of Medicine in this restless and rapidly changing world. We physicians are privileged people who carry on in peace and war, using our training and energy to keep people well and to heal the sick. We must, of course, select a few from our number who will give us true representation in conference with the various professional and other groups which make up the governing bodies of a democratic country.

I was surprised to learn when I looked into the matter, that physicians have actually gone on strike to attain certain objectives. This was not in this country or in Canada.* Provision was probably made for the care of the seriously ill when the physicians left their posts, but this recourse to the procedure used by the less vital members of the community is not to my mind consistent with the highest tradition of our profession. There are probably more effective and more dignified ways of maintaining the correct position of medicine and attaining objectives consistent with our professional responsibilities.

I have spent nearly thirty-five years in medical research. A consideration of recent findings or of unsolved problems is not what I wish to discuss

---

*[This comment, made in 1955, is of interest in view of the widely publicized disagreement in 1962 between the medical profession and the Government of the province of Saskatchewan, Canada.]

here today. I was brought up as I have told you, in a medical household where very frequently the assistance of all the members was required to help my father in some emergency arising in his widely dispersed general practice. The distance to be covered, the financial status of the patients or their value to the community were never factors in the effort made to help them.

One of my father's friends who is also mine, Dr. Charles Armstrong of Robbinston, Maine, tells his patients, "You had better appreciate me, ladies and gentlemen, I am the last of the country doctors."

My own contribution was probably of little benefit to these patients. I remember giving an anaesthetic in a farm house, when I was twelve years old, and was duly impressed with my importance till I learned that my father sometimes let patients pour on the ether for themselves. Their state of consciousness automatically controlled the rate of supply!

With this background it is perhaps surprising that I have never engaged in actual medical practice. After graduating in medicine in Toronto and doing postgraduate work in England, Germany, and Denmark, I became certain that research had a far greater attraction for me than the care of patients. But I have missed the satisfaction that the cure of an individual patient brings.

Most of our work over the years has been related to insulin and diabetes, heparin and thrombosis, to the vitamin choline, and to cirrhosis of the liver. During the last war, of course, our interests were focused on military problems such as the preparation of dried blood serum, a study of night vision, motion sickness, and a whole host of problems that assume great importance during an emergency. Many of our researches brought us into intimate contact with the problem of world health and since the last war a considerable part of my interest has been directed towards the problem of undernutrition.

Undernutrition, i.e., partial starvation, affects one billion people in various parts of the world. The cure of this condition is well known and one of the greatest problems affecting the world is to provide more good protein for the underdeveloped countries. I have discussed many of the medical aspects of this central world problem on various occasions and in many countries. You all know the main factors confronting organizations which are attempting to improve this dire situation—lack of money, lack of education, lack of food, lack of knowledge. In what order should these be attacked and corrected? There can never be a contented world while these lacks exist in the *majority* of the people. We must realize the economic and social upheaval which is caused by curing the sick and greatly increasing the survival rate.

In the more privileged countries we have also the problem of an aging population. What should be the medical attitude on the grave problems raised by situations such as these? Medical opinion will not be divided on the necessity of developing to the full our knowledge of how to care most effectively for older people. We must realize that the advance of medical knowledge prolongs the lives not only of the productive and mentally fit, but also of those who are at the opposite end of the scale.

I am sure we will all agree that medical men should always do their utmost not only to develop new curative measures—the first half of this century has witnessed more therapeutic triumphs than any previous fifty years—but should make great efforts to keep our statesmen, economists, and the public informed of the true state of affairs, so that wise decisions can be made on world problems, many of which have more medical aspects than are usually recognized.

The physician should never allow himself to be placed in a position where he is obligated or forced to do less than his utmost to relieve human distress. The physician must continue to play an important part in world affairs, but he should make his fellows realize that his tradition, his training, and his firmly rooted determination all force him to make the fullest use of his privileged position to improve the health and lengthen the lives of as many people as possible. This is his primary concern and if the results of his success do sometimes socially, economically, or politically disturb the existing balance of things, the remedy for this situation should not force upon the medical man any diminution or interference with his humanitarian efforts. He should do his utmost in co-operation with nutritionists and social workers, economists and statesmen, but his path of duty, while not less difficult, is simpler than theirs.

Any Convocation Address which does not give good advice to the Graduating Class is, of course, a hopeless failure. It matters not that the staff of your own University has given you the same advice over the years.

One of the worst sensations in the world is to finish an important race with the knowledge that you did not put everything you had to give into it. The most important race for each one of us is our life. I hope each one of you will have a long and productive one. Plan it well and at the most important points, run yourself fully out. A few of you may crack under the strain, but this should not deter individuals with a higher resistance to fatigue and stress from giving everything they have at the proper time, in order to make their *full* contributions. I trust you will be rewarded in proportion to your contribution to the public good, and will remember that many rewards and satisfactions are not related to material wealth.

Do not let your muscles atrophy from disuse, or become overladen with adipose tissue. Exercise your muscles (in moderation) and your lungs and your hearts, but most important of all, do not let the cells of your *brain* atrophy from disuse. Your university education has taught you how to prevent this disastrous condition. It is insidious in onset because as the brain cells atrophy the appreciation of what is happening also decreases—a very vicious cycle thus becomes established.

The condition can be prevented by selecting some subject—related or unrelated to your principal interest. Only a small corner of the subject is necessary but you must resolve that you will read and *think* about this, that you will *study* it and keep abreast of the advances, in so far as you are able, for as long as you live.

Part V: EPILOGUE

Epilogue

The selection of the papers to be reprinted brought clearly to my mind all my former colleagues and graduate students with whom I have worked over the last forty-two years. These scientists are now in some thirty different countries and the accounts of their visits to us and ours to them have been carefully preserved in my wife's diary. My visits to England would not be the same without my former mentors, Sir Henry Dale and Professor A. V. Hill in London. Over the years I have had many good discussions of our mutual scientific interests with Professor Frank Young of Cambridge. Professor Joseph Hoet in Belgium has been a friend and scientific associate since 1925. I will not single out any one of my many former graduate students who are now in the United States but it is a pleasure to see a number of them each year when I am lecturing in that country. My work with the American Diabetes Association has provided many of my most valued friendships.

Graduate students and former colleagues from my departments are associated with most of the universities in Canada. In Halifax, at Dalhousie University, my old friend Beecher Weld is Chairman of the Department of Physiology and L. B. Macpherson is the Assistant Dean of the Faculty of Medicine. In the province of Quebec, Dr. E. Pagé holds professorial rank at the University of Montreal and Dr. Pierre Potvin at Laval. Dr. Omand Solandt, now Vice-President of the Canadian National Railways, in charge of research, spends some time at McGill University in the Department of Physiology headed by my friend Professor F. C. MacIntosh. At Queen's University in Kingston, Ontario, J. M. R. Beveridge is Chairman of the Department of Biochemistry, and R. E. Semple is Associate Professor in the Department of Physiology, under Professor Harold Ettinger. Dr. G. E. Hall, President of the University of Western Ontario and Dr. G. E. Manning of the same university, were graduate students in my department but did their research work entirely with Banting. At the University of Saskatchewan, my former associates, L. B. Jaques and C. S. McArthur, occupy the Chairs of Physiology and Biochemistry respectively.

Toronto has been my home for nearly fifty years. It has provided countless friendships and the University of Toronto has given me great opportunities. The comradeship and loyalty of the heads of the seven sections in the Department of Physiology and the seven in the Banting and Best Department of Medical Research obviously provide one of the greatest satisfactions a man could have. The names of many appear on the papers which have been selected for this volume: Haist, Monkhouse, Campbell, Rappaport, Scott, Clarke, Sirek, Franks, Lucas, Baer, Wrenshall, Salter, Logothetopoulos, and Baker.

My former graduate students Edward Sellers and Kenneth Fisher are Chairmen of the Departments of Pharmacology and of Zoology, respectively. J. B. Firstbrook has returned to Toronto as an Associate Professor in my first department, Physiological Hygiene.

Several former colleagues have carried the investigative attitude into the clinical field. Dr. A. L. Chute heads the Department of Pediatrics at the Toronto Hospital for Sick Children, a worthy successor to my late friend Dr. Alan Brown. Dr. W. Stanley Hartroft has recently become Director of the Research Institute at the same Hospital and Dr. Donald Fraser is active in the investigation of rare metabolic disorders.

The Connaught Medical Research Laboratories under Dr. J. K. W. Ferguson, and the School of Hygiene under Dr. Andrew Rhodes, include many of my colleagues and close friends, some dating back to the earliest part of the twenty years during which I was intimately associated with those institutions. I would mention particularly David Scott, Milton Brown, Donald MacLean, Albert Fisher, Peter Moloney, Neil McKinnon, and R. D. Defries. I recall with deep affection the late Dr. J. G. FitzGerald and Dr. D. T. Fraser. All these men and wonderful colleagues in other departments have made Toronto the most attractive place in which to live and work.

BIBLIOGRAPHY

Bibliography

The numbers in square brackets refer to Papers in this volume.

1. ABDERHALDEN, E., and PAFFRATH, H., 1925. Arch. ges. Physiol. Pflügers 207: 228. [37]
2. ABEL, J. J., 1926. Crystalline insulin. Proc. Nat. Acad. Sci. 12: 132–6. [29; 30]
3. ABEL, J. J., and KUBOTA, S., 1919. J. Pharmacol. Exp. Therap. 13: 243. [50]
4. ACHELIS, J. D. VON, and HARDEBECK, K., 1955. Deut. med. Wochschr. 80: 1452. [16]
5. ADDIS, T., POO, L. J., LEW, W., and YUEN, D. W., 1936. J. Biol. Chem. 113: 497. [39]
6. ADDISON, T., 1836. Guy's Hosp. Rep. 1: 476. [44]
7. ALLEN, F. M., 1913. Glycosuria and Diabetes. Boston: W. M. Leonard. [7]
8. —— 1913. (see p. 480, ref. 7). [16]
9. —— 1921. Am. J. Physiol. 54: 451. [5]
10. ALLEN, F. M., STILLMAN, E., and FITZ, R., 1919. Total dietary regulation in the treatment of diabetes. Monograph No. 11, New York: Rockefeller Inst. Med. Research. [7; 14]
11. ALLES, G. A., 1934. The physiological significance of choline derivatives. Physiol. Rev. 14: 276–307. [37]
12. ANDERSON, G. E., MONACO, R. N., PERFETTO, A. J., and TERMINE, C. M., 1957. Physiologic role for glucagon. Diabetes 6: 239–47. [31]
13. ANDERSON, R. J., 1930. J. Am. Chem. Soc. 52: 1607 [42]
14. ANITSCHKOW, N., and CHALATOW, S., 1913. Ueber experimentelle Cholesterinsteatose und ihre Bedeutung für die Entstehung einiger pathologischer Prozesse. Zentr. allgem. Pathol. u. pathol. Anat. 24: 1–9 [36]
15. ANON. (Editorial), 1944. J. Am. Med. Assoc. 124: 1062. [17]
16. ——1946. Naval medical research. J. Can. Med. Services, 3: 311–409. [1; 59]
17. —— (Editorial), 1956. Glucagon. Brit. Med. J. 2: 288 [31]
18. ARNOZAN [C.L.X.], and VAILLARD [L.], 1884. Arch. de Physiol. norm. et Path. Ser. 3, 3: 287. [4; 29]
19. ARNSTEIN, H. R. V., 1950. Biochem. J. 47: xviii. [48]
20. ARNSTEIN, H. R. V., and NEUBERGER, A., 1953. Biochem. J. 55: 259. [48]
21. ARTOM, C., 1951. Mechanism of action of lipotropic factors in animals. In Trans. 10th Conf. on Liver Injury, pp. 62–90. Josiah Macy Foundation. [48]
22. —— 1953. J. Biol. Chem. 205: 101. [48]
23. —— 1955. J. Biol. Chem. 213: 681. [48]
24. —— 1955. Federation Proc. 14: 174. [48]
25. ASHBY, J. S. 1922–23. Am. J. Physiol. 67: 77. [13]
26. ASHMORE, J., CAHILL, G. F., JR., EARLE, A. S., and ZOTTU, S., 1958. Diabetes 7: 1. [23]
27. ASHMORE, J., CAHILL, G. F., JR., and HASTINGS, A. B., 1956. Metabolism 5: 774. [23]
28. ASHWORTH, C. T., 1947. Proc. Soc. Exp. Biol. Med. 66: 382. [44]
29. ATWATER, W. O., and BENEDICT, F. G., 1902. Mem. Nat. Acad. Sci. 8: 231. [44]
30. AUDOVA, A., and WAGNER, R., 1924. Klin. Wochschr. 3: 231. [11]
31. BABKIN, B., 1923. Brit. J. Exp. Pathol. 4: 310. [11]
32. BAER, E., and KATES, M., 1950. J. Am. Chem. Soc. 72: 942. [48]
33. BAER, E., and MAURUKAS, J., 1955. J. Biol. Chem. 212: 25. [48]
34. BAER, E., MAURUKAS, J., and RUSSELL, M., 1952. J. Am. Chem. Soc. 74: 152. [48]
35. BAERNSTEIN, H. D., 1932. J. Biol. Chem. 97: 663. [41]

36. BAILEY, C. H., 1916. J. Exp. Med. 23: 69   [36]
37. BAKER, S L., DICKENS, F., and DODDS, E. C., 1924. Brit. J. Exp. Pathol. 5: 327. [13]
38. BALL, E. G., and BARRNETT, R. J., 1960. Diabetes 9: 70.   [31]
39. BANG, I., 1913. Der Blutzucker, p. 85. Wiesbaden. [8]
40. BANTING, F. G., and BEST, C. H., 1922. J. Lab. Clin. Med. 7: 251. [1; 5; 7; 9; 15; 29; 30]
41. —— 1922. J. Lab. Clin. Med. 7: 464. [9; 13; 30]
42. BANTING, F. G., BEST, C. H., COLLIP, J. B., CAMPBELL, W. R., and FLETCHER, A. A., 1922. Can. Med. Assoc. J. 12: 141. [9]
43. BANTING, F. G., BEST, C. H., COLLIP, J. B., HEPBURN, J., and MACLEOD, J. J. R., 1922. Trans. Roy. Soc. Can. 16, Sect. V: 35. [1; 30]
44. BANTING, F. G., BEST, C. H., COLLIP, J. B., and MACLEOD, J. J. R., 1922. Trans. Roy. Soc. Can. 16, Sect. V: 27. [1; 9; 30]
45. —— 1922. Trans. Roy. Soc. Can. 16, Sect. V: 42. [1; 30]
46. BANTING, F. G., BEST, C. H., COLLIP, J. B., MACLEOD, J. J. R., and NOBLE, E. C., 1922. Trans. Roy. Soc. Can. 16, Sect. V: 31. [1; 30]
47 —— 1922. Trans. Roy. Soc. Can. 16, Sect. V: 39. [1; 9; 30]
48. —— 1922. Am. J. Physiol. 62: 162. [8]
49. BANTING, F. G., BEST, C. H., and MACLEOD, J. J. R., 1922. Am. J. Physiol. 59: 479P. [1; 29]
50. BARGER, G., and DALE, H. H., 1910. J. Chem. Soc. 97: 2592. [50]
51. —— 1910–11. J. Physiol. (London) 41: 499. [50]
52. BARRETT, H. M., BEST, C. H., MACLEAN, D. L., and RIDOUT, J. H., 1939. J. Physiol. (London) 97: 103. [14]
53. BARRETT, H. M., BEST, C. H., and RIDOUT, J. H., 1938. J. Physiol. (London) 93: 367. [48]
54. BARRETT, H. M., MACLEAN, D. L., and CUNNINGHAM, J. G., 1938. J. Ind. Hyg. 20: 360. [40]
55. BARRETT, J. F., 1935. Biochem. J. 29: 2442. [57]
56. BARRON, M., 1920. The relation of the islets of Langerhans to diabetes with special reference to cases of pancreatic lithiasis. Surg. Gynecol. Obstet. 31: 437–48. [4]
57. BEARDWOOD, J. R., 1944. Am. J. Digest. Diseases 11: 345. [17]
58. BEESTON, A. W., and CHANNON, H. J., 1936. Biochem. J. 30: 280. [41]
59. BEESTON, A. W., CHANNON, H. J., and WILKINSON, H., 1935. Biochem. J. 29: 2659. [38]
60. BEHRENS, O. K., and BROMER, W. W., 1958. Glucagon. Vitamins and Hormones 16: 263–301. [21]
61. BELLOWS, J. G., and CHINN, H., 1943. Arch. Ophthalmol. 30: 105. [48]
62. BENEDICT, S. R., 1911. J. Am. Med. Assoc. 57: 1193. [21]
63. BERNARD, CLAUDE, 1855–56. Leçons de physiologie expérimentale appliquée à la médecine. Paris: Baillière. [29]
64. BERNARD, R., and DEMERS, J. M., 1949. Can. J. Research, E. 27: 281. [48]
65. BERSON, S. A., and YALOW, R. S., 1958. Insulin antagonists, insulin antibodies and insulin resistance. Am. J. Med. 25: 155–9. [30]
66. BERTHET, J., SUTHERLAND, E. W., and MAKMAN, M. H., 1956. Metabolism 5: 768. [23]
67. BERTRAM, F. VON, BENDFELDT, E., and OTTO, H., 1955. Deut. med. Wochschr. 80: 1455. [16]
68. BEST, C. H., 1926. Proc. Roy. Soc. (London), B 99: 375. [1]
69. —— 1929. J. Physiol. (London) 67: 256. [1; 52]
70. —— 1938. Heparin and thrombosis. Brit. Med. J. 2: 977–81. [53]
71. —— 1950. Protection of liver and kidney by dietary factors. Federation Proc. 9: 506–11. [46]
72. —— 1952. The insulin content of the pancreas. Diabetes 1: 155–7. [29]
73. —— 1953. Early experiences with choline—a retrospect. Nutrition Rev. 11: 321–3. [48]
74. —— 1956. The lipotropic agents in the protection of the liver, kidney, heart,

and other organs of experimental animals. Proc. Roy. Soc. (London), B *145*: 151–69. [1]

75. —— 1956. Reminiscences of the discovery of insulin. Diabetes *5*: 64–7. [24]
76. —— 1959. Preparation of heparin and its use in the first clinical cases. Circulation *19*: 79–86. [1]
77. —— 1959. Metabolic problems involving the pancreas, choline, insulin, and glucagon. *In* Ciba Foundation 10th anniversary symposium on significant trends in medical research, pp. 164–95, ed. G. E. W. Wolstenholme *et al.* London: J. and A. Churchill. [31]
78. BEST, C. H., and CAMPBELL, J., 1936. J. Physiol. (London) *86*: 190. [1; 39; 40; 48]
79. BEST, C. H., and CHANNON, H. J., 1935. Biochem. J. *29*: 2651. [38; 47; 48]
80. BEST, C. H., CHANNON, H. J., and RIDOUT, J. H., 1934. J Physiol. (London) *81*: 409. [1; 37; 38; 40; 48]
81. BEST, C. H., COWAN, C., and MacLEAN, D. L., 1938. J. Physiol. (London) *92*: 20. [56]
82. BEST, C. H., DALE, H. H., DUDLEY, H. W., and THORPE, W. V., 1926–27. J. Physiol. (London) *62*: 397. [1; 51; 52]
83. BEST, C. H., DALE, H. H., HOET, J. P., and MARKS, H. P., 1926. Proc. Roy. Soc. (London), B*100*: 55. [1]
84. BEST, C. H., FERGUSON, G. C., and HERSHEY, J. M., 1933. J. Physiol. (London) *79*: 94. [48]
85. BEST, C. H., HAIST, R. E., and RIDOUT, J. H., 1939. J. Physiol. (London) *97*: 107. [1]
86. BEST, C. H., HARTROFT, W. S., LUCAS, C. C., and RIDOUT, J. H., 1949. Brit. Med. J. *2*: 1001. [46; 48]
87. —— 1955. Brit. Med. J. *1*: 1439. [47; 48]
88. BEST, C. H., HARTROFT, W. S., and SELLERS, E. A., 1952. Gastroenterology *20*: 375. [45]
89. BEST, C. H., and HERSHEY, J. M., 1932. J. Physiol. (London) *75*: 49. [34; 36]
90. BEST, C. H., HERSHEY, J. M., and HUNTSMAN, M. E., 1932. Am. J. Physiol. *101*: 7P. [48]
91. —— 1932. J. Physiol. (London) *75*: 56. [1; 35; 36]
92. BEST, C. H., HOET, J. P., and MARKS, H. P., 1926. Proc. Roy. Soc. (London), B *100*: 32. [12]
93. BEST, C. H., HOFFMAN, F., LUCAS, C. C., and TALESNIK, J., 1946–47. J. Physiol. (London) *105*: 27P. [48]
94. BEST, C. H., and HUNTSMAN, M. E., 1932. J. Physiol. (London) *75*: 405. [1; 36; 42; 43; 47; 48]
95. —— 1935. J. Physiol. (London) *83*: 255. [1; 38; 47; 48]
96. BEST, C. H., HUNTSMAN, M. E., McHENRY, E. W., and RIDOUT, J. H., 1935. J. Physiol. (London) *84*: 38P. [37]
97. BEST, C. H., HUNTSMAN, M. E., and SOLANDT, O. M., 1932. Trans. Roy. Soc. Can. *26*, Sect. V: 175. [48]
98. BEST, C. H., HUNTSMAN, M. E., and YOUNG, F. G., 1935. J. Physiol. (London) *85*: 8P. [48]
99. BEST, C. H., JEPHCOTT, C. M., and SCOTT, D. A., 1932. Am. J. Physiol. *100*: 285. [1]
100. BEST, C. H., and LUCAS, C. C., 1943. Choline—chemistry and significance as a dietary factor. Vitamins and Hormones *1*: 1–51. [48]
101. —— 1950. Choline malnutrition. *In* Clinical Nutrition, pp. 561–85, ed. N. Jolliffe *et al.* New York: Hoeber, Inc. (2nd. ed. 1962, pp. 227–60). [48]
102. BEST, C. H., LUCAS, C. C., PATTERSON, J. M., and RIDOUT, J. H., 1946. Biochem. J. *40*: 368. [42; 44; 46; 48]
103. —— 1951. Biochem. J. *48*: 452. [45]
104. BEST, C. H., LUCAS, C. C., and RIDOUT, J. H., 1953–54. The lipotropic factors. Ann. N. Y. Acad. Sci. *57*: 646–53. [48]
105. BEST, C. H., LUCAS, C. C., RIDOUT, J. H., and PATTERSON, J. M., 1950. J. Biol. Chem. *186*: 317. [46]

106. BEST, C. H., and McHENRY, E. W., 1930. J. Physiol. (London) 70: 349. [37]
107. —— 1931. Histamine. Physiol. Rev. 11: 371–477. [1]
108. BEST, C. H., MACLEAN, D. L., and RIDOUT, J. H., 1934–35. J. Physiol. (London) 83: 275. [37]
109. BEST, C. H., and PARTRIDGE, R. C., 1928. Proc. Roy. Soc. (London), B 103: 218. [49]
110. —— 1929. Proc. Roy. Soc. (London), B 105: 323. [1]
111. BEST, C. H., and RIDOUT, J. H., 1933. J. Physiol. (London) 78: 415. [1; 36; 38]
112. —— 1935. J. Physiol. (London) 84: 7P. [38]
113. —— 1939–40. J. Physiol. (London) 97: 489. [47; 48]
114. BEST, C. H., and SCOTT, D. A., 1923. Trans. Roy. Soc. Can. 17, Sect. V: 87. [13]
115. —— 1923. J. Am. Med. Assoc. 81: 382. [1; 13]
116. —— 1923. J. Metabolic Research 3: 177. [13]
117. BEST, C. H., SCOTT, D. A., and BANTING, F. G., 1923. Trans. Roy. Soc. Can. 17, Sect. V: 81. [13]
118. BEST, C. H., SMITH, R. G., and SCOTT, D. A., 1924. J. Biol. Chem. 59: xxx. [13]
119. —— 1924. Am. J. Physiol. 68: 161. [13]
120. BEVERIDGE, J. M. R., and LUCAS, C. C., 1945. J. Biol. Chem. 157: 311. [44]
121. BEVERIDGE, J. M. R., LUCAS, C. C., and O'GRADY, M. K., 1944. J. Biol. Chem. 154: 9. [45; 47]
122. —— 1945. J. Biol. Chem. 160: 505. [45; 46; 47; 48]
123. BICKEL, A., and COLLAZO, J. A., 1923. Deut. med. Wochschr. 49: 1408. [11]
124. BIEDL, A., and KRAUS, R., 1909. Wien. klin. Wochschr. 22: 363. [53]
125. BISSINGER, E., and LESSER, E. J., 1926. Biochem. Z. 168: 398. [11; 12]
126. BISSINGER, E., LESSER, E. J., and ZIPF, K., 1923. Klin. Wochschr. 2: 2233. [11; 12]
127. BIZZOZERO, J., 1882. Arch. pathol. Anat. u. Physiol. Virchows 90: 261. [55]
128. BLATHERWICK, N. R., MEDLAR, E. M., BRADSHAW, P. J., POST, A. L., and SAWYER, S. D., 1931–32. Proc. Soc. Exp. Biol. Med. 29: 345. [36]
129. —— 1932. J. Biol. Chem. 97: xxxiii; 100: xviii; 103: 93. [36]
130. BLISS, C. I., 1949–50. The design of biological assays. Ann. N.Y. Acad. Sci. 52: 877–88. [15]
131. BLOOR, W. R., PELKAN, K. F., and ALLEN, D. M., 1922. J. Biol. Chem. 52: 191. [23; 47]
132. BLOTNER, H., 1945. Arch. Internal Med. 75: 39. [17]
133. —— 1946. Studies in glycosuria and diabetes mellitus in selectees. J. Am. Med. Assoc. 131: 1109–14. [17]
134. BLOTNER, H., HYDE, R. W., and KINGSLEY, L. V., 1943. New. Engl. J. Med. 229: 885. [17]
135. BLUMBERG, H., MACKENZIE, C. G., and SELIGSON, D., 1942. Federation Proc. 1: 187. [48]
136. BODONG, A., 1905. Arch. exp. Pathol. Pharmakol. 52: 242. [Foreword to Paper 53]
137. BOLLMAN, J. L., MANN, F. C., and MAGATH, T. B., 1925. Am. J. Physiol. 74: 238. [11]
138. BONDY, P. K., and CARDILLO, L. R., 1956. J. Clin. Invest. 35: 494. [20]
139. BORDET, J., and GENGON, O., 1901. Ann. Inst. Pasteur 15: 129. [53]
140. BORNSTEIN, J., and LAWRENCE, R. D., 1951. Brit. Med. J. 1: 732. [15]
141. —— 1951. Brit. Med. J. 2: 1541. [29]
142. BORSOOK, H., and DUBNOFF, J. W., 1947. J. Biol. Chem. 171: 363. [48]
143. BOSTRÖM, L., 1944. In Laborationsteknik för sjukhus (Laboratory Technique for Hospitals) (see p. 57). Stockholm: Norstedt. [19]
144. BOXER, G. E., and STETTEN, DEWITT, JR., 1944. J. Biol. Chem. 153: 617. [48]
145. BOYD, W., 1947. Textbook of Pathology, 5th ed. (see p. 623). Philadelphia: Lea and Febiger. [43]
146. BRADLEY, H. C., 1922. Autolysis and atrophy. Physiol. Rev. 2: 415–39. [51]

147. BRAND, E., 1946–47.   Ann. N.Y. Acad. Sci. 47: 187.   [29]
148. BRIGGS, A. P., 1922.   J. Biol. Chem. 53: 13.   [34]
149. BROCK, J. F., 1953–54.   Survey of the world situation on kwashiorkor.   Ann. N.Y. Acad. Sci. 57: 696–713.   [45]
150. BROCK, J. F., and HANSEN, J. D. L., 1956.   Am. J. Clin. Nutrition 4: 286.   [47]
151. BROCK, J. F., HANSEN, J. D. L., HOWE, E. E., PRETORIUS, P. J., DAVEL, J. G. A., and HENDRICKSE, R. G., 1955.   Kwashiorkor and protein malnutrition.   Lancet 2: 355–60.   [47]
152. BROWN, E. M., JR., DOHAN, F. C., FREEDMAN, L. R., DeMOOR, P., and LUKENS, F. D. W., 1952.   Endocrinology 50: 644.   [21]
153. BRUGSCH, T., and HORSTERS, H., 1924.   Biochem. Z. 147: 150.   [13]
154. —— 1930.   Arch. exp. Pathol. Pharmakol. 148: 295.   [13]
155. BUCKLEY, G. F., and HARTROFT, W. S., 1955.   Arch. Pathol. 59: 185.   [48]
156. BURN, J. H., and DALE, H. H., 1922.   Med. Research Council (Brit.) Spec. Rep. Ser. no. 69.   [52]
157. —— 1924.   J. Physiol. (London) 59: 164.   [10; 11; 12]
158. —— 1926.   J. Physiol. (London) 61: 185.   [50; 52]
159. BURNS, J. L., and HARTROFT, W. S., 1949.   Am. J. Ophthalmol., 32: Part II, 79. [48]
160. BUTTS, J. S., and DEUEL, H. J., JR., 1933.   J. Biol. Chem. 100: 415.   [39]
161. CAMPBELL, J., 1938.   Endocrinology 23: 692.   [1; 39]
162. —— 1955.   Diabetogenic actions of growth hormone.   In International Symposium on the Hypophyseal Growth Hormone, 270–85, ed. R. W. Smith Jr., et al.   New York: McGraw-Hill.   [30]
163. CAMPBELL, J., and BEST, C. H., 1938.   Lancet 1: 1444.   [14]
164. —— 1956.   Physiologic aspects of ketosis.   Metabolism 5: 95–113.   [30]
165. CAMPBELL, W. R., GRAHAM, R. R., and ROBINSON, W. L., 1939.   Trans. Assoc. Am. Physicians 54: 304.   [14]
166. CAMPBELL, R. M., and KOSTERLITZ, H. W., 1948.   J. Biol. Chem. 175: 989.   [45]
167. —— 1949–50.   J. Endocrinol. 6: 308.   [45]
168. —— 1952.   Biochim. Biophys. Acta 8: 664.   [45]
169. CAMPBELL, W. R., and MACLEOD, J. J. R., 1924.   Insulin.   Medicine 3: 195–308. [11; 12]
170. CANNON, W. B., and MENDENHALL, W. L., 1914.   Am. J. Physiol. 34: 225.   [54]
171. CANNON, P. R., STEFFEE, C. H., FRAZIER, L. J., ROWLEY, D. A., and STEPTO, R. C., 1947.   Federation Proc. 6: 390.   [47]
172. CANTONI, G. L., 1952.   J. Am. Chem. Soc. 74: 2942.   [48]
173. —— 1953.   J. Biol. Chem. 204: 403.   [48]
174. CARDEZA, A. F., 1950.   Rev. soc. arg. biol. 26: 150.   [29]
175. CARLSON, A. J., and DRENNAN, F. M., 1911.   Am. J. Physiol. 28: 391.   [5]
176. CASSELMAN, W. G. B., and WILLIAMS, G. R., 1954.   Nature 173: 210.   [48]
177. CASTRO-MENDOZA, H., JIMÉNEZ DÍAZ, C., and VIVANCO, F., 1947.   Rev. clin. españ. 27: 176.   [48]
178. CAVALLERO, C., and MALANDRA, B., 1953.   Acta Endocrinol. 13: 79.   [20; 21]
179. CHAIKOFF, I. L., 1942.   The application of labelling agents to the study of phospholipid metabolism.   Physiol. Rev. 22: 291–317.   [48]
180. CHAIKOFF, I. L., and CONNOR, C. L., 1940.   Proc. Soc. Exp. Biol. Med. 43: 638.   [44; 48]
181. CHAIKOFF, I. L., CONNOR, C. L., and BISKIND, G. R., 1938.   Am. J. Pathol. 14: 101.   [44]
182. CHAIKOFF, I. L., and FORKER, L. L., 1950.   Endocrinology 46: 319.   [19]
183. CHAIN, E. B., 1959.   Recent studies on carbohydrate metabolism.   Brit. Med. J. 2: 709–19.   [31]
184. CHALATOW, S. S., 1912.   Arch. pathol. Anat. u. Physiol. Virchows 207: 452. [36]
185. CHAMBERS, W. H., 1938.   Undernutrition and carbohydrate metabolism.   Physiol. Rev. 18: 248–96.   [14]
186. CHANG, H. C., and GADDUM, J. H., 1933.   J. Physiol. (London) 79: 255.   [37]
187. CHANNON, H. J., and EL SABY, M. K., 1932.   Biochem. J. 26: 2021.   [36]

188. CHANNON, H. J., LOACH, J. V., LOIZIDES, P. A., MANIFOLD, M. C., and SOLIMAN, G., 1938. Biochem. J. 32: 976. [41; 47]
189. CHANNON, H. J., MANIFOLD, M. C., and PLATT, A. P., 1938. Biochem. J. 32: 969. [41]
190. —— 1940. Biochem. J. 34: 866. [48]
191. CHANNON, H. J., MILLS, G. T., and PLATT, A. P., 1943. Biochem. J. 37: 483. [47]
192. CHANNON, H. J., PLATT, A. P., LOACH, J. V., and SMITH, J. A. B., 1937. Biochem. J. 31: 2181. [42]
193. CHANNON, H. J., and SMITH, J. A. B., 1936. Biochem. J. 30: 115. [42]
194. CHANNON, H. J., and WILKINSON, H., 1935. Biochem. J. 29: 350. [38; 47; 48]
195. CHANUTIN, A., and FERRIS, E. B., 1932. Arch. Internal Med. 49: 767. [43]
196. CHANUTIN, A., and LUDEWIG, S., 1933. J. Biol. Chem. 102: 57. [36]
197. CHARGAFF, E., and OLSON, K. B., 1937. J. Biol. Chem. 122: 153. [53]
198. CHARLES, A. F., and SCOTT, D. A., 1933. J. Biol. Chem. 102: 425, 431. [53; 54]
199. —— 1934. Trans. Roy. Soc. Can. 28, Sect. V: 55. [53; 54]
200. —— 1936. Biochem. J. 30: 1927. [1; 53; 54]
201. CHEN, K. K., ANDERSON, R. C., and MAZE, N., 1946. Proc. Soc. Exp. Biol. Med. 63: 483. [30]
202. CHRISTENSEN, K., 1942. Arch. Pathol. 34: 633. [43; 48]
203. CLARK, A. H., 1919. Johns Hopkins Hosp. Reports 18: 229. [9]
204. CLARKE, H. T., GILLESPIE, H. B., and WEISSHAUS, S. Z., 1933. J. Am. Chem. Soc. 55: 4571. [42]
205. COCHRANE, W., 1960. Idiopathic infantile hypoglycemia and leucine sensitivity. Metabolism 9: 386–99. [31]
206. COLLAZO, J. A., HÄNDEL, M., and RUBINO, P., 1954. Deut. med. Wochschr. 50: 747. [11]
207. COLLIP, J. B., 1922. Trans. Roy. Soc. Can. 16, Sect. V: 28. [1; 9; 30]
208. —— 1922–23. Proc. Soc. Exp. Biol. Med. 20: 321. [13]
209. —— 1923. Nature 111: 571. [13]
210. —— 1923. Trans. Roy. Soc. Can. 17, Sect. V: 39. [13]
211. —— 1923. Trans. Roy. Soc. Can. 17, Sect. V: 45. [13]
212. —— 1922–23. Am. J. Physiol. 63: 391P. [13]
213. —— 1923. J. Biol. Chem. 55: xxxix. [13]
214. —— 1923. J. Biol. Chem. 56: 513. [13]
215. —— 1923. J. Biol. Chem. 57: 65. [13]
216. —— 1923–24. J. Biol. Chem. 58: 163. [13]
217. —— 1926–27. Proc. Soc. Exp. Biol. Med. 24: 731. [13]
218. CONN, J. W., 1940. Interpretation of the glucose tolerance test. Am. J. Med. Sci. 199: 555–64. [17]
219. CONNOR, C. L., and CHAIKOFF, I. L., 1938. Proc. Soc. Exp. Biol. Med. 39: 356. [44]
220. COPELAND, D. H., and SALMON, W. D., 1946. Am. J. Pathol. 22: 1059. [48]
221. CORI, C. F., 1923–24. Proc. Soc. Exp. Biol. Med. 21: 417. [11]
222. —— 1923–24. Proc. Soc. Exp. Biol. Med. 21: 419. [11]
223. —— 1925. J. Pharmacol. Exp. Therap. 25: 1. [12]
224. CORI, C. F., and CORI, G. T., 1926. J. Biol. Chem. 70: 557. [14]
225. —— 1947. Polysaccharide phosphorylase. In Les Prix Nobel en 1947, pp. 216–35. Stockholm: Norstedt, 1949. [30]
226. CORI, C. F., CORI, G. T., and GOLTZ, H. L., 1923. J. Pharmacol. Exp. Therap. 22: 355. [10]
227. CORI, C. F., CORI, G. T., and PUCHER, G. W., 1923. J. Pharmacol. Exp. Therap. 21: 377. [11]
228. CORI, G. T., 1925. Am. J. Physiol. 71: 708. [13]
229. —— 1925. J. Cancer Research 9: 408. [13]
230. CORI, G. T., and CORI, C. F., 1927. J. Biol. Chem. 72: 615. [14; 39]
231. CRAFOORD, C., 1937. Acta Chir. Scand. 79: 407. [53]
232. CRAMER, W., DICKENS, F., and DODDS, E. C., 1926. Brit. J. Exp. Pathol. 7: 299. [13]

233. Crist, R. H., Murphy, G. M., and Urey, H. C., 1934. J. Chem. Phys. 2: 112. [40]
234. Cruickshank, E. W. H., 1913–14. J. Physiol. (London) 47: 1. [6]
235. Curtis, A. C., and Newburgh, L. H., 1927. Arch. Internal Med. 39: 828. [41]
236. Daft, F. S., Sebrell, W. H., and Lillie, R. D., 1941. Proc. Exp. Soc. Biol. Med. 48: 228. [44]
237. Dale, H. H., 1923. A lecture on the physiology of insulin. Lancet 1: 989–93. [9; 12]
238. —— 1926. The pancreas and insulin. In Lectures on Certain Aspects of Biochemistry, pp. 47–90 (see p. 73). London: University of London Press. [12]
239. —— 1929. Some chemical factors in the control of the circulation. Lancet 1: 1233–7. [52]
240. Dale, H. H., and Dudley, H. W., 1921–22. J. Pharmacol. Exp. Therap. 18: 27. [50]
241. —— 1929–30. J. Physiol. (London) 68: 97. [52]
242. Dale, H. H., and Laidlaw, P. P., 1910–11. J. Physiol. (London) 41: 318. [50; 52]
243. —— 1918–19. J. Physiol. (London) 52: 355. [50]
244. Dale, H. H., and Richards, A. N., 1918–19. J. Physiol. (London) 52: 110. [50]
245. Dale, H. H., and Schuster, E. H. J., 1927–28. J. Physiol. (London) 64: 356. [52]
246. Dann, M., and Chambers, W. H., 1930. J. Biol. Chem. 89: 675. [14]
247. Davidson, I. W. F., Salter, J. M., and Best, C. H., 1957. Nature 180: 1124. [1; 22]
248. Davis, J. N. P., 1953–54. The pathology of dietary liver disease in tropical Africa. Ann. N.Y. Acad. Sci. 57: 714–21. [47]
249. Deren, M. D., 1937. J. Lab. Clin. Med. 22: 1138. [17]
250. Dianzani, M. U., 1955. Biochim. Biophys. Acta 17: 391. [48]
251. Dible, J. H., 1932. J. Pathol. Bacteriol. 35: 451. [39; 45]
252. Dible, J. H., and Libman, J., 1934. J. Pathol. Bacteriol. 38: 269. [45]
253. Dick, F., Hall, W. K., Sydenstricker, V. P., McCollum, W., and Bowles, L. L., 1952. Arch. Pathol. 53: 154. [45]
254. Dickinson, W. L., 1890. J. Physiol. (London) 11: 566. [Foreword to Paper 53]
255. Dingemanse, E., 1928. Arch. exp. Pathol. Pharmakol. 128: 44. [13]
256. Dirscherl, W., 1931. Z. physiol. Chem. 202: 116. [13]
257. Dohan, F. C., and Lukens, F. D. W., 1947. Federation Proc. 6: 97. [30]
258. —— 1948. Endocrinology 42: 244. [21]
259. Doisy, E. A., Somogyi, M., and Shaffer, P. A., 1923. J. Biol. Chem. 55: xxxi. [9]
260. Donohue, W. L., 1948. J. Pediatrics 32: 739. [29]
261. Doyon, M., 1912. Rapports du foie avec la coagulation du sang. J. physiol. et pathol. gén. 14: 229–40. [53]
262. Drabkin, D. L., 1945. Science 101: 445. [29]
263. Drennan, F. M., 1911. Am. J. Physiol. 28: 396. [9]
264. Drury, A. N., and Szent-Györgyi, A., 1929–30. J. Physiol. (London) 68: 213. [37]
265. Drury, D. R., Wick, A. N., and Sherrill, J. W., 1954. Diabetes 3: 129. [20]
266. Dubin, H. E., and Corbitt, H. B., 1923–24. Proc. Soc. Exp. Biol. Med. 21: 16. [13]
267. Duchek, A., 1853. Prag. Vjschr. 3: 104, cited by Ruge (see p. 252. ref. 656). [44]
268. Dudley, H. W., 1923. Biochem. J. 17: 376. [9]
269. Dudley, H. W., Laidlaw, P. P., Trevan, J. W., and Boock, E. M., 1923. J. Physiol. (London) 57: xlvii. [12]
270. Dudley, H. W., and Marrian, G. F., 1923. Biochem. J. 17: 435. [11; 12]
271. Duff, G. L., McMillan, G. C., and Wilson, D. C., 1947. Proc. Soc. Exp. Biol. Med. 64: 251. [21]

272. DUFF, G. L., and TORESON, W. E., 1951.   Endocrinology 48: 298.   [21; 29]
273. DUNN, J. S., SHEEHAN, H. L., and McLETCHIE, N. G. B., 1943.   Lancet 1: 484. [30]
274. DURLACHER, S. H., MEIER, J. R., FISHER, R. S., and LOVITT, W. V., 1954.   Am. J. Pathol. 30: 633P.   [48]
275. EADIE, G. S., and MACLEOD, J. J. R., 1923.   Am. J. Physiol. 64: 285.   [9]
276. EADIE, G. S., MACLEOD, J. J. R., and NOBLE, E. C., 1925.   Am. J. Physiol. 72: 614. [11]
277. EBERTH, J. C., and SCHIMMELBUSCH, C., 1886.   Arch. pathol. Anat. u. Physiol. Virchows 103: 39; 105: 456.   [54; 55]
278. ECKSTEIN, H. C., 1952.   J. Biol. Chem. 195: 167.   [48]
279. EFFKEMANN, G., and HEROLD, L., 1935.   Z. ges. exp. Med. 96: 195.   [39]
280. EISLER, M., and PORTHEIM, L., 1924.   Biochem. Z. 148: 566.   [13]
281. ELLIS, R. W. B., 1931.   Arch. Disease Childhood 6: 285.   [14]
282. ELRICK, H., 1955.   Discussion on influence of growth hormone on human metabolism. In International Symposium on the Hypophyseal Growth Hormone, pp. 561–8, ed. R. W. Smith Jr., et al.   New York: McGraw-Hill.   [20]
283. —— 1956.   Nature 177: 892.   [20]
284. ELRICK, H., HLAD, C. J., ARAI, Y., and SMITH, A., 1956.   J. Clin. Invest. 35: 757. [20]
285. ELRICK, H., HLAD, C. J., and WITTEN, T., 1955.   J. Clin. Invest. 34: 1830.   [20]
286. ELWYN, D., WEISSBACH, A., HENRY, S. S., and SPRINSON, D. B., 1955.   J. Biol. Chem. 213: 281.   [48]
287. ELWYN, D., WEISSBACH, A., and SPRINSON, D. B., 1951.   J. Am. Chem. Soc. 73: 5509.   [48]
288. ENGEL, R. W., COPELAND, D. H., and SALMON, W. D., 1947–48.   Ann. N.Y. Acad. Sci. 49: 49.   [48]
289. ENGEL, R. W., and SALMON, W. D., 1941.   J. Nutrition. 22: 109.   [43; 48]
290. ENTENMAN, C., CHAIKOFF, I. L., and FRIEDLANDER, H. D., 1946.   J. Biol. Chem. 162: 111.   [48]
291. ERICKSON, B. N., AVRIN, I., TEAGUE, D. M., and WILLIAMS, H. H., 1940.   J. Biol. Chem. 135: 671.   [42]
292. EULER, U. S. VON, and GADDUM, J. H., 1931.   J. Physiol. (London) 72: 74. [37]
293. EVANS, M., and HAIST, R. E., 1951.   Am. J. Physiol. 167: 176.   [29]
294. EWINS, A. J., and LAIDLAW, P. P., 1910–11.   J. Physiol. (London) 41: 78.   [51; 52]
295. EZRIN, C., SALTER, J. M., OGRYZLO, M. A., and BEST, C. H., 1958.   Can. Med. Assoc. J. 78: 96.   [1]
296. FAJANS, S. S., and CONN, J. W., 1954.   Diabetes 3: 296.   [30]
297. FALKENHAUSEN, M. F. VON, 1925.   Arch. exp. Pathol. Pharmakol. 109: 249.   [19]
298. FERGUSON, J. H., 1934.   Am. J. Physiol. 108: 670.   [55]
299. FISHER, N. F., and McKINLEY, E. B., 1923–24.   Proc. Soc. Exp. Biol. Med. 21: 248.   [13]
300. FISHER, N. F., and NOBLE, B. E., 1923.   Am. J. Physiol. 67: 72.   [13]
301. FLOSDORF, E. W., STOKES, F. J., and MUDD, S., 1940.   J. Am. Med. Assoc. 115: 1095.   [58]
302. FOLCH, J., and WOOLLEY, D. W., 1942.   J. Biol. Chem. 142: 963.   [42]
303. FOLIN, O., 1930.   J. Biol. Chem. 86: 173.   [19]
304. FOLIN, O., and WU, H. J., 1920.   J. Biol. Chem. 41: 367.   [17]
305. FORSCHBACH, J., 1909.   Arch. exp. Pathol. Pharmakol. 60: 131.   [9]
306. —— 1909.   Deut. med. Wochschr. 35: 2053.   [9]
307. FRANK, E., HARTMANN, E., and NOTHMANN, M., 1925.   Klin. Wochschr. 4: 1067. [12]
308. FRANK, E., NOTHMANN, M., and WAGNER, A., 1924.   Klin. Wochschr. 3: 581. [10]
309. FRANKE, H., and FUCHS, J., 1955.   Deut. med. Wochschr. 80: 1449.   [16; 30]
310. FRANZ, F., 1903.   Arch. exp. Pathol. Pharmakol. 49: 342.   [Foreward to Paper 53]

311. FREUND, E., 1888. Med. Jahrb. (Wien), Ser. 3, 3: 259. [53]
312. FREY, E. K., and KRAUT, H., 1928. Arch. exp. Pathol. Pharmakol. 133: 1. [37]
313. FRY, E. G., 1937. Endocrinology 21: 283. [39]
314. FUNK, C., and CORBITT, H. B., 1922–23. Proc. Soc. Exp. Biol. Med. 20: 422. [13]
315. FÜRTH, O. VON, and SCHWARZ, C., 1911. Biochem. Z. 31: 113. [9]
316. FURUSAWA, K., HILL, A. V., and PARKINSON, J. L., 1927–28. Proc. Roy. Soc. (London), B 102: 29. [49]
317. GAVIN, G., and McHENRY, E. W., 1941. J. Biol. Chem. 139: 485. [42]
318. GAVIN, G., McHENRY, E. W., and WILSON, M. J., 1933. J. Physiol. (London) 79: 234. [37]
319. GEMMILL, C. L., and HAMMAN, L., JR., 1941. Bull. Johns Hopkins Hosp. 68: 50. [31]
320. GILLESPIE, R. J. G., and LUCAS, C. C., 1958. Can. J. Biochem. Physiol. 36: 307. [44]
321. GLASER, E., and WITTNER, L., 1924. Biochem. Z. 151: 279. [13]
322. GLYNN, L. E., HIMSWORTH, H. P., and LINDAN, O., 1948. Brit. J. Exp. Pathol. 29: 1. [45; 48]
323. GODLOWSKI, Z., 1933. Wien. med. Wochschr. 83: 1034. [53; 54]
324. GOLDBLATT, H., LYNCH, J., HANZAL, R. F., and SUMMERVILLE, W. W., 1934. J. Exp. Med. 59: 347. [43]
325. GOMES DA COSTA, S. F., 1931. Compt. rend. soc. biol. 107: 85. [22]
326. GOMORI, G., 1941. Am. J. Pathol. 17: 395. [15; 21]
327. —— 1950. Am. J. Clin. Pathol. 20: 665. [21]
328. GORNALL, A. G., and BARDAWILL, C. J., 1952. Can. J. Med. Sci. 30: 256. [23]
329. GOTTSCHALK, A., 1924. Deut. med. Wochschr. 50: 538. [13]
330. GRAAF, REGNER DE, 1671. Traité de la nature et de l'usage du suc pancréatique (Leiden). Transl. by C. Pack. London: N. Brook, 1676. [29]
331. GREAVES, R. I. N., and ADAIR, M. E., 1939. J. Hygiene 39: 413. [58]
332. GRIFFITHS, M., 1941. J. Physiol. (London) 100: 104. [29]
333. GRIFFITH, W. H., 1942. Choline. In Biological Action of the Vitamins, pp. 169–84, ed. E. A. Evans, Jr. Chicago: University of Chicago Press. [46]
334. GRIFFITH, W. H., and MULFORD, D. J., 1941. J. Am. Chem. Soc. 63: 929. [46]
335. GRIFFITH, W. H., and WADE, N. J., 1939. J. Biol. Chem. 131: 567. [43; 48]
336. GUGGENHEIM, M., 1912. Therap. Monatsch. 26: 795; 1914, 28: 174. [50]
337. —— 1924. Die biogenen Amine; 2nd ed.; Berlin: Springer. [37]
338. GUGGENHEIM, M., and LÖFFLER, W., 1916. Biochem. Z. 72: 303. [52]
339. GUTFREUND, H., 1948. Biochem. J. 42: 544. [29]
340. GYÖRGY, P., 1954. On some aspects of protein nutrition. Am. J. Clin. Nutrition 2: 231–42. [48]
341. GYÖRGY, P., and GOLDBLATT, H., 1939. J. Exp. Med. 70: 185. [48]
342. —— 1940. J. Exp. Med. 72: 1. [43; 48]
343. —— 1949. J. Exp. Med. 90: 73. [48]
344. HAHN, P. F., 1943. Science 98: 19. [48; 53]
345. HAIST, R. E., 1944. Factors affecting the insulin content of the pancreas. Physiol. Rev. 24: 409–44. [29; 30]
346. —— 1959. Islet cell function. Ann. N.Y. Acad. Sci. 82: 266–86. [30]
347. HAIST, R. E., CAMPBELL, J., and BEST, C. H., 1940. The prevention of diabetes. New Engl. J. Med. 223: 607–15. [1; 15; 18]
348. HAIST, R. E., EVANS, M., KINASH, B., BRYANS, F. E., and ASHWORTH, M. A., 1949. Factors affecting the volume of the islands of Langerhans. Proc. Am. Diabetes Assoc. 9: 53–62. [29]
349. HAIST, R. E., RIDOUT, J. H., and BEST, C. H., 1939. Am. J. Physiol. 126: 518P. [14]
350. HAM, A. W., 1940. Arch. Pathol. 29: 731. [43]
351. HAM, A. W., and HAIST, R. E., 1941. Am. J. Pathol. 17: 787. [21]
352. HANDLER, P., 1946. J. Nutrition 31: 621. [43]
353. —— 1948. J. Biol. Chem. 173: 295. [48]

354. Handler, P., and Bernheim, F., 1949. Proc. Soc. Exp. Biol. Med. 72: 569. [48]
355. —— 1950. Am. J. Physiol. 162: 189. [48]
356. Hanke, M. T., and Koessler, K. K., 1920. J. Biol. Chem. 43: 543. [51]
357. —— 1925. J. Biol. Chem. 66: 495. [52]
358. Hare, M. L. C., 1928. Biochem. J. 22: 968. [51; 52]
359. Harper, A. E., Benton, D. A., Winje, M. E., and Elvehjem, C. A., 1954. J. Biol. Chem. 209: 159. [45]
360. —— 1954. J. Biol. Chem. 209: 171. [48]
361. Harper, A. E., Monson, W. J., Benton, D. A., and Elvehjem, C. A., 1953. J. Nutrition 50: 383. [45; 47]
362. Harper, A. E., Monson, W. J., Benton, D. A., Winje, M. E., and Elvehjem, C. A., 1954. J. Biol. Chem. 206: 151. [45; 47]
363. Harrop, G. A., Jr., and Benedict, E. M., 1922–23. Proc. Soc. Exp. Biol. Med. 20: 430. [11]
364. Hartroft, W. S., 1948. Brit. J. Exp. Pathol. 29: 483. [43; 48]
365. —— 1950. Anat. Record 106: 61. [45; 48]
366. —— 1950. The escape of lipid from fatty cysts in experimental dietary cirrhosis. In Trans. 9th Conf. on liver injury, pp. 109–50. New York: Josiah Macy Foundation. [48]
367. —— 1953. Arch. Pathol. 55: 63. [48]
368. —— 1953–54. The sequence of pathologic events in the development of experimental fatty liver and cirrhosis. Ann. N.Y. Acad. Sci. 57: 633–45. [48]
369. —— 1954. Anat. Record 119: 71. [48]
370. —— 1955. Am. J. Pathol. 31: 381. [15]
371. Hartroft, W. S., and Best, C. H., 1947. Science 105: 315. [48]
372. —— 1949. Brit. Med. J. 1: 423. [1; 48]
373. Hartroft, W. S., and Ridout, J. H., 1951. Am. J. Pathol. 27: 951. [1; 48]
374. Hartroft, W. S., Ridout, J. H., Sellers, E. A., and Best, C. H., 1952. Proc. Soc. Exp. Biol. Med. 81: 384. [48]
375. Hartroft, W. S., and Sellers, E. A., 1952. Am. J. Pathol. 28: 387. [48]
376. Hartroft, W. S., and Wrenshall, G. A., 1953. Federation Proc. 12: 390. [15]
377. —— 1955. Diabetes 4: 1. [15; 16]
378. Hatcher, R. A., and Wolf, C. G. L., 1907. J. Biol. Chem. 3: 25. [11]
379. Hausberger, F. X., and Ramsay, A. J., 1953. Endocrinology 53: 423. [21]
380. Haycraft, J. B., 1883–84. Proc. Roy. Soc. (London), 36: 478. [Foreword to Paper 53]
381. Hedenius, P., and Wilander, O., 1936. Acta Med. Scand. 88: 443. [53; 54]
382. Hédon, E., 1909. Compt. rend. soc. biol. 66: 621. [4; 9]
383. —— 1909. Compt. rend. soc. biol. 66: 699; 67: 792. [9]
384. —— 1910. Arch. intern. Physiol. 10: 192. [9]
385. Hepburn, J., and Latchford, J. K., 1922. Am. J. Physiol. 62: 177. [10]
386. Herbert, F. K., and Bourne, M. C., 1930. Biochem. J. 24: 299. [17]
387. Hershey, J. M., 1930. Am. J. Physiol. 93: 657P. [34; 42]
388. Hershey, J. M., and Soskin, S., 1931. Am. J. Physiol. 98: 74. [1; 34; 42; 48]
389. Heymans, J. F., and Heymans, C., 1927. Compt. rend. soc. biol. 96: 719. [13]
390. Hill, A. V., 1927–28. Proc. Roy. Soc. (London), B 102: 380. [49]
391. Himsworth, H. P., 1935. Diet and the incidence of diabetes mellitus. Clin. Sci. 2: 117–48. [14]
392. —— 1948. Nutrition and liver disease. Sci. Progr. 36: 577–86. [44]
393. —— 1949. The syndrome of diabetes mellitus and its cause. Lancet 1: 465–72. [17]
394. Hjärre, A., 1927. Arch. f. Tierheilk. 57: 1. [15]
395. Honorato, C. R., and Vadillo, N. I., 1944. Bol. soc. biol. Santiago, Chile 2: 3. [43]
396. Horowitz, N. H., and Beadle, G. W., 1943. J. Biol. Chem. 150: 325. [42]
397. Horowitz, N. H., Bonner, D., and Houlahan, M. B., 1945. J. Biol. Chem. 159: 145. [42]
398. Hoshi, T., 1926. Tohoku J. Exp. Med. 7: 422, 446. [13]

399. Houssay, B. A., 1947. The role of the hypophysis in carbohydrate metabolism and in diabetes. *In* Les Prix Nobel, 1947, pp. 129–36. Stockholm: Norstedt, 1949. [30]

400. —— 1951. Brit. Med. J. 2: 505. [29]

401. Houssay, B. A., Brignone, R. F., and Mazzocco, P., 1946. Rev. soc. arg. biol. 22: 195. [15]

402. Houssay, B. A., Foglia, V. G., Smyth, F. S., Rietti, C. T., and Houssay, A. B., 1942. J. Exp. Med. 75: 547. [15]

403. Hove, E. L., and Copeland, D. H., 1954. J. Nutrition 53: 391. [48]

404. Howard, J. M., Moss, N. H., and Rhoads, J. E., 1950. Intern. Abstr. Surg. 90: 417. [29]

405. Howell, W. H., 1922–23. Am. J. Physiol. 63: 434P. [53]

406. —— 1924–25. Am. J. Physiol. 71: 553. [53]

407. —— 1928. Bull. Johns Hopkins Hosp. 42: 199. [53; 54]

408. Howell, W. H., and Holt, E., 1918–19. Am. J. Physiol. 47: 328. [53]

409. Howell, W. H., and McDonald, C. H., 1930. Bull. Johns Hopkins Hosp. 46: 365. [54]

410. Howland, G., Campbell, W. R., Maltby, E. J., and Robinson, W. L., 1929. J. Am. Med. Assoc. 93: 674. [29]

411. Huss, Magnus, 1852. Alcoholismus chronicus. Leipzig and Stockholm. (Cited by Ruge, see p. 252, ref. 656.) [44]

412. Hutchinson, H. B., Smith, W., and Winter, L. B., 1923. Biochem. J. 17: 683, 764. [13]

413. Ibrahim, J., 1909. Biochem. Z. 22: 24. [5; 7]

414. Ingle, D. J., 1941. Endocrinology 29: 838. [29]

415. Ingle, D. J., Beary, D. F., and Purmalis, A., 1954. Proc. Soc. Exp. Biol. Med. 85: 432. [20]

416. Ingle, D. J., Nezamis, J. E., and Humphrey, L. M., 1953. Proc. Soc. Exp. Biol. Med. 84: 232. [20]

417. Issekutz, B. von, 1924. Biochem. Z. 147: 264. [12]

418. Ivy, A. C., and Fisher, N. F., 1924. Am. J. Physiol. 67: 445. [13]

419. Jacobi, H. P., and Baumann, C. A., 1942. J. Biol. Chem. 142: 65. [48]

420. Jacobi, H. P., Baumann, C. A., and Meek, W. J., 1941. J. Biol. Chem. 138: 571. [48]

421. Jacobs, H. R. D., 1931. J. Lab. Clin. Med. 16: 901. [54]

422. Jacoby, C., 1904. Deut. med. Wochschr. 30: 1786. [Foreword to Paper 53]

423. Jaffé, E. R., Wissler, R. W., and Benditt, E. P., 1950. Am. J. Pathol. 26: 951. [48]

424. Jaques, L. B., 1940. J. Biol. Chem. 133: 445. [1; 53]

425. Jaques, L. B., Fidlar, E., Feldsted, E. T., and Macdonald, A. G., 1946. Can. Med. Assoc. J. 55: 26. [1; 53]

426. Jaques, L. B., and Waters, E. T., 1940. Am. J. Physiol. 129: 389P. [53]

427. —— 1940–41. J. Physiol. (London) 99: 454. [53]

428. Jephcott, C. M., 1931. Trans. Roy. Soc. Can. 25, Sect. V: 183. [13; 14]

429. John, H. J., 1943. Variation and interpretation of glucose tolerance tests. Southern Med. J. 36: 624–35. [17]

430. Johnson, B. C., Mitchell, H. H., Pinkos, J. A., and Morrill, C. C., 1951. J. Nutrition 43: 37. [48]

431. Jorpes, E., 1935. Biochem. J. 29: 1817. [53]

432. ——1939. Heparin in the Treatment of Thrombosis. 1st ed., 1939; 2nd ed., 1946. London: Oxford University Press. [Foreword to Paper 53] [53]

433. Joslin, E. P., and Lombard, H. L., 1936. Diabetes epidemiology from death records. New Engl. J. Med. 214: 7–9. [17]

434. Joslin, E. P., Root, H. F., White, P., Marble, A., and Bailey, C. C., 1946. The treatment of diabetes mellitus. 8th ed.; Philadelphia: Lea and Febiger. [17]

435. Jukes, T. H., and Williams, W. L., 1954. Vitamin B_{12}: biochemical systems. *In* The Vitamins: 1: 421–43, ed. W. H. Sebrell, Jr., and R. S. Harris. New York: Academic Press. [48]

436. Kamimura, N., 1917. Mitt. med. Fak. Univ. zu Tokyo 17: 95. [4]

437. KAPLAN, A., and CHAIKOFF, I. L., 1936. J. Biol. Chem. *116*: 663. [39]
438. KASPER, J., and JEFFREY, I. A., 1944. Am. J. Clin. Pathol. *14*: Tech. Sect. 8: 117. [17]
439. KATZ, L. N., and STAMLER, J., 1953. Experimental Atherosclerosis. Springfield: Charles C. Thomas. [48]
440. KAUFMANN, E., 1927. Z. ges. exp. Med. *55*: 1. [13]
441. —— 1928. Z. ges. exp. Med. *60*: 285; *62*: 147, 154, 739. [13]
442. KAY, H. D., and ROBISON, R., 1924. Biochem. J. *18*: 1139. [11]
443. KELLER, E. B., RACHELE, J. R., and DU VIGNEAUD, V., 1949. J. Biol. Chem. *177*: 733. [48]
444. KELLY, H. G., RAO, P. T., and JACKSON, R. L., 1955. Insulin requirements of children with diabetes mellitus maintained in good control. Am. J. Diseases Children *89*: 31–41. [15]
445. KENDALL, A. I., 1927. J. Infect. Diseases *40*: 689. [51; 52]
446. KENNEDY, E. P., 1956. The biological synthesis of phospholipids. Can. J. Biochem. Physiol. *34*: 334–48. [48]
447. KÉPINOV, L., and LEDEBT-PETIT DUTAILLIS, S., 1927. Compt. rend. soc. biol. *96*: 371; *97*: 25. [13]
448. —— 1929. Arch. intern. physiol. *31*: 310. [13]
449. KERR, R. B., and BEST, C. H., 1937. Am. J. Med. Sci. *194*: 149. [28]
450. KESTEN, H. D., SALCEDO, J., JR., and STETTEN, D., JR., 1945. J. Nutrition *29*: 171. [48]
451. KIMBALL, C. P., and MURLIN, J. R., 1923–24. J. Biol. Chem. *58*: 337. [30; 31]
452. KIMURA, T., and TANAKA, T., 1931. Trans. Japan Pathol. Soc. *21*: 370. [36]
453. KING, E. J., 1932. Biochem. J., *26*: 292. [47]
454. —— 1951. Micro-analysis in Medical Biochemistry. 2nd ed. p. 23. London: J. and A. Churchill. [23]
455. KING, E. J., and WOOTTON, I. D. P., 1956. Micro-analysis in Medical Biochemistry. 3rd ed. p. 83. London: J. and A. Churchill. [23]
456. KINGSLEY, G. R., 1940. J. Biol. Chem. *133*: 731. [23]
457. KINSELL, L. W., BROWN, F. R., FRISKEY, R. W., and MICHAELS, G. D., 1956. Science *123*: 585. [16]
458. KIRKBRIDE, M. B., 1912. J. Exp. Med. *15*: 101. [4]
459. KLEINER, I. S., 1919. J. Biol Chem. *40*: 153. [4; 7; 9]
460. KNOWLTON, F. P., and STARLING, E. H., 1912–13. J. Physiol. (London) *45*: 146. [4; 9; 30]
461. KOCHAKIAN, C. D., 1937. Endocrinology *21*: 750. [19]
462. KOCHAKIAN, C. D., and MURLIN, J. R., 1935. J. Nutrition *10*: 437. [19]
463. —— 1936. Am. J. Physiol. *117*: 642. [19]
464. KOESSLER, K. K., and HANKE, M. T., 1919. J. Biol. Chem. *39*: 497. [52]
465. —— 1919. J. Biol. Chem. *39*: 521. [50]
466. —— 1924. J. Biol. Chem. *59*: 889. [52]
467. KOLFF, W. J., 1946. The Artificial Kidney. Kampden, Holland: J. H. Kok. 1947. New Ways of Treating Uraemia. London: J. and A. Churchill. [53]
468. KOLFF, W. J., and BERK, H. Th. J., 1944. Acta Med. Scand. *117*: 121. [53]
469. KORNER, A., 1960. Biochem. J. *74*: 471. [31]
470. KOSTER, S., 1930. Archiv. ges. Physiol. Pflügers *224*: 212. [29]
471. KOZUKA, K., 1927. Tohoku Exp. Med. *9*: 130. [13]
472. KRAHL, M. E., 1957. Speculations on the action of insulin, with a note on other hypoglycemic agents. Perspectives in Biology and Medicine *1*: 69–96. [31]
473. KRAUT, H., FREY, E. K., and WERLE, E., 1930. Z. physiol. Chem. *189*: 97. [37]
474. KREMIANSKY, J., 1868. Arch. pathol. Anat. u. Physiol. Virchows *42*: 321–51 (see p. 340). [44]
475. KUHN, R., and BAUR, H., 1924. Münch. med. Wochschr. *71*: 541. [11]
476. LABARRE, J., 1927. Arch. intern. physiol. *29*: 238, 257. [13]
477. —— 1927. Compt. rend. soc. biol. *96*: 193, 196; 1928, *98*: 859. [13]
478. LAGUESSE, E., 1893. Compt. rend. soc. biol. Ser. 9, *5*: 819. [29]
479. —— 1911. J. physiol. et pathol. gén. *13*: 5. [4]
480. LÁNCZOS, A., 1934–35. Arch. ges. Physiol. Pflügers *235*: 422. [39]

481. LANE, M. A., 1907–8. Am. J. Anat. 7: 409. [4; 29]
482. LAUFBERGER, W., 1924. Klin. Wochschr. 3: 264. [12]
483. ——— 1924. Z. ges. exp. Med. 42: 570. [12]
484. LANGERHANS, P., 1869. Beiträge zur mikroskopischen Anatomie der Bauchspeichel-
       drüse. Berlin: G. Lange. Transl. by H. Morrison. Baltimore: Johns Hopkins
       Press, 1937. [29]
485. LAWRENCE, R. D., 1924. Brit. Med. J. 1: 516. [10]
486. ——— 1936. Brit. Med. J. 1: 526. [17]
487. ——— 1947. Symptomless glycosurias: differentiation by sugar tolerance tests.
       Med. Clin. N. America 31: 289–97. [17]
488. LAWRENCE, R. D., MADDERS, K., and MILLAR, H. R., 1930. Brit. J. Exp. Pathol.
       11: 117. [13]
489. LAZARUS, S. S., and VOLK, B. W., 1958. Glycogen infiltration ("hydropic degene-
       ration") in the pancreas. Arch. Pathol. 66: 59–71. [21]
490. ——— 1958. Endocrinology 63: 359. [1; 21]
491. LEATHES, J. B., and RAPER, H. S., 1925. The Fats. London: Longmans Green
       and Co. [34]
492. LÉPINE, R., 1909. Le diabète sucré. Paris: F. Alcan. [9]
493. LESSER, E. J., 1924. Biochem. Z. 153: 39. [12]
494. ——— 1924. Die innere Sekretion des Pankreas. In Handb. d. Biochemie d.
       Mensch. u. Tiere, vol. 9, pp. 159–228, ed. Carl Oppenheimer. Jena: Gustav
       Fischer. [12]
495. LEVENE, P. A., and ROLF, I. P., 1927. J. Biol. Chem. 74: 713. [34]
496. LEVINE, R., and GOLDSTEIN, M. S., 1955. On the mechanism of action of insulin.
       Recent Progr. in Hormone Research 11: 343–80. [30]
497. LEVINE, S. A., GORDON, B., and DERICK, C. L., 1924. J. Am. Med. Assoc. 82:
       1778. [49]
498. LEVINE, H., and SMITH, A. H., 1927. J. Biol. Chem. 75: 1. [39]
499. LEWASCHEW, S. W., 1886. Arch. mikroskop. Anat. 26: 453. [4]
500. LEWIS, G. N., and MACDONALD, R. T., 1933. J. Am. Chem. Soc. 55: 3057. [40]
501. LI, C. H., and EVANS, H. M., 1948. The biochemistry of pituitary growth
       hormone. Recent Progr. in Hormone Research 3: 3–44. [30]
502. LI, T. H., 1941. Chinese J. Physiol. 16: 9. [48]
503. LILLIE, R. D., ASHBURN, L. L., SEBRELL, W. H., DAFT, F. S., and LOWRY, J. V.,
       1942. Public Health Rep. (U.S.) 57: 502. [44; 45; 48]
504. LILLIE, R. D., DAFT, F. S., and SEBRELL, W. H., 1941. Public Health Rep.
       (U.S.) 56: 1255. [44]
505. LINTZEL, W., and FOMIN, S., 1931. Biochem. Z. 238: 438. [42]
506. LINTZEL, W., and MONASTERIO, G., 1931. Biochem. Z. 241: 273. [42]
507. LITWACK, G., HANKES, L. V., and ELVEHJEM, C. A., 1952. Proc. Soc. Exp. Biol.
       Med. 81: 441. [45]
508. LOGOTHETOPOULOS, J., and SALTER, J. M., 1960. Diabetes 9: 31. [21]
509. LOGOTHETOPOULOS, J., SHARMA, B. B., SALTER, J. M., and BEST, C. H., 1959.
       New Engl. J. Med. 261: 423. [21; 30]
510. LONG, C. N. H., and LUKENS, F. D. W., 1936. J. Exp. Med. 63: 465. [30]
511. LOUBATIÈRES, A., 1957. The mechanism of action of the hypoglycemic sulfona-
       mides: a concept based on investigations in animals and in human beings. Ann.
       N.Y. Acad. Sci. 71: 192–206. [30]
512. ——— 1959. General pharmacodynamics of the hypoglycemic arylsulfonylureas.
       Ann. N.Y. Acad. Sci. 74: 413–18. [30]
513. LOWRY, J. V., ASHBURN, L. L., DAFT, F. S., and SEBRELL, W. H., 1942. Quart. J.
       Studies Alc. 3: 168. [44]
514. LOWRY, J. V., ASHBURN, L. L., and SEBRELL, W. H., 1945. Quart. J. Studies Alc.
       6: 271. [48]
515. LOWRY, J. V., DAFT, F. S., SEBRELL, W. H., ASHBURN, L. L., and LILLIE, R. D.,
       1941. Public Health Rep. (U.S.) 56: 2216. [44; 48]
516. LUCAS, C. C., and RIDOUT, J. H., 1948. Proc. Can. Physiol. Soc., 12th Annual
       Meeting, p. 25. [43; 48]
517. ——— 1955. Can. J. Biochem. Physiol. 33: 25. [45; 47; 48]

518. LUKENS, F. D. W., 1958.   Federation Proc. *17:* 100.   [1]
519. —— 1959.   Pancreas: insulin and glucagon. Ann Rev. Physiol. *21:* 445–74.   [30]
520. LUNDBERG, E., 1924.   Compt. rend. soc. biol. *91:* 418.   [13]
521. LUSTIG, B., and LANGER, A., 1931.   Biochem. Z. *242:* 320.   [23]
522. McARTHUR, C. S., 1946.   Science *104:* 222.   [42]
523. McARTHUR, C. S., LANG, J. M., and LUCAS, C. C., 1945.   Can. Chem. Process Ind. *29:* 100 (216).   [42]
524. MacCALLUM, W. G., 1909.   Bull. Johns Hopkins Hosp. *20:* 265.   [4]
525. McCOLLUM, E. V., and SIMMONDS, N., 1918.   J. Biol. Chem. *33:* 55.   [41]
526. McCORMICK, N. A., and MACLEOD, J. J. R., 1923.   Trans. Roy. Soc. Can. *17,* Sect. V: 63.   [11]
527. MacFARLAND, M. L., and McHENRY, E. W., 1945.   J. Biol. Chem. *159:* 605.   [45]
528. McHENRY, E. W., 1935.   J. Physiol. (London) *85:* 343.   [37]
529. MacKAY, E. M., and BARNES, R. H., 1937.   Am. J. Physiol. *118:* 525.   [39]
530. MacKENZIE, C. G., CHANDLER, J. P., KELLER, E. B., RACHELE, J. R., CROSS, N., and DU VIGNEAUD, V., 1949.   J. Biol. Chem. *180:* 99.   [48]
531. McKIBBIN, J. M., THAYER, S., and STARE, F. J., 1944.   J. Lab. Clin. Med. *29:* 1109.   [48]
532. MacLEAN, D. L., and BEST, C. H., 1934.   Brit. J. Exp. Pathol. *15:* 193.   [1; 48]
533. MacLEAN, D. L., RIDOUT, J. H., and BEST, C. H., 1937.   Brit. J. Exp. Pathol. *18:* 345.   [41]
534. MacLEAN, H., and MacLEAN, I. S., 1927.   Lecithin and Allied Substances.   London: Longmans Green and Co.   [34]
535. McLEAN, J., 1916.   Am. J. Physiol. *41:* 250.   [1; 53]
536. MACLEAN, N., and OGILVIE, R. F., 1955.   Diabetes *4:* 367.   [16]
537. MACLEOD, J. J. R., 1920.   Physiology and Biochemistry in Modern Medicine.   3rd ed., St. Louis: C. V. Mosby.   [30]
538. —— 1922.   Insulin and diabetes.   Brit. Med. J. *2:* 833–4.   [9]
539. —— 1924.   Insulin.   Physiol. Rev. *4:* 21–68.   [10; 12]
540. MACLEOD, J. J. R., and PEARCE, R. G., 1912–13.   Zentr. Physiol. *26:* 1311.   [4]
541. —— 1913.   Am. J. Physiol. *32:* 184.   [30]
542. MACLEOD, J. J. R., and PRENDERGAST, D. J., 1921.   Trans. Roy. Soc. Can., Sect. V. *15:* 37.   [6]
543. McMEANS, J. W., 1915–16.   J. Med. Research *33:* 475.   [36]
544. MACPHERSON, H. T., 1946.   Biochem. J. *40:* 470.   [29]
545. MADISON, L. L., and UNGER, R. H., 1958.   J. Clin. Invest. *37:* 631.   [31]
546. MAJOOR, C. L. H., 1947.   J. Biol. Chem. *169:* 583.   [23]
547. MALLOY, H. T., and EVELYN, K. A., 1937.   J. Biol. Chem. *119:* 481.   [23]
548. MANN, F. C., 1920.   Am. J. Physiol. *51:* 182P.   [6]
549. MANN, G. V., ANDRUS, S. B., McNALLY, A., and STARE, F. J., 1953.   J. Exp. Med. *98:* 195.   [47; 48]
550. MANTEGAZZA, P., 1869.   Gazz. med. lombarda; 1871, Ann. univ. di medicina (quoted by Bizzozero, J., see ref. 127).   [55]
551. MARKOWITZ, J., and RAPPAPORT, A. M., 1951.   The hepatic artery. Physiol. Rev. *31:* 188–204.   [48]
552. MARKOWITZ, J., RAPPAPORT, A. M., and SCOTT, A. C., 1949.   Proc. Soc. Exp. Biol. Med. *70:* 305.   [48]
553. MARKS, H. H., 1946.   Statistics of diabetes.   New Engl. J. Med. *235:* 289–94.   [17]
554. MARKWARDT, F., 1957.   Z. physiol. Chem. *308:* 147.   [Foreword to Paper 53]
555. MARSHALL, F. W., 1930–31.   The sugar content of the blood in elderly people.   Quart. J. Med. *24:* 257–84.   [17]
556. MARTIN, A. J. P., and SYNGE, R. L. M., 1941.   Biochem. J. *35:* 1358.   [29]
557. MASON, E. C., 1924.   Surg., Gynecol. Obstet. *39:* 421.   [53; 54]
558. —— 1924–25.   J. Lab. Clin. Med. *10:* 203.   [53; 54]
559. MAYER, J., BATES, M. W., and DICKIE, M. M., 1951.   Science *113:* 746.   [15]
560. MELLANBY, J., 1909.   J. Physiol. (London) *38:* 441.   [Foreword to Paper 53]

561. MERING, J. VON, and MINKOWSKI, O., 1889–90.   Arch. exp. Pathol. Pharmakol. 26: 371.   [4; 7; 15; 30]
562. METZ, R., 1960.   Diabetes 9: 89.   [31]
563. MICHAELIS, L., 1930.   J. Biol. Chem. 87: 33.   [52]
564. MILLER, M., and CRAIG, J. W., 1956.   Metabolism 5: 162.   [16]
565. MILLER, B. F., and VAN SLYKE, D. D., 1936.   J. Biol. Chem. 114: 583.   [19]
566. MILNE, J., 1947.   J. Biol. Chem. 169: 595.   [23]
567. MIRSKY, I. A., 1956.   The role of insulinase and insulinase inhibitors.   Metabolism 5: 138–43.   [30]
568. MIRSKY, I. A., DIENGOTT, D., and DOLGER, H., 1956.   Science 123: 583.   [16]
569. MIRSKY, I. A., PERISUTTI, G., and DIENGOTT, D., 1956.   Metabolism 5: 156.   [16]
570. MIRSKY, I. A., PERISUTTI, G., and JINKS, R., 1956.   Proc. Soc. Exp. Biol. Med. 91: 475.   [16]
571. MITCHELL, H. H., 1935.   J. Nutrition 10: 311.   [44]
572. MITCHELL, H. H., and CURZON, E. G., 1940.   Quart. J. Studies Alc. 1: 227.   [44]
573. MOHNIKE, G. VON, and WITTENHAGEN, G., 1957.   Deut. med. Wochschr. 82: 1556.   [23]
574. MOLONEY, P. J., and COVAL, M., 1955.   Biochem. J. 59: 179.   [30]
575. MOLONEY, P. J., and FINDLAY, D. M., 1923.   J. Biol. Chem. 57: 359.   [9]
576. —— 1924.   J. Phys. Chem. 28: 402.   [9]
577. MOON, V. H., 1934.   Experimental cirrhosis in relation to human cirrhosis.   Arch. Pathol. 18: 381–424.   [44]
578. MOSENTHAL, H. O., and BARRY, E., 1949.   Criteria for and interpretation of normal glucose tolerance tests.   Proc. Am. Diabetes Assoc. 9: 277–99.   [17]
579. MOSES, C., LONGABAUGH, G. M., and GEORGE, R. S., 1950.   Am. J. Physiol. 163: 736P   [48]
580. MOTT, F. W., and HALLIBURTON, W. D., 1899.   The physiological action of choline and neurine.   Phil. Trans. Roy. Soc. (London), B. 191: 211–67 (see pp. 216, 242).   [50]
581. MOTTRAM, V. H., 1909.   J. Physiol. (London) 38: 281.   [39]
582. MOYER, J. H., and WOMACK, C. R., 1950.   Glucose tolerance: a comparison of 4 types of diagnostic tests in 103 control subjects and 26 patients with diabetes.   Am. J. Med. Sci. 219: 161–73.   [17]
583. MULFORD, D. J., and GRIFFITH, W. H., 1942.   J. Nutrition 23: 91.   [46]
584. MURLIN, J. R., and KRAMER, B., 1913.   J. Biol. Chem. 15: 365.   [4; 7; 9]
585. MURRAY, G. D. W., 1939–40.   Heparin in thrombosis and embolism.   Brit. J. Surgery 27: 567–98.   [Foreword to Paper 53]
586. MURRAY, G. D. W., and BEST, C. H., 1938.   Heparin and thrombosis: the present situation.   J. Am. Med. Assoc. 110: 118–9.   [56]
587. MURRAY, G. D. W., DELORME, E., and THOMAS, N., 1947.   Arch. Surg. 55: 505.   [53]
588. —— 1948.   J. Am. Med. Assoc. 137: 1596.   [53]
589. MURRAY, G. D. W., JAQUES, L. B., PERRETT, T. S., and BEST, C. H., 1936.   Can. Med. Assoc. J. 35: 621.   [1; 53; 55]
590. ——1937.   Surgery 2: 163.   [53; 56]
591. MYERS, V. C., and BAILEY, C. V., 1916.   J. Biol. Chem. 24: 147.   [4]
592. NASH, T. P., 1925.   J. Biol. Chem. 66: 869.   [12]
593. NATIONAL HEALTH SURVEY, 1935–36.   The magnitude of the chronic disease problem in the United States.   Preliminary reports sickness and medical care series.   Bulletin No. 6, United States Public Health Service, Washington, 1938.   [17]
594. NATIONAL INSTITUTE FOR MEDICAL RESEARCH.   Department of Biological Standards, Hampstead, London, N.W.3. 1942–44.   Memorandum on a provisional international standard for heparin, 1942.   Quart. Bull. League of Nations 10: 151.   [53]
595. NELSON, N., 1944.   J. Biol. Chem. 153: 375.   [17]
596. NEUMANN, A. L., KRIDER, J. L., JAMES, M. F., and JOHNSON, B. C., 1949.   J. Nutrition 38: 195.   [48]

597. Newburgh, L. H., Conn, J. W., Johnston, M. W., and Conn, E. S., 1938. A new interpretation of diabetes mellitus in obese, middle-aged persons: recovery through reduction of weight. Trans. Assoc. Am. Physicians 53: 245–57.   [14; 17]

598. Niño-Herrera, H., Harper, A. E., and Elvehjem, C. A., 1954. J. Nutrition 53: 469.   [45]

599. Nothmann, M., 1925. Ueber die Verteilung des Insulin im Organismus des Normalen und pankreasdiabetischen Hundes. Arch. exp. Pathol. Pharmakol. 108: 1–63.   [13]

600. —— 1926. Klin. Wochschr. 5: 297.   [13]

601. Nyiri, W., 1926. Arch. exp. Pathol. Pharmakol. 116: 117.   [57]

602. Oehme, C., 1913. Arch. exp. Pathol. Pharmakol. 72: 76.   [52]

603. Okey, L., 1932–33. Proc. Soc. Exp. Biol. Med. 30: 1003.   [36]

604. —— 1933. J. Biol. Chem. 100: lxxv.   [36]

605. Oliver, G., and Schäfer, E. A., 1895. J. Physiol. (London) 18: 277.   [50]

606. Opie, E. L., 1901. Diabetes mellitus associated with hyaline degeneration of the islands of Langerhans of the pancreas. Johns Hopkins Hosp. Bull. 12: 263–4.   [4]

607. Osborne, W. A., and Vincent, S., 1900. J. Physiol. (London) 25: 283.   [50]

608. Page, I. H., and Brown, H. B., 1952. Circulation 6: 681.   [48]

609. Page, I. H., and Corcoran, A. C., 1948. Experimental Renal Hypertension. American Lecture Series. Springfield: Charles C. Thomas.   [48]

610. Paldrock, A., 1896. Arbeiten des Pharm. Inst. zu Dorpat 13: 64.   [Foreword to Paper 53]

611. Partos, A., 1929. Archiv. ges. Physiol. Pflügers 221: 562.   [13]

612. Patek, A. J., Jr., 1947. Evaluation of dietary factors in treatment of Laennec's cirrhosis of liver. J. Mt. Sinai Hosp. 14: 1–7.   [44]

613. Patterson, S. W., and Starling, E. H., 1913–14. J. Physiol. (London) 47: 137.   [4; 9; 30]

614. Paulesco, N. C., 1921. Compt. rend. soc. biol. 85: 555.   [4; 7]

615. Pemberton, H. S., and Cunningham, L., 1925. Lancet 2: 1222.   [10]

616. Penau, H., and Simonnet, H., 1925. Bull. soc. chim. biol. 7: 17.   [13]

617. Perlman, I., and Chaikoff, I. L., 1939. J. Biol. Chem. 127: 211.   [42]

618. Pflüger, E., 1906. Glycogène. In "Dictionnaire de Physiologie," vol. 7. ed. C. R. Richet.   [11]

619. —— 1907. Arch. ges. Physiol. Pflügers 118: 265.   [7]

620. Piazza, E. U., Goodner, C. J., and Freinkel, N., 1959. A re-evaluation of in vitro methods for insulin bio-assay. Diabetes 8: 459–65.   [30]

621. Piccaluga, N., and Cioffari, S., 1925. Compt. rend. soc. biol. 93: 1118.   [22]

622. Plough, I. C., Patek, A. J., and Bevans, M., 1952. J. Exp. Med. 96: 221.   [48]

623. Pollak, L., 1926. Arch. exp. Pathol. Pharmakol. 116: 15.   [13]

624. Popielski, L., 1909. Arch. ges. Physiol. Pflügers 128: 191.   [50]

625. Quick, A. J., 1935. J. Biol. Chem. 109: lxxiii.   [23]

626. —— 1936. Am. J. Physiol. 116: 535.   [53]

627. Ramalingaswami, V., Sriramachari, S., and Patwardhan, V. N., 1954. Ind. J. Med. Sci. 8: 433.   [45]

628. Rao, P. T., and Jackson, R. L., 1953. Insulin and nutritional requirements of children with diabetes mellitus in good control. Read at the Thirteenth Annual Meeting of the American Diabetes Association, May 31, 1953 (see also ref. 444).   [15]

629. Rappaport, A. M., 1955. Trans. 5th Conf. on shock and circulatory homeostasis pp. 273, 297. New York: Josiah Macy Jr. Foundation.   [48]

630. Rappaport, A. M., Borowy, Z. J., Lougheed, W. M., and Lotto, W. N., 1954. Subdivision of hexagonal liver lobules into a structural and functional unit. Anat. Record. 119: 11–27.   [48]

631. Redenbaugh, H. E., Ivy, A. C., and Koppanyi, T., 1925–26. Proc. Soc. Exp. Biol. Med. 23: 756.   [13]

632. Reed, C. I., 1925. Am. J. Physiol. 74: 79.   [53]

633. —— 1928–29. J. Lab. Clin. Med. 14: 243.   [54]

634. Rees, M. W., 1946. Biochem. J. 40: 632.   [29]

635. REINECKE, R. M., BALL, H. A., and SAMUELS, L. T., 1939. Proc. Soc. Exp. Biol. Med. *41*: 44. [20]
636. RENNIE, J., and FRASER, T., 1907. Biochem. J. 2: 7. [7; 9]
637. RICHARDS, T. W., and SHIPLEY, J. W., 1912. J. Am. Chem. Soc. *34*: 599. [38]
638. RICHARDSON, K. C., and YOUNG, F. G., 1937. J. Physiol. (London) *91*: 352. [29]
639. —— 1938. Lancet *1*: 1098. [21]
640. RICKETTS, H. T., PETERSEN, E. S., STEINER, P. E., and TUPIKOVA, N., 1953. Spontaneous diabetes mellitus in the dog. Diabetes 2: 288–94. [15]
641. RICKETTS, H. T., WILDBERGER, H. L., and SCHMID, H., 1957. Long term studies of the sulfonylureas in totally depancreatized dogs. Ann. N.Y. Acad. Sci. 71: 170–6. [23]
642. RIDOUT, J. H., LUCAS, C. C., PATTERSON, J. M., and BEST, C. H., 1952. Biochem. J. *52*: 79. [45]
643. —— 1954. Biochem. J. *58*: 297. [45; 46; 47]
644. RIDOUT, J. H., PATTERSON, J. M., LUCAS, C. C., and BEST, C. H., 1954. Biochem. J. *58*: 306. [48]
645. RINGER, M., 1923–24. J. Biol. Chem. *58*: 483. [11; 12]
646. RITTENBERG, D., and SCHOENHEIMER, R., 1935. J. Biol. Chem. *111*: 169. [40]
647. RITTENBERG, D., and SCHOENHEIMER, R., 1937. J. Biol. Chem. *121*: 235. [40]
648. RODRIGUEZ-CANDELA, J. L., 1953. Inhibitory effect of pancreas extract and H-G factor on the insulin glucose uptake of the isolated diaphragm. *In* Ciba Foundation colloquia on endocrinology 6: 233–41. ed. G. E. W. Wolstenholme. London: J. and A. Churchill. [20]
649. ROKITANSKY, CARL, 1849. A Manual of Pathological Anatomy, vol. 2 (see p. 145). London: Sydenham Society. [44]
650. ROSE, W. C., OESTERLING, M. J., and WOMACK, M., 1948. J. Biol. Chem. *176*: 753. [47]
651. ROSE, W. C., and RICE, E. E., 1939. J. Biol. Chem. *130*: 305. [48]
652. ROSE, W. C., SMITH, L. C., WOMACK, M., and SHANE, M., 1949. J. Biol. Chem. *181*: 307. [46]
653. ROSE, B., WEIL, P. G., and BROWNE, J. S. L., 1941. Can. Med. Assoc. J. *44*: 442. [58]
654. ROSENMUND, K. W., and KUHNHENN, W., 1923. Z. Lebens-Untersuch. u. Forsch. *46*: 154. [36]
655. ROWNTREE, L. G., and SHIONOYA, T., 1927. J. Exp. Med. *46*: 7. [55]
656. RUGE, P., 1870. Arch. pathol. Anat. u. Physiol. Virchows *49*: 252. [44]
657. RUIZ, C. L., SILVA, L. L., and LIBENSON, L., 1930. Rev. soc. arg. biol. 6: 134. [30]
658. SAKAMI, W., and WELCH, A. D., 1950. J. Biol. Chem. *187*: 379. [48]
659. SALMON, W. D., and COPELAND, D. H., 1953–54. Liver carcinoma and related lesions in chronic choline deficiency. Ann. N.Y. Acad. Sci. *57*: 664–77. [48]
660. SALTER, J. M., and BEST, C. H., 1953. Brit. Med. J. 2: 353. [1; 22]
661. SALTER, J. M., DAVIDSON, I. W. F., and BEST, C. H., 1957. Can. J. Biochem. Physiol. *35*: 913. [1; 22]
662. —— 1957. Diabetes 6: 248. [1; 21; 22]
663. SALTER, J. M., DE MEYER, R., and BEST, C. H., 1958. Brit. Med. J. 2: 5. [1]
664. SALTER, J. M., EZRIN, C., LAIDLAW, J. C., and GORNALL, A. G., 1960. Metabolism 9: 753. [31]
665. SANDMEYER, W., 1895. Z. Biol. *31*: 12. [7]
666. SANGER, F., 1949. Some chemical investigations on the structure of insulin. Cold Spring Harbor Symposia Quant. Biol. *14*: 153–60. [29]
667. SANGER, F., THOMPSON, E. O. P., and KITAI, R., 1955. Biochem. J. *59*: 509. [30]
668. SAUBERLICH, H. E., 1953. Federation Proc. *12*: 263. [45; 48]
669. SCHAFFER, N. K., and LEE, M., 1935. J. Biol. Chem. *108*: 355. [39]
670. SCHAMBYE, P., 1957. Physiological and toxicological study of various hypoglycemic substances in normal and depancreatized dogs. Ann. endocrinol. (Paris) *18*: 174–83. [23]

671. —— 1957. Diabetes 6: 146. [23]
672. Schayer, R. W., 1959. Catabolism of physiological quantities of histamine *in vivo*. Physiol. Rev. 39: 116–26. [1]
673. Schlotthauer, C. F., and Millar, J. A. S., 1951. Diabetes mellitus in dogs and cats. J. Am. Vet. Med. Assoc. 118: 31–5. [15]
674. Schmidt, A., 1892. Zur Blutlehre. Leipzig: Vogel. [53]
675. Schmidt-Mülheim, A., 1880. Arch. Anat. u. Physiol. p. 33. [53]
676. Schmitz, A., and Fischer, A., 1933. Z. physiol. Chem. 216: 264. [53]
677. Schoenheimer, R., and Rittenberg, D., 1935. J. Biol. Chem. 111: 175. [40]
678. —— 1936. J. Biol. Chem. 114: 381. [40]
679. Schultze, Erich, 1892. Ueber die Verwendung von Blutegelextract bei der Transfusion des Blutes. Thesis Greifswald. [Foreword to Paper 53]
680. Schulze, W., 1900. Arch. mikroskop. Anat. 56: 491. [29]
681. Schuster, E. H. J., 1924. J. Physiol. (London) 59: 94. [12]
682. Scott, D. A., 1934. Biochem. J. 28: 1592. [29; 30]
683. —— 1939. Crystalline insulin. Endocrinology 25: 437–48. [29]
684. Scott, D. A., and Charles, A. F., 1933. J. Biol. Chem. 102: 437. [53; 54; 57]
685. Scott, D. A., and Fisher, A. M., 1935. J. Pharmacol. 55: 206. [1]
686. —— 1938. Am. J. Physiol. 121: 253. [14; 15]
687. —— 1938. J. Clin. Invest. 17: 725. [14]
688. Scott, E. L., 1911–12. Am. J. Physiol. 29: 306. [5; 7; 9]
689. Scow, R. O., Wagner, E. M., and Cardeza, A., 1957. Endocrinology 61: 380. [1]
690. Scow, R. O., Wagner, E. M., and Ronov, E., 1958. Endocrinology 62: 593. [1]
691. Sellers, E. A., and You, R. W., 1949. Science 110: 713. [48]
692. —— 1951. J. Nutrition. 44: 513. [48]
693. —— 1952. Biochem. J. 51: 573. [48]
694. Shaffer, P. A., and Hartmann, A. F., 1920–21. J. Biol. Chem. 45: 365. [4]
695. Shaffer, P. A., and Somogyi, M., 1933. J. Biol. Chem. 100: 695. [14]
696. Shikinami, Y., 1928. Tohoku J. Exp. Med. 10: 560. [13]
697. Shils, M. E., Friedland, I., and Stewart, W. B., 1954. Proc. Soc. Exp. Biol. Med. 87: 473. [45; 48]
698. Shils, M. E., and Stewart, W. B., 1953. Abstr. 19th Intern. Physiol. Congr., p. 758. Montreal, Canada. [45]
699. —— 1954. Proc. Soc. Exp. Biol. Med. 85: 298. [45; 48]
700. —— 1954. Proc. Soc. Exp. Biol. Med. 87: 629. [45; 48]
701. Shionoya, T., 1927. J. Exp. Med. 46: 19. [53; 54; 55]
702. Siekevitz, P., and Greenberg, D. M., 1950. J. Biol. Chem. 186: 275. [48]
703. Sigma Chemical Co., 1958. Tech. Bull. No. 505. [23]
704. Silberstein, F., Freud, J., Révész, T., and Schneid, B., 1927. Z. ges. exp. Med. 55: 56. [22]
705. Simola, P. E., 1927. Ann. Acad. Sci. Fennicae 29: 23. [13]
706. Sinclair, R. G., 1930. J. Biol. Chem. 88: 575. [40]
707. Singal, S. A., Hazan, S. J., Sydenstricker, V. P., and Littlejohn, J. M., 1953. J. Biol. Chem. 200: 867. [45; 47; 48]
708. Singal, S. A., Sydenstricker, V. P., and Littlejohn, J. M., 1949. Federation Proc. 8: 251. [47]
709. Sirek, A., 1957. Nature 179: 376. [1]
710. Sirek, A., Sirek, O. V., Hanus, Y., Monkhouse, F. C., and Best, C. H., 1959. Diabetes 8: 284. [1[
711. Sirek, A., Sirek, O. V., Logothetopoulos, J., and Best, C. H., 1959. Histologic studies on tolbutamide treated dogs. Metabolism 8: 577–84. [1]
712. Sirek, A., Sirek, O. V., Monkhouse, F. C., and Best, C. H., 1957. Rev. Can. Biol. 16: 515. [23]
713. Smetana, H. F., Keller, T. C., and Dubin, I. N., 1953. Rev. Gastroenterology 20: 227. [48]
714. Smith, P. K., Trace, J., and Barbour, H. G., 1936. J. Biol. Chem. 116: 371. [40]

715. SNEDECOR, G. W., 1946. Statistical Methods. 4th ed.; Ames: Iowa State College Press. [16]
716. SNEDECOR, J. G., DeMEIO, R. H., and PINCUS, I. J., 1955. Proc. Soc. Exp. Biol. Med. 89: 396. [20]
717. SOBIN, S. S., 1946. Am. J. Physiol. 146: 179. [43]
718. SOBIN, S. S., and LANDIS, E. M., 1947. Am. J. Physiol. 148: 557. [43]
719. SOLANDT, D. Y., and BEST, C. H., 1938. Lancet 2: 130. [48; 53]
720. ——— 1939. Nature 144: 376. [48]
721. ——— 1940. Lancet 1: 1042. [48]
722. SOLANDT, D. Y., NASSIM, R., and BEST, C. H., 1939. Lancet 2: 592. [1; 53]
723. SOLANDT, D. Y., and ROBINSON, F. L., 1938. J. Sci. Instr. 15: 268. [57]
724. SOMMELET, M., and FERRAND, M., 1924. Bull. soc. chim. (Paris) Ser. 4, 35: 446. [42]
725. SOMOGYI, M., 1945. J. Biol. Chem. 160: 61, 69. [17]
726. ——— 1952. J. Biol. Chem. 195: 19. [21]
727. SÖRENSEN, S. P. L., 1907. Biochem. Z. 7: 45. [51]
728. SPELLBERG, M. A., and LEFF, W. A., 1945. J. Am. Med. Assoc. 129: 246. [17]
729. SPERRY, W. M., and WEBB, M., 1950. J. Biol. Chem. 187: 97. [47]
730. SRIRAMACHARI, S., and RAMALINGASWAMI, V., 1953. Indian J. Pediat. 20: 1. [45]
731. SSOBOLEW, L. W., 1902. Arch. path. Anat. u. Physiol. Virchows 168: 91. [4]
732. STADIE, W. C., 1958. Is the metabolism of peripheral tissues affected by the arylsulfonylureas? Diabetes 7: 61-3. [30]
733. STARLING, E. H., 1920. Principles of human physiology. 3rd ed.; London: J. and A. Churchill. [30]
734. STAUB, HANS, 1924. Insulin. Berlin: J. Springer. [10]
735. STEKOL, J. A., WEISS, S., SMITH, P., and WEISS, K., 1953. J. Biol. Chem. 201: 299. [48]
736. STEKOL, J. A., WEISS, S., and WEISS, K. W., 1952. Arch. Biochem. Biophys. 36: 5. [48]
737. STERN, L., and ROTHLIN, E., 1919-20. J. physiol. et pathol. gén. 18: 441. [50]
738. STETTEN, DeWITT, JR., 1941. J. Biol. Chem. 138: 437. [42]
739. STETTEN, DeWITT, JR., and SALCEDO, J., JR., 1944. J. Biol. Chem. 156: 27. [48]
740. STEWART, G. N., and ROGOFF, J. M., 1918. Am. J. Physiol. 46: 90. [8]
741. STOKER, S. B., 1934. J. Physiol. (London) 82: 8P. [54]
742. STOKSTAD, E. L. R., 1954. Pteroylglutamic acid: biochemical systems. In The Vitamins, vol. 3: pp. 124-42, ed. W. H. Sebrell, Jr., and R. S. Harris. New York: Academic Press. [48]
743. SWEENEY, J. S., 1927. Arch. Internal Med. 40: 818. [17]
744. SYMPOSIUM ON DISORDERS OF CARBOHYDRATE METABOLISM, 1959. Am. J. Med. 26: 659-714. [31]
745. TABOR, E. C., and FRANKHAUSER, K. H., 1950. Detection of diaebtes in a nutrition survey. Public Health Rep. (U.S.) 65: 1330-5. [17]
746. TARDING, F., and SCHAMBYE, P., 1958. Endokrinologie 36: 222. [23]
747. TEJNING, S., 1947. Dietary factors and quantitative morphology of the islets of Langerhans. Acta med. Scand. Suppl. 198: 1-154. [29]
748. THALHIMER, W., 1937-38. Proc. Soc. Exp. Biol. Med. 37: 641. [53; 57]
749. ——— 1939. Proc. Soc. Exp. Biol. Med. 41: 230. [58]
750. THALHIMER, W., SOLANDT, D. Y., and BEST, C. H., 1938. Lancet 2: 554. [1; 53]
751. THORPE, W. V., 1928. Biochem. J. 22: 94. [52]
752. TOENNIES, G., BENNETT, M. A., and MEDES, G., 1943. Growth 7: 251. [48]
753. TREADWELL, C. R., 1945. J. Biol. Chem. 160: 601; 1948, 176: 1141, 1149. [46]
754. TREADWELL, C. R., GROOTHUIS, M., and ECKSTEIN, H. C., 1942. J. Biol. Chem. 142: 653. [47]
755. TREADWELL, C. R., TIDWELL, H. C., and GAST, J. H., 1944. J. Biol. Chem. 156: 237. [46; 47]
756. TREVAN, J. W., 1927. Proc. Roy. Soc. (London), B. 101: 483. [14]
757. TREVAN, J. W., and BOOCK, E., 1926. League of Nations Health Organization, C.H. 398: 47. [14]

758. Tristram, G. R., 1946.   Biochem. J. 40: 721.   [29]

759. Tronstad, L., Nordhagen, J., and Brun, J., 1935.   Nature 136: 515.   [40]

760. Tucker, H. F., and Eckstein, H. C., 1937.   J. Biol. Chem. 121: 479.   [1; 41; 47; 48]

761. —— 1938.   J. Biol. Chem. 126: 117.   [41; 48]

762. Tucker, H. F., Treadwell, C. R., and Eckstein, H. C., 1940.   J. Biol. Chem. 135: 85.   [48]

763. Tyberghein, J. M., Halsey, Y. D., and Williams, R. H., 1956.   Proc. Soc. Exp. Biol. Med. 92: 322.   [23]

764. Van Itallie, T. B., Morgan, M. C., and Dotti, L. B., 1955.   J. Clin. Endocrinol. and Metabolism 15: 28.   [20]

765. Van Slyke, D. D., 1917.   J. Biol. Chem. 32: 455.   [6]

766. Vaughan, M., 1957.   The effect of tolbutamide on glucose production by the liver in vitro.   Ann. N.Y. Acad. Sci. 71: 112–17.   [23]

767. Verney, E. B., and Starling, E. H., 1922.   J. Physiol. (London) 56: 353.   [52]

768. du Vigneaud, V., 1952.   A Trail of Research. Ithaca, N.Y.: Cornell University Press.   [48]

769. du Vigneaud, V., Chandler, J. P., Moyer, A. W., and Keppel, D. M., 1939.   J. Biol. Chem. 128: cviii.   [41]

770. —— 1939.   J. Biol. Chem. 131: 57.   [48]

771. du Vigneaud, V., Dyer, H. M., and Kies, M. W., 1939.   J. Biol. Chem. 130: 325.   [48]

772. du Vigneaud, V., Sifferd, R. H., and Sealock, R. R., 1933.   J. Biol. Chem. 102: 521.   [29]

773. Vincent, S., and Curtis, F. R., 1926.   The nature of the depressor substance or substances in tissue extracts. Lancet 1: 1142–3.   [50]

774. Vincent, S., Dodds, E. C., and Dickens, F., 1925.   Quart. J. Exp. Physiol. 15: 313.   [13]

775. Vincent, S., and Sheen, W., 1903.   J. Physiol. (London) 29: 242.   [50]

776. Virchow, R., 1863.   Cellular Pathology.   Lecture 10, transl. from 2nd ed. original by F. Chance (see p. 230). Philadelphia: Lippincott.   [55]

777. Waldschmidt-Leitz, E., Stadler, P., and Steigerwaldt, F., 1929.   Z. physiol. Chem. 183: 39.   [Foreword to Paper 53]

778. Wang, C., Hegsted, D. M., Lapi, A., Zamcheck, N., and Black, M. B., 1949.   J. Lab. Clin. Med. 34: 953.   [45]

779. Warren, Shields, 1938.   The Pathology of Diabetes Mellitus. 2nd ed.; Philadelphia: Lea and Febiger.   [29]

780. Waters, E. T., Markowitz, J., and Jaques, L. B., 1938.   Science 87: 582.   [53]

781. Waugh, D. F., 1946.   J. Am. Chem. Soc. 68: 247.   [29]

782. Weber, G., and Cantero, A., 1958.   Metabolism 7: 333.   [23]

783. Weichselbaum, T. E., 1946.   Am. J. Clin. Pathol. 16: Tech. Sect. 10, p. 40.   [23]

784. Weil, R., and Stetten, De Witt, Jr., 1947.   J. Biol. Chem. 168: 129.   [1; 48]

785. Weinman, E. O., Chaikoff, I. L., Entenman, C., and Dauben, W. G., 1950.   J. Biol. Chem. 187: 643.   [48]

786. Welch, A. D., and Landau, R. L., 1942.   J. Biol. Chem. 144: 581.   [42]

787. Welch, A. D., and Nichol, C. A., 1952.   Water-soluble vitamins concerned with one- and two-carbon intermediates.   Ann. Rev. Biochem. 21: 633–86.   [46; 48]

788. Welch, M. S., Irving, L., and Best, C. H., 1935.   Can. Chem. Met. 19: 66.   [48]

789. Welch, M. S., and Welch, A. D., 1938.   Proc. Soc. Exp. Biol. Med. 39: 5.   [48]

790. Welch, W. H., 1920.   Thrombosis, Papers and Addresses, vol. 1, p. 110. Baltimore: Johns Hopkins Press.   [54; 55]

791. Weld, C. B., 1944.   Can. Med. Assoc. J. 51: 578.   [48]

792. Whipple, A. O., 1952.   Can. Med. Assoc. J. 66: 334.   [29]

793. Widström, G., and Wilander, O., 1936.   Acta Med. Scand. 88: 434.   [54]

794. Wilander, O., 1939.   Studien über Heparin. Skand. Arch. Physiol. 81: Supp. 15: 3–89.   [53]

795. Wilder, R. M., 1952.   Hypoglycemia.   Diabetes 1: 183–7.   [29]

796. Wilder, R. M., Allan, F. N., Power, M. H., and Robertson, H. E., 1927. J. Am. Med. Assoc. 89: 348. [29]
797. Wilgram, G. F., Best, C. H., and Blumenstein, J., 1955. Federation Proc. 14: 163. [48]
798. —— 1955. Proc. Soc. Exp. Biol. Med. 89: 476. [48]
799. Wilgram, G. F., and Hartroft, W. S., 1955. Brit. J. Exp. Pathol. 36: 298. [48]
800. Wilgram, G. F., Hartroft, W. S., and Best, C. H., 1954. Brit. Med. J. 2: 1. [48]
801. —— 1954. Science 119: 842. [48]
802. Wilgram, G. F., Lewis, L. A., and Blumenstein, J., 1955. Circulation Research 3: 549. [48]
803. Wilkerson, H. L. C., and Krall, L. P., 1947. J. Am. Med. Assoc. 135: 209. [17]
804. Wilson, J. W., 1951. Cancer Research 11: 290. [48]
805. —— 1953–54. Hepatomas produced in mice by feeding bentonite in diet. Ann. N.Y. Acad. Sci. 57: 678–83. [48]
806. Wilson, W. D., 1950. Bull. Intern. Assoc. Med. Museums 31: 216. [47]
807. —— 1952. Am. Assoc. of Anatomists Abstr. Anat. Record 112: 468. [15]
808. Winje, M. E., Harper, A. E., Benton, D. A., Boldt, R. E., and Elvehjem, C. A., 1954. J. Nutrition 54: 155. [45]
809. Winter, L. B., and Smith, W., 1923. J. Physiol. (London) 57: xl; 1925, 60: v. [13]
810. Winzler, R. J., 1955. In Methods of Biochemical Analysis 2: p. 290, ed. David Glick. New York: Interscience. [23]
811. Wissler, R. W., Eilert, M. L., Schroeder, M. A., and Cohen, L., 1954. Arch. Pathol. 57: 333. [48]
812. Witzleben, H. D. von, 1925. Klin. Wochschr. 4: 2115. [22]
813. Woerner, C. A., 1938. Anat. Record 71: 33; 1939, 75: 91. [29]
814. Wrenshall, G. A., 1951. Studies on the extractable insulin of human pancreas. Ph.D. Thesis, University of Toronto. [16]
815. Wrenshall, G. A., Bogoch, A., and Ritchie, R. C., 1952. Diabetes 1: 87. [15; 16; 29; 30]
816. Wrenshall, G. A., Collins-Williams, J., and Hartroft, W. S., 1949. Am. J. Physiol. 156: 100. [16]
817. Wrenshall, G. A., Hartroft, W. S., and Best, C. H., 1954. Diabetes 3: 444. [16]
818. Wrenshall, G. A., and Hetenyi, G., Jr., 1959. Successive measured injections of tracer as a method for determining characteristics of accumulation and turnover in higher animals with access limited to blood. Metabolism 8: 531–43. [31]
819. Wright, I. S., Marple, C. D., and Beck, D. F., 1948. Anticoagulant therapy of coronary thrombosis with myocardial infarction. J. Am. Med. Assoc. 138: 1074–9. [53]
820. Yalow, R. S., and Berson, S. A., 1960. Plasma insulin in man. Am. J. Med. 29: 1–8. [31]
821. Young, F. G., 1937. Lancet 2: 372. [1; 30]
822. —— 1953. Discussion of R-Candela's paper (see [648], pp. 241–2). [20]
823. Yuasa, D., 1928. Beitr. pathol. Anat. u. allgem. Pathol. 80: 570. [36]
824. Zahn, F. W., 1875. Arch. pathol. Anat. u. Physiol. Virchows 62: 81; 1884, 96: 1. [54]
825. Zeffren, J. L., and Sherry, S., 1957. Metabolism 6: 504. [23]
826. Zilversmit, D. B., Entenman, C., and Chaikoff, I. L., 1948. J. Biol. Chem. 176: 193. [48]
827. Zuelzer, G., 1908. Z. exp. Pathol. Therap. 5: 307. [9]
828. Zunz, E., and LaBarre, J., 1927. Arch. intern. physiol. 29: 265; 1929, 31: 20. [13]
829. —— 1927. Compt. rend. soc. biol. 96: 421, 708, 710, 1045; 1928, 99: 335. [13]
830. Zurhelle, E., 1910. Experimentelle Untersuchungen über die Beziehungen der Infektion und der Fibringerinnung zur Thrombenbildung im strömenden Blut. Beit. pathol. Anat. u. allgem. Pathol. 47: 539–70. [54; 55]

Lightning Source UK Ltd.
Milton Keynes UK
UKHW030612210722
406167UK00006B/688